Fisch and Spehlmann's EEG Pr

Fisch and Spehlmann's EEG Primer

Basic Principles of Digital and Analog EEG

Third Revised and Enlarged Edition

BRUCE J. FISCH, M.D.

Professor of Neurology
Director, Comprehensive Epilepsy Program and
Clinical Neurophysiology Laboratories
Louisiana State University School of Medicine
New Orleans, LA 70112, USA

ELSEVIER

Amsterdam – Lausanne – New York – Oxford – Shannon – Singapore – Tokyo

ELSEVIER

Radarweg 29 P.O. Box 211, 1000 AE Amsterdam, The Netherlands
The Boulevard, Langford Lane, Kidlington, Oxford, OX5 1GB, UK

First edition 1981
Reprinted 1982, 1985, 1987 (twice), 1988 (twice), 1990
Second edition 1991
Reprinted 1993, 1994 (twice), 1996, 1997, 1998
Third revised and enlarged edition 1999
Reprinted 2002, 2005, 2006 (twice), 2007, 2008

British Library Cataloguing in Publication Data
A catalogue record is available from the British Library.

ISBN: 978-0-444-82148-5 (PB)

Transferred to Digital Print 2009
Printed and bound in Singapore

Library of Congress Cataloging-in-Publication Data
Fisch, Bruce J.
   Fisch and Spehlmann's EEG primer. – 3rd printing, rev. and enl. / Bruce J. Fisch.
      p. cm
   Rev. ed. of EEG primer / R. Spehlmann. C1991.
   Includes bibliographical references and index.
   ISBN 0-444-82147-3 (hardbound : alk. paper) – ISBN 0-444-82148-1
(pbk. : alk. paper)
   1. Electroencephalography.   I. Spehlman, Rainer, 1931 - EEG
Primer. II. Title: EEG primer.
   [DNLM: 1. Electroencephalography.   WL 150 F528s]
RC386.6.E43S64 1991
616.8 047547--dc20
DNLM/DLC
for Library of Congress

The paper used in this publication meets the requirements of ANSI/NISO Z39.48-1992 (Permanence of Paper).

This book is dedicated to Susan, Ian and Paul and to my parents, June and Charles

Preface to the Third Edition

Remarkable changes in electroencephalography have occurred since the last edition of the EEG Primer. The advantages of information processing and cost have made digital EEG the clear choice for routine recording and interpretation. Important strides have also been made in elucidating the underlying physiology of EEG rhythms and epileptiform activity. Although quantitative statistical EEG analysis still does not have a clear clinical role, valid research applications abound.

The third edition of the EEG Primer continues to be organized according to EEG patterns. This unique approach for an EEG textbook has been retained because it mirrors the natural process of EEG interpretation: electroencephalographers are confronted first by patterns. Careful analysis of the electroencephalographic information is then combined with clinical information to provide a final assessment of brain function and to help formulate the differential diagnosis. Although almost all EEG findings are etiologically non-specific, some patterns are highly associated with certain disorders. In other instances the anatomical (topographic) distribution of EEG patterns serves to limit the diagnostic possibilities.

As in the last edition, controversial or unresolved areas of EEG have been avoided and I have also tried to avoid the insertion of any personal, but as yet unproven, beliefs about EEG. In this age of increasing 'information overload' I have focused the EEG Primer on practical information derived from convincing studies and the consensus of opinion by my colleagues in North America and around the world. However, the EEG Primer also contains sufficient information to make it an effective laboratory manual. The EEG correlates of most neurological disorders can be easily accessed through the index, and the appendices include the American Clinical Neurophysiology Society EEG guidelines and the international glossary of EEG terminology.

The most important purpose of a Preface, of course, is to thank those who have contributed in various ways to the final work. Dr. Omkar Markand at Indiana University introduced me to electroencephalography. Drs. Donald Klass, Barbara Westmoreland, Frank Sharbrough, and Jack Grabow at the Mayo Clinic provided me with an unparalleled fellowship experience in EEG. Indeed, at the time of my fellowship there were fewer neurophysiological procedures than today and in retrospect I am ever more grateful that I was allowed to focus on EEG. They also generously allowed me to enlist the help of the technologists in various projects, a vital resource for anyone in training. I will always be grateful to have spent time with these towering figures of clinical electroencephalography.

Once again, I am especially grateful to my good friend and colleague Dr. Timothy Pedley who shared his unique understanding of EEG and academic medicine with me. Equally important, he gave me the opportunity to pursue my interests in EEG as a young faculty member at Columbia University. I am also grateful to Dr. Jerome Engel who has always been supportive and who assisted me in becoming the editor of the second edition of the EEG Primer. A very special thanks to Dr. Austin Sumner, the chairman of Neurology at Louisiana State University School of Medicine, whose consistent support has allowed me and my colleagues to establish the first comprehensive epilepsy center in New Orleans and the central Gulf south region. Lastly, I want to thank all of our clinical neurophysiology fellows who have helped me to see electroencephalography from the perspective of the student year after gratifying year.

Bruce J. Fisch, M.D.

Introduction

The steps involved in recording an EEG are illustrated in Fig. 0.1 and described in Chapters 1–7 comprising Part A of this text.

(1) *The source* of the EEG is electrical activity generated by nerve cells in the cerebral cortex in response to cortical processing and various kinds of input, including that from pacemakers of rhythmical activity in the depth of the brain. These fluctuating potentials summate and conduct to the scalp where they can be recorded as the scalp EEG.

(2) *Recording electrodes* usually consist of small metal cups or disks that are attached to the scalp so that they make good mechanical and electrical contact. They cover the surface of the head at regular intervals.

(3) *Digital and analog EEG instruments* receive electrical input from the scalp electrodes which are connected to an input board. Digital EEG instruments contain differential amplifiers in the input board. In analog EEG instruments the cable of the input board terminates at the input selector switches which are used to select a pair of electrodes, or a calibration voltage, as the input of each recording channel. The input is connected to differential amplifiers which increase the size of the electrical potential differences between the two electrodes and reject interference simultaneously affecting both electrodes. High and low frequency filters are used to reduce the size of very slow and very fast potential changes and to emphasize clinically important electrical activity in the medium frequency range. A 60 Hz filter can eliminate the most common electrical interference in EEG recordings, namely that from power lines, if it cannot be eliminated by other means. The amplified electrical potentials are used to display the signal on a computer monitor or drive an ink pen, or other writing devices, up and down on chart paper which is pulled along at a constant speed.

(4) *Spatial analysis* of the EEG is a critical part of EEG interpretation that involves the application of electrical principles of differential amplification and volume conduction. It allows the EEG reader to determine the cortical location of observed waveforms.

(5) *The product* of the recording, namely the clinical EEG record, must satisfy a number of technical requirements to be acceptable. Requirements for routine clinical recordings differ from those for recordings from infants and small children, for all-night sleep recordings, for recordings in cases of suspected cerebral death and for recordings transmitted by telephone.

(6) *Artifacts* are pen deflections that are not due to cerebral activity and may come from such extracerebral activity as eye movements, heart beat and muscle contraction or from electrical interference, malfunctioning recording electrodes, or defects of the EEG machine. They must be eliminated or clearly explained to avoid confusion with cerebral activity.

(7) *Special methods of recording and analyzing the EEG,* including digital signal analysis and topographic mapping, are used to answer questions which cannot be answered by the conventional method of examining the pages of a routine recording.

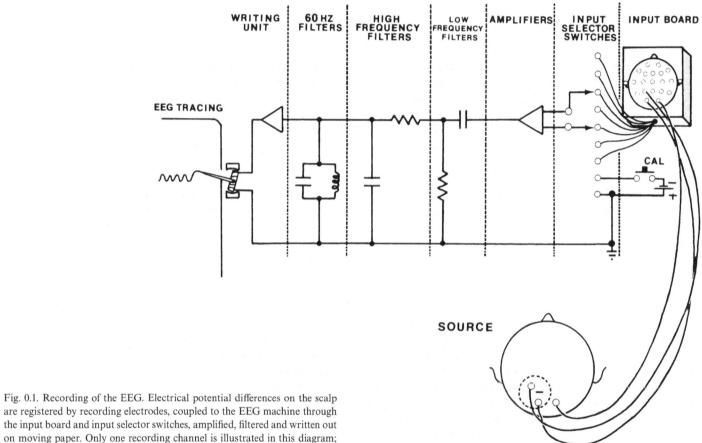

Fig. 0.1. Recording of the EEG. Electrical potential differences on the scalp are registered by recording electrodes, coupled to the EEG machine through the input board and input selector switches, amplified, filtered and written out on moving paper. Only one recording channel is illustrated in this diagram; most machines have 8 or more channels.

X

Contents

Part B: The normal EEG

Part C: The abnormal EEG

Part A

Technical background

1 The source of the EEG

SUMMARY

(1.1) *The EEG is generated by cortical nerve cell inhibitory and excitatory postsynaptic potentials.* These postsynaptic potentials summate in the cortex and extend to the scalp surface where they are recorded as the EEG. In addition to postsynaptic potentials, *intrinsic cell currents* produced by activation of ionic channels probably also contribute to the EEG, although their role has not been clearly established. Although *nerve cell action potentials* were originally thought to be the source of the EEG, they have a much smaller potential field distribution (less penetration into the extracellular space) and are much shorter in duration than postsynaptic potentials (about 1 ms compared to postsynaptic potentials of 15 to more than 200 ms). Action potentials, therefore, do not contribute significantly to either scalp or clinical intracranial EEG recordings.

(1.2) *Rhythmical cortical EEG activity arises from an interaction between the thalamus and cortex.* Many thalamic, thalamocortical and cortical neurons have intrinsic oscillatory firing properties that allow them to participate in cellular networks that generate rhythmic EEG activity. Sleep spindles are currently among the best understood of the rhythmic EEG activities. During sleep thalamic pacemaker cells in the nucleus reticularis of the thalamus stimulate thalamocortical cells which send excitatory impulses to the cortex. When the pacemaker cells within the nucleus reticularis are surgically or pharmacologically isolated their spindle activity continues whereas sleep spindle activity in the cortex and other structures ceases.

Desynchronization is the loss of rhythmical activity. It results from: (1) alterations in subcortical pacemaker activity (e.g., pacemaker cells of the nucleus reticularis in the thalamus fire tonically during desynchronization and in rhythmic bursts when producing sleep spindles), (2) alterations in systems that project diffusely to the cortex from the brainstem and basal forebrain areas (e.g., activation by ascending cholinergic systems produces a desynchronized EEG pattern), or (3) direct suppression or injury to any of the components of rhythmic cellular networks (i.e., damage to the subcortical pacemaker, thalamocortical, corticocortical, or cortical networks).

(1.3) Scalp electrodes record mainly the *summated postsynaptic potentials* of neurons in the underlying cortex, favoring slow, simultaneous, potential changes generated in large cortical areas of pyramidal cells oriented in parallel at 90° to the plane of the scalp surface. The tissue lying between the generating cells and the recording electrode through which electrical current must flow (e.g., brain, CSF, skull, and scalp) forms an electrical *volume conductor*. The volume conductor greatly modifies the amplitude and morphology (shape) of the cortical signal before it reaches the recording electrodes. The amplitude of potentials recorded directly from the cortex is typically 2 to 58 times greater than that seen in scalp electrodes depending on: (1) the degree of postsynaptic potential synchronization, (2) the orientation of the pyramidal cells to the scalp surface, and (3) the size of the area of participating cortex. The larger the area of cortex generating the potential, the less attenuation there is at the scalp.

The EEG is mainly generated by pyramidal cell postsynaptic potentials that form an extracellular cortical dipole layer. This dipole layer parallels the surface of the cortex projecting opposite electrical polarities towards the cortical surface compared to the innermost layers of the cortex. The scalp electrodes see only those potentials that are aimed at them and conducted from the cortical surface to the scalp.

The scalp electrode that is closest to the cortical generator does not always record the maximal potential. This is explained by the *solid angle theorem* of volume conduction.

1.1 THE GENERATOR OF THE EEG

The EEG is represented as a graph of voltage versus time where the y (vertical) axis is voltage and the x (horizontal) axis is time. Voltage at any given instant is always (for purely technical reasons to be discussed later) obtained as the difference in voltage between at least 2 electrode sites on the body, at least one of which is placed on the scalp. Thus, the operational definition of the EEG is that *the EEG is the difference in voltage between two different recording locations plotted over time*. This simple definition is actually seen to apply to all clinical bioelectrical recording techniques (ECG, EMG, ENG, etc.). The interpretational definition of the EEG is that it consists of *inhibitory and excitatory postsynaptic potentials of pyramidal cells generated in the cortex of the brain*.

The EEG signal that arises from thousands of synchronized pyramidal cell postsynaptic potentials is greatly modified by the time it reaches the recording electrode on the scalp. The factors that modify the original signal are:

(a) the electrical conductive properties of whatever tissues lie between the electrical source and the recording electrodes (e.g., brain parenchyma, dura, CSF, skull, scalp),

(b) the orientation of the electrical generator to the recording electrode (i.e., to what extent the generator is 'aimed towards' the electrode), and

(c) the conductive properties of both the recording electrodes and the scalp–electrode interface (the size of the electrodes, the electrical properties of the materials the electrode is constructed from, and the resistance to current flow produced by the junction of the electrode and scalp).

The process of current flow through the tissues between the electrical generator and the recording electrode is referred to as *volume conduction*. It is important for the electroencephalographer to have some understanding the effect of volume conduction on the original signal in order to create a mental picture of the original signal source. In this way the electroencephalographer can estimate the anatomical localization of a particular EEG activity. *Indeed, one of the more important and challenging aspects of learning electroencephalography is not pattern recognition. It is the ability to mentally reconstruct the most plausible 3-dimensional picture of current sources from the '2-dimensional' information provided by the EEG (4.8).*

There are 2 important factors (one biophysical and one physiological) that limit EEG interpretation. First, for any scalp recorded EEG signal there are an infinite number of source or sources within the volume of the brain that can explain, or 'fit,' the scalp recorded signal. Therefore, one or more generators in different locations in the brain can produce the same EEG findings at the scalp. This means it is theoretically impossible to know the location of the EEG generator in the brain with only scalp recorded EEG information. This is referred to as the *inverse problem*. In contrast, if the anatomical source, intensity and orientation of the electrical generator in the brain are known, then the EEG findings in scalp electrodes can be accurately predicted. This is referred to as the *forward problem*. However, it is the inverse problem that the electroencephalographer is confronted with in clinical practice. Because the localization of EEG sources within the brain is so important, the search for methods to help solve the inverse problem (referred to as *source localization*) is currently a central theme in EEG research (4.8). Fortunately, in routine EEG practice a formally trained electroencephalographer can greatly narrow the number of possible solutions to the inverse problem.

The second factor that limits interpretation is that EEG signal abnormalities do not always localize to the area of the brain where the main pathological attack is taking place. That is, an abnormal cortical signal may occasionally appear at a distance from the most prominent functional or structural damage. For example, the substance of a large structural lesion (e.g., tumor, stroke, etc.) is typically electrically silent. However, bordering tissue involved in EEG generation produces the abnormal activity seen. Indeed, in some cases EEG abnormalities recorded over the middle and anterior temporal areas may occur in the setting of a structural abnormality that more directly involves deep hemispheric structures or the frontal, parietal or posterior temporal lobes.

The cellular activity that produces the EEG consists mainly of cortical postsynaptic potential changes that alter the electrical charge across the pyramidal cell membrane (Fig. 1.1). Cortical neurons, like other nerve cells, have a resting electrical charge (membrane potential), that is the difference in the electrical potential between the interior of the cell and the extracellular space. The resting potential fluctuates as a result of impulses arriving from other neurons at synapses located on the cell body and its processes.

Such impulses generate relatively sustained local postsynaptic potentials that cause electrical current flow along the membrane of the cell body and dendrites. These changes can reduce the membrane potential to a critical level at which the membrane loses its charge completely, generating an action potential of brief duration that is propagated along the axon. The varying EEG signal is produced by the temporal and spatial summation of electrical currents that arise from postsynaptic potentials.

In addition to postsynaptic potentials there are intrinsic cellular currents mediated by ionic channels that produce high amplitude, long duration, extracellular potentials. It is highly likely that these extracellular potentials contribute to the EEG. Intrinsic cellular currents arise in neocortical cells undergoing burst firing with prolonged afterhyperpolarization potentials. Burst firing (a discharge consisting of a cluster of action potentials) with an afterhyperpolarization potential produces an event much longer in duration than a synaptic potential. Burst firing also tends to occur in synchrony with

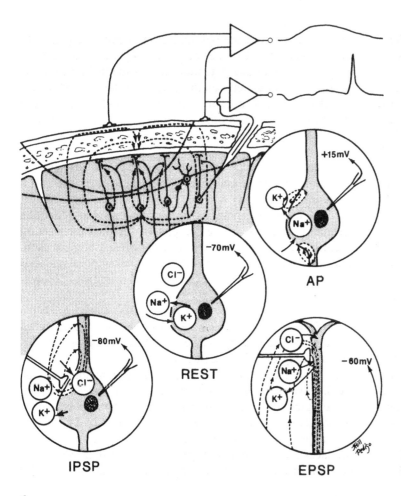

AP

+15mV

REST

−70mV

IPSP

−80mV

EPSP

−60mV

Fig. 1.1. The generation of the EEG by the cerebral cortex. Scalp electrodes record potential differences that are caused by postsynaptic potentials in the cell membrane of cortical neurons. The closed loops of the lighter dashed lines represent the summation of extracellular currents produced by the postsynaptic potentials; the open segments of heavier dashed lines connect all points having the same voltage level. The two scalp electrodes are at different voltage levels and record this difference, as it changes with time, in the form of a wave, which is indicated by the first of the two tracings at the upper right. A simultaneous recording made with a microelectrode from a single cortical neuron is indicated by the second tracing and bears no close relation to the scalp EEG. The round insets show the major ionic and electrical events at single neurons. REST: the uneven distribution of ions across the cell membrane, partly maintained by the semipermeable membrane, partly by the active extrusion of sodium ions and intrusion of potassium ions, causes a steady potential difference of about 65 mV which can be recorded with an intracellular microelectrode. IPSP: an inhibitory postsynaptic potential is caused by activation of an inhibitory synapse on the cell body, which transiently increases the permeability of the postsynaptic membrane to an influx of chloride (and in some cases also an efflux of potassium) ions and thereby increases the membrane potential, generating electrical current flow of decreasing intensity along the cell membrane. EPSP: an excitatory postsynaptic potential, caused by activation of an excitatory synapse on a dendritic process of the neuron, causes a nonselective increase of permeability to ions including sodium and thereby transiently decreases the membrane potential locally, generating current flow which tends to depolarize the membrane of the cell body. AP: an action potential is initiated at the axon hillock of the cell body by the summation of excitatory postsynaptic potentials which reduce the membrane potential by at least 10 mV to a critical level at which point the membrane suddenly becomes freely permeable to all ions so that the membrane potential momentarily collapses and reverses; local current flow depolarizes neighboring membrane parts and results in the propagation of an action potential along the membrane spreading radially from the cell body through the axon and dendritic tree.

other neurons in the same cell population. Both of these characteristics are important for generating potentials recordable at the scalp. In contrast to postsynaptic potentials and intrinsic cellular currents, isolated action potentials actually contribute little or nothing to the recorded EEG.

1.1.1 *The resting potential* of a neuron usually measures approximately –65 mV (varying from –40 to –80 mV in different nerve cells) and is negative on the inside of the cell membrane with respect to the outside. It is the result of (a) passive and (b) active properties of the cell membrane. (a) The passive properties are those which do not require metabolic energy. They result from unequal permeability of the membrane to sodium, potassium, chloride and other ions (Fig. 1.1). Diffusion and electrical gradients tend to drive ions in or out of the cell so that they distribute unevenly on both sides of the membrane. This uneven distribution contributes to a steady difference of electrical potential at rest. (b) Active properties require metabolic energy to counteract leakage of ions across the membrane; leaking ions are continuously transported against diffusional and electrical gradients back to concentrations appropriate for resting conditions. Most important is the sodium-potassium pump that actively transports sodium out of the cell and potassium into the cell. The concentration of sodium is maintained at about 10 times higher outside the cell than inside. Conditions which disrupt cerebral metabolism, such as anoxia or ischemia, may reduce or abolish this pumping action of the membrane, causing reduction of the membrane potential and increased excitability or complete collapse of neuronal function.

1.1.2 *Postsynaptic potentials* in nerve cells are caused by impulses (action potentials) arriving from other neurons via axons which terminate in a specialized contact zone, or synapse, located on the cell body or its processes. The impulse in the afferent neuron causes release of a neurotransmitter substance from its nerve terminal that diffuses across the synaptic cleft to the postsynaptic neuronal membrane patch where it interacts with a specialized receptor. The interaction produces a transient change in permeability to certain ions in the membrane portion near the synapse; this causes a local change in the resting potential or a postsynaptic potential (PSP). An excitatory postsynaptic potential (EPSP, Fig. 1.1) is a transient partial reduction in membrane potential which is usually due to an increased local permeability to sodium and potassium ions. Because sodium is a positively charged ion on the outside of the cell, its entry into the cell makes the negative intracellular resting potential less negative (i.e., partially depolarizes the cell). In contrast, an inhibitory postsynaptic potential (IPSP, Fig. 1.1) is a transient increase in intracellular negativity produced by the entry of negatively charged chloride ions into the cell or the exit of potassium ions from the cell. Even though the inside of the cell is relatively negative, the higher concentration of chloride outside the cell leads to an influx of chloride ions when the chloride channels are opened by the inhibitory postsynaptic potential. Inhibitory postsynaptic potentials also may involve an increase in permeability to potassium ions. The potentials generated at inhibitory synapses on different parts of the cell are thus summated and hyperpolarize the cell making it less likely to fire. The potential difference between the postsynaptic membrane portion and the other parts of the neuronal membrane causes an electrical current to flow along the neuronal membrane and to change the membrane potential of the cell body. Postsynaptic potentials alter the neuronal membrane potential by several millivolts and last over 100 ms.

1.1.3 *Action potentials* occur when the neuronal membrane is depolarized beyond a critical level or threshold (Fig. 1.1). This threshold is lowest at the junction of the cell body and the axon, or the axon hillock. A depolarization of the resting potential by at least 10 mV triggers a self-limited sequence of events consisting of a brief increase of the membrane permeability to sodium and potassium ions which leads to a sudden collapse, brief reversal and quick restitution of the membrane potential. This electrical change is the action potential; it has an amplitude of about 110 mV and lasts only about 1 ms. It is referred to as an all or none phenomenon because it does not vary in amplitude. By depolarizing and inducing the same sequence of events in neighboring membrane parts, the action potential flows as a wave of excitation over the cell membrane; it travels from the axon hillock down to the dendritic terminal where the depolarization releases neurotransmitter from the cell and causes an EPSP or IPSP to occur in other neurons.

The action potential itself causes only a very brief local current that does not penetrate far into the extracellular space. The amount of neurotransmitter released by the action potential depends only on the number of action potentials that are produced per second.

1.1.4 *Summation of electrical potential changes in the cortex* occurs mainly at the vertically oriented large pyramidal cells of the cortex. These neurons are especially suited for this role for several reasons.
(a) The dendrites of the pyramidal cells extend through nearly all layers of the cortex, guiding the flow of currents generated by postsynaptic potentials at either the cell body in the deep layers of the cortex or at dendrites in the more superficial layers through the entire thickness of the cortex.
(b) Cortical pyramidal cells are closely packed into functional vertical columns each containing several hundred cells oriented parallel to each other, facilitating spatial summation of the currents generated by each neuron towards the cortical surface.
(c) Groups of these neurons receive similar input and respond to it with potential changes that produce electrical currents of similar direction and timing. One afferent axon may contact several thousand cortical pyramidal neurons.
(d) The input to a pyramidal cell is magnified by the number

of synapses on each cell. Each pyramidal cell contains over 100,000 synapses.

The currents generated by these neurons summate in the extracellular space as indicated in Fig. 1.1. Most of the current is limited to the cortex. However, a small fraction penetrates through the meningeal coverings, spinal fluid and skull to the scalp where it causes different parts of the scalp to be at different potential levels. These potential differences, of usually only 10 to 100 μV, can be recorded between two electrodes and constitute the EEG.

Although the EEG is a result of individual neuronal potential changes, microelectrode activity from individual cortical cells correlates poorly with the ongoing EEG activity. This is partly because an extremely large number of potentials summate to produce the EEG. Furthermore the summating effects of volume conduction help to obscure the overlapping contributions (temporal dispersion) of individual neurons (see 1.3).

Interestingly, the normal geometry of synaptic distributions over the pyramidal cell makes it impossible to know whether an EEG event at the scalp is due to an inhibitory or excitatory postsynaptic potential. This is because excitatory and inhibitory synapses at opposite ends of a vertically oriented cortical pyramidal nerve cell can produce the same polarity potential changes at the cortical surface.

The biophysical explanation for this phenomenon is relatively straightforward. As mentioned in (1.1.2), the postsynaptic potential creates a cellular circuit of current. In the case of an EPSP, this current flows into the cell at the synapse as sodium ions enter the cell. The current then proceeds through the cell, emerges at a distance from the synapse, and then returns to the synapse in the extracellular space. Although EPSPs and IPSPs induce opposite polarity changes (with opposite directions of current flow), if the EPSPs and IPSPs are located at opposite ends of the vertical pyramidal cell, then the circuit of current flow seen by a surface EEG electrode will appear to have the same polarity whether it is caused by an EPSP or IPSP. Therefore, *if an excitatory and an inhibitory synapse are located at opposite ends of a vertically oriented pyramidal cell, both will produce the same polarity EEG change at the cortical surface.* Although there is technically no way to know if a given EEG waveform is generated by inhibitory or excitatory postsynaptic potentials (or various combinations of both), the inhibitory or excitatory generators of certain waveforms can sometimes be inferred from experimental information. For example, the spike component of the spike and slow wave pattern seen in patients with seizure disorders is known to be generated by excitation (e.g., the paroxysmal depolarizing shift) and the slow wave by inhibition.

1.2   RHYTHMICAL EEG ACTIVITY

Although one might expect that the complex neuronal activities of the brain would result in irregular EEG waves, the hu-

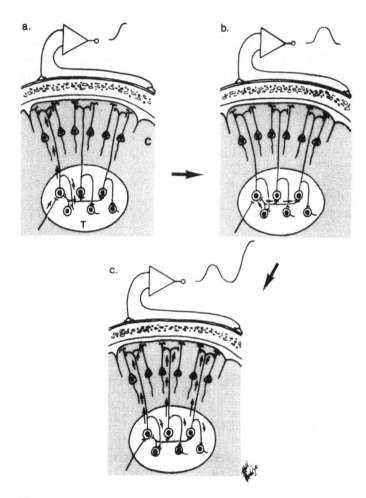

man EEG, recorded during wakefulness or sleep, commonly contains rhythmical activity (e.g., the alpha rhythm, mu rhythm, sleep spindles). Current understanding of the mechanisms responsible for the production of rhythmical EEG activity is based largely on animal experimentation. These experiments have shown that:

(a) slow frequency repetitive stimulation of nonspecific nuclei of the medial and intralaminar thalamus produces rhythmical cortical activity in a widespread distribution that resembles barbiturate induced rhythmical spindle shaped activity (the so-called *recruiting response*);

(b) repetitive stimulation of specific nuclei of the lateral thalamus produces rhythmical cortical activity over more localized areas (the so-called *augmenting response*) cor-

Fig. 1.2.   Steps in the production of rhythmical EEG activity in the cortex (C) as proposed by the original facultative pacemaker theory. (a) A thalamocortical relay neuron (TCR) in the thalamus (T) is excited by an afferent neuron and sends an impulse simultaneously to cortical neurons and to an inhibitory thalamic interneuron. Postsynaptic potentials of cortical neurons generate the first deflection in the cortical EEG. (b) The output of the inhibitory thalamic interneuron suppresses the activity of several TCR neurons. The resultant disappearance of postsynaptic cortical activity represents the end of the first deflection of the cortical EEG. (c) Several TCR interneurons, simultaneously released from inhibition by interneurons, send synchronous impulses to cortical neurons, causing another larger deflection of the cortical EEG. Simultaneous impulses to larger numbers of inhibitory thalamic interneurons initiate the next cycle of rhythmical activity.

responding in distribution to the thalamocortical pathways for primary sensory information;

(c) transection of the brainstem below the level of the thalamus has little influence on sleep spindles or barbiturate induced spindle-like activity, but destruction of the thalamus obliterates such activity;

(d) following surgical isolation of the cortex from the thalamus rhythmical activity persists in the thalamus whereas little evidence of such activity is recorded at the cortex;

(e) thalamic neurons in the nucleus reticularis continue to demonstrate rhythmic bursting activity (7–14 Hz) after they have been surgically or pharmacologically isolated (by synaptic blockade, in vitro), whereas similar rhythmic activity in the cortex and in target structures of the nucleus reticularis ceases;

(f) the similarity between 2 EEG alpha rhythms (i.e., the coherence) is greater between nearby cortical areas than between thalamic and cortical areas; but in experiments in dogs, for example, the pulvinar nucleus of the thalamus shows greater coherence with cortical activity than other thalamic areas;

(g) delta (< 4 Hz) waveforms in sleep occur with greatest amplitude in cortical layer V and correlate with periods of reduced pyramidal cell neuron activity.

These observations have led to the prevailing view that, in most cases, EEG rhythmicity begins with cortical activation or pacing by thalamic pacemaker cells. However, the cellular mechanism that is responsible for the pacing activity itself remains unknown.

Two leading models of how the thalamus interacts with the cortex to induce rhythmicity have been proposed. The first, and oldest, proposed by Andersen and Andersson (1968) is referred to as the *facultative pacemaker theory*.

According to this theory, thalamocortical cells send fibers to the cortex as well as giving off branches that turn back and end on thalamic inhibitory interneurons (Fig. 1.2a). The firing of one or a few thalamocortical neurons, in addition to affecting a few cortical neurons, excites thalamic inhibitory interneurons via recurrent collateral fibers (Fig. 1.2a). The output of the interneurons inhibits a large number of thalamocortical cells (Fig. 1.2b). At the end of the period of inhibition, the pool of thalamocortical neurons overshoots into excitation, giving off a synchronized volley which is again distributed both to cortical neurons and to inhibitory thalamic interneurons (Fig. 1.2c). The interneurons inhibit an even larger number of thalamocortical neurons, thus generating another cycle of rhythmical discharges. Theoretically, interneurons that have an inhibitory action lasting a tenth of a second could cause periodic synchronous inhibition and rebound excitation of thalamocortical neurons at about 10 times a second (in the frequency range of alpha activity). The projection of those impulses to the cortex at the same rate would thus induce postsynaptic potentials and a 10 Hz rhythmical EEG activity.

More recent work has demonstrated the presence of cells in

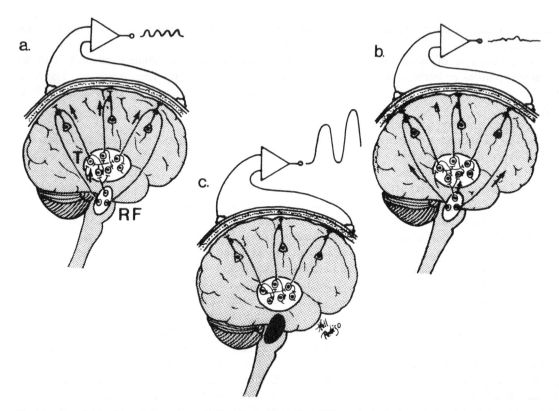

Fig 1.3. Postulated effect of the mesencephalic reticular formation (RF) on rhythmical cortical activity induced by a thalamic pacemaker (T). (a) Rhythmical activity is generated by the pacemaker system in the absence of strong activating impulses from the reticular formation. (b) Activating impulses from the reticular formation to the cortex and the thalamus abolish rhythmical cortical activity. (c) Lesions destroying or inactivating the reticular formation or its rostral connections result in the appearance of rhythmical slow waves, presumably caused by release of synchronizing centers from a tonic desynchronizing input by the reticular formation.

the nucleus reticularis of the thalamus that have intrinsic pacemaker properties responsible for the EEG sleep spindle pattern. The nucleus reticularis is a thin layer of neurons covering much of the anterior, ventral and lateral surfaces of the thalamus. These cells release the inhibitory transmitter GABA in rhythmic bursts of depolarizations that are directed to the neurons of the dorsal thalamus and rostral brainstem. The pacemaker cells stimulate the thalamocortical cells of the thalamus, which then produce rhythmic excitation in the cortex. The excitatory thalamocortical cells have the intrinsic property of producing bursts of depolarizations as a rebound response to each inhibitory stimulus of the pacemaker cells. The rhythmic pacing activity within the nucleus reticularis continues when the cells are surgically or pharmacologically isolated. Not only thalamocortical cells, but other thalamic, neocortical, and hippocampal cells that contain excitatory amino acids also have the intrinsic property of producing burst discharges. The burst discharges occur during periods of behavioral non-arousal whereas more continuous firing patterns occur during periods of arousal. The burst discharge consists of a sudden series of action potentials followed by a prolonged afterhyperpolarization. Burst firing is associated with rhythmical EEG patterns whereas transition to a steady firing pattern is associated with a cessation of rhythmical activity. Individual cell bursts usually occur in synchrony with bursting activity in other cells within the same neuronal network population.

Cortical rhythmicity depends, in part, on networks within the cortex itself. Cortical to cortical connections are more abundant than thalamic to cortical connections. Animal experimentation has shown that the rhythmical activity of one cortical area may correlate more closely with the rhythmical activity of another cortical area than with similar activity in the thalamus. Finally, computer modeling experiments based on cortical neuronal recordings suggest that although single cortical cell recordings may not show rhythmical activity, EEG rhythmicity may occur as the result of a complex interaction among large numbers of such cortical cells (Traub et al., 1989). Such population or network behavior reveals that prominent potentials may arise at the cortical surface with little obvious correlation with individual cell activities.

In summary, EEG rhythmicity appears to be dependent on interactions between the cortex and thalamus, both of which have certain structural and functional properties that lend themselves to the production of rhythmical activity. The thalamus is essential for generating or pacing rhythmical activities, whereas the cortex produces virtually all of the recordable potentials at the scalp and provides a synchronous output in response to thalamic input. Thus, certain rhythmical activities, such as sleep spindles, may be abolished by lesions involving either thalamic structures or cortical structures directly, or by involving only subcortical areas that interrupt thalamic input to the cortex.

The interruption of rhythmical activity, also referred to as *desynchronization* of the EEG, has been shown to occur in response to activation of ascending cholinergic projections of the basal forebrain and brainstem and projections from the raphe nuclei and locus ceruleus. These neuronal groups receive input from practically all sensory systems and cortical areas and send their output to the entire cortex through direct connections and relays in the diencephalon (Fig. 1.3a). Rhythmical activity is thereby interrupted through a direct effect on cortical neurons and indirectly through the modulation of thalamic neurons that participate in the pacing of cortical rhythms. As mentioned above, at the cellular level desynchronization is accompanied by a transition from a burst firing pattern to a more continuous or single spike pattern. Desynchronization is enhanced by behavioral arousal and suppressed by non-REM sleep (i.e., stages I, II, III and IV sleep). Abnormal rhythmical EEG patterns, such as the alpha coma pattern, occur in the setting of widespread injury (such as anoxia or brain trauma) to the ascending neuronal systems that would otherwise produce arousal and desynchronization.

1.3 RECORDING OF ELECTRICAL POTENTIALS WITH SCALP ELECTRODES

As previously stated, electrodes on the scalp record mainly the summated electrical changes of the underlying cortex; they may also rarely record some potential changes generated in distant parts of the brain, as well as potential changes produced outside the brain (i.e., artifacts). The amplitude of the recorded potentials depends on the intensity of the electrical source, on its distance from the recording electrodes, its spatial orientation, and on the electrical resistance and capacitance of the structures between the source and the recording electrode. These factors favor the recording of potential changes which (a) occur near the recording electrodes, (b) are generated by cortical dipole layers that are oriented towards the recording electrode at a 90° angle to the scalp surface, (c) are generated in a large area of tissue, and (d) rise and fall at rapid speed.

The EEG recorded with scalp electrodes differs from that recorded simultaneously with electrodes placed directly on the underlying cortex (also referred to as the 'electrocorticogram' or 'ECoG'). The scalp EEG is of lower amplitude and is by comparison somewhat distorted in shape. Generally, faster frequencies are attenuated more than slower ones. Very fast and brief potential changes may be lost completely in scalp recordings or may be picked up only over their production site or near skull defects, whereas slower potentials tend to be conducted farther and thus recorded over greater distances.

Comparisons of simultaneous scalp and cortical recordings of normal activity suggest that at least 6 cm^2 of cortex with synchronous activity is needed to create a reliably recorded scalp potential. Higher intensity, highly synchronized potentials, such as epileptiform spikes, can occasionally be recorded at the scalp with the activation of somewhat smaller areas of cortex. These filtering effects depend in part on the electrical properties of structures between cortex and scalp electrodes. The amplitude of the scalp EEG may decrease as a result of either: (a) an increase of the overall electrical impedance between the source and the recording electrodes, for instance an increase in the thickness of the skull, which reduces the flow of currents between the source and the recording electrodes, or (b) a decrease in the impedance at different stages across the path of these currents, as may occur with a collection of subdural blood or cerebrospinal fluid that shunts ('short-circuits') the currents before they reach the recording electrodes.

Even though the scalp EEG reflects local potential changes, cortical potentials of very similar shape and timing over wide parts of the brain may be triggered by more localized cerebral disorders. This process has been called 'projection' and the resulting rhythms have been called 'projected rhythms' or 'rythmes à distance.' Because the pacemaker for bilateral synchronous discharges was originally presumed to be located at the center of the brain, the term 'centrencephalic' was used. Although these rhythms may be induced by the action of distant centers, the recorded EEG is generated by cortex near the recording electrodes, not by distant or subcortical sites. Moreover, although it is clear that most widespread rhythms are secondarily generated from initiating sites in the thalamus, it is also clear that bilateral synchronous activity may arise from cortical lesions, particularly those that produce epileptiform activity.

Scalp electrodes only rarely record potentials generated at distant sites. This is illustrated by the observation that scalp electrodes over a large area of cortex with completely abolished function will generally show complete absence of electrical activity. In addition, individual epileptiform spikes generated solely by the hippocampus within the temporal lobe never appear in simultaneous scalp recordings and very rarely in direct subtemporal cortical recordings. Rarely, some types of high amplitude activity, such as slow waves or cortical spikes arising from a large cortical area, are conducted electrically through the volume of the interposed brain tissue. They then may appear in scalp electrodes at considerable distance, intermixed with the EEG representing more proximal cortical activity. Electrical conduction also accounts for the appearance of EEG potentials at scalp electrodes ipsilateral to hemispherectomies.

Aside from placing electrodes directly in the cortex, the alternatives for improving the detection of cortical potentials include: (1) changing the spatial filtering characteristics of the recording electrodes by changing their physical size, (2) changing the spatial filtering characteristics by altering the combinations of electrodes placed in any one amplifier (e.g., change of montage; Chapter 4), and (3) increasing sampling at the scalp surface by placing additional scalp electrodes, creating smaller interelectrode distances. Sampling can be increased to the point where electrodes are placed one electrode diameter apart from each other. This has led some manufacturers to develop electrode scalp nets for rapid placement of up to 128 electrodes at a time. It has also led to the relatively recent development of a newer system of electrode placement in which the nomenclature for electrode placement has been expanded to include more than double the previous number of electrodes (the 10–20 versus the modified 10–20 system; 2.3). In routine practice at least 21 scalp electrodes are used for EEG recording.

Potentials that are generated by sources other than the brain that are picked up by scalp electrodes and recorded together with the EEG are referred to as *artifacts* (6). For instance, scalp electrodes located over muscle frequently record muscle fiber activity. Movements of the eyes, tongue and other large and electrically charged structures also generate changing electrical fields, which are recorded by scalp electrodes. Heart muscle contraction can induce potential changes at scalp electrodes similar to the potential changes recorded in the electrocardiogram. Strong sources of alternating current near the recording site may interfere with the recording.

The transmission of a signal through a volume conductor occurs nearly at the speed of light. Therefore, similar appearing waveforms that occur in different or non-adjacent scalp locations without any difference in their time of appearance most likely arise from the same cortical generator. In contrast, those that appear with any measurable time delay between them must involve transsynaptic conduction and cannot arise from the same cortical cells. Since transsynaptic transmission may occur within milliseconds, such distinctions can only be made using digital EEG systems. Analog EEG systems do not display signals with sufficient time resolution to distinguish timing differences of several milliseconds between different recording channels.

REFERENCES

Abraham, K. and Ajmone Marsan, C. (1958) Patterns of cortical discharges and their relation to routine scalp electroencephalography. Electroenceph. Clin. Neurophysiol. 10: 447–461.
Andersen, P. and Andersson, S.A. (1968) Physiological Basis of the Alpha Rhythm. Appleton, New York.
Andersen, P. and Andersson, S.A. (1974) Section IV. Thalamic origin of cortical rhythmical activity. In: A. Rémond (Ed.), Handbook of Electroenceph. Clin. Neurophysiol., Vol. 2C. Elsevier, Amsterdam, pp. 90–118.
Ball, G.J., Gloor, P. and Thompson, C.J. (1977) Computed unit-EEG correlations and laminar profiles of spindle waves in the electroencephalogram of cats. Electroenceph. Clin. Neurophysiol. 43: 330–345.
Burgess, R.C. (Ed.) (1991) Localization of neural generators. J. Clin. Neurophysiol. 8.
Buser, P. (1987) Thalamocortical mechanisms underlying synchronized EEG activity. In: A.M. Halliday, S.R. Butler and R. Paul (Eds.), A Textbook of Clinical Neurophysiology. Wiley, New York, pp. 595–622.
Buzsaki, G. and Traub, R. (1997) Physiological basis of EEG activity. In: J. Engel, Jr. and T.A. Pedley (Eds.), Epilepsy: A Comprehensive Textbook. Lippincott-Raven Publishers, Philadelphia, pp. 819–830.
Cooper, R., Winter, A.L., Crow, H.J. and Walter, W.G. (1965) Comparison of subcortical, cortical and scalp activity using chronically indwelling electrodes in man. Electroenceph. Clin. Neurophysiol. 18: 217–228.

Creutzfeldt, O. and Houchin, J. (1974) Section I. Neuronal basis of EEG-waves. In: A. Rémond (Ed.), Handbook of Electroenceph. Clin. Neurophysiol., Vol. 2C. Elsevier, Amsterdam, pp. 5–55.

Gabor, A.J. (1978) Physiological Basis of Electrical Activity of Cerebral Origin. Grass Instrument Co., Quincy, MA (available on request).

Gloor, P. (1985) Neuronal generators and the problem of localization in electroencephalography: Application of volume conductor theory to electroencephalography. J. Clin. Neurophysiol. 2: 327–354.

Goldensohn, E.S. (1979) Neurophysiological substrates of EEG activity. In: D. Klass and D. Daley (Eds.), Current Practice of Clinical Neurophysiology. Raven, New York, pp. 421–440.

Kellaway, P., Gol, A. and Proler, M. (1966) Electrical activity of the isolated cerebral hemisphere and isolated thalamus. Exp. Neurol. 14: 281–304.

Lagerlund, T. (1996) Volume conduction. In: J. Daube (Ed.), Clinical Neurophysiology. F.A. Davis, Philadelphia, pp. 29–39.

Leissner, P., Lindholm, L.E. and Petersén, I. (1970) Alpha amplitude dependence on skull thickness as measured by ultrasound technique. Electroenceph. Clin. Neurophysiol. 29: 392–399.

Llinás, R.R. (1988) The intrinsic electrophysiological properties of mammalian neurons: insight into the central nervous system. Science 242: 1654–1664.

Lopes da Silva, F. (1987) Dynamics of EEGs as signals of neuronal populations: models and theoretical considerations. In: E. Niedermeyer and F. Lopes da Silva (Eds.), Electroencephalography: Basic Principles, Clinical Applications and Related Fields. Urban and Schwarzenberg, Baltimore, pp. 15–28.

Metherate, R. and Ashe, J. (1993) Ionic flux contributions to neocortical slow waves and nucleus basalis-mediated activation: whole-cell recordings in vivo. J. Neurosci. 13: 5312–5323.

Nunez, P.L. (1981) Electric Fields of the Brain: The Neurophysics of EEG. Oxford University Press, New York.

Nunez, P.L. (1995) Neocortical Dynamics and Human EEG Rhythms. Oxford University Press, New York.

Pedley, T.A. and Traub, R.D. (1990) Physiological basis of the EEG. In: D.D. Daly and T.A. Pedley (Eds.), Current Practice of Clinical Electroencephalography, Second Edition. Raven Press, New York, pp. 107–137.

Pfurtscheller, G. and Cooper, R. (1975) Frequency dependence of the transmission of the EEG from cortex to scalp. Electroenceph. Clin. Neurophysiol. 38: 93–96.

Schlag, J. (1974) Section V. Reticular influences on thalamo-cortical activity. In: A. Rémond (Ed.), Handbook of Electroenceph. Clin. Neurophysiol., Vol. 2C. Elsevier, Amsterdam, pp. 119–134.

Speckman, E.J. and Elger, C.E. (1993) Introduction to the neurophysiological basis of the EEG and DC potentials. In: E. Niedermeyer and F. Lopes da Silva (Eds.), Electroencephalography: Basic Principles, Clinical Application and Related Fields. Williams and Wilkins, Baltimore, pp. 15–26.

Steriade, M. (1993) Cellular substrates of brain rhythms. In: E. Niedermeyer and F. Lopes da Silva (Eds.), Electroencephalography: Basic Principles, Clinical Application and Related Fields. Williams and Wilkins, Baltimore, pp. 27–62.

Steriade, M., Curro Dossi, R. and Nunez, A. (1991) Network modulation of a slow intrinsic oscillation of cat thalamocortical neurons implicated in sleep delta waves: cortically induced synchronization and brainstem cholinergic suppression. J. Neurosci. 11: 3200–3217.

Traub, R.D., Miles, R. and Wong, R.K.S. (1989) Model of the origin of rhythmic population oscillations in the hippocampal slice. Science 243: 1319–1325.

2 Recording electrodes

SUMMARY

Recording electrodes transfer electrical potentials at the recording site to the input of the recording machine.

(2.1) *Electrode types* most commonly used in clinical EEG are metal discs or cups attached to the scalp and other recording sites. Needle scalp electrodes are no longer recommended for routine clinical use. Nasopharyngeal and sphenoidal electrodes require special insertion procedures and are used in some laboratories in addition to scalp electrodes in an attempt to record the EEG from the undersurface of the temporal lobe.

(2.2) *Electrical properties* determine whether recording electrodes can couple potential changes from the head to the input of the EEG machine without distortion. Electrodes should have a surface made of gold, chlorided silver or other materials that do not interact electrically with the scalp. Electrode application should create an electrical contact with impedances between 100 and 5000 Ω. Electrodes with much higher impedances can attenuate the recording and cause 60 Hz artifact; impedances of less than 100 Ω are usually the result of accidental short-circuits between electrodes. Polarization and bias potentials develop at the interface between electrode and tissue and can be minimized by careful technique and the use of proper electrode metals.

(2.3) *Placement of electrodes* should cover the entire head evenly and be reproducible between subjects and laboratories. This is accomplished using the international 10–20 system or more recently, the modified 10–20 system. The 10–20 system uses measurements between bony landmarks on the skull to determine the coordinates for 21 recording electrodes. The modified 10–20 system duplicates the 10–20 system but has provisions for additional electrodes and is now the preferred system of electrode placement. Fewer electrodes may be used in infants.

(2.4) *Recording non-cerebral potentials* is useful for detecting and identifying artifacts that contaminate the EEG as well as for monitoring other body functions such as eye movements, axial muscle tone, respiration, and motor activity. Whenever the technologist encounters spontaneous abnormal movements, additional electrodes or monitors should be placed that will display the movements and allow them to be correlated with the ongoing EEG.

2.1 ELECTRODE SHAPES AND APPLICATION METHODS

Electrodes consist of a conductor attached to a wire that leads to a plug that is inserted into the input of the recording machine. Scalp electrodes are applied after determining their precise scalp location and after preparing the scalp to reduce electrical impedance. Metal surface electrodes should be cleansed with a solution of an antiseptic soap after each use. Nasopharyngeal electrodes should be autoclaved; penetrating electrodes used on patients with contagious diseases should be discarded after use. Special handling and cleaning procedures must also be used for surface electrodes in patients at special

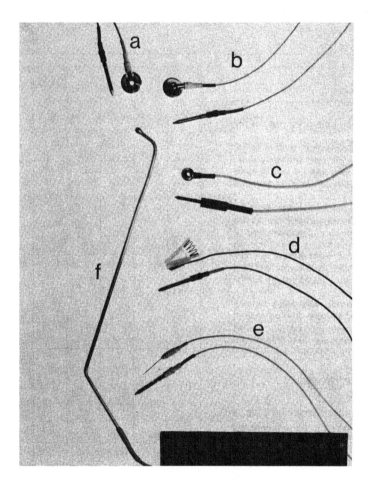

risk for contagious diseases such as AIDS, viral hepatitis or Creutzfeldt–Jakob disease.

2.1.1 *Metal disc and cup electrodes* usually have diameters of 4–10 mm (Fig. 2.1). Smaller or larger electrodes do not make stable mechanical and electrical contact with the scalp. An insulated lead wire is attached to each electrode. The insulation of each wire has a different color for easy identification of each electrode. Mechanical and electrical problems are reduced if the insulations of the lead wires are attached to each other in the form of a stranded cable from which the leads separate only at the two ends. Before electrodes are applied, the application site is determined by measurements (2.3) and prepared by wiping with alcohol or abrasive electrolyte gels (such as Omni Prep).

Several methods may be used to attach electrodes to the scalp. The collodion technique has the advantage of giving very stable recordings with relatively few artifacts. It is the only available method for long term recording. In this technique, cup electrodes with a central hole are placed onto the prepared scalp site and held in place with a stylus while a few drops of collodion are applied around the edge of the elec-

---

Fig. 2.1. Various types of extracranial EEG electrodes, shown with their connector plugs and part of their lead wires. (a) Large metal cup electrode with a central hole. (b) Large metal cup electrode without hole. (c) Small metal cup electrode with central hole. (d) Clip electrode. (e) Needle electrode. (f) Nasopharyngeal electrode.

trode and spread onto the scalp. The spreading and drying of the collodion may be facilitated by a stream of compressed air guided through a tube around the stylus. After the electrode is securely attached, the stylus is removed and the cup is filled with conductive jelly which is injected with a blunt hypodermic needle inserted through the central hole of the cup. If cup electrodes without a central hole are used, they are filled with conductive paste before application to the scalp. Some laboratories place small pieces of gauze soaked with collodion over the electrodes to hold them in place. Electrodes are removed by dissolving the collodion with acetone. Because of the chemicals involved, the collodion method should not be used in areas that have limited ventilation or explosion hazards such as infant isolettes or operating rooms.

Another method of applying electrodes uses a paste that can both hold the electrode in place and provide good electrical contact. After preparation of the scalp site, a piece of this adhesive conductive paste is placed on the scalp and the electrode is pressed into the center of the paste until it makes firm contact. Electrodes with a central hole allow the paste to escape through the hole so that the rim of the cup sits firmly on the scalp. A gauze pad or cotton ball may be placed over the electrode to hold it more securely in place and to delay drying of the paste. This method is fast, but electrodes tend to lose good mechanical and electrical contact more readily than when they are applied with collodion.

Other methods of applying disc or cup electrodes involve the use of: (a) paraffin wax, (b) suction electrodes, or (c) headbands, straps or caps which hold an entire set of electrodes in place. These methods generally give less satisfactory results than the other methods described above.

Metal disc or cup electrodes may be placed around the eyes, on the chest or other parts of the body to monitor electrical potentials which are generated by eye movements, heart beat, respiration, muscle contraction or body movements that often contaminate the EEG (4.3). While EEG scalp electrodes may be used to monitor the occurrence of extracerebral activity, they introduce some distortion and special electrodes are required if faithful recordings of such activity are desired.

2.1.2 *Clip electrodes* are sometimes used for recordings from the earlobes. The clips should contain cups or discs made from the same materials as the scalp electrodes to avoid electrical problems caused by recording from dissimilar electrodes.

2.1.3 *Needle electrodes* are sharp wires, usually made of steel or platinum. They are inserted into the superficial layers of the scalp after thorough disinfection of the insertion site. The advantage of fast application is outweighed by the disadvantages of pain, possible infection and unfavorable electrical characteristics. Some laboratories still use these electrodes for emergency recordings from comatose patients, but most electroencephalographers feel they should not be used. Needle electrodes are frequently used during intraoperative recording and in association with intracranial electrode recording.

2.1.4 *Nasopharyngeal electrodes* are used in addition to scalp electrodes by some laboratories in patients who are suspected of having epileptiform activity in the basal parts of the temporal lobe but who do not show such activity in scalp recordings.

Nasopharyngeal electrodes are made of a conducting wire embedded in rigid plastic that has a z-shape to fit the path of insertion. The tip is an uninsulated 2–5 mm diameter metal ball. One electrode is inserted through each nostril, slid backwards along the bottom of the nasal cavity near the midline, and then rotated outward. This places the tip against the roof of the nasopharynx and very close to the skull at the base of the middle cerebral fossa, i.e. close to the tip of the temporal lobe. Because the insertion can cause discomfort, gagging and slight injury to the mucous membranes, it is often done by a physician using a local anesthetic spray.

It is important to recognize that nasopharyngeal electrode recordings occasionally produce artifacts that mimick epileptiform spikes and sharp waves. Thus, epileptiform activity occurring exclusively at the nasopharyngeal electrode should be considered artifact until proven otherwise. The main advantage of nasopharyngeal recordings is to emphasize or clarify activity also recorded at other electrode sites. In this regard, however, it is also important to recognize that certain benign patterns, such as small sharp spikes, may be greatly amplified icy nasopharyngeal recordings. This amplification frequently leads readers unfamiliar with nasopharyngeal recordings to mistakenly identify pseudoepileptiform patterns as abnormal epileptiform patterns.

2.1.5 *Sphenoidal electrodes* are used to detect epileptiform activity in the temporal lobes. This electrode consists of a flexible wire with an uninsulated tip which is placed near the sphenoidal wing through a cannula inserted through the temporal and masseter muscles. Electrode placement can be checked by X-ray. The electrodes can be left in place for several days of serial EEG recordings without danger of breaking or injury to the patient. (For a more detailed explanation of electrode placement refer to the references at the end of the chapter.)

Sphenoidal electrodes are mainly of value for distinguishing between mesial and lateral temporal epileptogenic sources. They rarely increase the likelihood of detecting temporal epileptiform discharges, particularly if surface electrodes recorded with long interelectrode distances are placed near the sphenoidal electrode insertion points, or if so-called true anterior temporal surface electrodes are used (2.3.2). Their usefulness is mainly due to the typical distribution of temporal lobe epileptiform spikes, shown in Fig. 2.2.

2.1.6 *Electrocorticographic ball or wick electrodes* are used during some neurosurgical procedures, usually excision of epileptogenic foci, to record the ECoG from the exposed cortical surface. These electrodes consist of metal balls or saline-soaked cotton wicks which may be mounted on springs and held in place by swivel joints for easy placement.

2.1.7 *Subdural and epidural electrodes* are used to localize epileptiform activity and to map cortical function. They consist of sheets or single column strips of evenly spaced disc electrodes (usually made of platinum or stainless steel) embedded in a thin layer of flexible translucent Silastic rubber. The sheets are inserted through a craniotomy opening, whereas the strips consisting of single rows of electrodes can also be introduced into the epidural or subdural space through a burr hole. Once the electrodes are in place, the underlying cortical activity can be recorded by connecting the electrode leads to the input board of any routine EEG machine. In addition, the subdural electrodes can be used to stimulate the underlying cortex by applying an electrical current to individual electrodes. The results of stimulation, which typically include involuntary movements, sensory manifestations, or various forms of aphasia, are used to map the locations of critical cortical functions so they may be spared during cortical resection.

2.1.8 *Depth electrodes* are used for EEG recording, to define the targets for surgical destruction, and for placement as stimulating electrodes for the treatment of movement disorders. EEG recording depth electrodes consist usually of a bundle of fine wires that terminate at different cylindrical contacts along the length of the depth electrode and thus allow for recordings from different depths. As with subdural electrodes, platinum metal is used for MRI compatability. The insertion of depth electrodes is stereotactically guided by determining the position of the target in a three-dimensional reference system using a frame attached to the head. The trajectory coordinates of the head frame are matched to MRI and CT images for precise placement into targeted brain structures. So-called 'frameless' stereotaxy currently lacks precision for the routine implantation of depth electrodes.

2.2 ELECTRICAL PROPERTIES OF RECORDING ELECTRODES

Good recording electrodes should couple the electrical potential changes at the recording site to the input of the recording machine without distortion. To obtain such high fidelity recordings, one must (1) choose recording electrodes of suitable material; (2) measure electrode resistance to ascertain electrical continuity between the two ends of the electrode if in doubt; (3) measure electrode impedance after every electrode application and during the recording to evaluate the electrical contact between electrode and scalp; and (4) avoid electrode polarization and bias potentials.

2.2.1 *Electrode materials* should be those which do not interact chemically with the electrolytes of the scalp. Electrodes coated with gold, silver chloride, tin or platinum are satisfactory.

2.2.2 *Electrode resistance,* or opposition to direct current

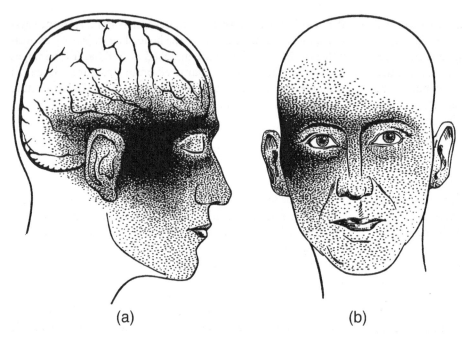

(a)   (b)

Fig. 2.2.   The stippled area shows the approximate distribution of right temporal lobe epileptiform spike activity over the surface of the head. Note that the best areas for recording are behind the outer canthus of the eye, over the area of the inferior zygomatic arch (where sphenoidal electrode insertion is located), superior to the zygomatic arch (where so called true anterior temporal electrodes are placed) and immediately anterior to the ear (the auricular electrodes A1 and A2 often detect a higher amplitude spike than do F7 and F8). Reproduced from Gibbs and Gibbs, 1952.

flow, is measured when a break in the electrical continuity between electrode, lead wire and connector plug is suspected. This measurement is made while the electrode is not attached to the scalp. The two uninsulated ends of the electrode are connected to an ohmmeter which passes a weak direct current through the electrode. The resistance of an intact electrode should measure no more than a few ohms.

2.2.3 *Electrode impedance,* or opposition to alternating current flow, is measured after an electrode has been applied to the recording site to evaluate the contact between electrode and scalp. The impedance of each electrode should be measured routinely before every EEG recording and should be between 100 and 5000 Ω. Electrode impedance is measured with an impedance meter that passes a weak alternating current from the electrode selected for testing through the scalp to all other electrodes connected to the meter (Fig. 2.3). The measured impedance reflects mainly that of the selected electrode, the other electrodes offering multiple return pathways with negligible total impedance.

An alternating current is used for this measurement for two reasons: (a) Alternating current is more representative of the alternating potential changes recorded in the EEG, especially if it alternates at about 10 Hz, a common frequency of EEG potential changes; the opposition to current alternating at this frequency may differ from that to alternating current of other frequencies and, especially from that to direct current. (b)

Passage of direct current through an electrode attached to the scalp can electrically polarize the interface between electrode and skin and thereby lead to distortion of subsequent EEG recordings.

Most EEG machines have provisions for testing electrode impedance during the recording. This is done by injecting a weak alternating current of constant intensity through a pair of electrodes connected to the input of a recording channel. This causes a pen deflection in that channel with an amplitude proportional to the sum of the impedances of the two electrodes. If the deflection indicated has an unacceptably high or low impedance, the faulty electrode of the pair must be identified by pairing each electrode with another electrode of acceptable impedance and repeating the current injection.

Very high or very low impedance is undesirable. Very low impedance acts like a shunt between the recording electrodes and effectively short-circuits the EEG potential differences. It is practically impossible to reduce electrode impedance to less than a few hundred ohms without there being an abnormal pathway of conduction between the electrodes across the scalp. An electrode showing very low impedance may be making contact with another electrode because of an excess of electrolyte jelly or paste, or because of saline or sweat forming a conductive bridge between the electrodes on the scalp. Such an electrode should be inspected, cleaned, and reapplied or exchanged if necessary.

Very high impedance is undesirable mainly because con-

a.　　　　　　　　　　　　　　　　　　　　　　　b.

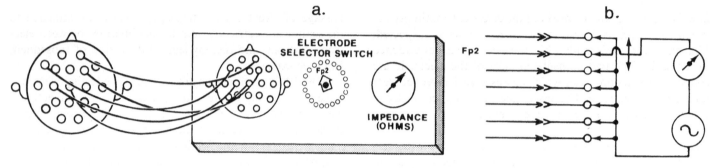

Fig. 2.3.   Measurement of electrode impedance. (a) Diagram of the input board with receptacles for the connectors from scalp electrodes (left), selector switch designating electrode Fp2 for impedance measurement (middle), and impedance meter (right). (b) Electrical circuit used for impedance measurement: a weak alternating current is passed through the impedance meter to the electrode selected for measurement (Fp2) and its contact with the scalp (not shown); the current is returned through a combination of all other scalp electrodes. The impedance of the selected electrode is read from the impedance meter; the impedance of the return path is negligible relative to that of the electrode being tested.

necting an electrode of very high impedance and one of lower impedance to the input of a differential amplifier causes an imbalance which favors the recording of 60 Hz interference* (3.4). Electrodes showing high impedance readings should be checked for good mechanical and electrical contact and the junctions of the lead wire with the metal disc or cup and with the plug terminal should be inspected for possible breaks.

2.2.4   *Electrode polarization and bias potentials* may occur

---
* Interference has a frequency of 50 Hz in countries using alternating current of that frequency.

and distort EEG recordings even when mechanical and electrical recording conditions seem good.

Fortunately, the effect of these phenomena on the routine clinical EEG is usually negligible using modern electrodes, methods of electrode application and recording machines. *Polarization* results from current flow across the interface between electrode and tissue. The current carries positive ions to the more negative part of the junction and negative ions to the more positive part. This build-up of ions polarizes the electrode so that it favors current flow in one direction and resists flow in the opposite direction, thereby distorting the recording of alternating EEG potentials. Polarization is kept to a minimum by: (a) a fairly large contact area between electrode and scalp that keeps current density at any one point low; (b) high impedance amplifier inputs that keep the current (amperage) flowing through the electrodes during the recording low; and (c) avoidance of steady current flow, especially that used to measure electrode resistance. With these precautions, it is not necessary to use non-polarizable electrodes such as chlorided silver electrodes for routine clinical EEG recordings, although such electrodes are necessary for other purposes, especially for faithful recording of very slowly changing or steady potential differences.

Bias potentials result from the exchange of metal ions and electrolytes in the absence of current flow. They interfere with EEG recordings only when they are not steady. Steady bias potentials cause blocking of amplifiers that occurs in analog EEG instruments immediately after switching to a new selection of electrodes. The effect of bias potentials can be minimized by using (a) electrodes of pure metals with clean surfaces which reduce ion exchange and (b) electrodes of the same kind at the inputs of each amplifier; this neutralizes electrical differences caused by bias potentials.

2.3 ELECTRODE PLACEMENT

2.3.1 *The international 10–20 system* of electrode placement provides for uniform coverage of the entire scalp. It uses the distances between bony landmarks of the head to generate a system of lines which run across the head and intersect at intervals of 10 or 20% of their total length. Electrodes are placed at the intersections. The use of the 10–20 system assures symmetrical, reproducible electrode placements and allows a more accurate comparison of EEGs from the same patient and from different patients, recorded in the same or different laboratories. The system is flexible: additional electrodes, which may be needed to accurately localize an abnormality, can be incorporated by further subdividing the distances between intersections using the nomenclature of the modified 10–20 system.

The standard set of electrodes for adults (Fig. 2.4) consists of 21 recording electrodes and one ground electrode. The recording electrodes are named with a letter and a subscript. The letter is an abbreviation of the underlying region: prefrontal or frontopolar (Fp), frontal (F), central (C), parietal (P), occipital (O) and auricular (A). The subscript is either the letter z, indicating zero or midline sagittal placement, or a number, indicating lateral placement. Odd numbers refer to electrodes on the left, even numbers refer to electrodes on the right side of the head. The numbers increase with increasing distance from the anterior posterior midline of the head. The inferior frontal electrodes F7 and F8 are often called 'anterior temporal' electrodes because they fairly faithfully record activity from the anterior temporal area.

Exact measurements are needed to precisely determine the placement of each recording electrode. Measurements are best made with a metric measuring tape of cloth or plastic. A grease pencil is used to mark electrode locations and the intermediate measurements needed to determine them. The measurements refer to three bony landmarks of the skull: (1) the inion, or the bony protruberance in the middle of the back of the head, (2) the nasion, or the bridge of the nose directly under the forehead, and (3) the preauricular point, or the depression of bone in front of the ear canal. Measurements are made in a sequence of five steps (Fig. 2.4). Although the older nomenclature of the 10–20 system is used in the following description, readers are encouraged to adopt the newer terminology of the modified 10–20 system in which T3 and T4 are renamed T7 and T8 and T5 and T6 are renamed P7 and P8.

Step 1: The distance between nasion and inion is measured along the midline.

Along this line, the frontopolar point, Fp, is marked at 10% above the nasion. Frontal (Fz), central (Cz), parietal (Pz) and occipital (O) points are marked at intervals of 20% of the entire distance leaving 10% for the interval between O and inion. The midline points Fpz and Oz are used only for intermediate measurements but routinely receive no electrode.

Step 2: The distance between the two preauricular points across Cz is measured. Along this line, the transverse position for the central points C3 and C4 and the temporal points T3 and T4 are marked 20 and 40% respectively from the midline.

Step 3: The circumference of the head is measured from the occipital point (O) through the temporal points T3 and T4 and the frontopolar points Fp. The longitudinal measurement for Fp1 is located on that circumference, 5% of the total length of the circumference to the left of Fpz. The longitudinal measurements for F7, T3, T5, O1, O2, T6, T4, F8, Fp2 are at distances of 10% of the circumference.

Step 4: The longitudinal distance from Fp1 and Fp2 through C3 and C4 to O1 and O2 is measured on each side. The midpoints of these distances give the longitudinal coordinates of C3 and C4. The midpoints between Fp1 and C3 on the left, and Fp2 and C4 on the right give the longitudinal coordinates for F3 and F4. The midpoints between C3 and O1 on the left, and C4 and O2 on the right give the longitudinal coordinates for P3 and P4.

Step 5: Measurements from F7 to F8 through Fz define the transverse coordinates for F3 midway between F3 and Fz, and for F4 midway between Fz and F8; measurements from T5 to T6 through Pz define the transverse coordinates for P3 midway between T5 and Pz and for P4 midway between Pz and T6.

Electrodes are placed at Fz, Cz and Pz, at all lateral points designated above, on or near both ears in positions called A1 and A2 or on the mandibular angles (4.2.4) in positions called M1 and M2, and on the point chosen for the ground electrode, usually in the middle of the head or over one of the mastoids. The use of a smaller number of electrodes in routine EEG is

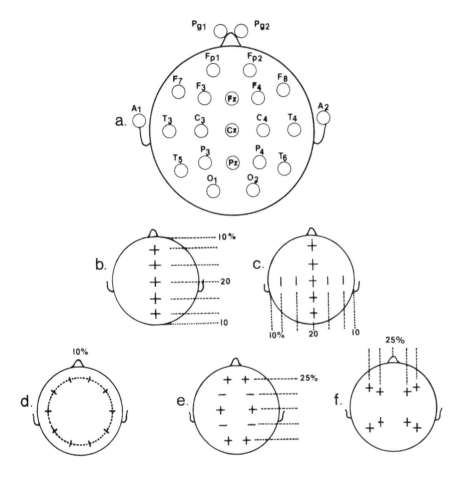

now considered substandard. If needed, additional electrodes may be placed midway between these recording electrodes. In some cases, scalp lesions, skull asymmetries or other abnormalities may make it impossible to place electrodes in the positions of the 10–20 system. In these cases, electrodes should be placed as closely as possible to these positions and as symmetrically as possible on the two sides using the modified 10–20 system of placement. The deviations from standard placement should be indicated in a diagram on the EEG record. Other electrode placements may be used for EEG recordings from small infants and for monitoring of extracerebral activity such as eye movements, heart beat, respiratory or other movements (4.3).

2.3.2 *True anterior temporal electrodes.* Because interictal epileptiform activity frequently emanates from the anterior temporal lobe, some laboratories occasionally use additional electrode placements that are closer

Fig. 2.4. Placement of recording electrodes. (a) Electrode names and placements in the international 10–20 system. (b–f) Steps in determining the electrode placements as described in the text.

MODIFIED COMBINATORIAL NOMENCLATURE

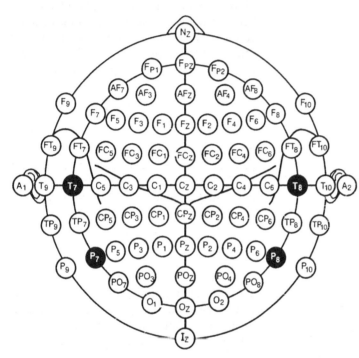

Fig. 2.5. Modified expanded '10–20' system as proposed by the American Clinical Neurophysiology Society. See also Appendix II.

to the anterior temporal region than F7 and F8 (see Fig. 2.2 for the typical distribution of anterior temporal spikes). Often these are placed according to the recommendation by Silverman (1960) and are referred to as *true anterior temporal electrodes.* Although these electrodes are often labeled as T1 and T2, according to the international 10–20 system, T1 and T2 would be placed between F7 and T3, and F8 and T4, respectively. The positions for so-called true anterior temporal electrodes are located by first finding an imaginary line between the external auditory canal and the lateral canthus of the eye. The point along that line that is anterior to the external auditory canal by 1/3 the distance of the total line is then located. The electrode is placed 1 cm directly above that point.

2.3.3 *Modified 10–20 system.* The placement of additional electrodes to those routinely employed in the 10–20 system may be indicated to: (1) improve the localization of ictal or interictal epileptiform activity; (2) increase spatial resolution for special studies using computerized EEG signal analysis; or (3) detect highly localized evoked potentials. The American Clinical Neurophysiology Society has developed new guidelines for extending the 10–20 system of electrode placement. In order to create a logical nomenclature, four electrodes, T3, T4, T5 and T6, have been renamed T7, T8, P7, and P8, respectively (Fig. 2.5). The American Clinical Neurophysiology Society guidelines that explain renaming of these electrodes and the placement of the additional electrodes have been reproduced in Appendix II.

2.4 RECORDING NON-CEREBRAL POTENTIALS

2.4.1 *Eye movements* are often monitored so that they can be distinguished clearly from frontal or anterior temporal cerebral potentials. Eye movements are usually recorded in two channels; monitoring in one channel is less reliable. If two channels are available, one electrode is placed slightly above and to the side of one eye and connected to input 1 of the first channel (E1). A second electrode is placed slightly below and to the side of the other eye (E2) and connected to input 1 of the second channel. Input 2 of both channels is connected to the same reference electrode on the ear or mastoid (e.g., E1–A2 and E2–A2). This arrangement of electrodes forces all eye movements to produce pen or waveform deflections in opposite directions (phase reversals, 4.2) between the 2 channels of recording, whereas any deflections that are in the same direction do not arise from eye movement. If only one channel is used for monitoring of eye movements, electrodes E1 and E2 are connected to input 1 and input 2 of that channel. The recording will not distinguish between horizontal and vertical eye movements or between eye movements and EEG.

Eye movement monitoring is also used to detect REM sleep during multiple sleep latency testing (MSLT; 7.7) and polysomnography (7.6). The finding of two or more REM episodes during separate naps of the MSLT is highly suggestive of narcolepsy when coupled with the appropriate clinical findings (e.g., daytime sleepiness and cataplexy). However, distinguishing REM sleep from drowsiness or brief wakefulness during arousal from sleep can sometimes be difficult. Eye movement monitoring that differentiates lateral from vertical eye movements can help with this distinction because REM sleep usually contains prominent lateral eye movements, whereas arousal and wakefulness usually contain more prominent vertical eye movements. If one electrode is placed above and between the eyes (Fz), one electrode is placed below and to the right of the right eye (OD) and a third electrode is placed below and to the left of the left eye (OS), then these electrodes can be used to create the following 2 channels of recording: OD–Fz and OS–Fz. This arrangement of electrodes forces all lateral eye movements to produce deflections in the 2 channels that are opposite in direction whereas all vertical eye movements and frontal lobe EEG potentials will produce deflections in the 2 channels that are in the same direction.

2.4.2 *Heart beat* may be monitored by connecting an amplifier to an EEG electrode placed on the neck or the chest and to another electrode at some distance away. If electrodes with long lead wires are available, standard ECG electrode positions on the extremities may be used.

2.4.3 *Respiration* is best monitored by simultaneously recording respiratory body movements and air flow. Respiratory movement may be recorded with a piezoelectric crystal transducer belt placed around the chest and the abdomen, or in special circumstances a pressure-sensitive balloon in the esophagus may be used to monitor subtle intrathoracic pressure changes. Respiratory air flow is routinely monitored using thermal sensitive detectors taped under the nostrils that register air flow from both nose and mouth. While EEG electrodes cannot monitor respiration, they may be of some use in identifying ventilator artifact in EEG recordings. For this purpose, EEG electrodes attached to the patient may be taped or looped around parts of the respiratory equipment which move with respiration (e.g., the ventilator tubing). This should result in recording of movement artifact corresponding with inspiration and expiration.

2.4.4 *Muscle activity* can be monitored with EEG electrodes placed over the center of a muscle. To monitor tonic muscle activity in sleep, a channel is devoted to a pair of electrodes placed on the neck below the chin at equal distances of at least 1–2 cm from the midline. This provides a measurement of submental muscle tone and is useful for determining whether REM sleep (in which there is an absence of muscle tone and EMG artifact) is present. Needle electrodes inserted into a muscle may also be used to record local muscle activity that can be displayed on an EEG tracing within the limitations of the high frequency response or paper speed of an analog EEG instrument.

2.4.5 *Movement* caused by tremor, myoclonus or convulsive twitching may be monitored by electrodes placed on the moving body parts; such monitoring is likely to indicate the occurrence of movements, but the type of movement must be described on the recording by the technologist.

2.4.6 *Blood pressure, body temperature, eye position, blood oxygen saturation and other slowly changing or sustained activities* require special electrodes or transducers and can be recorded only with EEG instruments and polygraphs equipped with directly coupled amplifiers.

REFERENCES

American EEG Society Guidelines in EEG and Evoked Potentials (1986) Report of the committee on infectious diseases. J. Clin. Neurophysiol. 3 (Suppl. 1): 38–42.
Binnie, C.D. (1987) Recording techniques: montages, electrodes, amplifiers and filters. In: A.M. Halliday, S.R. Butler and R. Paul (Eds.), A Textbook of Clinical Neurophysiology. Wiley, Chichester, pp. 3–22.
Binnie, C.D., Rowan, A.J. and Gutter, T.H. (1982) A Manual of Electroencephalographic Technology. University Press, Cambridge.
Binnie, C.D., Marston, D., Polkey, C.E. and Amin, D. (1989) Distribution of temporal spikes in relation to the sphenoidal electrode. Electroenceph. Clin. Neurophysiol. 73: 403–409.
Blume, W., Buva, R. and Okazaki, H. (1974) Anatomic correlates of the 10–20 electrode placement system in infants. Electroenceph. Clin. Neurophysiol. 36: 303–307.
Broughton, R., Hanley, J., Quanbury, A.O. and Roy, O.Z. (1976) Section 1. Electrodes. In: A. Rémond (Ed.), Handbook of Electroenceph. Clin. Neurophysiol., Vol. 3A. Elsevier, Amsterdam, pp. 5–27.
Cooper, R., Osselton, J.W. and Shaw, J.C. (1981) Electrodes. In: EEG Technology. Butterworth, London, pp. 15–29.

Geddes, L.A. (1972) Electrodes and the Measurement of Bioelectric Events. Wiley, New York.

Gibbs, F.A. and Gibbs, E.L. (1952) Atlas of Electroencephalography. Volume 2. Addison-Wesley, Reading, MA, p. 164.

Grings, W.W. (1974) Recording of electrodermal phenomena. In: R.F. Thompson and M.M. Patterson (Eds.), Bioelectric Recording Techniques, Vol. IC. Academic Press, New York and London, pp. 273–296.

Harner, P.F. and Sannit, R. (1974) A Review of the International Ten-Twenty System of Electrode Placement. Grass Instrument Co., Quincy, MA.

Homan, R.W., Herman, J. and Purdy, P. (1987) Cerebral location of international 10–20 system electrode placement. Electroenceph. Clin. Neurophysiol. 66: 376–382.

Ives, J.R. and Gloor, P. (1978) Update: chronic sphenoidal electrodes. Electroenceph. Clin. Neurophysiol. 44: 789–790.

Jasper, H.H. (1958) The ten–twenty electrode system of the International Federation. Electroenceph. Clin. Neurophysiol. 10: 371–375.

Lehtinen, L.O.J. and Berstrom, L. (1970) Naso-ethmoidal electrode for recording the electrical activity of the inferior surface of the frontal lobe. Electroenceph. Clin. Neurophysiol. 29: 303–305.

Lesser, R.P., Lüders, H., Klem, G., Dinner, D.S., Morris, H.H., Hahn, J.F. and Wyllie, E. (1987) Extraoperative cortical functional localization in patients with epilepsy. J. Clin. Neurophysiol. 4: 27–54.

Lüders, H., Lesser, R.P., Dinner, D.S., Morris, H.H., Wyllie, E. and Godoy, J. (1988) Localization of cortical function: new information from extra-operative monitoring of patients with epilepsy. Epilepsia 29 (Suppl. 2): S56–65.

Mavor, H. and Hellen, M.K. (1964) Nasopharyngeal electrode recording. Am. J. EEG Technol. 4: 43–50.

Picton, T.W. and Hillyard, S.A. (1972) Cephalic skin potentials in electroencephalography. Electroenceph. Clin. Neurophysiol. 33: 419–424.

Sannit, T. (1963) The ten–twenty system: footnotes to measuring technique. Am. J. EEG Technol. 3: 23–30.

Silverman, D. (1960) The anterior temporal electrode and the ten–twenty system. Electroenceph. Clin. Neurophysiol. 12: 735–737.

Sperling, M.R. and Engel, Jr., J. (1986) Sphenoidal electrodes. J. Clin. Neurophysiol. 3: 67–74.

Venables, P.H. and Martin, I. (1967) Skin resistance and skin potential. In: P.H. Venables and I. Martin (Eds.), A Manual of Psychophysiological Methods. North-Holland, Amsterdam, pp. 53–102.

Wieser, H.G., Elger, C.E. and Stodieck, S.R.G. (1985) The foramen ovale electrode: a new recording method for the preoperative evaluation of patients suffering from mesio-basal temporal epilepsy. Electroenceph. Clin. Neurophysiol. 61: 314–322.

Zablow, L. and Goldensohn, E.S. (1969) A comparison between scalp and needle electrodes for the EEG. Electroenceph. Clin. Neurophysiol. 26: 530–533.

3 Digital and analog EEG instruments: parts and functions

SUMMARY

(3.1) *The electrode input board* of an analog EEG instrument receives the wires from the electrodes on the patient's head and relays the EEG by cable to the electrode selector switches and amplifiers. In contrast, the input board of a *digital* EEG instrument not only receives the EEG signal from the electrode wires, it also amplifies the signal before sending it by cable to the computer and monitor.

(3.2) Analog EEG instrument *input selector switches* are used to select the input to each amplifier. Digital EEG instrument electrode selection is performed by software manipulation (see 3.25).

(3.3) *Calibration pulses* of known voltage are used to measure the amplitude of EEG potentials and to test the functioning of the amplifiers and penwriters in analog systems. The calibration signal is a square wave pulse whose output at the penwriter shows the effects of the filters and amplifier gain. Digital instruments often require the user to input a known amplitude signal using a separately purchased signal generator. *Analog EEG biocalibration* can be performed by connecting the same electrode pair to the inputs of all amplifiers for a brief trial recording in order to verify that the scalp to amplifier interface is working adequately in all channels. *Digital EEG biocalibration* is similarly performed by displaying the same electrode pair in each channel of recording; however, some commercial systems currently display the output of only one amplifier as if it truly represents all the amplifiers.

(3.4) Each *channel of EEG recording* is produced by the output of one *differential amplifier*. Each differential amplifier has two input terminals. EEG amplifiers increase only the difference in voltage between the input terminals; identical voltages appearing at the two inputs are not amplified and create a flat line output. EEG amplifiers are constructed so that *if input 1 becomes more negative than input 2, the signal deflects upward.* *If input 1 becomes more positive than input 2, then the signal deflects downward.*

(3.5) *Analog filters* reduce the amplitude of signals of selected frequencies. A low and a high frequency filter are used to remove very slow and very fast waves in order to select the spectrum of frequencies which has the greatest clinical significance (0.5–30 Hz).

(3.6) *Penwriting units* of analog EEG instruments are driven by the amplified and filtered potential changes recorded at the scalp. The pens move up and down, writing on chart paper that is moving horizontally at an even speed of 30 mm/s.

(3.7) *Analog to digital conversion* converts a continuously varying voltage (i.e., analog signal) into a series of discrete numerical values. The number of digital values used for each second of analog signal is referred to as the *sampling rate*. If the sampling rate is not at least twice as fast as the fastest frequency contained in the analog signal, then the digital signal will create frequencies that are not present in the analog signal *(Nyquist theorem)*. The misrepresentation of the analog signal caused by sampling at too slow a rate is referred to as *aliasing*.

(3.8) *Digital signal display* can take the form of any readable output that a computer can produce, including paper or a monitor screen. Routine visualization of digital EEG for clinical interpretation should be performed using a large, high resolution, computer screen. It should be possible to display 1 s of recording across a monitor screen width of no less than 25 mm (vs. 30 mm/s for paper analog EEG) using at least 100 data points. Vertical spacing between channels should be at least 15 mm. However, higher standards should be sought by those purchasing new equipment.

(3.9) *Digital filtering*, like analog filtering, involves the suppression of waveforms in selected frequency ranges. The ranges selected are similar to those used in analog recording.

(3.10) *Montage reformatting* is the retrospective changing of the display montage. Digital EEG instruments store the original digital EEG in a common reference montage. During review other reference montages are created simply by subtracting or adding channels together.

(3.11) *Data storage* requirements of digital EEG vary depending on the design of the digital EEG system software. The storage hardware should provide for rapid access to old records for comparison with subsequent recordings and in most instances should have a shelf life of at least 10 years. DVD or CD are examples of adequate storage media.

(3.12) *Electrical safety* issues that electroencephalographers and clinical neurophysiologists must be familiar with include leakage current, grounding, micro and macro shock, and ground loops.

INTRODUCTION

This chapter contains a detailed description of both analog and digital EEG instruments. Both are described together because they share many components. Indeed, a digital EEG instrument is in reality an analog EEG system combined with an analog to digital signal converter and personal computer equipped with specialized monitor display software. Although the visual clarity of the waveform displays produced by commercially available digital instruments is not yet as good as the older pen and ink writers (or even analog oscilloscopic monitors), there are a number of compelling reasons to abandon the analog technology. First, digital EEG makes available a number of extremely useful tools for clinical interpretation, including retrospective montage, filter, and gain selection. Second, digital processing reduces the cost of instrumentation and storage space and reduces record retrieval time. Finally, digital EEG makes possible the routine application of a variety of complex signal processing tasks such as spectral analysis, automated seizure detection, statistical quantitative analysis, and spatial graphical displays of EEG activity (topographic analysis). Indeed, the only potential drawback to this shift in technology is that electroencephalographers may need to devote some time to understand digital technology and the limitations of digital signal processing. This point is underscored by recent and continuing experience with the misguided application of quantitative EEG, particularly in the medical and legal areas of psychiatry and head injury (Epstein, 1994; Fisch and Pedley, 1989).

As with any new technology, it is important that digital EEG instruments provide a recording that is at least as informative as the analog instruments they are intended to replace. Thus, new recording systems should be able to meet the standards such as those described by the American Clinical Neurophysiology Society (ACNS; formerly the American EEG Society). If similar standards cannot be applied then neither can well established methods of interpretation. As with penwriter recordings the digital system should allow for the entry of identifying relevant historical information and should be capable of performing instrumental and bioelectrical calibrations at the beginning and end of the recording. The recording should contain all of the technologist's notations as they would be entered in a routine recording and the technologist should be able to enter comments after the recording is completed. Montage, filter, and sensitivity settings should be displayed and the display should be adequate for visual review (American EEG Society digital EEG guidelines, 1994). If these simple requirements cannot be met then the electroencephalographer is better off using a conventional analog system for routine recording.

3.1 THE ELECTRODE PANEL

As one observes a patient undergoing EEG recording they will notice that the electrode wires extend from the patient's head into a box at the bedside. The box is an *electrode input board* (also referred to as an *input board, input box,* or *jackbox*). The female connectors at the ends of the electrode lead wires are plugged into male receptacles in the *input panel* (also referred to as a *jackbox,* or *input box*). For safety purposes the ends of electrode leads are female. This makes it impossible to plug them into power sockets or make direct contact between the patient and other current sources. Each receptacle is labeled with a symbol that indicates the location of the electrode on the head. To aid in selecting the correct receptacle, they are often arranged in a diagram representing the head. Additional receptacles may be used for additional electrode placements. The wires from each receptacle in the input panel run in a cable to the EEG instrument. The input panel either contains an impedance meter or has connections for such a meter so that electrode impedance can be measured without unplugging the electrode wires from the electrode input panel.

Because electrode lead wires should be no longer than 1 m (to minimize electrical interference), the input board is kept near the patient. Indeed, the shorter the distance of the conducting wire between the scalp electrode and the analog amplifier, the lower the electrical interference. In digital EEG instruments the analog amplifiers are typically in the input board whereas in analog instruments the amplifiers are in the chassis of the penwriting instrument. However, even in the case of analog EEG instruments, the cable from the input panel to the EEG machine may be much longer than the wires between the patient's head and the input panel because it is electrically shielded and less likely to pick up interference. In laboratories using an electrically shielded recording room for the patient, the input board must stay in that room; if the EEG analog or digital instrument is located outside the shielded room, the cable is fed through an opening in the shielding to rest of the EEG instrument.

3.2 ANALOG EEG INSTRUMENT INPUT SELECTOR SWITCHES

All analog EEG instruments have individual selector switches for each channel as well as a master selector switch. These switches are used to connect each channel to either: (a) the calibration signal, (b) one or more recording electrodes, or (c) the ground of the amplifier.

3.2.1 *Individual channel selector switches* may consist of mechanical rotary, push button, or slide switch with over 21 contact positions. Alternatively, individual electrodes for each channel may be programmed for each channel using a monitor screen with a moveable cursor.

3.2.2 *A master electrode selector switch* is used to connect a specific combination of electrodes (montage) to the input terminals of all amplifiers at once. A hard-wired or programmable master switch has only one setting for each combination and can reduce the time spent in selecting individual channel switches; this is useful for routine recordings using standard electrode combinations.

3.2.3 *Channel input selections* are of four types. (a) The calibration position connects the source of the calibration signal to the amplifier input. (b) Any receptacle of the input board, except that of the ground electrode, can be connected to any amplifier input. The same electrode may be selected at the input of more than one amplifier. However, if the same electrode is selected at both available inputs of the same amplifier, the inputs are short-circuited and closed, and the penwriter displays a flat line. (c) Combinations of two or more electrodes can be selected at one input to an amplifier. This selection of multiple electrodes, which are physically joined to the same amplifier input, is most often used to create an 'average reference.' The term 'average' is used because each individual electrode will contribute equally to the voltage signal recorded from their combination. (d) Ground can be selected as an input to an amplifier, connecting that input to the ground of the amplifier and effectively closing the input regardless of whether or not the ground is connected to the patient.

3.3 ANALOG AND DIGITAL CALIBRATION

Calibration in clinical EEG has two main purposes: (a) to determine the voltage of EEG potentials by comparing them to a potential of known voltage; and (b) to verify the integrity of each channel by demonstrating that all channels amplify and filter the same signal in the same way. Both purposes are served by the most commonly used calibration procedure of applying standard voltage pulses simultaneously to the input of all amplifiers. The functioning of the amplifiers can also be compared using the patient's EEG as a calibration signal.

3.3.1a *Analog instrumental calibration.* For analog EEG instruments a negative potential of pre-selected voltage is applied to the input of an amplifier using a calibration switch mounted in the analog instrument (Fig. 3.3). The calibration signal that is sent to the amplifiers and filters is in the shape of a square wave. This shape is then modfied by the effects of the amplifier gain setting (i.e., the amount of amplification) and the high and low frequency filters and the 60 cycle notch filter before it reaches the penwriter. The high frequency filter affects the steepness of the initial pen deflection of the square wave pulse (causing it to have a more rounded appearance) whereas the low frequency filter causes the pen to drift back to baseline. Only the initial deflection represents the amplitude of the calibration voltage, and even when the calibration voltage is sustained, the pen gradually drifts back to the baseline as the result of the low frequency filter (3.5.1). When the calibration voltage is turned off after the pen has reached baseline, the pen is suddenly deflected in the opposite direction and to the same amplitude as at the beginning of the calibration pulse. For routine calibration, a series of such deflections is recorded in all channels.

The pen deflection of the analog instrument is used to determine if the voltage output of the amplifier and penwriter are properly calibrated. The *sensitivity* setting of the analog instrument consists of a switch or push button that is rated in units of *microvolts per millimeter of pen deflection*. The calibration pulse voltage switch can also be set to different levels, but is commonly set to deliver a signal of 50 μV to the amplifier. The *standard sensitivity setting for analog EEG is 7 μV/mm.* If a 50 μV calibration signal is delivered to the amplifier and the sensitivity setting is 7 μV/mm, then the pen should deflect a distance of (1 mm/7 μV × 50 μV) = 7.14 mm. The EEG technologist may then apply a ruler to EEG paper to verify that the pen deflection arising from the calibration signal is correct. At the end of a routine recording it is good practice to apply the calibration signal at each of the sensitivity settings used during the recording. In this way it can be verified that the amplifiers and penwriters were calibrated for all sensitivity settings used during recording.

3.3.1b *Digital instrumental calibration.* Calibration for digital EEG instruments is performed with either an external signal generator that can be interfaced with the electrode input board or digital instrument computer chassis, or an internal signal generator housed within the instrument. The signal generator should create a sine wave signal whose frequency and voltage can be selected by the technologist. The frequency should be in the range of EEG activity (> 0 Hz to 70 Hz). The digital EEG software should contain a voltage cursor that allows the user to determine the voltage of individual waveforms. This cursor is then applied to the known signal from the signal generator to determine if the system is properly calibrated.

3.3.2 *Analog and digital biocalibration.* The patient's EEG may be used to compare the performance of all amplifiers and, more importantly, test the integrity of the entire recording system. To obtain a wide range of relatively high amplitude EEG frequencies for this comparison, a frontopolar electrode and a contralateral occipital electrode are usually selected as input 1 and input 2, respectively, for each and every amplifier. The frontopolar electrode (e.g., Fp1) usually contains high amplitude slow waveforms caused by eyeblink artifact whereas the occipital electrode (e.g., O2) usually contains 8–13 Hz alpha activity. In addition to routine biocalibration, biocalibration is performed to verify the integrity of any special electrodes or devices being used to record non-cerebral activity. For example, if the technologist is monitoring eye movements and nasal airflow, then at the beginning of the recording the patient would be requested to move their eyes in all directions and then to breath in and out. The results of those maneuvers are then be used to calibrate, or verify, the accuracy of the eye movements and air flow.

3.4 AMPLIFIERS

EEG amplifiers are designed to serve two main functions: *differential discrimination* and *amplification*. *Discrimination* is the ability of the amplifier to reveal differences in electrical potential between amplifier electrode inputs 1 and 2 while rejecting potentials which are common to the inputs (referred to as *common mode rejection*); *amplification* increases the size of potential differences to a level at which they can either drive the

pens of the analog EEG instrument or the analog to digital converter of the digital EEG instrument.

3.4.1 *Discrimination.* Each amplifier of the EEG machine has two input terminals named 'input 1' and 'input 2' (formerly called 'grid 1' and 'grid 2' after the grids in vacuum tubes). Potential changes, or signals, applied to each terminal are amplified to the same degree but in opposite direction with reference to the ground of the amplifier. This is done by inverting the polarity of the signal applied to input 2 so that it is effectively subtracted from the signal applied to input 1. This mode of operation is called *differential* or *balanced* amplification. The differential amplifier therefore only amplifies the *difference* between the incoming signals in inputs 1 and 2. All bioelectrical recording devices use differential amplification because, as described below, this allows the amplifier to remove electrical noise from the amplified signal. Amplifiers that do not subtract one input from another are referred to as *single ended amplifiers* because they compare the difference between a single input and the electrical ground, which has a voltage close to zero. Although single-ended amplifiers are inadequate for the initial amplification of bioelectrical signals, they are used to further amplify bioelectrical signals that have already undergone amplification by differential amplifiers.

The polarity of the output signal of a differential amplifier thus depends not only on the polarity of the input signal but

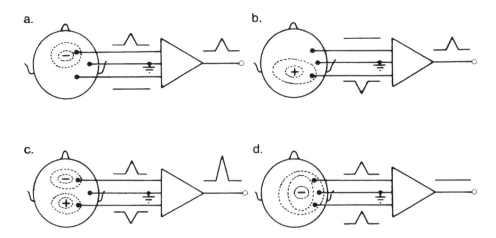

Fig. 3.1.   Differential amplification of simple signals, applied to input 1 (top input at the triangular amplifier symbol) and input 2 (bottom input) with respect to an electrical zero level at the ground connection (middle input). Electrical changes at scalp electrodes are indicated by fields on the head diagram; a change towards negative in an electrode is indicated by an upward deflection of the signal above or below the electrode lead; a change towards positive is indicated by a downward deflection. The same polarity convention is used for the signals at the amplifier output which represent pen deflections. (a) A negative signal at input 1 causes an upgoing pen deflection. (b) A positive signal at input 2 is inverted at the ground level and also causes an upgoing pen deflection. (c) Two signals of equal size but opposite polarity appearing simultaneously at both inputs are added to each other and cause a pen deflection twice the size of that caused by each potential alone. (d) Two signals of equal size and the same polarity applied simultaneously to both inputs are subtracted from each other and cause no pen deflection.

also on the input terminal to which it is applied. EEG machines are wired so that greater negativity at input 1 than at input 2 causes an upward deflection of the signal from baseline, whereas greater negativity at input 2 than at input 1 causes a downward deflection. Stated another way, greater positivity at input 2 compared to input 1 causes an upward deflection of the signal, whereas greater positivity at input 1 compared to input 2 causes a downward deflection of the signal. *Because upward and downward deflections of the EEG signal in a single channel of recording do not reveal which input (or*

41

electrode) is active, up or down deflections in a single channel should not be called 'negative' or 'positive.'

The results of differential amplification are illustrated by four examples in Fig. 3.1.

(a) A negative signal applied to input 1 causes an upward deflection at the output.
(b) A positive signal applied to input 2 also causes an upward deflection at the output.
(c) Two signals of opposite polarity applied simultaneously to each input produce an output that represents the sum of the outputs caused by either signal alone.
(d) Two signals of the same amplitude, polarity and timing applied to both inputs are subtracted from each other and produce no output. Such signals are said to be in 'common mode.'

The four examples in Fig. 3.1 show potentials of identical shape, amplitude and timing. Potentials with these shapes are not actually produced by the brain but they provide a useful illustration for more complicated conditions, such as those shown in Fig. 3.2. A change of potential affecting both electrodes to a different degree causes an output with an amplitude that equals the difference between the potentials at both inputs. For instance, if the absolute potential (i.e., voltage) at input 1 becomes negative 100 μV and negative 50 μV at input 2, then the amplifier input 'sees' a potential difference

between the inputs that equals negative 50 μV ($-100 - -50 = -100 + 50 = -50$; Fig. 3.2a and b). Potential changes involving both inputs that occur at slightly different times may result in a composite waveform that is longer in duration with more phases (i.e., up and down deflections) than that which occurred at either of the two input electrodes (Fig. 3.2c and d).

It soon becomes apparent that in differential amplification *one type of output can be the result of an infinite variety of different kinds of input*. The methods used to deduce the most likely inputs (i.e., the polarity, distribution and relative amplitude of the electrical potentials at each electrode), based on the output, are discussed in the next chapter.

To reiterate, *discrimination* between signals is the process of amplifying signal differences between inputs and rejecting identical (i.e., common mode) signals that appear at both amplifier input signals (i.e., common mode rejection). Discrimination is often expressed as a *ratio of the differential and common mode amplification of an amplifier*. This ratio can be determined for any amplifier by: (1) applying a signal differentially (i.e., different signals between inputs) at a voltage which produces a measurable output, and (2) applying an identical signal at both input 1 and 2 (i.e., a common mode signal) at a voltage that produces the same amplitude of output as the differential signal. The *common mode rejection ratio* is the ratio of the common mode input voltage over the output voltage.

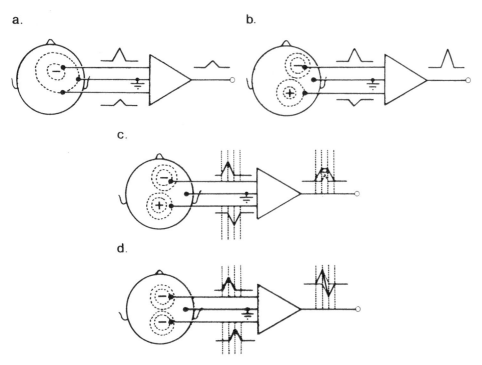

Fig. 3.2. Differential amplification of signals of different amplitude (a and b) and timing (c and d). Symbols are the same as in Fig. 3.1. (a) Simultaneous appearance of a negative potential at input 1 and of a negative potential of half its size at input 2 causes an upgoing pen deflection half the size of that produced by the potential at input 1 alone. (b) Simultaneous appearance of a negative signal at input 1 and of a positive signal of half its size at input 2 causes an upgoing pen deflection of an amplitude 1.5 times that produced by the signal at input 1 alone. (c) Appearance of a negative signal at input 1 followed by appearance of a positive signal of the same size at input 2 causes a sustained upgoing pen deflection. (d) Appearance of a negative signal at input 1 followed by a negative signal of the same size at input 2 causes a diphasic pen deflection of a longer total duration and of a faster falling phase than that caused by either signal alone.

Good EEG instruments have amplifiers with high discrimination, or *common mode rejection* ratios, of 10,000 or more.

The point of differential amplification is to eliminate electrical potentials that do not come from the brain. Potentials from the brain are usually not evenly distributed over the scalp; these differences in potential are amplified and appear in the EEG. In contrast, electrical interference typically affects all scalp electrodes in the same manner and is usually eliminated by common mode rejection. This is true especially of 60 Hz interference. Unfortunately, differential amplification alone cannot always distinguish between cerebral activity and artifact because many artifacts produce different potentials at different scalp electrodes. But the failure of discrimination to eliminate common mode artifact is usually due to either: (a) unequal impedance of the recording electrodes or (b) absence of an effective ground connection to the patient.

Impedance is the resistance of a part of circuit to the passage of an alternating current. *Resistance* is the inability of a part of a circuit to allow the passage of a direct (constant voltage) current. Because all EEG signals are varying (not *direct current; DC)* the main concern is resistance to varying or alternating current flow (i.e., impedance). *Unequal impedance of the recording electrodes* at the two inputs to an amplifier causes potentials of equal amplitude on the scalp to appear with different amplitude at the inputs. This difference in signal amplitude will then be amplified and appear at the output. The most

common example of unequal electrode impedance is the appearance at the output of 60 Hz (or 50 Hz in some countries) artifact from alternating current sources. The amplitude of the artifact depends on the severity of the impedance imbalance and the strength of the interference signal. The interference is weak in most EEG laboratories, but may be strong when recordings are made in unshielded locations such as patient rooms, intensive care units and operating rooms; minor imbalances of electrode impedances may then become critical.

The most common cause of an impedance imbalance serious enough to interfere with recording is the partial or complete loss of contact between electrode and scalp. This results in an output reflecting only the difference between a single input (the remaining scalp electrode) and the ground electrode which has been placed on the patient. If the ground electrode has been placed near the eyes, the technologist will be quickly alerted to the problem of a poorly attached or unattached scalp electrode because its input will be replaced by eye movement artifact that is extremely easy to spot in the recording. For this reason, the patient ground electrode is usually placed at Fpz so that the presence of abnormally distributed eye movements can be used by the technologist and electroencephalographer to identify defective electrode contacts. Such *ground recordings* usually arise from poor electrode attachment to the scalp. But they may also be the result of any interruption of electrode contact, including a broken electrode wire or failure to plug the electrode into the input board.

If the amplifier ground is not connected to the patient and one of the two input electrodes is not connected to the patient, the output represents the difference between cerebral potential changes and the entirely unrelated potential level of the amplifier ground (or depending on the commercial system it may be related to some combination of the remaining electrodes). This may produce a true monopolar or 'single-ended' recording but it has little value because the loss of common mode rejection results in a recording that is obscured by interference.

Absent or ineffective ground connection to the patient does not preclude recording of potential differences between input 1 and 2. However, the inputs float without reference to the potential level at which the amplifier inverts input 2 to subtract it from input 1. An amplifier with floating input is therefore more likely to 'see' signals which are equal with reference to the patient's head as being different and to therefore amplify artifacts which would be rejected if the amplifier had an effective ground connection to the patient's head. As pointed out in Section 3.12, the only purpose of the ground electrode is to reduce electrical interference. It does not protect the patient and in certain situations actually increases the risk of electrical shock.

Rejection of cerebral potentials. Discrimination cancels cerebral potentials that are in common mode. EEG potential changes which appear at exactly the same time and have exactly the same shape and amplitude over all parts of the head would therefore escape detection in recordings from scalp electrodes and would require recordings between one electrode over the head and another electrode elsewhere on the body. In practice this is not encountered. Even widespread potential changes differ slightly in shape, amplitude and timing at some scalp recording sites. However, the closer the input 1 and input 2 recording electrodes are on the scalp the more they see the same cerebral activity and the more cancellation between them will occur.

3.4.2 *Amplification.* The amplifier increases the voltage difference between the inputs so that the voltage of the output can be used to drive the pens of the analog EEG instrument or analog to digital converter of the digital EEG instrument. EEG and evoked potential amplifiers boost the voltage of the biological signal from microvolts to volts. Amplification is characterized in terms of *sensitivity* and *gain*.

As noted above, *sensitivity* is the ratio of input voltage to the signal deflection it produces. Sensitivity is measured in microvolts per millimeter (μV/mm) of pen deflection in analog EEG instruments. A commonly used sensitivity is 7 μV/mm. At this sensitivity, a calibration signal of 50 μV causes a pen deflection of about 7 mm. Note that a sensitivity setting of higher numerical value means a lower amplification recording. A sensitivity setting of 10 μV/mm will make a calibration signal look smaller than a sensitivity setting of 7 μV/mm.

Conversely, decreasing the setting from 10 to 7 μV/mm increases the output of the amplifier.

The sensitivity of each channel can be adjusted between high values of 1 or 2 μV/mm and low values of at least 1000 μV/mm. These adjustments are made on analog instruments with switches that increase the sensitivity stepwise by factors of no more than two. A variable control permits equalizing the sensitivity between channels precisely; equalization should be necessary only rarely. In addition to these individual sensitivity controls for each channel, most EEG instruments have a master sensitivity switch that controls the sensitivity of all channels.

Because sensitivity can be directly determined by applying a calibration pulse and measuring the pen deflection, sensitivity rather than gain is usually used to describe amplification by EEG instruments.

Gain is the ratio of signal voltage obtained at the output of the amplifier to the signal voltage applied at the input. For instance, an amplifier set to give an output voltage of 10 V for an input of 10 μV is said to have a gain of 1 million; and this is the usual maximum gain of EEG analog amplifiers. Gain is sometimes expressed in decibels, the number of decibels amounting to 20 times the logarithmic of the gain. For instance, a gain of 10 equals 20 dB, a gain of 100 equals 40 dB, and a gain of 1 million equals 120 dB. In contrast to sensitivity, gain is defined so that it increases with increasing amplification (sensitivity and gain are inversely proportional). However, gain is not a useful measure in clinical EEG because the output to input voltage ratio of the amplifier is not directly measured.

3.5 FILTERS

Filters are used to exclude waveforms of relatively high or low frequency from the EEG so that waveforms in the most important range (1–30 Hz) can be recorded clearly and without distortion. The filters receive the EEG signal after it has passed from the differential amplifier to a second, single-ended, amplifier. After passing through each filter the signal is amplified again by single-ended amplifiers.

The effect of a filter is often illustrated and specified in terms of its action on electronically generated sine or square waves (Fig. 3.3). Filters affect any component of the EEG to the extent that it rises or falls with a slope corresponding with that of the sine wave frequency that is being filtered out (Fig. 3.3, right). In this section much of the information provided applies to both analog and digital filters, particularly the nomenclature and the effects of filters on signals. Moreover, all digital EEG instruments initially filter the analog signal using analog filters. Additional information specific to digital filtering is presented in 3.9.

EEG instruments have three kinds of analog and digital filters. (1) The *low frequency filter* reduces the amplitude of slow waves. (2) The *high frequency filter* reduces the amplitude of fast waves. (3) The *notch filter* selectively reduces the amplitude of waves in a narrow frequency range in order to remove electrical line interference. In North America the notch filter is set at the mains frequency of 60 Hz, the frequency of the most common electrical artifact*. Perhaps the most difficult concept to grasp initially is that *filters are not absolute. That is, they do not perfectly remove or preserve all frequencies above or below their individual settings, but provide a continuum of gradual filtering* (see below).

The *low frequency filter* is also often referred to as a *high pass filter,* because it allows the higher frequencies to pass through the amplifier to the final recording without being attenuated. Similarly, the *high frequency filter* is often referred to as a *low pass filter,* because it allows the lower frequencies to remain and attenuates the higher frequencies. The *notch filter* allows both higher and lower frequency waveforms that are above the selected frequency setting of the filter to pass without significant attenuation. Analog EEG instruments provide control over each of these three filter actions by individual channel controls permitting different selections for each channel and by a master switch that allows selection of the same settings for all channels. Digital EEG instruments, which have evolved directly from the analog systems, emulate the analog systems by providing software controlled filter switches for

individual channels and for all channels simultaneously as a master command during data acquisition.

Digital software controlled filtering can also be used retrospectively for viewing after the EEG has been acquired.

3.5.1   Digital and analog *low frequency filters* can be characterized by their effects either on sine waves as a *low frequency filter cutoff frequency*, or on square pulses as a *time constant.*

The low filter frequency setting specifies the *cutoff frequency* at which sine waves are reduced in amplitude by a set percentage. This percentage of attenuation of the unfiltered signal is the same regardless of the cutoff setting. Thus, a low frequency filter that is set at 1 Hz will reduce the amplitude of a 1 Hz sine wave by the same percentage as a low frequency filter set at 5 Hz will reduce the amplitude of a 5 Hz sine wave. Figs. 3.3 and 3.4 show the effects of different analog filter settings on sine waves of different frequencies. The first four channels in each figure were recorded with low filter frequencies of 0.1, 0.3, 1 and 5 Hz. These filters, manufactured by Grass Corp. Instruments, are set to reduce the amplitude of the cutoff frequency sine waves by 20% or 2 dB. *Most manufacturers provide a 30.3% or 3 dB attenuation at the cutoff frequency.* In the figure sine waves of lower frequency are reduced more, and sine waves slightly above the cutoff frequency are reduced by less than 20%. As a result, a sine wave of 0.3 Hz is nearly abolished by a filter setting of 5 Hz, severely reduced by a setting of 1 Hz, and reduced by 20% by a setting of 0.3 Hz. It can be recorded

---

* A 50 Hz filter is used in countries using a power line frequency of 50 Hz.

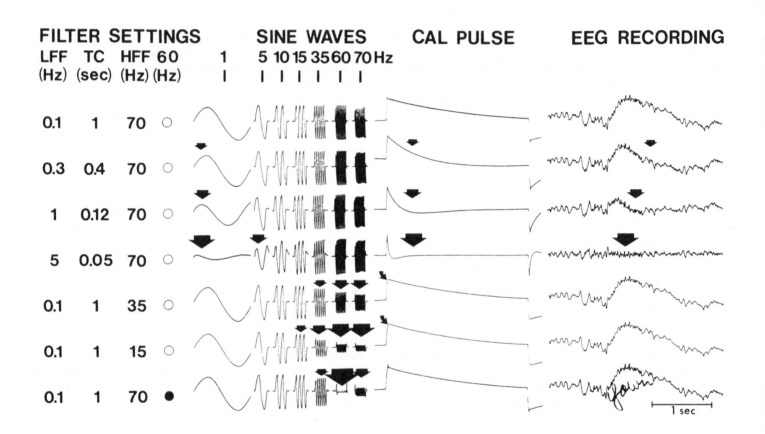

FILTER SETTINGS				SINE WAVES	CAL PULSE	EEG RECORDING
LFF (Hz)	TC (sec)	HFF (Hz)	60 (Hz)	1 5 10 15 35 60 70 Hz		
0.1	1	70	○			
0.3	0.4	70	○			
1	0.12	70	○			
5	0.05	70	○			
0.1	1	35	○			
0.1	1	15	○			
0.1	1	70	●			1 sec

48

without amplitude distortion only with a filter setting well below 0.3 Hz. Similarly, a low frequency filter setting of 5 Hz will nearly abolish a signal as low as 0.2 Hz, severely reduce the amplitude of a 3 Hz signal, only reduce by 20% the amplitude of a 5 Hz signal, slightly reduce the amplitude of a 10 Hz signal, and have little or no effect on a 20 Hz signal.

The relationship between the amplitude and the frequency of sine waves at different filter settings is summarized in the diagram at the bottom of Fig. 3.4. Here, each curve on the left side represents one low frequency filter setting and shows the amount of reduction of amplitude of waves having frequencies below the medium range. This figure again makes it clear that *filters of EEG machines eliminate frequencies gradually and in both directions*: waveforms of frequencies below the low filter cutoff frequency are not entirely eliminated and waveforms slightly above that frequency are also attenuated.

The time constant describes the effect of the low frequency filter on square pulses. The time constant is the time required for the pen to fall 63% from the peak of the deflection produced when a steady voltage, such as a calibration square wave pulse, is applied to the input of the amplifier (Fig. 3.5a). The time constant can be easily measured in EEG recordings by drawing a horizontal line at about one-third (37%) of the height of the calibration signal; the time constant is the time elapsed on the x-axis from the beginning of the calibration pulse to the intersection of the horizontal line with the falling phase of the calibration signal (Fig. 3.5a). Fig. 3.3 shows the effect of different low frequency filter settings on square pulses. These settings are indicated both in terms of low filter

---

◄ Fig. 3.3.   The effect of different filter settings on sine waves of various frequencies, a calibration pulse and a segment of EEG recording. The same signals are applied to the inputs of all channels; therefore, the differences in the outputs, enhanced by arrows, are due to the different filter settings used in each channel. Filter settings are indicated at the left margin. Low frequency filter settings are given both in terms of low filter frequency (LFF) representing the frequency at which sine waves are reduced by 20% in amplitude, and in terms of the corresponding time constant (TC). High frequency filter settings are indicated in terms of high filter frequency (HFF) representing the frequency at which sine waves are reduced in amplitude by 20%. The 60 Hz filter is used only in the last channel. Channels 1–4 show the effect of increasing the low filter frequency, or of decreasing the time constant: the amplitude of sine waves of low frequency is progressively reduced, the calibration pulse returns to baseline faster, and slow waves are reduced in the EEG. Channels 5 and 6 show the effect of decreasing the high frequency filter: sine waves of high frequency are reduced in amplitude, the calibration pulse is rounded off at its tip, and fast waves in the EEG are reduced in amplitude and increased in duration as compared with channels 4 and 7, although this effect is less noticeable here than in tracings containing fast activity of higher amplitude (Fig. 6.2, parts 1 and 2). The last channel shows the effect of the 60 Hz filter: sine waves of 60 Hz are eliminated and those at 35 and 70 Hz are reduced in amplitude, the calibration pulse shows a barely visible deformation in the rising and falling phase, and the EEG tracing loses the slight amount of superimposed 60 Hz activity which is recognizable as the 'hum' or thickness of the tracing in channel 4 and reduced by the high frequency filter settings used in channels 5 and 6; this effect is better appreciated in tracings containing more 60 Hz artifact (Fig. 6.3, part 1).

frequencies and of time constants on the left side of the figure. Note that an increase in the time constant means that waves of lower frequency are amplified without distortion, i.e., a long time constant, or a time constant of high numerical value, corresponds with a reduced filtering effect on waves of low frequency. *A mnemonic to remember this relationship is to consider the time constant as the width of a doorway that allows waveforms to pass into the recording according to their width (i.e., wavelength or duration).* The wider the door (longer the time constant) the more fat waveforms (slow, longer duration) can get into the recording. The most commonly used low frequency time constant settings fall in the range of 1–0.03 s.

The values of time constants and low frequency filter cutoff frequencies can be calculated from each other. The time constant (TC) in a simple network of resistors and capacitors is related to the low filter frequency by the equation $TC = 1/2\pi f$, where f is the frequency at which the amplitude is attenuated by 30.3% or 3 dB. This means that time constants of 1, 0.3, 0.1 and 0.03 s, used in most EEG instruments, correspond with 30.3% amplitude attenuation (cutoff frequency) at frequencies of 0.16, 0.53, 1.6 and 5.3 Hz. The low frequency settings producing 20% attenuation at 0.1, 0.3, 1 and 5 Hz, used in some other instruments, correspond with time constants of 1, 0.4, 0.12 and 0.035 s.

The extreme lower limit of low frequency filtering results from the design of EEG instruments. Most instruments are not designed to record very slow or very long sustained potential changes. Their inputs do not have direct coupling which is needed to conduct potential changes of 0 Hz (direct current, DC). Instead, they are coupled through *capacitors* which process alternating current signals (AC). Direct coupling is not used in clinical EEG because cerebral activity of very low frequency does not contain diagnostic information (except perhaps during ictal seizure recording) and it is extremely difficult to record over long periods of time because of the instability of the electrical properties of skin, electrodes, amplifiers and other electrical components.

Electrical construction of low frequency analog filters involves the placement of a capacitor (C) in the path of the signal (Fig. 3.5a) which is separated from ground by a resistor (R). *Capa-*

Fig. 3.4. The effect of different filter settings on the amplitude of sine waves that have frequencies representative of the spectrum of frequencies recorded in the ▶ EEG. Top: sine waves of logarithmically increasing frequency are recorded with filter settings which are indicated at the left margin in the same notation as used for Fig. 3.3. Filter settings for both high and low frequencies are changed between channels 1 and 4 so that the amplitude of slow and fast waves progressively decreases; the 60 Hz filter is used in channel 4. Arrows indicate the frequencies at which the amplitude is reduced by 20%; dotted lines project these values to the graph below. Bottom: a graph of filter settings is derived from the recording in the top part and relates the amplitude of sine waves, in percent of total amplification (vertical axis on left), to the wave frequency (horizontal axis with logarithmic scale at bottom). Each curve corresponds with a setting of the low frequency filter (LFF), high frequency filter (HFF) or 60 Hz filter and indicates the reduction in amplitude of sine waves at that setting.

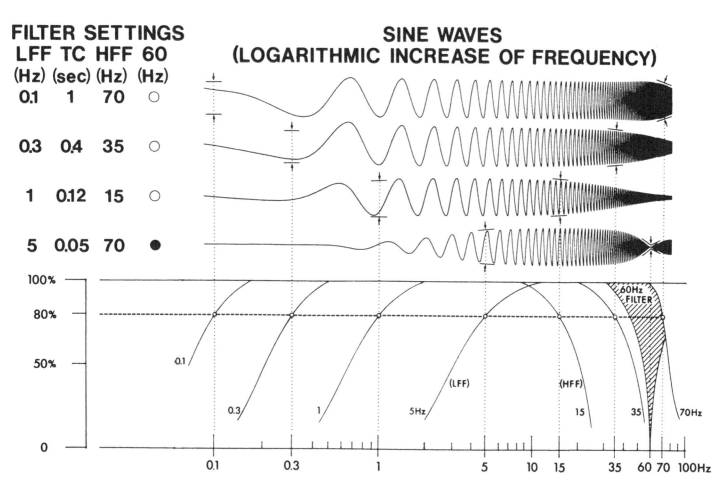

FILTER SETTINGS

LFF (Hz)	TC (sec)	HFF (Hz)	60 (Hz)
0.1	1	70	○
0.3	0.4	35	○
1	0.12	15	○
5	0.05	70	●

**SINE WAVES
(LOGARITHMIC INCREASE OF FREQUENCY)**

60Hz FILTER

0.1

0.3

1

(LFF)

5Hz

(HFF)

15

35

70Hz

100%

80%

50%

0

0.1   0.3   1   5   10 15   35   60 70 100Hz

51

citance is the property of current flow that occurs when an extremely high resistance insulator (like air) is placed in the path of current flow. A capacitor consists of a conductor-insulator-conductor assembly in which the conductors are composed of metal electrode plates separated by an insulating material. When the voltage in the circuit is turned on, a charge builds on the electrode plates on either side of the insulator. When the voltage is turned off it can be shown using a meter that the charge of the plates on either side of the insulator remains. More charge can be stored by increasing the area (size) of the conducting elements (i.e., electrode plates) on either side of the insulator or by decreasing the distance between the electrode plates. The more charge the capacitor (also referred to as a condensor) can hold the higher the capacitance. Capacitance also increases according to the conductive property of the insulating material, the *dielectric constant*. As the dielectric constant increases, capacitance increases. The quantitative expression of capacitance is the *farad*.

Capacitors are ideal for filtering alternating signals because they offer very high impedance (i.e., resistance to alternating signals) at zero cycles (DC), but their impedance decreases as the signal frequency increases. Thus, if a capacitor is placed in the direct path of current flow it will filter out slower frequencies more than faster frequencies (i.e., creating a low frequency filter or high pass filter). If instead the capacitor is placed between the current path and ground it will 'siphon off' or allow faster frequencies to be removed to ground and only the slower frequencies will pass (i.e., creating a high frequency or low pass filter). The circuit in Fig. 3.5a shows a low frequency filter (high pass filter). It has a time constant (TC) which is TC = R × C (where R is resistance and C is capacitance) and a low frequency reduction of 3 dB or 30.3% at a frequency of f = 1/2 πrR × C.

3.5.2 *The high frequency filter* reduces the size of fast waves. Its effect is specified by the frequency of waves which are reduced by a fixed fraction, for instance 30.3% or 3 dB, or 20% or 2 dB (depending on the manufacturer). Figs. 3.3 and 3.4 show the effects of high frequency filter settings of 15, 35 and 70 Hz which reduce the amplitude of sine waves at these frequencies by 20% or 2 dB. Sine waves above the cutoff frequencies are reduced more, but sine waves slightly below the cutoff are also reduced, even though by less than 20%. These relations are summarized by the curves on the right side of the diagram at the bottom of Fig. 3.4.

The middle part of Fig. 3.3 shows the effects of high frequency filters on square waves used for calibration. Square waves contain high frequency components at their vertical departure and return to baseline. The filtering of high frequencies is easiest to see in the rise time of the calibration pulses. This effect is barely visible at the normally slow speed of EEG recordings but causes the tips of the calibration square wave pulses to become slightly rounded (curved arrows in Fig. 3.3). This effect becomes more obvious with very low settings of the high

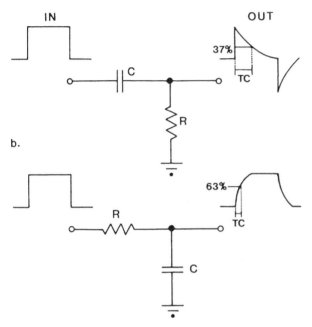

a.

IN   OUT

37%

C

R

TC

b.

R

63%

TC

C

Fig 3.5. Circuits of simple low and high frequency filters made of a capacitor (C) and a resistor (R). (a) Low frequency filter consists of a capacitor in the signal path and a resistor connection to ground. The time constant (TC) of this circuit is defined as the time required for a steady input voltage to drop to 37% of its original amplitude at the output and equals the product of R × C. (b) High frequency filter consists of a resistor in the signal path and a capacitor connection to ground. The time constant of this circuit is defined as the time required for the output voltage to rise to 63% of a sudden input voltage and is also equal to the product of R × C.

frequency filter and very high recording speeds, but measurement of the time constant of the rising phase (TC in Fig. 3.5b) is not practical with the recording methods used in conventional analog EEG.

High frequency filters must be set to include frequencies faster than those usually considered important in clinical EEG. Although most waveforms over 35 Hz are of little clinical interest, the use of high frequency filters set at that value can distort non-cerebral potentials to the extent that they appear to be cerebral in origin. This is especially true of muscle activity, a common contaminant consisting of fast waves that are not usually completely eliminated by filtering. Instead, filtered muscle activity is reduced in amplitude and appears to have longer duration waveforms. Filtered muscle activity may therefore appear to be much more difficult to distinguish from cerebral activity (e.g., beta activity or epileptiform spikes) than unfiltered muscle activity (Fig. 6.2).

Digital EEG instruments commonly use a steeper high frequency analog filter than low frequency filter (e.g., 6–24 dB vs. 3 dB). Removing high frequency activity with an analog filter prior to digitizing the EEG eliminates unnecessary high frequency components and reduces demand on the sampling rate of the analog to digital converter (see 3.7). The *limit of high frequency* recording in analog EEG systems is due to the design of the writing units; the oscillographic penwriters cannot be driven to write much faster than 70 Hz without significant distortion.

Electrical construction of high frequency filters includes a capacitor (C) to shunt high frequencies from the signal path to ground (Fig. 3.5b). The circuit in Fig. 3.5b reduces the amplitude of waves of a frequency of $f = 1/2 \, \pi r R \times C$ by 30.3% or 3 dB.

3.5.3 *Phase shift.*

It is important to note that filters also distort the time relation between waves of frequencies near the cutoff frequency, each filter delaying or advancing these waves by different amounts of time. This is referred to as a *phase shift* or *phase distortion* because a phase of the waveform appears to be advanced or delayed in time. The low frequency filter which affects the rapidity of the return to baseline of a long duration waveform or square wave pulse actually moves the peak of a slow waveform backwards in time. In contrast, the high frequency filter that affects the rapidity of the initial deflection from baseline of a square wave pulse acts to move the peak of the faster waveform later in time. Phase shift caused by filters increases as the filter acts more strongly on the waveform. Phase shift due to filtering becomes important in the interpretation of timing differences between events in the millisecond range, such as the spread of an epileptiform spike over the scalp or in latency measurements of evoked potential waveforms.

3.5.4

The 60 Hz filter helps to eliminate the most common type of electrical artifact, namely interference from devices powered by alternating current. This filter sharply reduces the amplitude of sine waves of 60 Hz (a 50 Hz filter is used in countries using a power line frequency of 50 Hz), but it cannot accomplish this without also reducing the amplitude of waveforms of neighboring frequencies to some extent (Figs. 3.3 and 3.4). Although sine waves of 60 Hz are not produced by the brain in scalp recordings, the 60 Hz filter should not be used routinely because 60 Hz interference is a useful warning sign of poor electrode contact or an improper input selection. These technical problems could be missed or their detection delayed if the 60 Hz filter is used indiscriminately. The 60 Hz filter should therefore be used only in the full knowledge of what it may obscure and after all other efforts to eradicate the cause of the interference have been exhausted.

In some instances, particularly in noisy recording environments created by other equipment, interference may occur at some frequency other than 60 (or 50) Hz. The mains current passing through other electrical components (such as electrical motors) changes the frequency of the interference. In such cases it may be necessary to disconnect the other instruments from the wall sockets or to use other EEG instrument filters to eliminate noise.

3.6   ANALOG WRITING UNITS

3.6.1   *Analog writing devices* serve to convert the output of the amplifiers into a vertical movement. In most analog EEG instruments, this is accomplished with an *oscillographic pen-writer*. An oscillograph consists of a galvanometer coil which is mounted in the field of a permanent magnet so that the coil rotates in response to the electrical potential changes coming from the amplifier output. The shaft of the galvanometer coil protrudes above the writing surface and holds the writing device that moves up and down on the EEG paper with excursions corresponding with the amplitude of the electrical potential changes. The most common writing devices are pens consisting of a metal tube filled with ink from an inkwell. Other writing devices include ink jets, carbon paper, and light or heat sensitive (thermal) paper.

Curvilinear distortion results from the arc-like movement of oscillograph pens around their axis. The deviation from rectilinear movement causes faulty representation of both vertical and horizontal coordinates (Fig. 3.6). The vertical deflection is neither strictly straight nor strictly proportional to the applied voltage. The horizontal position of a deflected pen depends on the degree of the vertical deflection. This makes a higher deflection seem to occur later in time than a simultaneous deflection of lower amplitude. Both types of distortion increase with the amplitude of the deflection and distort the shape and amplitude of every curvilinear EEG writeout to some degree.

Vertical and horizontal pen alignments should be routinely inspected and adjusted (Fig. 3.7). The pens must have equal distance from each other and point exactly in the direction of the paper movement. The pens must also be aligned so that a signal appearing in all channels at the same time deflects the pens on the same vertical line on the paper. If one pen protrudes to the left or right of the others, a signal written by that pen will seem to have occurred earlier or later than a signal written at the same time by the other pens. Faulty pen alignment occurs in the following situations:

(1)   If the horizontal spacing between the pen tips is uneven (Fig. 3.7b), a pen may have been damaged or moved out of its seat; if this is not the case, the pen may have rotated away from its correct position on the galvanometer shaft and should be rotated to the correct position by readjusting its seat on the shaft.

(2)   If the horizontal spacing between the pens changes suddenly when they are connected to the amplifier outputs (i.e., the oscillograph is turned on, Fig. 3.7c), the electrical potential level of the output is at fault and should be reset by adjusting the *electrical zero potential level (bias) of the amplifier outputs*. Minor steps of the baseline may appear during everyday operation and are tolerable if they are not much larger than the width of the ink tracing (Fig. 3.7a and e). Transient pen deflections may appear suddenly when the amplifier inputs are opened immedi-

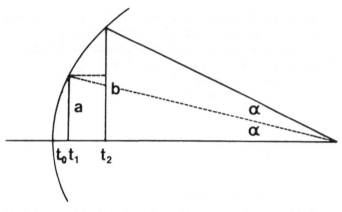

Fig. 3.6. Distortions of the EEG by curvilinear meriting movements of pens. The circular movement of the pen around the shaft causes the tracing to deviate from rectangular coordinates both in the horizontal and vertical dimensions. Horizontal error: a pen deflection to the height indicated by line a or b seems to occur at times t_1 and t_2 even though it is synchronous with t_0. Vertical error: the amplitude of b, even though caused by a pen deflection twice that of a, is not twice the amplitude of a.

ately after changing the selection of recording electrodes at the input and are usually due to electrode bias potentials (2.2.4).

(3) If the tips of the pens at rest are not aligned in a straight vertical line on the paper (Fig. 3.7d), the pens deviating from this line can be moved left or right into the correct position by adjusting the position of the pen seat in the EEG instrument. Before making this adjustment, one should be sure that the deviation is not due to bent or damaged pens.

3.6.2 *The paper transport,* that pulls the paper from a folded stack in a storage bin within the analog instrument, moves it at an even speed under the writing pens and across a surface where the ink dries and the record can be inspected and labeled for at least several seconds before it moves into another storage bin where it is folded again. Most instruments use the internationally recommended paper speed of 3 cm/s and usually have additional faster and slower speeds. EEG paper is often imprinted with vertical lines every 3 cm, corresponding with 1 s at regular speed; these intervals may be subdivided. Many EEG instruments have time markers producing a pen deflection in an extra channel every 1 s. This should generate intervals of the same length as those printed on the chart paper if the paper is moving at the speed of 3 cm/s.

Physically, the paper transport consists of a motor with gear shift and friction rollers which pull the margin of the paper. The transport mechanism may give rise to the following problems:

(1) If the paper slows or stops for a moment during the recording because of a momentary failure of the driving mechanism or because of a momentary resistance of the paper feed, the time base of the recording will be distorted: the pens will deflect up and down with little or

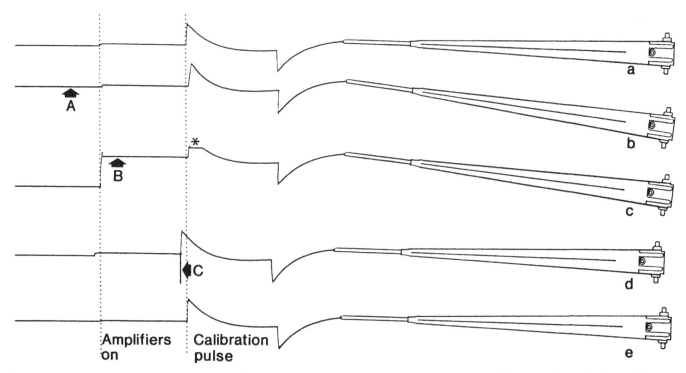

Amplifiers on   Calibration pulse

Fig. 3.7.   Pen misalignments. Pens a and e are normal: they write tracings that are properly spaced, show only minimal deflections when the amplifiers are turned on ('amplifiers on'), and do not distort the calibration pulse; the deflections of these pens fall on the same vertical line (dotted lines). Pen b writes a tracing that is displaced upward both before and after the amplifier output is connected to the pens (arrow A); this is due to a mechanical deviation from the zero line, usually caused by an improper adjustment of the pen on its shaft. Pen c writes a tracing that is displaced upward at the moment when the amplifiers are turned on (arrow B) and clips large signals in that direction (a); this is due to an electrical deviation from the zero line caused by faulty adjustment of the voltage level of the amplifier output. Pen d registers deflections that are displaced to the left (arrow C) and seem to occur earlier than those of the other pens; this horizontal deviation is usually due to improper alignment of the oscillograph or of the pen seat.

no movement to the side and create the impression of very fast and abnormal EEG transients, such as spikes. This artifact can be recognized by the very steep rises and falls of the pen deflections and by the fact that the same phenomenon occurs in all or most channels at the same time (Fig. 6.3).

(2) When stiff paper with sharp creases is not sufficiently stretched as it is pulled along under the pens, the pens may be bounced up and off the paper at each upward fold. This gives an interrupted, irregular tracing of all pens following each upward fold.

(3) The paper may run not on a straight course or it may track too close to the upper or lower edge. This can be corrected by adjusting the front or rear paper guides and rollers on the machine.

(4) The paper speed may vary due to defects of the friction rollers, gear shift or motor. This distorts the timing of the writeout and makes regular wave shapes appear irregular.

3.7 ANALOG TO DIGITAL CONVERSION

All digital instruments contain analog amplifiers and filters as described in the first half of this chapter. These components must first produce an EEG signal suitable for digital processing. Digital processing begins with the transformation of the continuous *analog* signal into a *digital* signal. The digital signal consists of a series of discrete, discontinuous data points separated by equal intervals of time. This transformation is performed by an *analog to digital converter,* or ADC. The ADC is literally an array of computer chips mounted on a circuit board that has inputs to receive the amplified analog EEG signal. It has 3 key attributes that determine how accurately the analog signal will be reproduced in digital form:
(1) the sampling rate (i.e., samples per second)
(2) the number of amplitude levels that can be resolved (characterized by the bit number), and
(3) the input voltage range (the range of voltage coming from the analog amplifiers that the ADC is set to analyze).

3.7.1 The number of digital points per second used to represent the analog signal is referred to as the *sampling rate* and the duration between each data point is referred to as the *dwell time*. If, for example, the ADC has a sampling rate of 100 Hz, each second of the digitized analog signal will contain 100 points each separated by a dwell time of 10 ms (1/100 s).

To represent a particular frequency, *the sampling rate must be at least twice the frequency of waveform to be resolved*. This is known as the *Nyquist theorem* and the critical sampling rate (2 times the fastest frequency in the signal) is referred to as the

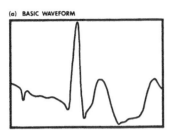

(a) BASIC WAVEFORM

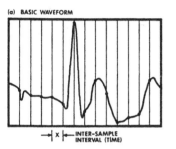

(a) BASIC WAVEFORM

→| x |← INTER-SAMPLE
INTERVAL (TIME)

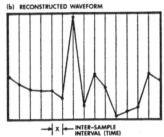

(b) RECONSTRUCTED WAVEFORM

→| x |← INTER-SAMPLE
INTERVAL (TIME)

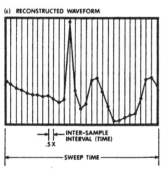

(c) RECONSTRUCTED WAVEFORM

→| |← INTER-SAMPLE
.5X   INTERVAL (TIME)

|←————— SWEEP TIME —————→|

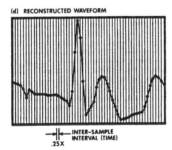

(d) RECONSTRUCTED WAVEFORM

→| |← INTER-SAMPLE
.25X   INTERVAL (TIME)

Nyquist rate. For example, if the fastest frequency in the signal is 100 Hz, then the sampling rate must be at least 200 Hz in order to detect it. Although a Nyquist rate of 200 Hz would accurately detect a 100 Hz sine wave, the waveform that would be represented by connecting the sampling points would be triangular rather than sinusoidal in appearance. A more accurate display of waveform morphology (shape) is produced by *oversampling* the frequency of interest (i.e., sampling at greater than the Nyquist rate). In practice it is helpful if the ADC sampling rate is at least 6 times faster than the fastest frequency to be presented for visual inspection. Otherwise the waveform morphology may be poorly represented making interpretation difficult. Fig. 3.8 illustrates the effects of increasing sampling rates on waveform morphology.

If the ADC samples the analog signal at a rate less than twice its frequency, then the analog signal will be misrepresented as slower frequency waveforms. This is referred to as *aliasing*.

Fig. 3.8. The effect of different *sampling rates* (*dwell times* or *sampling intervals* between samples) on signal resolution. a, upper center: the original analog signal; a, upper left: the original signal to be sampled at the intervals indicated by the vertical lines with a sampling interval of x. b: the result of sampling at intersample time x shows a failure to represent all waveform components. c: 0.5 x sampling interval produces a better representation of the original signal but the faster components are not seen. d: sampling at 0.25 x finally produces almost all the components of the original signal except for those waveforms whose duration is less than 2 of the sampling intervals. Adapted from Grass and Johnson (1980).

The concept of aliasing can be illustrated by imagining a waveform sampled at a rate equal to its frequency. If, for example, a 50 Hz sinusoidal waveform is sampled at 50 Hz, then the digital points will fall on the waveform at exactly the same point (e.g., at each peak only) of the waveform each time the wave is sampled. If a line is then drawn connecting each of the sampled points, the result is a flat line, falsely detected by the computer as a 0 Hz signal. Thus, a 50 Hz signal sampled at 50 samples/s creates a 0 Hz digital signal. As the sampling rate increases, digital waveforms slower than 50 Hz are created (falsely detected) until the sampling rate reaches 100 Hz and the 50 Hz analog signal is truly seen as a 50 Hz signal. Fig. 3.9 illustrates the effect of sampling a waveform at greater than twice its frequency (A) compared to sampling it at less than its frequency (B). The undersampled waveform creates a digital waveform (with a lower frequency) that does not exist in the original signal. Aliasing can be avoided by either: (1) increasing the sampling rate of the ADC until the Nyquist frequency is reached or exceeded, or (2) filtering the analog signal with a high frequency analog filter to remove all activity with a frequency faster than half the sampling rate of the ADC.

Some instruments offer variable sampling rates during digital data acquisition. The main advantage of variable sampling rates is to conserve storage space. If the fastest analog signal being digitized is, for example, 30 Hz, then the ADC can accurately sample the system at a much slower rate (Nyquist frequency = 60 Hz) than if the analog signal is 100 Hz (Nyquist frequency = 200 Hz). Fewer samples mean that less information needs to be stored and more storage space becomes available for storing a longer recording.

3.7.2   The amplitudes of digitized signals are quantified, or assigned to discrete non-overlapping amplitude levels by the ADC. The number of amplitude levels (amplitude resolution) that the ADC has available is expressed in terms of *bits*, where each bit is a power of two. For example, an 8-bit ADC has 2^8, or 256 amplitude levels that can be used to describe the signal (± 128 voltage levels). The computer registers amplitude changes only when the signal changes enough to reach the next amplitude level bin of the ADC. The ADC's amplitude resolution is therefore dependent on both its voltage range and the maximum number of bits of discrimination it can resolve.

To illustrate the concept of digital amplitude resolution, consider an ADC with 3 bits or 8 levels (3 bits$=2^3=8$) of amplitude discrimination and a voltage range of $+400$ to -400 μV. That many microvolts (800) spread over that many levels (8) will give the ADC 100 μV between each level of amplitude detection (8 levels spread over 800 μV; $+400$ to -400 μV). If the signal varies between 0 and $+99$ μV, no amplitude variation is detected. In contrast, if the signal varies over a much smaller range but that small range happens to vary between $+99$ and $+101$ μV, then an amplitude change is registered (for each variation between the 0–100 and the 101–200 μV bins).

Thus, ADCs with fewer bits make it more likely that relatively large changes can go undetected, and very small amplitude changes can be overrepresented. (The failure to detect an amplitude change is illustrated in Fig. 3.10 in which the amplitude sampling of a waveform is gradually increased until the digital representation is accurate.)

In the above example digital amplitude resolution could be improved by either: (1) setting the entire voltage range of the ADC to +100 to −100 μV, thereby allowing all 8 levels to be distributed in this range (i.e., each amplitude bin would then have a range of about 25 μV; 200/8); or (2) using an ADC with

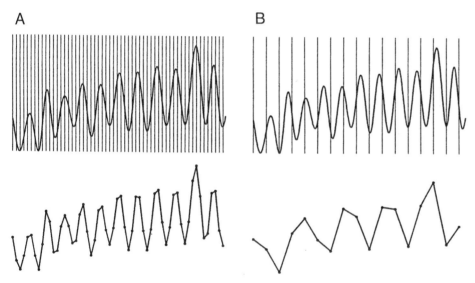

A   B

Fig. 3.9. Aliasing. A sinusoidal waveform is sampled at two different sampling rates. (A) The sampling rate is greater than twice the frequency of the waveform being sampled. This yields a true digital representation of the frequency of the analog waveform. (B) The sampling rate is less than twice the frequency of the waveform being sampled. This yields a false (aliased) digital representation of the analog waveform. Undersampling always results in aliasing and always produces a lower frequency waveform than that present in the original signal. From Goldensohn et al. (1998) with permission.

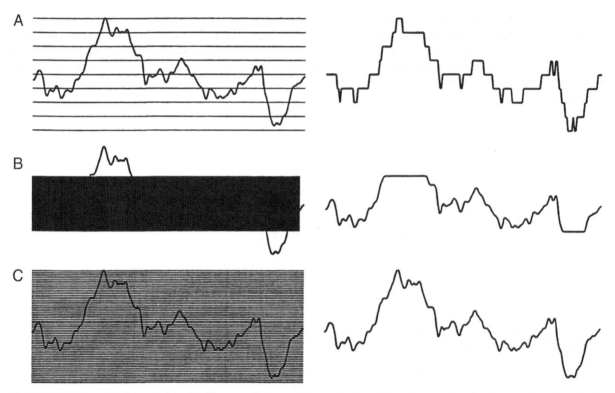

Fig. 3.10. Digital amplitude resolution. (A) The overrall range of the amplitude window is appropriate but the number of levels of amplitude discrimination (indicated by the horizontal lines) is too low. (B) The amplitude window is too narrow and the higher and lower peaks are cut off. The number of levels of amplitude discrimination for the other portions of the waveform are adequate. (C) The input window for amplitude range and the number of levels of amplitude discrimination are adequate to accurately represent the amplitude changes of the original analog signal. From Goldensohn et al. (1998) with permission.

a larger number of bits so that more amplitude levels would be available.

In actual practice the voltage range presented to the ADC by the analog EEG amplifiers is in volts (usually in the range of $+5$ to -5 V) rather than microvolts. ADCs used for EEG and evoked potential analysis should have at least 12-bit ($2^{12}=4096$ voltage levels spread over $+2048$ to -2048) amplitude discrimination.

Digitized signals can be converted back into analog signals by digital to analog converters (DAC). Like the ADC and other computer signal processing components, the DAC consists of computer processor chips mounted on a circuit board. The DAC is plugged into the computer and can then be connected to an analog display device (e.g., conventional pen writer EEG or oscilloscope) by cable.

3.8 THE SIGNAL DISPLAY

Although digital systems can easily output the recorded signal to a variety of display media (e.g., oscilloscopes, paper), in order to make use of the advantages of digital analysis, the most practical way of viewing the EEG is on a computer (monitor or flat panel display). The computer monitor that serves as the EEG display should approximate the quality and size of the visual image produced by a conventional pen writer output. For routine visual inspection a larger monitor screen is therefore preferable over a small one and 1 s of recording should occupy a screen width of at least 25 mm (routine EEG records at 30 mm/s). Each second of EEG displayed should contain at least 100 data points. These minimal requirements can be met with monitors that provide horizontal pixel representation of 1024 points. However, higher resolution is required to rival the quality of analog pen writers. Regardless of the number of channels displayed, vertical spacing between channels should be at least 15 mm (routine EEG recordings have approximately 20 mm separation). According to the American Clinical Neurophysiology Society the display should have a minimum of 2 pixels of resolution per vertical millimeter, but higher resolution monitors are available. A non-interlaced monitor is preferable for reducing screen flicker. To assess flicker on any monitor one should fixate on the frame of the monitor thereby engaging one's peripheral vision (cones of the central retina create fusion at a lower frequency than do rods). If the monitor appears to flicker then the refresh rate is too slow. Most commercial systems do not produce a 10 s page screen display with the same quality resolution as do analog pen-driven systems. However, when necessary visual resolution of waveforms can be significantly improved by displaying shorter epochs across the entire screen. In evaluating digital EEG display software it is important that the horizontal width of the screen be devoted to signal display and not various icons or alphanumerics. In summary, an adequate display monitor has high resolution, no flicker, and a large viewing area.

3.8.1 *Signal display duration.* The display resolution of individual waveforms can usually be improved by using the entire screen to display very short epochs of EEG. However, the main advantages of changing the display so that the entire monitor screen displays only 2–3 s of EEG are: (1) timing differences of waveforms between channels can be determined more precisely, and (2) very fast activity, such as 60 cycle interference, can be seen and identified with ease. The advantages of displaying a longer duration of time (e.g., compressing the EEG to 60 or 120 s of display on a single screen) are the same as those seen using a slow paper speed on a pen writing instrument: (1) the visualization of slowing is enhanced, (2) periodic or intermittent phenomena (such as suppression burst, tracé alternant or PLEDs) can be seen more easily, and (3) the record can be reviewed more rapidly when looking for known phenomena such as electrographic seizures (an approach often used during the review of epilepsy monitoring data).

Routine paper EEG provides a visual time discrimination of roughly 30 ms (paper speed of 33 ms/mm plus pen axis alignment error) whereas digital EEG may provide 10 ms resolution or better (e.g., 2 s of EEG sampled at 200 Hz presented on a 25–30 cm wide screen display). Time resolution is important for localizing the earliest occurrence of fast waveforms such as epileptiform spikes and evaluating the likelihood of transsynaptic vs. volume conduction of spikes between head regions.

3.8.2 *Signal display amplitude.* Digital EEG instruments display the amplitude scale as a vertical icon that provides a user selectable number of microvolts of vertical deviation. In addition, many vendors allow the user to select a waveform of interest and draw a line from peak to trough to get a numerical readout of the amplitude in microvolts. The accuracy of any system's amplitude scale can be tested using a signal wave generator (usually available from the hospital biomedical technology department). The output of the sine wave generator is decreased to the microvolt range and then connected to the electrode input of the digital EEG instrument headbox. The sine wave of known microvolt amplitude can then be compared to the digital EEG instrument's amplitude scale.

3.9 DIGITAL FILTERING

One of the great advantages of digital EEG analysis is that filtering adjustments can be performed retrospectively during EEG review. There are 3 common approaches to digital filtering: (1) *finite impulse response* (FIR), (2) *infinite impulse response* (IIR), and (3) frequency domain filtering using the *fast Fourier transform* (FFT). Most commercial EEG systems use FIR filtering during retrospective EEG review, because it is computationally much simpler and requires far less processing time than FFT filtering.

Both FIR and FFT filters have a distinct potential advantage over analog filtering in that they can be designed to preserve the timing of the phase of the signal. For example, a low frequency (high pass) *analog* EEG filter applied to a slow sine wave will displace the waveform backwards in time as the cutoff frequency setting of the filter is increased (Fig. 3.11). FIR and FFT filters can be designed to produce far less phase distortion. In comparing the FIR and FFT filters the FIR filter is computationally simpler than the FFT filter and the FIR filter can also more easily be applied to long duration signals than

A. High Pass Filter   B. Low Pass Filter

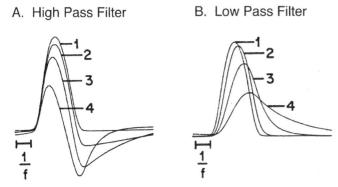

Fig. 3.11. The effect of analog filtering on the timing of waveforms. (A) The original signal (1) is passed through a low frequency filter (high pass) with an increasingly higher cutoff frequency (from 2 to 4). The low frequency filter displaces the peak backward in time as it decreases the overall amplitude of the signal. (B) The original signal (1) is passed through a high frequency filter (low pass filter) with increasingly lower cutoff frequency (from 2 to 4). The high frequency filter displaces the peak forward in time as it decreases the amplitude of the signal. Adapted from Ehle (1980) with permission.

can the FFT (see also under Frequency Domain Analysis). However, the FFT filter can provide a much sharper frequency cutoff.

Commercial systems rarely provide digital filters free of phase distortion. To determine the phase distortion in a particular system, adjacent channels of the same signal with different filter settings should be displayed to see if the waveforms appear to advance or retreat in time. Virtually all commercial systems allow for this kind of comparison.

The essential computational feature of FIR filtering is *amplitude averaging of adjacent digitized signal points*. Amplitude averaging is accomplished by the following steps:

(1)   The filter fixes on one point in the signal at a time.
(2)   As the filter is fixed on a particular point it computes an average amplitude of that point and the amplitudes of a specified number of points preceding and following that point.
(3)   The amplitude of the point the filter has fixed on is then reassigned the value of the average.
(4)   The filter is moved to the next adjacent digitized sample point and the process is repeated.

Thus, an FIR filter can be viewed as a moving average of digital sample points. The process described above creates a low pass filter (i.e., attenuation of faster frequencies). If the same number of points preceding and following the central point are used to create the average then phase distortion is minimized. The number of points that are averaged by the filter at any one time is referred to as the *order* of the filter. Such a filter will always have an order that is an odd number because it includes the central fixation data point (that is going to be reassigned the value of the average of the amplitudes) plus an equal number of preceding and following points. The higher the order of the filter, the longer the computation takes. The filter can also be 'shaped' so that equal weighting is given to each point and a true average is taken. Alternatively, the amplitudes of the points can be given a certain weight in the overall average, for example, with the points farthest away from the central point contributing less and less to the average. This has the effect of creating a wider low pass band (i.e., filtering out fewer fast frequencies). Reducing the order of the filter can also widen the low pass band.

As with analog filters, care must be taken in the application of digital filters. With low pass filtering muscle artifact can be made to appear as alpha activity or epileptiform spikes. With high pass filtering significant slowing or artifacts characterized by slow baseline shifts may be misinterpreted or missed altogether. Filtering can, however, be used to detect cerebral activity such as an electrographic seizure that would otherwise be obscured by muscle or movement artifact.

By combining the filter and amplitude settings in various ways it is possible to enhance the viewing of either fast or slow ac-

tivity. For example, if an asymmetry of beta activity (activity > 13 Hz) is suspected, then the low frequency filter cutoff can be raised from the standard setting of 1 Hz to 3 Hz to eliminate slower waveforms and the amplitude of the signal increased. Retrospective amplitude adjustments may be made to all channels of recording simultaneously or to individual channels. Individual channel adjustment can be useful for defining the presence of artifact. For example, if movement artifact is suspected but the ECG recording from chest electrodes shows no evidence of movement, then increasing the amplitude of the signal display of the ECG may reveal subtle changes consistent with movement at a particular time.

3.10 DIGITAL MONTAGE SELECTION AND MONTAGE REFORMATTING

In contrast to analog EEG instruments, digital EEG instruments allow for greater analysis of the regional distributions of individual waveforms over the scalp. One of the important tools for analyzing the spatial distribution of EEG over the scalp is montage reformatting. Digital EEG approaches to spatial analysis are discussed in greater detail in Chapter 4.

Perhaps the most difficult part of learning to read EEG, and the part that is most often not achieved during residency or technologist training, is localization. This, unfortunately, has resulted in the common misconception that EEG interpretation is simply a matter of pattern recognition. This is particularly disappointing when one realizes that many EEG phenomena that are novel to the interpreter can be properly classified or 'figured out' on the basis of localization.

The conventional spatial analysis of EEG requires the electroencephalographer to mentally construct the topography of the EEG. This is usually approached by combining views of the EEG from three or more montages. In routine paper EEG spatial analysis, the electroencephalographer makes the theoretical assumption that the EEG topography is similar at different times in the recording. Digital EEG circumvents this problem by virtue of montage reformatting which allows the same epoch to be analyzed using a variety of montages. Indeed, this is perhaps the greatest advantage of digital EEG.

Montage reformatting becomes surprisingly simple if it is recalled that the EEG signal from each channel is simply the subtraction of the activity in the electrode in input 2 from input 1. For example, when a technologist labels a channel montage as Fp1−A1 they have actually written a mathematical expression which states that the signal displayed will be Fp1 minus A1 (input 1 minus input 2). If a recording has been obtained from Fp1−A1 and F3−A1, then Fp1−F3 can be derived by subtracting F3−A1 from Fp1−A1 as follows:

$$(Fp1 - A1) - (F3 - A1) = Fp1 - A1 - F3 + A1 = Fp1 - F3.$$

Similarly, if a recording has been obtained from one channel with Fp1−F3 and one channel with F3−C3 then a recording of Fp1−C3 can be easily derived by adding the two channels:

$$(Fp1 - F3) + (F3 - C3) = Fp1 - F3 + F3 - C3 = Fp1 - C3.$$

As long as all the electrodes that are to be combined have been somehow be referred to each other in the original recording it is a simple matter to reconstruct any combination of montages, including more complex montages such as the common average reference and Laplacian (e.g., source derivation) montages. For this reason, commercial digital EEG systems store the EEG in a referential montage containing all electrodes. If the original recording montage does not incorporate a particular electrode, then a new montage cannot be derived that contains that electrode. Because montage reformatting is a simple mathematical operation, computers are able to reformat montages instantaneously.

3.11 DIGITAL DATA STORAGE AND TRANSMISSION

Whether the digitized EEG signal will be viewed on-line (e.g., in real time as during intraoperative recording) or off-line (e.g., retrospectively as in routine EEG analysis) the EEG should be stored for off-line review as well as for medicolegal purposes. The storage space required is dependent upon the amount of digitized information. The amount of digitized information is determined by the number of bits and the sampling rate of the ADC. One hour of EEG sampled and stored at 200 samples/s with 32 channels of recording (32 × 200 = 6400 samples/s) may require approximately 50 Mb/h of recording. The same recording stored at 400 samples/s would require 100 Mb/h. These figures vary from instrument to instrument depending on what information is stored with the signal, and what file format or data compression techniques are used. Most desktop computers contain storage devices that store in excess of several gigabytes. For more permanent storage the EEG may be copied from the hard drive to other storage devices or directly recorded onto other storage media.

Currently, compact disc (CD), DVD, or DAT (digital analog tape) are the most economical long term storage devices that offer the largest data capacity and quickest access for retrieval. These storage devices currently hold between 650 Mb and 5 Gb (1 Mb = 1 million bytes and 1000 Mb = 1 Gb). For example, a single DVD (digital video or versatile discs) can store about 4.7 Gb of information. DAT tape, previously the least expensive option, like all tape devices provides much slower access in recalling the EEG than a disc device because the tape must be advanced by the tape drive. Moreover, magnetic tape, like videotape, has a limited shelf life (7–10 years) which can be prolonged by periodically winding and rewinding the tape. CDs and DVDs reportedly can last up to 25 years, but their actual shelf life is unknown. It is reasonable to assume that before the next edition of this book that these

storage devices will be replaced by others that may or may not be compatible with the current technology. Unfortunately, most manufacturers of EEG instrumentation have failed to supply their customers with easy methods for upgrading stored EEGs to make them compatible with their latest devices. Digital EEG systems usually make it quite simple to also print out one or more pages of the record for 'hardcopy' storage. It is recommended that copies of several EEG pages containing any important findings be stored with the interpretive report. In some cases it may also be helpful to send copies with the report to the referring physician.

3.12 ELECTRICAL SAFETY

Physicians, technologists and others routinely involved in clinical neurophysiology, must continually address the issue of electrical safety. The main concern for patients and health care workers during bioelectrical recording is lethal electrical shock. However, another potentially lethal hazard is the explosion of flammable gas that can occur during the administration of general anesthesia in the operating room. A flammable gas explosion may result from the spark that occurs when the power switch of the EEG instrument is turned on if the EEG instrument is positioned next to a source of a flammable anesthetic gas.

The more common hazard of direct electrical shock is usually the result of one of the following three problems:

(1) a failure of grounding in the recording instrument or wall socket,
(2) improper use of patient grounding, or
(3) bringing electrodes into direct contact with the patient and strong electrical sources, such as the wall current.

Recently, electrode connectors have been changed from male to female because of several surprising cases in which non-EEG health care workers mistakenly plugged them directly into wall sockets electrocuting the patient. More typically, dangerous current that can flow through the patient arises from: (1) a short circuit within the instrument, or (2) capacitive or inductive leakage current within the instrument. Whether the current source is from a short circuit or leakage, danger to the patient almost always arises from either a failure of proper grounding or a misuse of grounding. Although it may seem paradoxical, *placing a ground electrode on the patient can only increase the danger of electrical shock (3.12.3). The only purpose of a ground electrode is to reduce noise contamination, not to protect the patient.*

3.12.1 *Macroshock* and *microshock*. The risk of exposure to electrical current depends on the path the current takes through the body. A 0.5–1 mA current at 60 Hz applied to dry skin is at the threshold of pain perception. A lethal 'macroshock' current (i.e., one that results in ventricular fibrillation) must exceed 100–300 mA. A much more dangerous situation arises in neonates and especially in patients in intensive care units with indwelling catheters, particularly cardiac catheters. Such patients have a low resistance pathway between the external current and the heart. Ventricular fibrillation or serious cardiac arrhythmia may result from 'microshock' currents of less than 100 μV.

3.12.2 *Short circuit and ground failure.* Each wall socket contains three color coded inputs:

(1) black (deadly), that carries the main voltage,
(2) white (neutral), that carries the voltage returning from the instrument, and
(3) green (safe), which is the ground that is in contact with the instrument chassis and earth ground.

Bioelectrical instrumentation should always be connected to a 3-pronged wall receptacle, never one that only accepts a 2-pronged plug. Two-pronged inputs contain only the 'hot' (black) and 'neutral' (white) connectors, whereas the ground (green) connection is used to protect against electrical shock. Under normal circumstances the chassis of the instrument is connected to the ground. If a short circuit in the instrument occurs that sends the wall current directly from the electronic components of the instrument to the chassis (outer covering) of the instrument, then if the instrument is connected to ground the current will shunt directly to ground. Risk from direct contact will be minimized because the current will flow preferentially to ground rather than through the person touching the instrument. Moreover, a fuse is always placed in the ground circuit that will break if excessive current flows through ground. The broken fuse will then cut all power to the instrument. However, there are two ways in which the ground system may fail:

(1) the green input of the wall receptacle becomes disconnected from ground, or
(2) the connection between the instrument chassis and ground becomes defective.

In either situation potentially lethal current may flow preferentially through the person touching the equipment. These situations can be easily avoided by periodically testing the equipment ground and wall receptacle ground. The equipment ground is tested with an ohmmeter by touching one probe to the ground prong of the power cord plug and the other to the chassis (or part of the chassis designated as a grounded site). The ohmmeter should show less than $0.1\ \Omega$ resistance. Otherwise, the instrument should be repaired before further use. Similarly, a simple inexpensive testing device is applied to the wall socket to determine if the ground is functioning properly and if the socket grips the plug with sufficient strength to form a firm, unexposed connection.

3.12.3 *Leakage current and ground failure.* In addition to a faulty connection between the mains current source and the chassis, unwanted current may also arise from capacitive and inductive sources. Capacitors are formed by two conductors separated by an insulator (3.5.1). Capacitors placed in a circuit will conduct alternating current. Faster frequencies are conducted more efficiently than slow frequencies. Indeed, this is the basis of analog filter construction (Fig. 3.5). One of the main sources of unwanted capacitance is the power cable between the instrument and the wall receptacle. The power cord contains 3 wires (one for each of the plug inputs) that are each separated by insulated covering. This creates a capacitor in which current can flow between the 3 wires (e.g., from the black 'hot' wire to the green ground wire). The longer the power cord, the greater the capacitance and the opportunity for additional current to flow which can then 'leak' into the instrument. Power cords are rated in capacitance per foot and are selected by the manufacturer to avoid excessive leakage current. Therefore, extension cords should never be used because they may raise leakage current to dangerous levels. For example, the leakage current produced by adding a 6 foot power extension cord will range from a minimum of $7\ \mu A$ up to $60\ \mu A$, depending on the construction of the cord (Tyner et al., 1983). In addition to the power cord, other components housed in the instrument (e.g., transformers) are potential sources of capacitive leakage current.

If a current is passed through electrical components (particularly coiled wires) it can create an electromagnetic field that may induce current flow in adjacent conductive materials. This unwanted inductance produces another potential source of leakage current. Fortunately this represents a less significant source of leakage current than capacitance. As with a short circuit, if either the instrumental or wall socket ground is not functioning properly and the patient comes in contact with a grounded object and either the instrument chassis or the ground electrode from the instrument, then the leakage current can flow through the patient. The hospital biomedical engineers should be requested to periodically test the instruments for leakage current.

3.12.4 *Current flow between unevenly grounded equipment.* If two different instruments are attached to the same patient and their ground levels are not the same, then any leakage current from one instrument may flow toward the patient through its ground electrode, through the patient, and into the ground electrode of the instrument that has a lower voltage ground level. This circuit of current flow is sometimes referred to as a *ground loop.* However, if only one instrument has a ground electrode attached to the patient, then the current is unlikely to flow from one instrument to the other. As an illustration, consider two instruments, A and B, that are attached to a patient. If instrument A has significant leakage current but the ground electrode from instrument A is not attached to the patient (and the patient is not touching the chassis of that instrument), then the leakage current may not be passed from instrument A through the patient to the ground electrode of instrument B. Alternatively, if instrument A's ground is attached to the patient but the ground of instrument B is not, then the leakage current will flow to the patient from instrument A only if there is a ground failure in instrument A as described in 3.12.1 or 3.12.2. To minimize the chances of current flow through the patient between two or more instruments that are unevenly grounded, the following rules should always be followed:

(1) Never attach a ground to the patient from more than one instrument at a time.
(2) Always plug all power cords from all instruments making contact with the patient into the same receptacle to increase the likelihood they all share the same ground level.
(3) When recording a patient who is attached to multiple instruments always use a current limiting device such as an isolation input panel.
(4) If the patient's bed needs to be grounded to reduce interference always ground it to the same wall socket being used by the other equipment.

The last rule refers to the situation in which excessive 60 cycle (or other mains cycle) interference is contaminating the recording due to excessive electromagnetic radiation from multiple electrical sources. In such a situation the technologist can often reduce or sometimes eliminate 60 cycle interference by connecting the patient's bed to a ground source with a wire. If the wire is connected to a ground that is at a lower level than the instrument ground, then current can pass through the patient the instant their body comes in contact with the metal parts of the bed. Although current can potentially flow between the instrument and any conducting pathway, including the EEG electrodes, following the above rules, obtaining periodic safety testing, and reducing ground electrode contact in potentially dangerous recording environments (e.g., ICU or OR) whenever possible are the most effective ways of ensuring the patient's safety.

REFERENCES

American Clinical Neurophysiology Society and American Academy of Neurology (1997) Assessment of digital EEG, quantitative EEG and EEG brain mapping. J. Clin. Neurophysiol. 49: 277–292.

American Electroencephalographic Society (1994) Guidelines for recording clinical EEG on digital media. J. Clin. Neurophysiol. 11: 114–115.

Barlow, J.S. (1986) Artifact processing in EEG data processing. In: A. Rémond (Ed.), Handbook of Electroencephalography and Clinical Neurophysiology, Vol. 2. Elsevier Science, Amsterdam.

Barlow, J.S., Kamp, A., Morton, H.B., Ripoche, A., Shipton, H. and Tchavdarov, D.B. (1978) EEG instrumentation standards (revised 1977). Report of the Committee on EEG Instrumentation Standards of the International Federation of Societies for Electroencephalography and Clinical Neurophysiology. Electroenceph. Clin. Neurophysiol. 45: 144–150.

Cooper, R., Osselton, J.W. and Shaw, J.C. (1981) EEG Technology, 3rd Edn. Butterworth, London.

Ebersole, J.S. (1997) EEG and MEG dipole source modeling. In: J. Engel, Jr. and T.A. Pedley (Eds.), Epilepsy: A Comprehensive Textbook, Vol. 1. Lippincott-Raven, Philadelphia, pp. 919–935.

Ehle, A.L. (1980) Instrumentation for evoked potentials. In: C.E. Henry (Ed.), Current Clinical Neurophysiology. Elsevier Science, Amsterdam, pp. 53–64.

Epstein, C.M. (1994) Computerized EEG in the courtroom. Neurology 44: 1566–1569.

Fisch, B.J. and Pedley, T.A. (1989) The role of quantitative topographic mapping of 'neurometrics' in the diagnosis of psychiatric and neurological disorders: the cons. Electroenceph. Clin. Neurophysiol. 73: 5–9.

Gevins, A.S. and Rémond, A. (Eds.) (1987) Methods of Analysis of Brain Electrical and Magnetic Signals. Handbook of Electroencephalography and Clinical Neurophysiology, Vol. 1 (Revised Series). Elsevier Science, Amsterdam.

Goldensohn, E.S., Legatt, A.D., Koszer, S. and Wolf, S.M. (1998) EEG Interpretation: Problems of Overreading and Underreading, 2nd Revised and Updated Edition. Futura, Armonk, New York.

Gotman, J. (1990) The use of computers in analysis and display of EEG and evoked potentials. In: D.D. Daly and T.A. Pedley (Eds.), Current Practice of Clinical Electroencephalography (2nd Edn.). Raven Press, New York, Chapter 3.

Grass, E.R. and Johnson, E. (1980) An Introduction to Evoked Response Signal Averaging. Grass Instruments, Quincy, MA.

Hopps, J.A. (1976) Shock hazards in electrophysiological recordings. In: A. Rémond (Ed.), Handbook of Electroencephalography and Clinical Neurophysiology, Vol. 3A. Elsevier, Amsterdam, pp. 75–79.

Lagerlund, T.D. (1996a) Electricity and electronics in clinical neurophysiology. In: J. Daube (Ed.), Clinical Neurophysiology. F.A. Davis, Philadelphia, pp. 3–17.

Lagerlund, T.D. (1996b) Digital signal processing. In: J. Daube (Ed.), Clinical Neurophysiology. F.A. Davis, Philadelphia, pp. 40–49.

Legatt, A.D. (1995) Impairment of common mode rejection by mismatched electrode impedances: quantitative analysis. Am. J. EEG Technol. 35: 296–302.

Lemos, M.L. and Fisch, B.J. (1991) The weighted average montage. Electroenceph. Clin. Neurophysiol. 79: 361–370.

McGee, F. (1981) EEG instrumentation. In: C.E. Henry (Ed.), Current Clinical Neurophysiology, Update on EEG and Evoked Potentials. Elsevier, Amsterdam, pp. 53–64.

Seeba, P.J. (1980) Electrical safety. Am. J. EEG Technol. 20: 1–13.

Seeba, P.J. (1984) Differential amplifiers and their limitations. Am. J. EEG Technol. 24: 11–23.

Tyner, F.S., Knott, J.R. and Mayer, Jr., W.B. (1983) Fundamentals of EEG Technology. Raven Press, New York.

Wong, P.K. and Lopes da Silva, F.H. (1997) EEG mapping and dynamic analysis. In: J. Engel, Jr. and T.A. Pedley (Eds.), Epilepsy: A Comprehensive Textbook, Vol. 1. Lippincott-Raven, Philadelphia, pp. 887–896.

4   Spatial analysis of the EEG

SUMMARY

(4.1) *Multichannel recordings* are used to determine the distribution of potential changes over the scalp. The lack of 'reference-free' information in EEG makes it necessary to use multiple differential electrode recording combinations to arrive at an estimate of the activity at any single electrode site. The combination of electrodes in inputs 1 and 2 of any one amplifier is known as the *derivation*. A *montage* consists of a combination of derivations using multiple channels of recording. Montages are *spatial filters*. Some montages are best suited for viewing highly localized activity over a limited area of the scalp and filtering out widespread waveforms that are *coherent* (i.e., occur simultaneously with similar amplitude and phase). Others are better for viewing widespread coherent waveforms than localized waveforms. Spatial analysis is critical for localizing abnormalities in the underlying cortex. Also, unlike pattern recognition, spatial analysis helps the novice to correctly classify cerebral potentials and artifacts never seen before.

(4.2) *Bipolar* derivations consist of a pair of electrodes located next to each other on the head (adjacent electrodes of the 10–20 system of placement 2.3) that are inserted into input 1 and 2 of the amplifier, respectively. *Bipolar montages* act as spatial filters that remove widespread coherent potentials from the recording. They are therefore best for analyzing low to medium amplitude waveforms that are highly localized. A single bipolar montage oriented in one direction (longitudinal or transverse) cannot be used to prove or disprove the existence of an interhemispheric asymmetry. A reference montage or another bipolar montage oriented at a 90° angle to the first montage is usually needed to verify an asymmetry.

(4.3) *Common electrode reference montages* consist of a series of derivations in which the same electrode is used in input 2 of each amplifier. Ideally, the input 2 reference electrode is at a distance from the source of the activity of interest so that it does not become intermixed with the activity occurring at the input 1 electrode. The reference electrode(s) may be placed at *cephalic* or *non-cephalic* (e.g., neck–chest) body locations. In contrast to the bipolar montage, widespread potentials that form similar, coherent waveforms are not filtered out of the recording. Highly localized low to medium amplitude activity that would be otherwise easily seen in a bipolar or other low spatial frequency filtering montages may be obscured by the higher amplitude more widely distributed activity seen in a reference montage.

(4.4) *The average reference montage* consists of a series of derivations in which all of the 10–20 electrodes are added together and placed in input 2 of every amplifier. The average reference montage produces a spatial filtering effect that is intermediate between the standard reference montage and the bipolar montage. In other words, there is less attenuation of widespread potentials than in the bipolar montage but more than in the common electrode reference montage. *As with all forms of reference montages, reference contamination occurs and can pose interpretational difficulties for the novice.*

(4.5) *The weighted average reference* montage is similar to the average reference montage in that the reference includes a combination of all scalp electrodes. It differs from the average reference montage because: (1) all the electrodes in input 2 do not contribute equally to the reference, (2) the input 1 electrode is not included in the input 2 average reference in a given channel, and (3) the reference potential varies dramatically from one derivation to the next. Electrodes are 'weighted' so that they contribute a larger percentage to the total reference the closer they are on the scalp to the input 1 (non-reference) electrode. Thus, the relative contributions of the reference electrodes vary from channel to channel depending on which electrode is in input 1. This creates a spatial filtering effect that is intermediate between the average reference and bipolar montages.

(4.6) *The Laplacian (or source derivation) montage* is similar to the weighted average reference montage but the reference usually includes only the nearest neighboring electrodes surrounding the input 1 electrode. This creates a more severe filtering of widespread, coherent waveforms. The Laplacian montage is therefore intermediate in filtering effects between the bipolar and weighted average reference montages.

(4.7) *Source localization* refers to various methods of calculating the precise anatomical location of a current source within the brain based on its distribution over the head. Source localization attempts to solve the *inverse problem* (1.1). In reality, there are an infinite number of possible solutions to the inverse problem (and therefore no way of knowing the single correct solution). However, a number of methods have been proposed that apply certain a priori assumptions (based on the principles of volume conduction and the assumed cortical origin of EEG) that provide an estimate of the most likely intracranial source of a scalp potential.

(4.8) *Montage display and design* guidelines of the American Clinical Neurophysiology Society (see Guidelines in Appendix II) recommend that every analog EEG recording be performed using a minimum of 3 basic montages: *longitudinal bipolar, transverse bipolar, and reference*. Digital instruments allow the user to display all of the derivations described above simultaneously to solve localization problems. All physicians and technologists should be familiar with the modified 10–20 system of electrode placement for those situations in which additional electrode placement would help to better localize or define a particular activity. Electrode derivations should be arranged in a consecutive series that run along either longitudinal (anterior to posterior) lines or transverse (left to right) lines.

(4.9) *Analysis of the topography of the EEG voltage field* over the scalp is an essential part of EEG interpretation. It requires the reader to be able to visualize the surface of the scalp as a spatial coordinate system in which the polarity and amplitude of the potential at each point in time at each electrode are seen as a 3-dimensional relief map of voltage peaks and valleys. Methods of computer assisted graphical mapping of EEG topography are described in Chapter 7.

4.1 MULTICHANNEL RECORDINGS

Spatial analysis of the distribution of EEG potentials over the scalp is the foundation upon which EEG interpretation is based. It is, unfortunately, often underemphasized in residency or technologist training programs. Unlike pattern recognition, spatial analysis is a deductive process that begins with the understanding that, in operational terms, the EEG is nothing more than the difference in voltage between different electrode inputs (head or body points) expressed over time. Differential amplification (3.4) allows for the recording of the EEG with the elimination of electrical interference, but because of differential amplification *the absolute potential value at any individual electrode can never be known.* Stated another way, even if the electrode in input 1 is placed on the scalp and electrode in input 2 is placed on the foot, the absolute potential at either electrode cannot be determined. This is because: (a) input 2 is subtracted from input 1, and (b) potentials from the brain or other body sources are transmitted by volume conduction throughout the body to both electrodes. This lack of 'reference-free' information (i.e., an ideal zero or ground potential reference recording) in EEG often makes it necessary to use multiple combinations of differential electrode recordings to arrive at an estimate of the activity in any single electrode.

Electrode recording combinations are referred to as *derivations* and *montages*. The selection of electrodes for inputs 1 and 2 for any one amplifier channel is referred to as the *derivation*. The combination of multiple derivations is referred to as a *montage*. Montages perform the function of *spatial filtering* because they filter out, to varying degrees, similarly shaped waveforms that are simultaneously and widely distributed over the scalp. Indeed, montages can be compared to different lens settings. Some montages (e.g., bipolar or Laplacian) are best suited for close-up viewing of highly localized activity, whereas others (e.g., reference) are better for distance viewing potentials that are widespread over the scalp. Because spatial analysis is so important in EEG interpretation, the most important advance in EEG technology in the last 20 years has been the routine application of EEG montage reformatting made possible by digital technology. There are currently 5 basic kinds of montages the EEG reader should be familiar with: bipolar, common electrode reference, average reference, weighted average reference, and Laplacian (source derivation).

4.2 BIPOLAR MONTAGES

Bipolar derivations consist of an adjacent pair of electrodes of the 10–20 system of electrode placement (2.3) inserted into inputs 1 and 2, respectively. *Bipolar montages* are formed by placing a series of linked bipolar derivations in straight lines (see Table 4.1), either longitudinally (anterior to posterior) or transversely (left to right) across the scalp. These derivations act as spatial filters that remove widespread potentials with similar amplitudes and phases (i.e., coherent waveforms) from the recording. *Bipolar montages are therefore best for analyzing low to medium amplitude waveforms that are highly localized.*

Bipolar montage derivations are arranged in a chain link fashion so that an electrode at input 2 of one amplifier is in input 1 of the amplifier in the next channel of recording (Fig. 4.1). In bipolar montages the localization of a cerebral potential is made according to the direction of waveform deflections between channels. An identical potential in input 2 of one channel and input 1 of the next channel causes waveform (or pen) deflections in opposite direction between those two channels. This reversal of phase is referred to as an *instrumental phase reversal* because it only occurs by virtue of the arrangement of the electrodes in successive channels and not because the polarity of the waveform produced by the brain is reversed in one head region compared to another. The latter would be referred to as a *true phase reversal* (4.9). Fig. 4.1a shows a bipolar montage recording of a relatively negative potential that has an instrumental phase reversal between the top channel and the next lower channel. The top channel shows a down-going deflection because it is connected to the electrode in input 2 that is near the negative potential, whereas the next channel, being connected to that electrode through input 1, shows an upgoing deflection. *Recall that in EEG recording if the electrode in input 1 is more negative than the electrode in* *input 2, then the waveform deflection will be upward. If the electrode in input 1 is more positive than the electrode in input 2, then the waveform deflection will be downward.*

The phase reversal shown in Fig. 4.1a does not indicate an actual reversal of polarity of the cerebral potential from one head region to the next (*true phase reversal*). It represents a

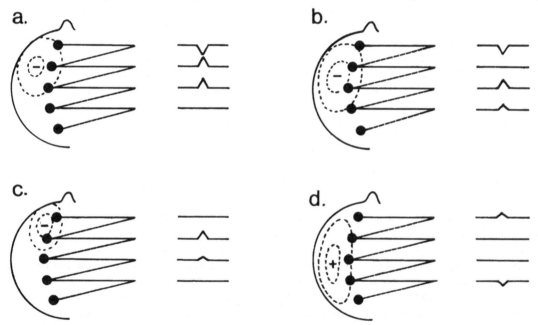

Fig. 4.1. Bipolar montages. a and b: localization of electrical potentials on the scalp by phase reversal; c and d: possible pitfalls of this method.

reversal in the direction of the waveform deflection created by configuration of the montage (hence an *instrumental* phase reversal). If the potential shown in Fig. 4.1a was positive instead of negative, all the waveform deflections in the figure would be in the opposite direction and the waveforms in the first two channels would then point away from each other instead of towards each other.

In the author's experience, many physicians who are learning to interpret EEG initially develop two fundamental misconceptions about polarity and phase reversal. The first is the belief that an upward deflection of the pen or waveform means that the scalp potential that caused the waveform was negative, and that a downward deflection was caused by a positive potential. *Remember, a waveform that points up is no more positive or negative than a waveform that points down. Polarity is totally dependent on which input of the differential amplifier the active electrode is in.* Thus, a positive scalp potential in the electrode of input 2 makes an upgoing deflection and a negative scalp potential in the electrode of input 1 makes the same upgoing deflection.

The second misconception is that a phase reversal is always an abnormal finding. This is partly the fault of the teacher who only invokes the concept of phase reversal in the setting of epileptiform spikes. *Instrumental phase reversals, like polarity, are simply the byproduct of the configuration of the bipolar montage and prominent normal examples can be found on virtually every page of a bipolar recording.*

True phase reversals are generated by the brain itself. True phase reversals are uncommon, but they are a characteristic feature of epileptiform spikes in benign rolandic epilepsy of childhood (with centromidtemporal spikes). *A true phase reversal can usually be identified by the presence of a single phase reversal in a reference montage or a double phase reversal in a bipolar montage.*

A potential having a maximum between two recording electrodes plugged into input 1 and input 2 of an amplifier (Fig. 4.1b) that produces the same potential in each of these electrodes causes no deflection in the output of that amplifier. However, a potential that is the same in two adjacent electrodes is detected in a bipolar montage because one or both of these electrodes is also connected to other electrodes in other channels which will show a phase reversal in relation to each other (see channels 1 and 3 in Fig. 4.1b).

Potentials that appear with greatest voltage in the last electrode in the chain of electrodes will produce waveform deflections in the chain of bipolar channels that are all in the same direction (i.e., no phase reversal). This has been referred to as the *end of the chain phenomenon*. In such an instance it can be reasonably assumed that the potential originates from the end of the chain of electrodes whose channel shows the highest amplitude waveform.

When a potential occurs between the last two electrodes in a chain and affects them equally then no output is seen in the channel that contains them both, whereas the remaining channels all show waveform deflections in the same direction (Fig. 4.1c). Finally, widespread potentials may be largely cancelled or produce phases that are opposite in direction in the opposite ends of the chain of channels (Fig. 4.1d). When uncertainties arise in bipolar montages during record review using digital instruments, other montages or derivations should be applied.

A final cautionary note about bipolar montages is that *they may not be reliable for assessing interhemispheric amplitude asymmetries unless the asymmetry is present in both the longitudinal and transverse bipolar montages.*

4.3 COMMON ELECTRODE REFERENCE MONTAGES

The common electrode reference montage consists of a series of derivations in which the same electrode is used in input 2 of each amplifier. Ideally, the input 2 reference electrode is at a distance from the source of the activity of interest, in a relatively 'quiet' location that is not *contaminated* by the activity at the input 1 electrode. Unlike the bipolar montage, the common electrode reference montage does not automatically filter out widespread potentials that have similar amplitudes and phases (i.e., coherent waveforms). It also produces a higher amplitude EEG recording because of longer interelectrode distances (there is less cancellation between the input 1 and 2 electrodes). Highly localized low to medium amplitude activity that would be easily seen in a bipolar montage may be obscured by the presence of intermixed, higher amplitude, widespread activity. There are two main categories of common electrode reference montages that are distinguished according to the placement of the reference electrodes on the body: *cephalic* and *non-cephalic*. Typical cephalic reference electrodes for the common reference electrode montage include A1 and A2

Fig. 4.2a shows a cephalic referential montage recording with the same potential as that recorded with a bipolar montage in Fig. 4.1a. Note that in the ideal common electrode referential montage, *the location of the maximal potential on the head is recognized by its amplitude, not by phase reversal.* That is, the channel which records the potential of highest amplitude is connected to the electrode nearest the cortical origin of the potential. If the output of two channels is of equal amplitude, the origin of the potential is usually located an equal distance from each of the two electrodes connected to input 1 of these channels (Fig. 4.2b). If several channels show a similar output, the potential affects input 1 of all these channels (Fig. 4.2c) to an equal degree. *If all channels show the same output then the activity is coming from the reference electrode itself until proven otherwise.*

Unlike the bipolar montage, the reference montage can give a better approximation of how the waveform shape might appear in a truly reference-free recording. However, it is sometimes difficult to find a cephalic reference electrode that is relatively inactive, or free of contamination from the cerebral potential in the input 1 electrodes. Moreover, potentials (cerebral or artifactual) at the reference electrode may sometimes

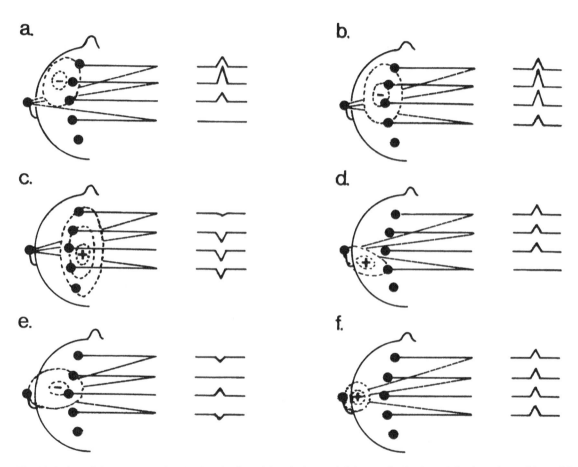

Fig. 4.2. Referential montages. a, b and c: localization of electrical potentials by amplitude of pen deflections; d, e and f: possible pitfalls of this method.

be large enough to overwhelm the recordings from all channels connected to that electrode. Difficulties in interpretation that may occur using common electrode cephalic reference montages are summarized as follows:

(1) A potential may affect only the reference electrode; for instance activity in the temporal lobe may appear as a transient positive potential at an ear electrode (A1 or A2) reference. This will produce a deflection in all channels connected through input 2 to this electrode (Fig. 4.2f) and may appear similar to a potential that does not involve the reference electrode (Fig. 4.2b).

(2) A potential located midway between the reference electrode and a scalp electrode may be cancelled in a channel connected to both these electrodes and appear in other channels that are connected to the reference electrode (Fig. 4.2d; this is similar to the appearance of Fig. 4.2a).

(3) A potential may be located between the reference electrode and some scalp electrodes so that, as in Fig. 4.2e, it appears as a contribution by input 1 in one channel, cancels between input 1 and 2 in another channel and appears with opposite polarity as a contribution by the reference electrode in the other channels.

The most widely used non-cephalic reference is the *neck–chest reference*. One electrode is placed at the sternal notch and a second electrode is placed at the base of the back of the neck. Both electrodes are joined together in input 2. Although this does minimize reference contamination by cerebral potentials, the ECG (which is a millivolt signal like EMG) may obscure the EEG signal (which is a microvolt signal) during the QRS complex. The point of placing one electrode on the neck and another on the chest is to try to cancel out the cardiac current vector of the R wave (the highest amplitude ECG scalp artifact) which normally is a positive wavefront moving from an anterior right to posterior left direction (6.1). The neck–chest reference is used routinely in some laboratories. With digital EEG it is more than reasonable to include it so that the reader always has the option of trying a non-cephalic reference during retrospective analysis.

Other approaches, including placing a ring of electrodes around the neck that cascade to a series of potentiometers, have been used to minimize ECG artifact. In the author's direct experience with several technical approaches there is no practical hardware solution to this problem. Using digital processing the ECG complex in a given channel can be extracted and then subtracted in subsequent portions of the recording. However, the amplitude of the ECG complex varies with the respiratory phase and blood pressure from moment to moment. Another approach to minimizing ECG in reference recording is to form a reference by adding two cephalic electrodes, each placed at the left and right earlobe, mastoid process, or angle of the mandible, respectively. This reduces ECG artifact by: (1) placing the reference electrodes closer to the scalp electrodes than the neck–chest reference so they 'see' the same ECG artifact and thereby cancel it, and (2) left–right reference cancellation of the cardiac vector (6.1). If other artifacts (e.g., muscle, movement, glossokinetic, etc.) can be minimized (usually in a cooperative patient), then only the problems of varying interelectrode distance and occasional reference contamination need to be dealt with.

4.4   AVERAGE REFERENCE MONTAGES

The average reference montage consists of a series of derivations in which all of the 10–20 electrodes are added together in input 2 of every amplifier to serve as a reference for each of the individual electrodes in input 1. If, for example, there are 19 scalp electrodes being recorded from, then all 19 would be combined together and placed in input 2 of every channel of recording. Each of the 19 electrodes would then contribute 1/19th of the total activity in input 2. Although the idea behind this reference is to minimize the contribution of any single electrode to the total reference output, a high (e.g., 150 μV) potential in one of the reference electrodes would still dominate the final value of the reference if the inputs from each of the other reference electrodes were relatively low (e.g., 5 μV each). Because the average reference usually contains all the scalp recording electrodes, the electrode in input 1 is compared against the other electrodes *and itself*. In the example of 19 recording electrodes, 1/19th of the activity in the input 1 electrode would be subtracted from the final output (the input 1 electrode cancels 1/19th of itself in the reference). In analog instruments the average reference electrodes are selectable and can be added or removed from the reference. This allows the technologist to increase the amplitude of activity of selected head regions (or reduce reference contamination from those same head regions) by removing the electrodes of those head regions from the reference. This is a feature which vendors of digital systems have been slow to implement. In general the average reference should contain at least 16 electrodes, but the intent of the montage is best served as the number of electrodes in the reference increases.

The average reference montage produces a spatial filtering effect that is intermediate between the common electrode reference montage and the bipolar montage; there is less attenuation of widespread potentials than in the bipolar montage but more than in the common electrode reference montage. This allows either localized or more diffusely distributed waveforms to be seen easily.

Some investigators have referred to the average reference montage as 'reference free.' This is true to the extent that the average reference montage does give an accurate reading of the relationship of voltage values between all the electrodes. Moreover, if the correct zero baseline potential at any given head region at any given moment could be known then an approximation of the true potential values at the different electrode sites could be calculated. This is, unfortunately, not the case in clinical applications. Because high amplitude potentials at even a few electrodes can contaminate the reference (assuming those electrodes are contained in the reference), the average reference montage should not be regarded by clinicians as reference free. For example, eye movement potentials that can be quite high in amplitude may appear prominently over the back of the head in the average reference montage because the electrodes that detect eye movements (Fp1, Fp2, F7, F8, F3, F4) 'contaminate' the reference. An eye blink potential will appear in the posterior electrode channels that is lower in amplitude and upside down compared to that seen in the anterior input 1 electrode channels. The upside down posterior activity does not arise in the occipital electrodes (as shown by non-cephalic reference recordings), instead it comes from the reference.

In the example shown in Fig. 4.3 an average reference recording of a vertex wave during stage I sleep shows the highest amplitude deflection in Cz. The Cz potential has a negative polarity (negativity in input 1 makes the pen deflect upward). There also appears to be a simultaneous waveform of opposite polarity arising from the temporal head region in electrodes Fp2, F8, T4. Thus, one interpretation of this is that vertex waves in sleep have a central negativity and temporal positivity (i.e., produce a true phase reversal or horizontal dipole over the scalp). The real explanation, however, is that the large negative potential over the central head regions 'contaminates' electrodes Fz, Cz, Pz, F3, F4, C3, C4, P3, and P4, all of which are in the average reference. Therefore, the waveform that appears in the temporal electrodes actually originates in the reference (AVG, input 2 of each amplifier). The proof of this conclusion is seen in the top channel, EKG1-AVG, in which the activity in the average reference is compared to an electrode on the chest. The negativity in the average reference is depicted between ECG complexes as a downward deflection (negativity in input 2 produces a downward deflection). The direct view of the distribution of the same vertex wave is shown in Fig. 4.4 in which all of the scalp electrodes are referred to a chest electrode. In this figure it can also be seen that the vertex wave does extend into the temporal head regions but it is negative (as at the vertex), not positive.

Although a high amplitude or widespread activity can contaminate the reference and produce a confusing picture, it is important to understand that in almost all cases, *the channel of the average reference that contains the highest amplitude waveform virtually always contains the input 1 electrode with the true maximal scalp potential.*

4.5 WEIGHTED AVERAGE MONTAGES

The weighted average reference montage is similar to the average reference montage except that the electrodes in input 2 do not contribute equally to the reference and the input 1 electrode is not included in the reference. The electrodes closer on the scalp to the input 1 electrode contribute more to the reference (have a greater 'weight') than the electrodes farther from the reference. Thus, the relative contributions of the reference electrodes vary from channel to channel, depending on which electrode is in input 1. In comparison to the average reference it reduces the possibility of a widespread activity contaminating the reference of

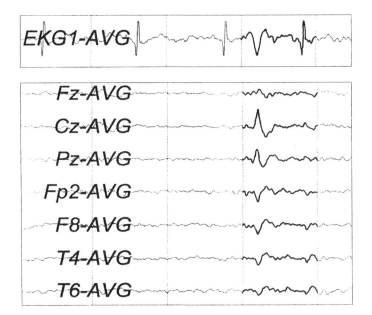

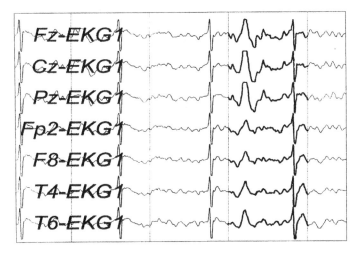

Fig. 4.3. Average reference recording of a vertex wave showing 'reference contamination' over the temporal head regions. The vertex potential in the temporal electrodes appears to be positive. In reality the vertex potential in the channels containing Fp2 and temporal electrodes is really arising from the average reference. The EKG1-AVG channel at the top of the figure demonstrates the negative potential arising from the AVG, average reference, by recording it with a non-cephalic chest reference (EKG1).

Fig. 4.4. Non-cephalic reference (EKG1) recording of the same vertex wave as in Fig. 4.3. The actual distribution of the vertex wave over the head is shown with negligible reference contamination. Notice that the negative vertex potential extends into the temporal electrodes.

all channels. The intention of the weighted average reference is to accurately demonstrate localized waveforms without creating reference contaminated waveforms. This is enhanced by using weighting factors based on actual scalp interelectrode distances. The weighting factors are usually calculated as inverse linear distances. The longer the distance from the input 1 electrode, the less the input 2 electrode will contribute to the reference. This creates a spatial filtering effect that is intermediate between the average reference and bipolar montages. The weighted average reference montage as originally described by Lemos and Fisch (1991) can be easily implemented on most commercial digital EEG systems using spreadsheet input described in their article.

4.6 LAPLACIAN MONTAGES

Laplacian montage design was first implemented by Hjorth (1975, 1980) who referred to it as *source derivation*. The Laplacian equation was originally applied to the study of thermal topography. Although it was originally derived to analyze a continuous process, it has been adapted to the analysis of the intermittent phenomenon such as spatial sampling of EEG. This is similar to analog to digital conversion but instead of creating sampling points of voltage over time each electrode site is a sample point for sampling voltage over space. In application the Laplacian montage design is similar in construction to the weighted average reference, but it is usually implemented using only the nearest neighboring electrodes surrounding the input 1 electrode. Ideally, the input 1 electrode is surrounded in a symmetric fashion by reference electrodes to create a local weighted average reference that approximates the mean potential gradient directed at the central (input 1) electrode. This is not possible for all input 1 electrodes of the 10–20 system because some are located at the edge of the scalp array and cannot be symmetrically surrounded by reference electrodes. Therefore, the Laplacian montage design cannot be uniform for all input 1 electrodes, it is always somewhat limited by so-called edge effects.

Like the weighted average reference, the contributions of the reference electrodes are linearly 'weighted' according to their distance from the input 1 electrode. This creates a more severe filtering of widespread waveforms. The Laplacian montage is therefore intermediate in filtering effects between the bipolar and weighted average reference montages. Most digital EEG instrument vendors now offer some version of the Laplacian montage. As with all other reference montages confusing pictures can still arise due to reference contamination. However, the Laplacian montage is extremely useful for filtering out widespread coherent waveforms and for emphasizing localized waveforms. It is frequently used in the evaluation of electrographic seizure topography.

4.7 SOURCE LOCALIZATION

Source localization refers to the process of calculating the precise anatomical location of a current source within the brain, using the distribution of potentials recorded from the scalp and other non-intracranial electrodes. This is referred to as solving the *inverse problem* or as simply *the inverse solution* (1.1). Although this is theoretically impossible, a number of approaches to the inverse problem have been proposed. Each applies certain reasonable assumptions about the anatomy of the volume conductor and the likely site of the generator(s). Although progress continues in this area of EEG research, the information provided by these methods is, at best, considered adjunctive and should never be used in isolation to make important clinical decisions (e.g., to identify the ictal onset zone of the brain for surgical removal). More progress towards the solution of the inverse problem has been made using an alternative technology, magnetoencephalography (MEG). MEG records intracellular neuronal magnetic currents (vs. extracellular electrical currents recorded by EEG) with reference-free recording (the reference is the magnetic field of the earth) and can more accurately localize detected sources within the brain. In contrast to electrical fields, the intervening tissues (CSF, skull, etc.) do not distort the magnetic fields between the generator and the detector. Currently, the widespread application of MEG is limited by its expense and its narrow clinical application to the presurgical evaluation of epilepsy.

4.8 MONTAGE DISPLAY AND DESIGN

The American Clinical Neurophysiology Society (see Guidelines in Appendix II) recommends that every EEG recording be performed using a minimum of 3 basic montages: *longitudinal bipolar (LB), transverse bipolar (TB),* and *reference (R).* In addition to the 3 basic montages recommended by the ACNS, there are special situations that require other montages. For example, neonatal recording routinely utilizes fewer scalp electrodes and includes the monitoring of respiration, submental EMG, and eye movements. Recording for electrocerebral inactivity requires the use of long interelectrode distances as well as movement and electrical interference monitoring.

Analog instrumentation requires that the technologist be able to change or customize montages as necessary during the actual recording. All technologists should be familiar with the modified 10–20 system of electrode placement for those situations in which additional electrode placement would help to better localize a particular activity. Those who use digital instruments have the advantage of being able to create a montage after the recording has been completed. Either a series of stored montage designs can be used to solve a particular localization or waveform identification problem, or the reader can design a better montage at the time of record review. Most digital instruments allow the user to rapidly change recording channel derivations using a mouse and drop down windows during review. For those with digital EEG this powerful advantage can be enhanced by the routine use of additional EEG electrodes (e.g., neck–chest reference) and physiological monitors (e.g., movement monitor).

Good montages fulfill a few simple requirements. As recommended by the ACNS for consistency between laboratories, montages should be displayed with left hemisphere electrode derivations placed above those on the right, and electrode derivations should be arranged in consecutive series running in either longitudinal anterior to posterior lines or transverse left to right lines. In addition, it is helpful to organize derivations in anatomical order as shown in Table 4.1, where the longitudinal bipolar montage is arranged so that as the reader scans the EEG from the top of the page to the bottom they see, in succession from top to bottom, the left temporal, left parasagittal, right parasagittal, and right temporal head regions. The transverse bipolar montage is also arranged anatomically in Table 4.1 so that the anterior head regions are at the top of the page and the posterior head regions are at the bottom. This topographic anatomical arrangement of derivations allows for quick orientation to the relative locations of the channels of recording on the scalp. The common electrode reference montage should maintain a long interelectrode distance between the reference electrode and all input 1 electrodes. Unlike the widely used ipsilateral ear reference montage in which all the electrodes are referred ipsilaterally to A1 or A2, a long interelectrode distance in every channel requires a combination of lateral and midline reference electrodes (as shown in the third montage from the left in Table 4.1). Otherwise, the montage will contain some channels in which the reference electrode forms bipolar derivations (e.g., T3-A1, or in the expanded 10–20 nomenclature, T7-A1).

4.9 ANALYSIS OF THE TOPOGRAPHY OF THE EEG VOLTAGE FIELD

Visualization of the topography of the EEG voltage field is a critical part of the mental process involved in routine EEG analysis and it is essential for accurate EEG interpretation. A mental image of the voltage topography of the EEG (i.e., the amplitude at any given point in time) is created by imagining the surface of the scalp as a spatial coordinate system in which the polarity and amplitude of the potentials at each electrode point in time are plotted as a 3-dimensional relief map. The illustrations in Fig. 4.5 show how the electrode chains laid along and across the head form a spatial coordinate system. The polarity and amplitude of the potentials at each point in the figure are depicted in the vertical direction. The output of all amplifiers at any instant can be used to plot an electrical field or voltage map in the form of a picture of mountains and valleys over different parts of the head. The examples in this chapter use only four channels to define the location of potentials in only one row in the antero-posterior direction. A more complete and accurate topographical picture would require additional electrodes, transverse electrode chains, and other referential montages. Fig. 4.5a shows an example of a negative potential plotted using a bipolar montage. The amplitude of each pen deflection is indicated by an arrow to the right of each recording and, because it represents the potential difference between adjacent electrodes, plotted halfway between the recording electrode locations. A line connecting the tips of the arrows outlines the contour of the electrical field in this dimension. Fig. 4.5b shows the same

TABLE 4.1

Channel	LB	TB	CER	Ave	WAR	LR
1	Fp1-F7	F7-Fp	F7-Cz	F7-Ave	F7-WAR	F7-LR
2	F7-T3	Fp1-Fp2	T3-Cz	T3-Ave	T3-WAR	T3-LR
3	T3-T5	Fp-F8	T5-Cz	T5-Ave	T5-WAR	T5-LR
4	T5-O1	F7-F3	Fp1-A1	Fp1-Ave	Fp1-WAR	Fp1-LR
5	Fp1-F3	F3-Fz	F3-A1	F3-Ave	F3-WAR	F3-LR
6	F3-C3	Fz-F4	C3-A1	C3-Ave	C3-WAR	C3-LR
7	C3-P3	F4-F8	P3-A1	P3-Ave	P3-WAR	P3-LR
8	P3-O1	A1-T3	O1-A1	O1-Ave	O1-WAR	O1-LR
9	Fz-Cz	T3-C3	Fz-A2	Fz-Ave	Fz-WAR	Fz-LR
10	Cz-Pz	C3-Cz	Cz-A2	Cz-Ave	Cz-WAR	Cz-LR
11	FP2-F4	Cz-C4	Pz-A2	Pz-Ave	Pz-WAR	Pz-LR
12	F4-C4	C4-T4	Fp2-A2	Fp2-Ave	Fp2-WAR	Fp2-LR
13	C4-P4	T4-A2	F4-A2	F4-Ave	F4-WAR	F4-LR
14	P4-O2	T5-P3	C4-A2	C4-Ave	C4-WAR	C4-LR
15	Fp2-F8	P3-Pz	P4-A2	P4-Ave	P4-WAR	P4-LR
16	F8-T4	Pz-P4	O2-A2	O2-Ave	O2-WAR	O2-LR
17	T4-T6	P4-T6	F8-A2	F8-Ave	F8-WAR	F8-LR
18	T6-O2	T5-O1	T4-A2	T4-Ave	T4-WAR	T4-LR
19		O1-O2	T6-A2	T6-Ave	T6-WAR	T6-LR
20		O2-T6				

The 4 montages shown above are (from left to right) longitudinal bipolar (LB.18), transverse bipolar (TB.20), common electrode reference (CER.19), average reference (Ave.19), weighted average reference (WAR.19), and Laplacian reference (LR.19). The montages are arranged in topographic anatomical order. The common reference montage in the third column maintains at least 2 interelectrode distances between the reference and input 1 electrodes by using auricular and midline reference electrodes. The selection of A2 instead of A1 as reference for the midline electrodes is because A1 usually contains more ECG artifact than in A2. For the same reason A2 is often selected instead of A1 in polysomnography.

potential in a referential recording. The amplitude of each waveform deflection, representing the potential difference between each scalp electrode and the reference electrode, is indicated by an arrow to the right of the recordings and plotted as an elevation above each electrode. The contour of the potential derived from the referential recording is practically identical to the contour ob-

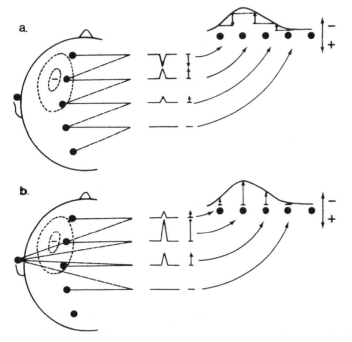

Fig. 4.5. Plotting the contour line of an electrical field along a chain of electrodes with bipolar (a) and referential (b) montages, both giving the same results. Arrows shown in the middle of the figure represent the pen deflections caused by the scalp potential; the arrows are used to plot the elevation of the potential above the horizontal electrode chain in the diagram on the right side of the figure. (a) In the bipolar montage, arrows in the diagram are drawn between scalp electrodes and with reference to adjacent arrows. (b) In the referential montage, arrows in the diagram are drawn above scalp electrode locations starting at a common baseline which represents the reference level.

tained from the bipolar recording. Points of equal potential levels may be connected with each other and these isopotential lines may be drawn either in a 3-dimensional view of peaks and valleys or in a 2-dimensional projection of isopotential lines on the surface of the head. Simple 2-dimensional views of isopotential lines can also be used to indicate the distribution of the electrical potentials (stippled lines in Figs. 4.1, 4.2 and 4.5).

A more complex situation arises when an EEG generator produces 2 opposite polarities over the scalp simultaneously. The term *dipole is* used to describe an electrical source (generator) that projects positive and negative electrical fields in opposite directions (one end, or pole, is negative and the opposite end is positive). All EEG potentials arise from the cortical dipole layer created by parallel neuronal columns. The cortical dipole layer has an orientation to the surface of the scalp that is vertical (radial), horizontal (tangential) or diagonal depending on where the columns lie along the gyri and sulci. The cortical dipole layer in the convexity of a gyrus or base of a sulcus points mainly in a radial direction towards the overlying scalp. In contrast, the cortical dipole layer in the wall of a sulcus points mainly in a tangential direction parallel to the surface of the overlying scalp. Other locations along the cortical surface produce diagonal dipoles of varying orientation. EEG potentials (positive or negative) are most likely to be detected by scalp electrodes if they have a radial orientation. Radial dipoles show only one polarity at the scalp surface because the opposite end of the dipole is directed 180° away from the overlying scalp surface towards the center of the brain. A common example of a radial dipole that almost always appears as a negative polarity waveform (negativity at the scalp surface) is the epileptiform spike or sharp wave, the positive end of the dipole points downward, away from the recording electrodes. If a dipole layer is located in the wall of a sulcus then it is oriented tangential (parallel) to the scalp surface. Depending on the area of cortex involved, the tangential dipole may either produce no detectable scalp potential or it may produce a *horizontal dipole* in which the opposite ends of the dipole appear simultaneously at 2 different scalp locations. This produces a *true phase reversal* (a double phase reversal in bipolar recordings and a single phase reversal in uncontaminated reference recordings; 4.2). Common examples of EEG activity that can be identified by their appearance as horizontal dipoles are small sharp spikes (SSS, also referred to as benign epileptiform transients of sleep, BETS; 19.4.4) and centromidtemporal epileptiform spikes of benign Rolandic epilepsy (benign epilepsy of childhood with centromidtemporal spikes, Chapter 17).

Small sharp spikes frequently occur with simultaneous opposite polarities located either over opposite hemispheres or in an antero-posterior direction within a single hemisphere. Epileptiform spikes that appear as horizontal dipoles in children and adolescents are almost pathognomonic for benign Rolandic epilepsy or the electrographic genetic trait of benign Rolandic epilepsy (Chapter 17). Rarely, horizontal dipole epileptiform spikes appear in association with structural abnormalities of cortical anatomy, for example in children with cerebral palsy. It is important to note, however, that the mere appearance of simultaneous and opposite polarity activity at different scalp locations does not necessarily mean that both potentials represent the opposite ends of the same dipole generator. Alternatively, it may mean that two or more generators that are anatomically distinct and opposite in polarity produce waveforms simultaneously by coincidence or because they are functionally linked.

An entire cortical dipole layer that generates a particular EEG activity rarely has a single direction of orientation to the scalp surface. Thus, any particular waveform of activity seen at the scalp surface is best viewed as an admixture of many cortical dipole columns with a variety of orientations to the scalp surface. Assuming that the cortical area of EEG generation is held constant, radially oriented dipoles have better representation at the scalp surface than dipoles with other orientations. However, the final waveform produced is almost always the result of summation and cancellation of dipoles that vary in their orientation to the overlying scalp.

4.10 SUMMARY

	Common reference	Average reference	Bipolar	Laplacian
Method	Voltage differences between each electrode in input 1 and an electrode in input 2 that is the same in all channels	Voltage difference between a single electrode in input 1 and and an average of all remaining 10–20 electrodes in input 2	Voltage differences between single, adjacent electrodes	Voltage differences between a single electrode and an average of all remaining electrodes weighted according to their distance from the electrode in input 1
Detection of localized neural current sources	Poor Acts as a spatial low pass filter to de-emphasize highly localized currents of low amplitude	Adequate High amplitude potentials (eye blinks, vertex waves) may contaminate the reference and appear falsely localized	Good Close electrode separation acts as a high pass spatial filter to emphasize localized currents	Excellent Acts as a spatial high pass filter to emphasize highly localized currents
Detection of widely distributed currents	Excellent Acts as a spatial low pass filter to emphasize widely distributed currents	Adequate Widely distributed currents are often detected but appear poorly localized due to reference contamination	Poor Close electrode separation acts as a high pass spatial filter and removes widely distributed currents	Poor Acts as a spatial high pass filter to remove widely distributed currents
Analysis of asymmetry	Good Reference electrode(s) must be symmetrically placed	Adequate Worsens as the asymmetry becomes widespread (due to reference contamination)	Adequate Reliable only if both transverse and longitudinal bipolar montages are used	Adequate to poor Worsens as the asymmetry becomes more widespread
Detection of electrode artifact	Excellent	Adequate High amplitude artifacts will contaminate the reference	Excellent Visual recognition facilitated by the appearance of phase reversals and the filtering of widespread waveforms	Adequate May involve channels containing adjacent electrodes

REFERENCES

American EEG Society (1994) Guidelines in EEG, 1–7,13 (Revised 1994). J. Clin. Neurophysiol. 11: 1–143 (see appendix in this volume).

Binnie, C.D. (1987) Recording techniques: montages, electrodes, amplifiers and filters. In: A.M. Halliday, S.R. Butler and R. Paul (Eds.), A Textbook of Clinical Neurophysiology. Wiley, New York, pp. 3–22.

Brazier, M.A.B. (1951) A study of the electrical fields at the surface of the head. Electroenceph. Clin. Neurophysiol. Suppl. 2: 38–52.

Burgess, R.C. (Ed.) (1991) Localization of neural generators. J. Clin. Neurophysiol. 8.

Burgess, R.C. and Collura, T.F. (1997) Polarity, localization, and field determination in electroencephalography. In: E. Wyllie (Ed.), The Treatment of Epilepsy: Principles and Practice, 2nd Edition. Williams and Wilkins, Baltimore, pp. 228–250.

Cooper, R., Osselton, J.W. and Shaw, J.C. (1981) EEG Technology, 3rd Edn. Butterworth, London.

Ebersole, J.S. (1994) Non-invasive localization of the epileptogenic focus by EEG dipole modeling. Acta Neurol. Scand. Suppl. 152: 20–28.

Gevins, A.S., Le, J., Martin, N.K. et al. (1994) High resolution EEG: 124-channel recording, spatial deblurring and MRI integration methods. Electroenceph. Clin. Neurophysiol. 90: 337–358.

Gloor, P. (1985) Neuronal generators and the problem of localization in electroencephalography: application of volume conductor theory to electroencephalography. J. Clin. Neurophysiol. 2: 327–354.

Goldman, D. (1950) The clinical use of the 'average' reference electrode in monopolar recording. Electroenceph. Clin. Neurophysiol. 2: 211–214.

Gregory, D.L. and Wong, P.K. (1984) Topographical analysis of the centrotemporal discharges in benign Rolandic epilepsy of childhood. Epilepsia 25: 705–711.

Hämäläinen, M., Hari, R., Ilmoniemi, R.J. et al. (1993) Magnetoencephalography: theory, instrumentation, and applications to noninvasive studies of the working human brain. Rev. Mod. Phys. 5: 413–496.

Henderson, C.J., Butler, S.R. and Glass, A. (1975) The localization of equivalent dipoles of EEG sources by the application of electrical field theory. Electroenceph. Clin. Neurophysiol. 39: 117–130.

Hjorth, B. (1975) An on-line transformation of EEG scalp potentials into orthogonal source derivations. Electroenceph. Clin. Neurophysiol. 39: 526–530.

Hjorth, B. (1980) Source derivation simplifies topographical EEG interpretation. Am. J. EEG Technol. 20: 121–132.

Hjorth, B. (1991) Principles for the transformation of scalp EEG from potential field into source distribution. J. Clin. Neurophysiol. 8: 391–396.

Hjorth, B. and Rodin, E. (1988) Extraction of 'deep' components from scalp EEG. Brain Topogr. 1: 65–69.

Homan, R.W., Herman, J. and Purdy, P. (1987) Cerebral location of international 10–20 system electrode placement. Electroenceph. Clin. Neurophysiol. 66: 376–382.

Jayakar, P., Duchowny, M., Resnick, T.J. and Alvarez, L.A. (1991) Localization of seizure foci: pitfalls and caveats. J. Clin. Neurophysiol. 8: 414–431.

Katznelson, R.D. (1981) EEG recording electrode placement and aspects of generator location. In: P.L. Nunez (Ed.), Electric Fields of the Brain. Oxford Univ. Press, London, pp. 176–213.

Klass, D.W. (1977) Symposium on EEG montages: Which, when, why and whither. Introduction. Am. J. EEG Technol. 17: 1–3.

Knott, J.R. (1985) Further thoughts on polarity, montages and localization. J. Clin. Neurophysiol. 2: 63–75.

Lagerlund, T.D. (1996a) Volume conduction. In: J. Daube (Ed.), Clinical Neurophysiology. F.A. Davis, Philadelphia, pp. 29–39.

Lagerlund, T.D. (1996b) Electrophysiologic generators in clinical neurophysiology. In: J. Daube (Ed.), Clinical Neurophysiology. F.A. Davis, Philadelphia, pp. 50–59.

Lemos, M.S. and Fisch, B.J. (1991) The weighted average montage. Electroenceph. Clin. Neurophysiol. 79: 361–370.

Lehmann, D. (1986) Spatial analysis of EEG and evoked potential data. In: F.

Duffey (Ed.), Topographic Mapping of Brain Electrical Activity. Butterworth, Boston, MA, pp. 29–62.

Lesser, R.P., Lüders, H., Dinner, D.S. et al. (1985) An introduction to the basic concepts of polarity and localization. J. Clin. Neurophysiol. 2: 46–61.

Lopes da Silva, F. and Van Rotterdam, A. (1993) Biophysical aspects of EEG and magnetoencephalogram generation. In: E. Niedermeyer and F. Lopes da Silva (Eds.), Electroencephalography: Basic Principles, Clinical Applications and Related Fields, Third Edition. Williams and Wilkins, Baltimore, pp. 78–91.

MacGillivray, B.B. (1974) Section 11. Derivations and montages. In: A. Rémond (Ed.), Handbook of Electroenceph. Clin. Neurophysiol., Vol. 3C. Elsevier, Amsterdam, pp. 22–57.

Magnus, O. (1961) On the technique of location by electroencephalography. Electroenceph. Clin. Neurophysiol. Suppl. 19: 1–35.

Morris, H.H., Lüders, H., Lesser, R.P., Dinner, D.S. and Klem, G.H. (1986) The value of closely spaced electrodes in the localization of epileptiform foci: a study of 26 patients with complex partial seizures. Electroenceph. Clin. Neurophysiol. 63: 107–111.

Nakasato, N., Levesque, M.F., Barth, D.S. et al. (1994) Comparisons of MEG, EEG, ECoG source localization in neocortical partial epilepsy in humans. Electroenceph. Clin. Neurophysiol. 91: 171–178.

Nunez, P.L. (1981) Electric Fields of the Brain. Oxford University Press, London, pp. 176–213.

Nunez, P.L. and Pilgreen, K.L. (1991) The spline-Laplacian in clinical neurophysiology: a method to improve EEG spatial resolution. J. Clin. Neurophysiol. 8: 397–413.

Offner, F.F. (1950) The EEG as potential mapping: the value of the average monopolar reference. Electroenceph. Clin. Neurophysiol. 2: 215–216.

Osselton, J.W. (1966) Bipolar, unipolar and average reference recording methods. I. Mainly theoretical considerations. Am. J. EEG Technol. 6: 129–141.

Osselton, J.W. (1969) Bipolar, unipolar and average reference recording methods. II. Mainly practical considerations. Am. J. EEG Technol. 9: 117–133.

Perrin, F., Pernier, J., Bertrand, O. et al. (1989) Spherical splines for scalp potential and current density mapping. Electroenceph. Clin. Neurophysiol. 72: 184–187.

Scherg, M. (1990) Fundamentals of dipole source potential analysis. In: F. Grandori, M. Hoke and G.L. Romani (Eds.), Auditory Evoked Magnetic Fields and Potentials. Advances in Audiology, Vol. 6. Karger, Basel, pp. 40–69.

Schneider, M. and Gérin, P. (1970) Une méthode de localisation des dipôles cérébraux. Electroenceph. Clin. Neurophysiol. 28: 69–78.

Sharbrough, F.W. (1977) The mathematical logic for the design of montages. Am. J. EEG Technol. 17: 73–83.

Tursky, B. (1974) Recording of human eye movements. In: R.F. Thompson and M.M. Patterson (Eds.), Bioelectric Recording Techniques, Vol. 1C. Academic Press, New York, pp. 99–135.

Van Oosterom, A. (1991) History and evolution of methods for solving the inverse problem. J. Clin. Neurophysiol. 8: 371–380.

Wong, P.K. (1991) Source modelling of the rolandic focus. Brain Topogr. 4: 105–112.

Yvert, B., Bertrand, O., Echallier, J.F. et al. (1996) Improved dipole localization using local mesh refinement of realistic head geometries: an EEG simulation study. Electroenceph. Clin. Neurophysiol. 99: 79–89.

5 The product of the recording: the clinical EEG record

SUMMARY

The clinical EEG record should contain a reasonable representation of the normal and abnormal patterns needed for clinical interpretation. To serve this purpose, the recording methods must meet certain general technical requirements. Special requirements apply in recordings from infants and small children, in all-night sleep recordings (polysomnography), in recordings evaluating suspected cerebral death, and in recordings transmitted by telephone. These requirements are described in 'Guidelines in EEG' issued by the American Clinical Neurophysiology Society.

(5.1) *General technical standards.* These standards apply, within certain technical limits, to both digital and analog EEG instruments. At least 21 recording electrodes should be placed according to the international 10–20 system, each with an electrical contact impedance of between 100 and 5000 Ω. The recording should have at least 8 channels and preferably more than 16. The sensitivity of the amplifiers should initially be set at 5–10 μV/mm and then adjusted as necessary. Filters should be set with the cutoff frequency (30% attenuation) of the low frequency filter at 1 Hz and the high frequency filter at 70 Hz. The record should be calibrated at the beginning and end by calibration pulses, an electrode test, and by a test recording using cerebral activity from the same electrode pair in all channels. Paper speed is routinely set at 3 cm/s. At least 20 min of artifact-free recording should be obtained during wakefulness. Wakefulness should *always* be clearly demonstrated by asking alerting questions (e.g., date, calculations) and recording the patient's responses on the record. In addition, recording during hyperventilation, photic stimulation and sleep should be performed when a seizure disorder is suspected.

The record should be labeled with the patient's name and age, date and time of the recording and other important information. During the recording, notations should be made to indicate the instrument settings, the patient's behavior and any event that could influence the recording or produce artifacts.

(5.2) *Standards for recordings from infants and small children* are the same as the general standards with a few exceptions. A smaller number of electrodes may be used in newborns. Eight-channel instruments are insufficient for newborns because recordings should include monitoring of eye movements, respiration, heart beat and muscle activity. Sensitivity and filter settings must be adjusted to display slower and larger potentials than are typical in adult recordings. Recordings in newborns usually require over 1 h to include a full cycle of quiet and active sleep. Labeling of the record must precisely reflect the patient's condition, position and all changes during the recording; the gestational and conceptional ages must be indicated for newborns.

(5.3) *Standards for recordings in cases of suspected cerebral death* are designed to produce a record that unequivocally answers the question whether or not any cortical activity is present. Electrocerebral inactivity (ECI), or electrocerebral silence, is defined as no EEG activity over 2 μV when recording from scalp electrode pairs 10 cm or more apart with interelectrode impedances under 10,000 Ω, but over 100 Ω. There are 10 minimum technical requirements for recording ECI (as described in Section 5.3). Recordings demonstrating the absence of electrocerebral activity should not be called 'flat', 'isoelectric' or 'linear' because, if done properly, they virtually always pick up activity from extracerebral sources. Telephone transmission should not be used for these recordings.

(5.4) *Standards for EEG transmission by telephone* require one fully trained technician and one fully equipped EEG instrument at both the transmitting and the receiving sites. The recordings at both sites should be identical and include all notes and comments made during the recording by the transmitting technician.

5.1 GENERAL TECHNICAL STANDARDS

Good clinical EEG recordings must satisfy many technical requirements. The American Clinical Neurophysiology Society has issued 'Guidelines in EEG and Evoked Potentials' (see reference at end of chapter) that contain minimum technical requirements for performing clinical electroencephalography. Eight of those guidelines apply specifically to EEG practice and have been reproduced in Appendix I. This chapter summarizes the 5 guidelines that discuss technical aspects of EEG and includes additional information that the author has found clinically useful.

5.1.1 *Electrode types.* Silver-silver chloride or gold electrodes are preferred, but adequate recordings can also be obtained with other electrode materials (e.g., tin). One should always, when possible, avoid mixing different kinds of electrodes in the same patient because of the likelihood of increasing electrical interference (due to impedance mismatches). In general, electrodes are best applied with collodion glue. The main advantages of collodion are that the electrodes remain firmly attached without changing position over time and are functional for long periods of time (hours). At the end of the recording electrodes are removed by dissolving the collodion glue with acetone. Because the fumes from acetone are potentially noxious, adequate ventilation is important and must always be kept in mind. For example, *if a young infant is in an isolette and cannot be at least partially removed from it and placed under warming lights then collodion and acetone should not be used.* In such circumstances electrode pastes should be substituted for collodion. Pastes are less desirable for routine use because they do not firmly anchor the electrodes to the head. In addition, paste is suboptimal for recordings lasting more than 30–60 min since drying of the paste will result in poor electrical contact.

5.1.2 *Electrode placements.* At least 21 recording electrodes should be used and placed according to the international 10–20 system. Additional electrodes may be placed between the standard electrodes to localize very circumscribed activity using the modified combinatorial 10–20 system nomenclature as proposed by the American Clinical Neurophysiology Society. A ground electrode should be added and connected to the ground input of the EEG instrument unless the patient is connected to ground through other electrical equipment and there is a potential for microshock hazard (3.12.1).

If electrode positions were not measured but only estimated, the terms '10–20 system' or 'modified 10–20 system' should not be used, but the term 'estimated 10–20 system' may be applied. Recordings that do not use the 10–20 system should define the relationship between the electrode placements used and those of the 10–20 system.

5.1.3 *Electrode impedance.* The impedance of disc electrodes should be checked routinely before every recording (2.2) and should not exceed 5000 Ω. Electrode impedances should not exceed 5000 Ω except in the case of needle electrodes where higher impedances cannot be avoided. Although the American Clinical Neurophysiology Society does not state a particular frequency of alternating current for impedance measurements, a frequency of about 10 Hz is most appropriate. Electrode impedance should also be checked when an unusual EEG pattern suggests the possibility of an artifact.

5.1.4 *Number of recording channels.* The EEG should be recorded on at least 8 channels at the same time. Sixteen or more channels are preferred because: (1) the likelihood of correctly localizing intermittent abnormalities increases with the number of recording channels; and (2) certain recordings (e.g., neonatal recordings) require additional channels for physiological monitoring.

5.1.5 *Montages.* Recordings should routinely include at least one longitudinal bipolar (LB), one transverse bipolar (TB), and one referential (R) montage as recommended by the American Clinical Neurophysiology Society (4.8). Additional montages should also be as simple as possible, easy to describe and easy to interpret. They should use electrodes along straight lines and with equal interelectrode distances. Activity from the front of the head should be displayed at the top of the record, activity from the back at the bottom. In addition, in North America left-sided leads should be placed

above right-sided leads for either alternating pairs of derivations or groupings of derivations.

5.1.6 *Sensitivity.* The sensitivity at the beginning of a routine recording should be set at 5–10 μV/mm for all channels. A commonly used sensitivity setting is 7 μV/mm which results in a pen deflection of about 7 mm for a calibration pulse of 50 μV/mm. The sensitivity of all channels should be adjusted during the recording so that the full range of the waveform (or pen deflection on analog instruments) is used to its best advantage: the EEG should be shown with good resolution and without blocking of waveforms on the computer monitor or on paper recordings.

5.1.7 *Filters.* During the recording, the low frequency filter should be routinely set at 1 Hz and the high frequency filter at 70 Hz. On most EEG instruments this corresponds to no more than a 30% (-3 dB) attenuation of activity at 1 Hz (i.e., a low frequency filter time constant setting of approximately 0.16 s) and 70 Hz. These settings therefore produce an increasing attenuation of activity below 1 Hz or above 70 Hz. They should be changed only to emphasize or clarify unusual EEG patterns. Changing filter settings should be a temporary maneuver, and the technician should write the new filter settings and the reason why they were changed on the record. It is important to be aware that changing filter settings may produce misleading results. For example, slow activity may be removed by setting the low frequency filter at a higher frequency. Setting the high frequency filter at a lower frequency than usual may give high frequency artifact (e.g., muscle artifact) the misleading appearance of cerebral potentials such as epileptiform spikes or fast background activity.

5.1.8 *Calibration.* Each record should be calibrated by applying known voltages to all channels at the beginning and the end of the recording. The calibration at the end should include calibration pulses recorded at each of the various combinations of sensitivity and filter settings used in the recording. The calibration pulses should have voltages strong enough to produce pen deflections of 7 mm or more, so that differences of 5% or more between channels can be detected; the pulses should not be so strong that they overdrive the pen deflection. Calibration pulses of different voltage need to be used for different sensitivity settings. If the amplitude, shape, horizontal and vertical alignment of the calibration pulses differ between channels, the cause for these differences must be determined and eliminated.

In addition to the square wave calibration, a biological calibration (also referred to as *biocalibration)* may be performed by recording the same electrode pair in every channel. For this purpose, a frontal and an occipital electrode provide a relatively high amplitude signal by virtue of the long interelectrode distance and will include a variety of frequencies (eye blinks, the alpha rhythm, etc.). Although this can be helpful for evaluating the pen, filter and amplifier functions, it should be recognized that a careful inspection of the square-wave ca-libration is actually a much more precise and measurable way of evaluating these components. Another useful procedure is the performance of an electrode test at the beginning and at the end of each recording. This may alert the technician to any abnormalities of electrode contact that have occurred since the time of application. It also informs the electroencephalographer whether or not the electrodes have been adequately applied and if good contact has been maintained throughout the recording.

5.1.9 *Paper speed.* A speed of 30 mm/s is recommended internationally and is used routinely in most laboratories. Slower speeds may also be used, for instance in neonatal recordings, or to emphasize slower waveforms. Faster speeds are helpful for evaluating fast events, such as time relationships between similar waves in different channels or 60 Hz artifact.

5.1.10 *Length of the recording.* Each montage should be recorded for at least 2 min. The waking record should contain at least 20 min of artifact-free recording at rest including brief periods when the eyes are open (11.1.6). This period does not include the time required for hyperventilation, photic stimulation and sleep recordings.

5.1.11 *Hyperventilation.* Overbreathing should be used routinely except when contraindicated by diseases of the heart and lungs, sickle cell disease (or trait), moyamoya disease, other cerebrovascular diseases associated with borderline cerebral blood perfusion, and acute cerebral disorders. The technician should explain and demonstrate hyperventilation, and note the quality of the patient's effort on the record. The EEG should be recorded during and for at least 1 min after hyperventilation or longer if hyperventilation induces abnormalities.

5.1.12 *Photic stimulation.* This activation procedure should be used whenever possible because it can induce diagnostically important abnormalities. It may, on rare occasions, induce seizures (which are almost always generalized); this may happen both in patients with a history of seizures and, extremely rarely, in patients without such a history. However, the development of seizures can usually be avoided if photic stimulation is stopped as soon as photoparoxysmal (epileptiform) activity appears.

Photic stimulation is performed with a stroboscopic lamp producing bright flashes of diffuse light. The lamp is placed approximately 30 cm from the patient's eyes. Flashes are given at varying rates typically including 1, 3, 5, 10, 13, 15, 17, 20 and 25 Hz in trains lasting about 10 s. Thorough testing includes periods when the eyes are closed, open, and while they are being opened and closed. The occurrence of each flash is monitored on a separate channel using a synchronizing pulse of the flash generator. The monitor pulse is displayed on a recording channel.

5.1.13 *Sleep.* A period of EEG recording during sleep should be obtained in addition to the 20 min waking baseline recording in patients with suspected or known convulsive disorders. To increase the chance of obtaining a sleep recording, many laboratories ask patients to avoid sleeping the night before the recording.

If sleep does not occur spontaneously, it may be induced with a sedative such as chloral hydrate. Chloral hydrate is preferred because, unlike benzodiazepines or barbiturates, minimum sedating doses usually do not induce excessive beta activity. Since patient sedation has obvious legal implications, patients should be accompanied by a responsible adult. After the test patients should also be instructed not to drive or to engage in other potentially dangerous activities.

5.1.14 *Special procedures* which are of risk to the patient should be carried out only for specific indications and then only in the presence of a qualified physician, in an environment with adequate resuscitation equipment, and with the informed consent of the patient, responsible relative or guardian.

5.1.15 *Labeling and editing of the record* is extremely important. Even a technically perfect EEG is useless without labeling and written comments by the technician. The technician must describe (a) the patient's medical characteristics, (b) the patient's behavior during the recording, (c) the montages, and (d) the instrument settings.

(a) *The description of the patient* should be written on the record and include at least the patient's name and age, the date and time of the recording, a list of all current medications, the time of the last meal, the name, amount and time of administration of any sedative taken during or shortly before the recording. Failure to document this information on the record can lead to serious medical and legal problems.

In addition to these minimum requirements, the technician should write down other important information. Cranial defects or abnormalities, scalp lacerations and contusions should be identified in a head diagram explaining the spatial relation between the abnormalities and the recording electrodes, especially where the abnormalities necessitated deviations from the electrode placements of the 10–20 system. The technician may obtain important information from the patient or the patient's chart and thus complement the information given by the referring physician. Items of special importance are a history and description of seizures, head injuries and significant diseases, the provisional diagnosis, reason for the EEG recording, abnormal laboratory test results, etc. Previous EEG recordings of the same patient should be available at the time of the interpretation.

(b) *The description of the patient during the recording.* The technician should indicate the patient's level of alertness, namely awake, drowsy, asleep or comatose, and any change of that level occurring during the recording. Unusual behavior such as restlessness, agitation, confusion, failure to cooperate, abnormal speech, hearing and vision should be noted.

The technician should try to recognize every movement of the patient, especially eye movements including eye blinks, eye opening and closing, movements of the face and head, swallowing, chewing, talking, coughing, sneezing, etc.; each movement should be indicated on the record at the time it occurs, especially if it causes an artifact in the recording. If there is any doubt whether an artifact is due to any such movement, the technician should ask the patient to repeat the movement and mark the request and the patient's response on the record. During the waking portion of the recording *the patient should always be asked alerting questions* such as the date and double digit calculations. This is necessary because mild normal background slowing due to drowsiness may occur even during commands to open and close the eyes or during hyperventilation. If the patient is unable to answer aforementioned questions correctly then simpler ones should be asked until a correct response is obtained. If seizure activity is suggested by a movement of the patient or by the appearance of epileptiform activity in the EEG, the technician should test the responsiveness of the patient by asking him how he feels and, if there is no answer, giving him a test word to remember. Later, when the patient is responsive, the technician should ask the patient if he or she remembers what was said. These questions and the answers should be written on the record. If epileptiform activity appears frequently or if it can be triggered by stimulation, the technician may ask the patient to count or to recite a nursery rhyme and note any interruptions by spontaneous or triggered epileptiform activity. A more precise measure of reactivity can be obtained by having the patient push a button in response to an auditory tone activated by the technician. Both the patient's and the technician's button presses are recorded on one of the EEG channels. In this way the technician can quickly test reactivity when unusual or epileptiform patterns occur. Most EEG equipment manufacturers offer auditory response testing devices as an option.

The technician should rate the patient's performance of hyperventilation as good, fair or poor. After hyperventilation, the patient should be asked how he felt during hyperventilation and, especially, whether hyperventilation reproduced or intensified any of his usual symptoms. The patient's response should be written on the chart.

In summary, the technician should continuously monitor the patient's behavior and document every movement and every word spoken during the recording. This is necessary because most artifacts can be positively identified only during the recording by correlating pen deflections with movements or other events. The technician is in the unique position of being able to make the diagnosis of a seizure by demonstrating a loss of responsiveness or documenting other, sometimes subtle, behavioral seizure manifestations during the occurrence of epileptiform activity in the EEG. The reader, if unaware of the patient's behavior, may be unable to identify many artifacts or to diagnose a seizure.

(c) *Description of montages.* The electrode combinations selected for each channel must be clearly indicated at the begin-

ning of each run. This may be done in one of several ways. (1) Abbreviations of the electrode placements used as input 1 and input 2 may be written for each channel as in Table 4.1. (2) Using a head diagram, the tracing of each channel may be connected to two electrode placements in the diagram; a solid line is commonly used to indicate the electrode connected to input 1, and a broken line is used to indicate the electrode connected to input 2; this method is used for many of the EEG illustrations in this text. (3) Electrode placements in the head diagram may be connected with arrows, each arrow being labeled with the number of the channel it represents and pointing from the electrode at input 1 to the electrode at input 2; this method is used in the illustration of montages in this text (Figs. 4.4 and 4.5). (4) Rubber stamps giving a list of the electrodes or a diagrammatic representation of a montage are used in some laboratories, but they can lead to errors more easily than other, less automatic methods. Montages should not be labeled with code names such as 'montage A' or 'run 1' because the meaning of the code may be unknown to the EEG reader.

(d) *Description of instrument settings.* The settings of master and individual channel switches controlling sensitivity and filters should be indicated at the beginning of each montage change and during calibration; the voltage of the calibration pulse must be identified. Every change of these settings and of chart speed must be indicated on the record when it is made and the affected channels must be clearly specified.

5.2 STANDARDS FOR PEDIATRIC RECORDINGS

Most of the general technical standards also apply to this age group. However, there are a few exceptions which are summarized in the guidelines of the American EEG Society on 'Minimum technical standards for pediatric electroencephalography' and are detailed below (see also 10.1).

5.2.1 *Electrode types.* Silver-silver chloride electrodes in the shape of a cup with a central hole for injection of conductive jelly (2.2.1) are best. Application with collodion is recommended because children are more likely than adults to move and produce artifacts. Collodion and acetone should *never* be used in isolettes and other areas with limited air circulation or explosion hazards; electrodes may be applied with electrode paste under these circumstances.

5.2.2 *Electrode placements.* Newborn infants, especially those with small heads, do not need the full number of electrodes prescribed by the 10–20 system. A minimum reduced array includes the following electrodes: Fp1, Fp2, C3, Cz, C4, T3, T4, O1, O2, A1 and A2. If the baby's earlobes are too small, mastoid electrodes M1 and M2 may be substituted for A1 and A2. Fp3 and Fp4 have been suggested as alternative placements to Fp1 and Fp2 because they are more anatomically correct; the frontal lobes of neonates and young infants occupy a relatively more posterior position in relation to Fp1 and Fp2 than in adults. Fp3 and Fp4 are placed midway between the Fp1 and F3 and Fp2 and F4 positions.

5.2.3 *Number of recording channels.* Instruments with only 8 channels are undesirable for recording neonates and young infants (i.e., patients less than 48 weeks conceptual age). Sixteen or more channels are preferred since 4 or more will be occupied by physiological monitors. Examples of montages are listed in Chapter 4 (Table 4.4).

5.2.4 *Montages.* Recordings from newborns need continuous monitoring of extracerebral electrical activity to identify alertness and sleep states and to recognize artifacts and abnormalities of breathing and heart rate. Most important is monitoring of respiration, eye movement, muscle tone (submental EMG monitor), and ECG (see also 10.1).

5.2.5 *Sensitivity.* The sensitivity needs to be adjusted more often in infants and young children; their EEG may have fairly high amplitude so that sensitivity needs to be reduced to 10 or 15 μV/mm. The sensitivity of channels monitoring extracerebral activity of newborns must be adjusted according to the output; eye movements and submental EMG should be recorded at 7 and 3 μV/mm respectively. For the respirogram, the sensitivity should be adjusted as necessary to yield a clear deflection with each respiration.

5.2.6 *Filters.* EEG recordings from infants should use time constants between 0.27 and 0.53 s, i.e. low filter frequency settings which reduce the amplitude of sine waves of 0.3–0.6 Hz by 30% (−3 dB). Eye movements should be monitored with the same filter settings. EMG (submental) recordings should be made with higher settings of the low frequency filter (about 5 Hz; time constant 0.03 s) and with the highest setting of the high frequency filter. Respiration should be monitored with very low settings of the low frequency filter.

5.2.7 *Length of the recording.* Newborns require usually over 1 h of recording to show a full cycle of both active sleep and quiet sleep. The chances of obtaining such a recording are best when the EEG is scheduled at feeding time and the baby is fed after application of the electrodes. Sedation should not be used to obtain a sleep record in newborns. Shorter recording periods than 1 h are acceptable only when the EEG is grossly abnormal; even then, a period of 1 h may be required to demonstrate the absence of variability.

Children may produce so many artifacts by moving and other mechanisms that satisfactory waking records of the length recommended for adults cannot be obtained; recordings during sleep may then provide the only useful information. In patients over 3 months of age, the technician should attempt to obtain recordings during wakefulness when the patient's eyes are open and when they are closed; passive eye closure, accomplished by placing the technician's hand over the patient's eyes, may be used to demonstrate the reactivity of EEG rhythms (11.1.6).

5.2.8 *Photic stimulation.* Flashes of 1–30 Hz should be used during wakefulness if indicated for activation in children. Repetitive photic stimulation is not useful for newborns.

5.2.9 *Labeling and editing the record.* In addition to the requirements described for EEG recordings in general, recordings from infants must state the baby's gestational age at birth and conceptional age, i.e., gestational age plus time since birth, in weeks, together with the chronological age since birth. Other relevant information, such as levels of blood gases and serum electrolytes, should be noted for the use of the electroencephalographer. Before recording EEGs of infants and young hospital patients, especially those requiring bedside recording, the technician should consult with the nursing staff concerning the patient's condition and any limitations on recording procedures. The patient's condition should be clearly indicated at the beginning of every montage and the position of head and eyelids of infants should be noted. Changes of position and other movements must be monitored as carefully as in adults. Stuporous or comatose patients and patients showing an invariant EEG pattern should be given vigorous visual, auditory and somatosensory stimulation. The stimuli and the patient's responses should be indicated on the recording paper at the time of their occurrence; absence of responses must also be noted. Infants should be stimulated only at the end of the recording period to avoid interruption of sleep cycles.

5.3 STANDARDS FOR RECORDINGS IN CASES OF SUSPECTED CEREBRAL DEATH

The EEG is an important tool for the evaluation of cerebral death, a diagnosis considered in victims of severe irreversible cerebral damage characterized by coma, absent or insufficient spontaneous respiration and absent brain stem reflexes. This diagnosis requires, amongst other criteria, repeated demonstrations of the absence of electrocerebral activity of over 2 μV/mm in amplitude. For adults and older children, electrocerebral inactivity (ECI) found in one recording is considered highly reliable for the determination of cortical death, unless the recording was made in the presence of either: (1) drugs depressing the central nervous system, (2) significant hypothermia, or (3) circulatory shock. However, younger children, especially those under 1 year of age, can survive longer periods of ECI without cerebral death. In such cases two recordings separated by a 24 h interval should be performed. ECI is defined by the American Clinical Neurophysiology Society as no EEG activity over 2 μV when recording from scalp electrode pairs 10 cm or more apart with interelectrode impedances under 10,000 Ω, but over 100 Ω.

Recording techniques in cases of suspected cerebral death must be designed to search for any trace of cerebral activity and take special precautions to avoid technical difficulties that could lead to the mistaken impression of absent cerebral activity. The American Clinical Neurophysiology Society has issued guidelines of 'Minimum technical standards for EEG recording in suspected cerebral death'; the guidelines are summarized and discussed here.

5.3.1 *Electrode placements. At least 8 scalp electrodes should be used* and placed in the frontopolar (Fp1, Fp2), central (C3, C4), temporal (T3, T4) and occipital (O1, O2) positions on both sides. Additional electrodes may be placed in the frontal (F3, F4) and parietal (P3, P4) areas, at the vertex (Cz) and on the earlobes (A1, A2), mastoids, mandibular angles or noncephalic reference points. A ground electrode should be added but not connected if other electrical equipment is attached to the patient (3.12). It is preferable whenever possible to employ a full set of recording electrodes (i.e., all 21 electrodes of the routine 10–20 system). Thus, the full set of recording electrodes should be applied at the start of the recording and an initial recording employing all of them is recommended.

5.3.2 *Electrode impedance. Interelectrode impedances should be under 5000 Ω and over 100 Ω.* The impedance of all electrodes should be similar to reduce the chance of artifacts caused by an imbalance of noise between input 1 and 2 of any amplifier.

5.3.3 *Testing the integrity of the recording system.* If a recording at low sensitivity settings and long interelectrode distances shows no electrocerebral activity, it is necessary to demonstrate that this is not due to a fault of the recording system. The recording of calibration pulses does not entirely exclude this possibility because it tests the recording system only between the inputs of the amplifiers and the monitor or penwriters whereas the fault may lie between the electrodes and the amplifier input. To test this part of the recording system, each electrode should be touched gently with a pencil or cotton swab during the recording; the electrode touched and the moment of touching should be indicated on the chart. Touching an electrode should create an artifact in the recording channels connected to that electrode. This artifact verifies that (a) the electrode is capable of recording, and (b) the correct electrode is selected for that channel.

5.3.4 *Interelectrode distances. Interelectrode distances of at least 10 cm should be used* because recording with shorter distances may attenuate amplitude. Referential montages may use the Cz electrode as the reference for long interelectrode distances. Ear reference recording nearly always contains too much ECG artifact to be useful. More than one montage should be used depending on how many recording channels are available. If occipital leads are difficult to attach or pick up movement artifact induced by artificial respiration, the combinations F7-T5, F3-P3, Fz-Pz, F4-P4 and F8-T6 may give better results.

5.3.5 *Sensitivity.* A sensitivity of at least *2 μV/mm*, or a lower sensitivity such as 1 μV/mm, should be used *for at least 30 min* (see below). This is very important because activity of 2 μV, i.e., the critical amplitude for electrocerebral silence, cannot be clearly distinguished at higher sensitivities. If possible a sensitivity setting of 1.5 or 1 μV/mm will allow the electroencephalographer to make a more confident assessment of low amplitude, and particularly slow frequency activity.

5.3.6 *Filters.* Filter settings should not attenuate any electrocerebral activity, especially very slow waves that are likely to occur in deep coma. Attempts should be made to record with low frequency filters set no higher than 1 Hz and with high frequency filters set no lower than 30 Hz. The 60 Hz filter should be used as needed.

5.3.7 *Additional monitoring techniques should be employed when necessary.* Because of the high sensitivity and wide interelectrode distances, recordings in suspected cerebral death are very likely to pick up artifacts. Possible sources of artifacts should be monitored. As a minimum, heart beat and movement should be included in the recordings.

5.3.8 *Stimulation of the patient.* The reactivity of the EEG of comatose patients should be tested by stimulation with sudden loud sounds and by stimuli that can produce pain in wakeful persons, for instance pressure on the nailbeds of the fingers or vigorous rubbing of the sternum. Flashes of bright light may also be used. The type and the moment of stimulation and the behavioral reaction of the patient, including the absence of a reaction, should be noted on the chart. The tracing may show different types of reactions: transient EEG activity may be induced in some patients who have no spontaneous EEG activity or extracerebral responses may be elicited (e.g., frontal potentials representing the retinal response to light flashes).

(a) *Artifacts arising from heartbeat* are very common and consist of ECG components, pulse waves and ballistic movements transmitted to the head and electrode wires.

(b) *Movement* of the patient may cause artifact that can be monitored with two electrodes on the back of the right hand, separated by 6–7 cm.

(c) *Respiratory artifact* should be monitored during at least part of the recording. Stopping the respirator momentarily may help to identify various kinds of respiratory artifact that cannot be eliminated.

(d) Electrical interference may be evaluated by connecting a resistor of 10,000 Ω between the inputs of one amplifier and placing it near the patient. This 'dummy patient' is representative of the electrical impedances of the EEG electrodes on the patient and can indicate the amount and type of interference from sources other than the patient.

(e) *Muscle artifact* may obscure the tracing. If it cannot be eliminated by repositioning of the patient or massaging the muscles near the contaminated recording electrode, a neuromuscular blocking agent such as pancuronium bromide (Pavulon) or succinylcholine (Anectine) may be used under the supervision of a physician.

(f) *Determining the presence of low amplitude rhythmical artifact* (e.g. ECG or pulse) can sometimes be made easier by overlaying two pages of the EEG and aligning identical channels in front of a bright light such as an X-ray viewing box. One page of EEG can then be moved relative to the other to inspect for the presence of superimposable repetitive waveforms.

5.3.9 *Recordings should be made only by a qualified technologist.* Recordings in cases of possible cerebral death should be made only by technicians who have had supervised instruction and recording experience in intensive care units and who work under the direct supervision of a qualified electroencephalographer.

5.3.10 *Repeat recordings.* If technical or other problems leave any uncertainty about the diagnosis of electrocerebral silence, the entire recording should be repeated after a few hours.

5.4 TELEPHONE TRANSMISSION

Recommendations for telephone transmission of EEGs have been included in the guidelines of the American EEG Society and in the report of the Committee on EEG Instrumentation Standards of the International Federation of Societies for EEG and Clinical Neurophysiology. The recommendations generally stipulate that technical standards of EEG recording should not be lowered by telephone transmission. This requires two fully trained technicians and two complete EEG recording instruments. The instruments should be connected so that the EEG at the transmitting site is completely and faithfully duplicated at the receiving site; at present, this requirement cannot be entirely fulfilled because currently used conventional telephone systems limit transmission of high frequencies for an 8-channel EEG to about 50 Hz and may introduce artifacts into recordings of low amplitude. However, these limitations may be acceptable in most cases. Specific recommendations for telephone transmission are listed below.

5.4.1 *Technicians* at both the transmitting and receiving laboratories should be fully trained and qualified EEG technicians. In addition, they should be familiar with telephone transmission techniques and, if possible, with each other's laboratories.

5.4.2 *Duplicate EEG records* should be produced. Recording a copy at the transmitting site is required so that the transmitting technician can correlate ongoing EEG activity with the patient's behavior and identify and eliminate artifacts. The requirement for a copy at the transmitting site may be eliminated in the future if acceptable alternative methods of monitoring the EEG at the transmitting site become available.

The comments of the transmitting technician, especially those that are vital for the identification of artifacts, should be transmitted simultaneously with the EEG to the receiving site. This can be done by signals in a standard code which temporarily replace the EEG recorded in one channel. Such a signaling system may be supplemented by intermittent voice communications between transmitting and receiving sites. A fail-safe code should be included to indicate technical problems, especially the loss of signal at the receiving site during transmission.

5.4.3 *Fidelity of the recording.* The tracing at the transmitting and receiving sites should be identical. As mentioned above, this is currently possible for recordings not including frequencies over 50 Hz and not consisting of very low amplitude activity.

5.4.4 *Cerebral death* cannot be evaluated appropriately by recordings transmitted over the telephone because artifacts from telephone networks may appear and obscure or mimic electrocerebral activity of low amplitude.

REFERENCES

American Clinical Neurophysiology Society (1994) Guidelines in EEG and Evoked Potentials, 1–7,13 (Revised 1994). J. Clin. Neurophysiol. 11: 1–143 (see appendix in this volume).

Alvarez, L.A., Moshe, S.L., Belman, A.L., Maytal, J., Resnick, T.J. and Keilson, M. (1988) EEG and brain death determination in children. Neurology 38: 227–230.

Ashwal, S. and Schneider, S. (1979) Failure of electroencephalography to diagnose brain death in comatose children. Ann. Neurol. 6: 512–517.

Bennett, D.R., Hughes, J.R., Korein, J., Merlis, J.K. and Suter, C. (1976) An Atlas of Electroencephalography in Coma and Cerebral Death. Raven Press, New York.

Chatrian, G.E. (1986) Electrophysiologic evaluation of brain death: a critical appraisal. In: M.J. Aminoff (Ed.), Electrodiagnosis in Clinical Neurology. Churchill-Livingstone, New York, pp. 669–736.

Green, J B. and Lauber, A. (1972) Return of EEG activity after electrocerebral silence: Two case reports. J. Neurol. Neurosurg. Psychiat. 35: 103–107.

Hanley, J.W. (1981) A step-by-step approach to neonatal EEG. Am. J. EEG Technol. 21: 1–13.

International Federation of Societies for Electroencephalography and Clinical Neurophysiology (1983) Recommendations for the Practice of Clinical Neurophysiology. Elsevier, Amsterdam.

Klem, G.H. (1979) Some problems of bedside EEG recording. Am. J. EEG Technol. 19: 19–29.

Lombroso, C.T. (1993) Neonatal EEG polygraphy in normal and abnormal newborns. In: E. Niedermeyer and F. Lopes da Silva (Eds.), Electroencephalography: Basic Principles, Clinical Applications and Related Fields, Third Edition. Williams and Wilkins, Baltimore, pp. 803–876.

Mizrahi, E.M. (1986) Neonatal electroencephalography: clinical features of the newborn, techniques of recording, and characteristics of the normal EEG. Am. J. EEG Technol. 26: 81–103.

Rechtschaffen, A. and Kales, A. (1968) A Manual of Standardized Terminology, Techniques and Scoring System for Sleep Stages of Human Subjects. U.S. Government Printing Office, Washington.

Report of the Task Force (1987) Guidelines for the determination of brain death in children. Neurology 37: 1077–1078.

Saunders, M.G. (1979) Minimum technical requirements for performing clinical electroencephalography: illustrative examples of principles on which some of the technical guidelines of the American EEG Society are based. In: D.W. Klass and D.D. Daly (Eds.), Current Practice of Clinical Electroencephalography. Raven Press, New York, pp. 7–26.

Stockard-Pope, J.E., Werner, S.S. and Bickford, R.G. (1992) Atlas of Neonatal Electroencephalography, 2nd Edn. Raven Press, New York.

6 Artifacts

SUMMARY

EEG artifacts are recorded signals that are non-cerebral in origin. They may be divided into one of two categories depending on their origin: *physiological artifacts* or *non-physiological artifacts.*

(6.1) *Physiological artifacts* arise from a variety of body activities that are either due to (1) *movements:* movements of the head, body, or scalp (e.g., pulsations of the scalp arteries, scalp muscle movement), (2) *bioelectrical potentials:* from moving electrical potentials within the body (such as those produced by eye, tongue and pharyngeal muscle movement), or elec-

trical potentials generated by the scalp muscles, heart or sweat glands, or (3) *skin resistance changes:* due to sweat gland activity, perspiration and vasomotor activity.

(6.2) and (6.3) *Non-physiological artifacts* arise from two main sources: (1) *external electrical interference* from other power sources such as power lines or electrical equipment, and (2) *internal electrical malfunctioning of the recording system,* arising from recording electrodes, electrode positioning, cables, amplifiers, pen motors or the paper drive.

6.1 ARTIFACTS FROM THE PATIENT

One of the most common pitfalls of EEG interpretation is to mistakenly identify non-cerebral potentials as originating from the brain. Although artifacts can often be recognized by their characteristic shape and distribution, in many cases artifacts can only be identified by the technologist during the recording. It is therefore essential that the technologist be skilled in the identification and elimination of artifacts. The patient and record must be closely observed throughout the recording and notations made whenever artifacts occur.

In many instances, artifacts can be immediately recognized by applying the following two rules of spatial analysis:

(1) Medium to high amplitude potentials that occur at only one electrode usually do not arise from the brain. Cortically generated potentials exhibit a physiological distribution over the scalp characterized by a potential maximum that gradually drops off in voltage with increasing distance across the scalp. Therefore, a prominent waveform that can only be recorded from one electrode is artifact until proven otherwise.

(2) Repetitive, irregular or rhythmical waveforms that appear simultaneously in unrelated head regions are usually not cerebral in origin. Evolving electrographic seizures or abrupt background abnormalities typically spread to involve adjacent electrodes. They do not jump to opposite ends of the head or to non-homologous (non-mirror image) areas of the opposite hemisphere.

6.1.1 *Blinking and other eye movements.* These movements cause potential changes that are picked up mainly by frontal electrodes, although they may extend into central and temporal electrodes. A simple but useful way of understanding eye movement artifact is to picture the front of the eye as a positive charge that either moves towards or away from the recording electrodes. The electrodes that record the largest potential change with vertical eye movements are Fp1 and Fp2 because they are placed directly above the eye. The electrodes that record the largest potential change with horizontal (lateral) eye movements are F7 and F8 because they are approximately lateral to the eyes. In a typical longitudinal bipolar montage an upward vertical eye movement (e.g., eye closure, eye blink) will produce a downward deflection in Fp1-F3 or Fp1-F7 because the positively charged cornea is moving towards Fp1 making it increasingly more positive (Figs. 6.1 and 6.3). If the eyes move to the left, in a lateral direction, then F7 will record the greatest increase in positivity and F8 will record the greatest negativity (in this case the negativity recorded by F8 is caused by a loss of positivity as the cornea moves away from it). Therefore the pen will deflect up in Fp1-F7 and down in F7-T3. The opposite will occur in Fp2-F8 and F8-T4. Notice that lateral eye movements make the aforementioned pairs of channels point in opposite directions (Fig. 6.1, example 5).

Rapid eye movements may cause jagged artifacts (Fig. 12.2). Muscle artifact may appear along with eye movements. Lateral eye movements may be preceded by a single sharp muscle potential sometimes referred to as a *lateral rectus spike*. Rarely, a lateral rectus spike in combination with the eye movement artifact may mimic abnormal epileptiform spike and wave activity.

Eye movement artifacts have long been believed to be due to movement of the eyeball which carries a steady electrical charge, the cornea being about 100 mV positive with respect to the retina. However, it seems that movement of this corneoretinal dipole is not necessary to produce blink artifacts: movements of the lids across the eyeball can produce a similar artifact. Moreover, some low amplitude eye movement artifacts can be recorded even after removal of the eye including cornea and retina, suggesting that movement of residual membranes deep in the orbit can cause artifacts.

Eye movement artifacts in the EEG can usually be identified by their frontal distribution, their symmetry and their characteristic shape. *The amplitude of vertical eye movements in longitudinal bipolar montages either remains the same or (more often) decreases in successive channels moving from anterior to posterior; the amplitude of vertical eye movements never increases in a more posteriorly located channel.* The frontal origin of eye movement artifacts may remain unclear in referential montages, particularly those using ear electrodes that may be contaminated by eye movements. Repetitive eye movements may mimic cerebral rhythms; slowly repetitive eye movements may closely resemble bilaterally synchronous frontal slow waves, and repetitive eye movements associated with lid flutter during eye closure may cause frontal rhythms of about 10 Hz. As a general rule, however, it is best to assume that *activity in the alpha frequency range localized to the frontopolar head regions is eye movement artifact until proven otherwise.*

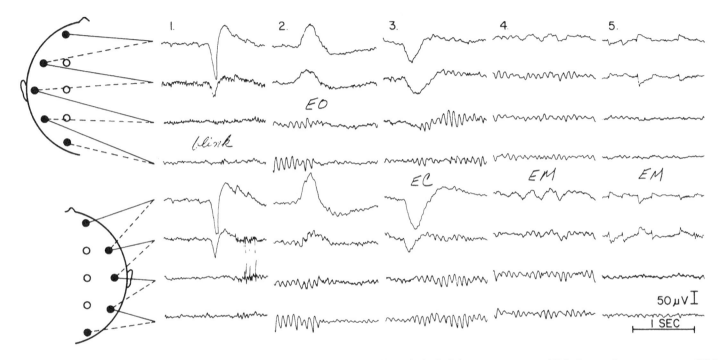

Fig. 6.1.   Eye movement artifacts. 1, blink, 2, eye opening (EO), 3, eye closing (EC), 4, rhythmical slow eye movements (EM), 5, saccadic eye movements (EM) preceded by spicules due to contraction of lateral eye muscles. Tracings show the technician's notations made during the recording to identify the cause of the artifacts.

Asymmetric eye movements usually occur under one of the following circumstances: (1) decreased movement of the eye or eyelid of one eye, (2) absence of an eye or destruction of the retina of one eye, (3) asymmetric electrode placement, or (4) a frontal skull defect. In the case of a missing part or breach of the frontal bone, the *eye movement artifact is lower in amplitude ipsilateral to the skull defect.* This is thought to occur by virtue of a shunting of the eye potential through the skull.

Eye movement artifacts can be identified during the recording by observing the patient and correlating eye blinks and movements with pen deflections. Even eye movements during eye closure can usually be seen through the eyelids. These movements can be further identified by their disappearance when the patient complies with the instruction to keep his eyes closed and still. If unable to do this, the patient may be told to place his fingertips on his eyes, or the technician may hold the eyelids and at the same time monitor eye movements felt through the eyelids. Taping cotton balls over the eyes may stop some eye movements but obscures observation of eye movements and interferes with recording the effect of other eye opening and closing on the EEG. If eye movements cannot be stopped and cannot be distinguished from frontal slow waves in the EEG, they may be monitored by electrodes placed near the eyes and linked so that eye movements can be distinguished from cerebral activity. Recordings from these linkages should be displayed simultaneously with, and next to, the recordings of frontal slow waves. Comparison of these recordings usually allows clear distinction between eye movement artifact and cerebral slow waves.

6.1.2 *Muscle artifact.* Muscle activity causes very short duration potentials that usually occur in clusters or periodic runs. If they recur as discrete potentials with the same shape and in the same distribution (Fig. 6.2), they may resemble cerebral

spike discharges except that most cerebral spikes are of much longer duration than muscle action potentials. If they recur in rapid bursts of discharges (Fig. 6.2), they can produce several different types of potentials that can merge and obscure the recording of cerebral activity. Muscle artifacts from scalp and face muscles occur mainly in the frontal and temporal regions but may be recorded by electrodes nearly anywhere on the head. Reducing the settings of the high frequency filter will reduce the amplitude of these fast potentials, but will also change their form (3.5.2) so that single muscle potentials may look more like spikes, and repetitive potentials may look like cerebral fast waves (Fig. 6.2).

Muscle artifact, even if not related to recognizable movement by the patient, is usually easily identified by its shape and repetition. It can be reduced and often eliminated by asking the patient to relax, drop the jaw or open the mouth slightly, or change position. Artifact from a single electrode can sometimes be stopped by gently pushing on that electrode, by stroking or massaging the skin near the electrode, or by reapplying the electrode. Reducing high frequency filter settings is only of limited value because of the aforementioned distortion.

A few specific conditions cause special electrographic patterns. Repetitive movements such as chewing, blinking or tremor may give rise to a combination of fast muscle and slow movement artifacts which may resemble cerebral discharges, especially if the combinations repeat with similar shape. Such rhythmical combinations may occur in *tremor of Parkinson's*

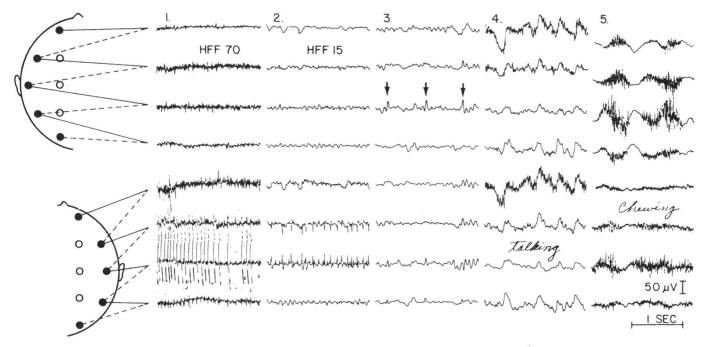

Fig. 6.2. Common artifacts generated by extracerebral physiological activity. 1: Continuous muscle artifact in all channels with superimposed intermittent muscle artifact of high amplitude in channels 6 and 7; the recording is made with a high frequency filter setting of 70 Hz. 2: Continuation of the recording shown in part 1, but with a high frequency filter setting of 15 Hz. 3: Heart beat artifacts (arrows). 4: Artifacts due to talking and frontal muscle contraction. 5: Compound artifact caused by chewing movements and associated muscle artifact.

disease, which is characterized by rhythmic 4–6 Hz waveforms that may appear in isolated electrodes or seem to have a phys-

iological distribution consistent with cerebral activity. Indeed, any monorhythmic theta pattern that occurs abruptly and

111

seems isolated from the rest of the ongoing background activity should raise the question of tremor artifact. On the other hand, seizures may lead to muscle activity so that a recording electrode picks up mixtures of cerebral seizure activity and muscle activity caused by the seizure.

Facial myokymia appears as a pseudoperiodic unilateral pattern of short bursts of 30–70 Hz muscle potentials (usually lasting less than 1 s) separated by 1–5 s intervals. Visible facial myokymia is usually recorded in Fp1 or Fp2. It may only be detected in temporal electrodes without visible signs in those cases in which only the vestigial auricular muscles innervated by the facial nerve are involved. Facial myokymia is often associated with brain stem lesions causing no other EEG signs

6.1.3 *Movement artifact.* Movements of the head and body or of the electrode wires can cause artifacts even if all electrodes make good mechanical and electrical contact. Movement artifacts are rhythmical in tremor, chewing and sucking (Fig. 6.2), breathing, or repetitive head movements, caused by the force of the blood rushing into the head (also referred to as cardioballistographic artifact).

Movement artifacts are usually easily recognized during the recording by their association with visible movements and should be identified by indicating the moment and kind of movement on the chart. Many movement artifacts can be abolished by asking the subject to stop moving. In persons who do not comply, for instance in restless or confused patients, infants and children, patients having seizures, tremors

or other movement disorders, the movements must be reduced as far as possible.

The main difficulty for the electroencephalographer occurs when the technologist has failed to document in writing on the record the occurrence of movements producing artifacts. Unfortunately, asking the technologist to try to recall if specific waveforms were associated with body movements is almost always a useless exercise. In addition to carefully observing the patient, the recording, and making frequent notations about movements, movements may be recorded and sometimes identified with special monitors (e.g., accelerometers). In addition, the ECG channel sometimes serves as an effective monitor for detecting gross body tremors and other movements.

6.1.4 *Electrocardiogram.* Potential changes generated by the heart are picked up in the EEG mainly in recordings with wide interelectrode distances, especially in linkages across the head and to the left ear, particularly in subjects who are overweight. The artifact may appear in all channels using a common reference, or only in one or a few channels. Small artifacts reflect mainly the R wave of the electrocardiogram (Fig. 6.2). Larger artifacts may reflect additional components of the electrocardiogram. Very large artifacts are often produced by interference from a cardiac pacemaker (Fig. 6.3). The R wave usually appears maximally over the left posterior head regions as a positive sharply contoured waveform and, with lower amplitude, over the right anterior head region as a negative waveform. This is because the main cardiac vector producing the R

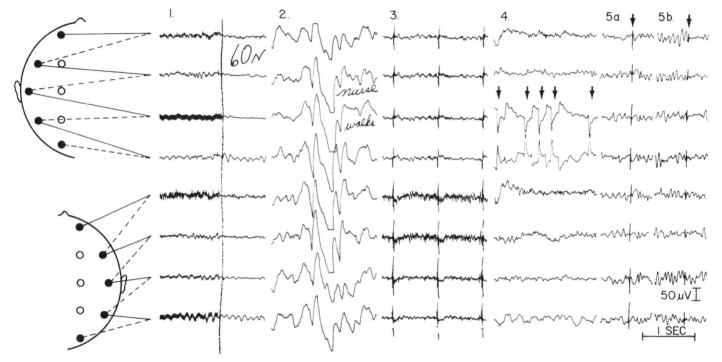

Fig. 6.3.   Non-biological artifacts. 1: 60 Hz interference before and after turning on the 60 Hz filter (60-). 2: Artifacts induced by a nurse walking near the patient. 3: Cardiac pacemaker artifacts. 4: 'Electrode popping' artifacts (arrows) from the left posterior temporal electrode making poor contact. 5a and 5b: 'Paper stop' artifacts (arrows) due to intermittent failure of paper drive.

wave is positive and directed diagonally from right to left and from anterior to posterior. Thus, in a longitudinal bipolar montage the ECG artifact, if present, appears as an upward deflection in T3-T5 and a downward deflection in T5-O1 (i.e.,

113

positivity at T5). If the head is turned, then the electrodes situated on the left and posterior with regard to the torso will still record the maximum positivity. The ECG artifact often changes amplitude and distribution as the patient breathes because breathing changes the position of the heart with respect to the head. *Premature ventricular contractions* are usually maximal over the posterior head regions but are greater in amplitude and duration than the normally conducted heart beat. *Their intermittent occurrence in the absence of an ECG monitor may give the impression of abnormal posterior sharp waves or rhythmic delta activity.* In contrast to most other artifacts, the heart beat artifact cannot usually be eliminated by corrective actions during the recording. It is rarely the only manifestation of a bad electrode contact and can therefore not usually be abolished by improving the contact or replacing the electrode. Referential recordings combining both ears as a reference tend to show less heart beat artifact than referential recordings to one ear. In approximately 80% of individuals a non-cephalic reference montage using a balanced neck to chest electrode pair as the reference will produce a recording free of ECG artifact. This consists of one electrode on the neck and one on the sternum, connected through a variable resistor that may be adjusted to null the ECG components affecting both these electrodes. If there is any doubt whether sharp waves are due to the heart beat artifact or to cerebral activity, the technician should record the heart beat in one channel and compare it with the timing of the suspected sharp waves.

If the heart beat has not been monitored during the recording and the EEG reader has difficulty in distinguishing heart beat artifact from cerebral activity, it is useful to measure the interval between clear heartbeat artifacts and apply this measure to subsequent suspicious events to determine whether they have equal intervals and therefore are likely due to heartbeat, or fall into the interval between events and are less likely of cardiac origin. However, this method may fail in extrasystoles and other cardiac arrhythmias, especially those altering the shape of the heartbeat artifact.

6.1.5 *Pulse wave artifact.* Periodic waves of smooth or triangular shape may be picked up by an electrode on or near a scalp artery as the result of pulse waves producing slight changes of the electrical contact between electrode and scalp. This is more likely to happen with electrodes in the frontal and temporal areas than with electrodes in the posterior head regions.

This artifact is recognized by its usually regular recurrence. If the heartbeat artifact is picked up in the same recording, it precedes the pulse wave artifact by a constant interval (Fig. 24.2). If necessary, the pulse wave artifact may be identified by simultaneous recording of the heartbeat. If it is eliminated by reapplication of the electrode at some distance from the pulsating artery, the new electrode position should be indicated on the chart.

6.1.6 *Skin potential.* There are 2 important artifacts that arise from skin changes. *Perspiration artifact* consists of slow waveforms that are usually greater than 2 s in duration. Perspiration alone causes slow shifts of the electrical baseline by changing the impedance or contact between the electrode and the skin. In addition, sweat gland activity produces slowly changing electrical potentials that are recorded by the electrodes. Less often rhythmic potentials are produced, particularly if stainless steel or unchlorided silver electrodes have been used. Perspiration artifact almost always appears in more than one channel, but may be lateralized or asymmetric. Therefore, very slow localized waveforms (greater than 2 s in duration) should never be considered unequivocal evidence of an underlying cerebral dysfunction unless accompanied by other changes such as slowing in the theta frequency range, or amplitude changes in the alpha and beta range. The simultaneous occurrence of perspiration artifact and generalized background slowing should always raise the question of hypoglycemia. Perspiration artifact can be reduced by cooling the patient and drying the scalp with a fan or alcohol.

The second less common artifact produced by the skin is the *sympathetic skin response* (SSR) also known as the galvanic skin response, or psychogalvanic skin response. The SSR consists of slow waves, each with a duration of 0.5–1 s (1–2 Hz), that last 1.5–2 s with 1–3 prominent phases (Fig. 6.4). The first phase may be negative or positive in polarity. The SSR represents an autonomic response produced by sweat gland and skin potentials mediated by unmyelinated cholinergic sympathetic fibers in response to a sensory stimulus or psychic event. It is more likely to be recorded as the environmental temperature increases. The SSR may be difficult to

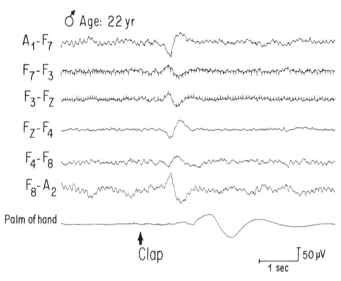

Fig. 6.4. Galvanic skin response. The galvanic skin response resulting from an alerting maneuver appears first over the scalp and then the palm due in part to the longer conduction time of autonomic pathways to the hand. This artifact may also occur with an asymmetric distribution. Courtesy of B.F. Westmoreland, Mayo Clinic.

identify correctly, particularly if it occurs in only one or two channels. Like other isolated delta wave artifacts its presence can be suspected if it is combined with normal background activity. It usually appears in the frontocentral channels in longitudinal bipolar montages and produces a characteristic triple phase reversal in transverse bipolar montages. SSR can

Bipolar montage

A₂-A₁

A₁-T₃

T₃-C₃

C₃-C₄

C₄-T₄

T₄-A₂

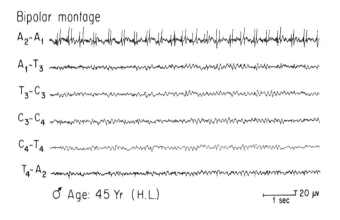

♂ Age: 45 Yr (H.L.)

$\vdash$ 1 sec ⅃ 20 μv

Referential montage

F_{P1}-A₂

F_{P2}-

F₃-

F₄-

C₃-

C₄-

A₂-A₁

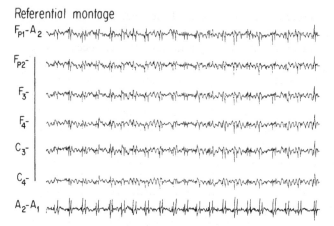

Fig. 6.5. Palatal myoclonus. Each involuntary movement of the pharynx and palate are marked by the fast paired deflections. The 10–20 electrode derivations that typically show this artifact best are those referenced to A1 and A2. This is clearly illustrated by the prominence of the artifact in the referential montage compared to the bipolar montage. Courtesy Dr. B.F. Westmoreland, Mayo Clinic.

be confirmed by simultaneous monitoring using one electrode placed on the palm (an area with abundant sweat glands) and one placed on the dorsum of the same hand. The skin should not be abraded during electrode application because damage to the skin can attenuate the response. A lower gain and longer time constant are used than in routine EEG recording.

6.1.7 *Movements of the tongue and other oropharyngeal structures.* These movements may produce intermittent or repetitive slow waves in a wide distribution, often with an apparent

maximum in longitudinal bipolar montages in the middle of the head. Tongue movement causes a 'glossokinetic' artifact because the tip of the tongue has a negative electrical charge with respect to the root. Tongue movement explains part of the artifacts generated by speaking, swallowing, chewing, sucking, sobbing, coughing and hiccoughing; movements of other structures probably contribute to these artifacts (Fig. 6.2) and account for those seen with sobbing. Artifacts from temporal, facial and scalp muscles may be mixed with the movement artifact. *Palatal myoclonus* causes rhythmical muscle artifacts at rates of about 60–120/min which are often only seen in referential montages to an ear electrode and persist in sleep (Fig. 6.5). A prominent evoked midline response from palatal myoclonus may occasionally appear as rhythmic sharp waves that are maximal at Cz or Pz that should not be mistaken for abnormal epileptiform activity.

Many of these artifacts may be identified during the recording if they are associated with visible movements and if they disappear when these movements stop. However, the identifi-cation of a glossokinetic artifact may be difficult if, for example, the mouth remains closed during tongue movements, or if it occurs with an asymmetric distribution (Fig. 6.6). Therefore, it is recommended that patients be routinely asked during the recording to repeat words that elicit tongue movements, such as 'lilt' or 'Tom Thumb' (Fig. 6.6).

6.1.8 *Dental restorations with dissimilar metals.* Dental fillings with dissimilar metals may produce spike-like artifacts

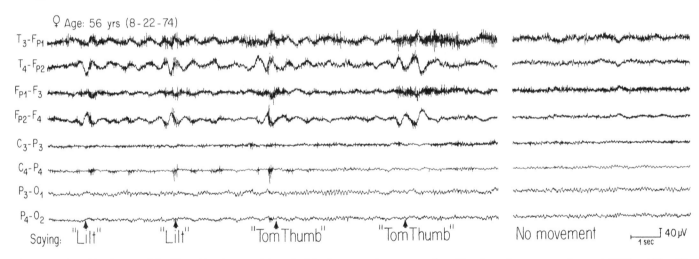

Fig. 6.6. Glossokinetic potentials. Glossokinetic potentials evoked for demonstration purposes by asking the patient to repeat the words 'Lilt' and 'Tom Thumb'. In longitudinal bipolar montages the artifact usually appears maximally in the anterior and posterior derivations. In some cases, as shown here, the artifact may have an asymmetric distribution. Courtesy Dr. D.W. Klass, Mayo Clinic.

117

whenever the metal pieces are moved against each other, for instance in chewing, swallowing or speaking.

6.2 INTERFERENCE

The most common artifact due to electrical interference comes from power lines and equipment. It has a frequency of 60 Hz in North America and of 50 Hz in many other countries. A slight amount of this interference is unavoidable wherever alternating current is used. While this background interference may be picked up by faulty electrodes and may appear in one or a few channels, inordinately strong interference can cause artifacts even with good recording electrodes and equipment; these artifacts are then likely to appear in all channels of all recordings made in the same recording room (Fig. 6.3). The artifacts may be introduced either electrostatically by unshielded power cables and regardless of current flow, or electromagnetically by strong currents flowing through cables and equipment such as transformers and electromotors. Electrostatic interference can be reduced by shielding the offending power cables and by using a shielded room for the recording; electromagnetic interference can be reduced by proper wiring of the power cables. Other types of interference include signals from nearby television stations, radio paging, telephone ringing, cardiac pacemakers (Fig. 6.3), or any movement of a charged body near the recording electrodes; electrostatic artifacts may be produced by a person walking through the recording room (Fig. 6.3) or by drops falling in an intravenous drip. However, modern EEG instruments have such high discrimination and input impedance that they reject all but the most powerful sources of interference from the environment. In setting up a laboratory, it is therefore not necessary to shield the recording room unless a trial recording from a patient or a 10,000 Ω resistor, placed at the prospective recording site, shows strong interference.

When recordings are made in an environment with much interference such as an intensive care unit or an operating room, the patient's head and the connections to the EEG instrument should be kept as far from power cables as possible. All electrode wires should be as short as possible and bound together in a single bundled cable. Electrode wires act as antennas for 60 Hz interference, especially when the individual wires are long or form loops. Any swaying of electrode wires and movement of tubing or of other charged objects should be minimized. Equipment other than the EEG instrument should be unplugged if feasible; even the respirator may be stopped for short periods to obtain artifact-free recordings or to determine the cause of interference.

6.3 ARTIFACTS ARISING FROM RECORDING ELECTRODES AND EQUIPMENT

6.3.1 *Artifacts arising from electrodes, electrode terminal board, input cable and selector switches.* Most artifacts in this category are distinguished from cerebral activity in that they differ radically from previously recorded activity, do not blend with other simultaneously recorded activity but seem to be superimposed on it, and appear only in channels connected to one electrode. However, not all of these artifacts are easily recognized. Although some of them have characteristic shapes, others lack such features and may resemble cerebral activity. A common artifact is 'electrode popping' which is due to a sudden change of electrode contact causing pen deflections which rise or fall abruptly and may mimic spike discharges (Fig. 6.3). Other electrode artifacts rise and fall more slowly and may resemble cerebral slow waves.

Identification and correction of artifacts in the distribution of one electrode requires checking electrical and mechanical continuity. Because the artifact is often due to faulty contact between the electrode and the scalp, the first step is to look at that junction: the electrode may be partly or completely detached, the lead wire may be broken, or the conductive paste or jelly may have dried up. As a next step, electrical impedance should be measured (2.2.3); if it is high, the electrode should be refilled with conductive jelly or paste, reapplied, or replaced if it is defective. If the artifact persists, the receptacle jack or the wiring of the input terminal board may be at fault; this can be investigated by changing the connections between electrodes and receptacles of the faulty channel so that the electrodes and the receptacles of that channel are presented in different channels: the electrodes of the faulty channel are connected to receptacles giving good recordings when con-

nected to other electrodes, and electrodes not giving artifacts when connected to other receptacles are connected to receptacles of the faulty channel. If the artifact changes channels corresponding with the electrodes from the faulty channel, one of these electrodes is at fault and can be identified by connecting the two electrodes to different channels and observing in which channel the artifact then appears. However, if the artifact remains at one receptacle, the input board or subsequent components of the recording channel may be at fault. In practice, the technician at this point or earlier will examine a piece of recording made while the inputs are closed. If the artifact persists under this condition, it arises from the recording instrument and should be investigated accordingly (6.3.2). However, if the artifact is present only when the input is open, and if an electrode fault has been excluded, the source of the artifact may be further determined by replacing the input board and input cable if replacements are available, and by checking the input terminals and selector switches if they are accessible.

6.3.2 *Artifacts arising from the recording instrument.* Like artifacts from the electrodes, artifacts from the instrument may often be recognized by the sudden appearance of waveforms very different from cerebral activity. The source of the artifacts can often be traced to one functional component of the instrument. Trouble shooting is facilitated by two features of modern EEG instruments. (a) Many components have indicator lights and electrical contact points with prescribed voltage readings which can be checked easily. (b) Components of individual channels are made of modules which can be exchanged. Artifacts due to faults of components that are common to all channels often cause lack of power or 60 Hz interference. Power failure may be caused by a faulty outlet or a blown fuse in the EEG instrument. If a replacement fuse also blows, the power supply may be at fault. Sixty hertz interference in all channels may be due to (a) a powerful source of interference in the recording room (6.2), (b) a faulty or absent connection of the subject with the ground of the EEG instrument (3.4.1), (c) defects in the power supply or other parts of the instrument.

Artifacts caused by components of individual channels appear only at the output of the defective channels and persist independently of the input selection. The causes of these problems can be traced by exchanging modular components of one channel with the corresponding components of another channel. For instance if 60 Hz artifact in one channel of an analog EEG instrument suggests a problem in its amplifier, this can be investigated by exchanging the amplifier for an amplifier of another channel not showing that artifact.

REFERENCES

Barlow, J.S. (1986) Artifact processing (rejection and minimization) in EEG data processing. In: F.H. Lopes da Silva, W. Storm van Leeuwen and A. Rémond (Eds.), Clinical Applications of Computer Analysis of EEG and other Neurophysiological Signals. Handbook of EEG, Vol. 2 (revised series). Elsevier, Amsterdam, pp. 15–64.

Beaussart, M. and Guiev, J.D. (1977) Section III. Artefacts. In: A. Rémond (Ed.), Handbook of Electroenceph. Clin. Neurophysiol., Vol. IIA. Elsevier, Amsterdam, pp. 80–96.

Bennett, D.R., Hughes, J.R., Korein, J., Merlis, J.K. and Suter, C. (1976) Atlas of Electroencephalography in Coma and Cerebral Death. Raven Press, New York.

Blume, W.T. (1982) Atlas of Pediatric EEG. Raven Press, New York.

Blume, W.T. and Kaibara, M. (1995) Atlas of Adult Electroencephalography. Raven Press, New York.

Brittenham, D. (1974) Recognition and reduction of physiological artifacts. Am. J. EEG Technol. 14: 158–165.

Espinosa, R.E., Lambert, E.H. and Klass, D.W. (1967) Facial myokymia affecting the electroencephalogram. Mayo Clin. Proc. 42: 258–270.

Espinosa, R.E., Klass, D.W. and Maloney, J.D. (1978) Contribution of the electroencephalogram in monitoring cardiac dysrhythmias. Mayo Clin. Proc. 53: 119–122.

Gordon, M. (1980) Artifacts created by imbalanced electrode impedance. Am. J. EEG Technol. 20: 149–160.

Harlan, W.L., White, P.T. and Bickford, R.G. (1958) Electric activity produced by eye flutter simulating frontal electroencephalographic rhythms. Electroenceph. Clin. Neurophysiol., 10: 164–169.

Kamp, A. and Lopes da Silva, F. (1987) Polygraphy. In: E. Niedermeyer and F. Lopes da Silva (Eds.), Electroencephalography: Basic Principles, Clinical Applications, and Related Fields. Urban and Schwarzenberg, Baltimore, pp. 681–686.

Klass, D.W. (1995) The continuing challenge of artifacts in the EEG. Am. J. EEG Technol. 35: 239–269.

Legatt, A. (1995) Impairment of common mode rejection by mismatched electrode impedances: quantitative analysis. Am. J. EEG Technol. 35: 296–302.

MacGillivray, B.B. (1974) Section IV. Artefacts, faults, and fault-finding. In: A. Rémond (Ed.), Handbook of Electroenceph. Clin. Neurophysiol., Vol.

3C. Elsevier, Amsterdam, pp. 88–102.

Pasik, P., Pasik, T. and Bender, M.B. (1965) Recovery of the electro-oculo-gram after total ablation of the retina in monkeys. Electroenceph. Clin. Neurophysiol. 19: 291–297.

Picton, T.W. and Hillyard, S.A. (1972) Cephalic skin potentials in electroence-phalography. Electroenceph. Clin. Neurophysiol. 33: 419–424.

Redding, F.K., Wandel, V. and Nasser, C. (1969) Intravenous infusion drop artifacts. Electroenceph. Clin. Neurophysiol. 26: 318–320.

Saunders, M.G. (1979) Artifacts: activity of noncerebral origin in the EEG. In: D.W. Klass and D.D. Daly (Eds.), Current Practice of Clinical Electroen-cephalography. Raven Press, New York, pp. 37–68.

Silbert, P.L., Roth, P.A., Kanz, B.S., Radhakrishnan, K. and Klass, D.W. (1994) Interference from cellular telephones in the electroencephalogram. Am. J. EEG Technol. 34: 6–12.

Stecker, M.M. and Patterson, T. (1998) Electrode impedance in neurophysio-logic recordings. 1. Theory and intrinsic contributions to noise. Am. J. EEG Technol. 38: 174–198.

Stephenson, W.A. and Gibbs, F.A. (1951) A balanced non-cephalic reference electrode. Electroenceph. Clin. Neurophysiol. 3: 237–240.

Stockard-Pope, J.E., Werner, S.S. and Bickford, R.G. (1992) Atlas of Neonatal Electroencephalography. 2nd Edn. Raven Press, New York.

Tyner, F.S., Knott, J.R. and Mayer, Jr., W.B. (1983) Fundamentals of EEG Technology. Raven Press, New York, pp. 280–311.

Westmoreland, B.F., Espinosa, R.E. and Klass, D.W. (1973) Significant pro-sopo-glossopharyngeal movements affecting the electroencephalogram. Am. J. EEG Technol. 13: 59–70.

Westmoreland, B.F. and Donat, J.F. (1998) The sympathetic skin response in the EEG. Am. J. EEG Technol. 38: 164–173.

7 Special methods of analysis and recording

SUMMARY

(7.1) *Quantitative EEG signal analysis* involves the transformation of the EEG signal into numerical values that can be used to examine selected EEG features. Once a specific feature of the EEG has been quantified, it can be displayed using various graphical methods such as topographic mapping or spectral trend monitoring. Other applications of quantitative analysis include automated event detection, intraoperative or ICU monitoring, and source localization. Normative databases of quantitative EEG features (such as the peak alpha rhythm frequency or amount of alpha reactivity, see Figs. 13.1 and 13.2) can be used for statistical comparisons in research studies. Statistical quantitative EEG analysis is not yet considered reliable as an independent measure of abnormal brain function for clinical purposes.

(7.2) *Topographic mapping* refers to the graphical display of the distribution of a particular EEG feature over the scalp or cortical surface. Advanced forms of topographic mapping attempt to display EEG activity as it might be seen at the cortical surface by superimposing a color or gray scale image of the EEG feature onto the cortical surface image taken from the subject's MRI (i.e., co-registration of the EEG and MRI images). More simplified forms of topographic mapping create a graphic display of an EEG feature over an imaginary head surface (see Fig. 7.2). All methods of topographic mapping depend heavily on montage construction (spatial filtering; Chapter 4).

(7.3) *Automated event detection* is a form of quantitative analysis in which certain signal characteristics are used to classify an EEG change. It is most commonly applied to the detection of electrographic seizures during epilepsy monitoring.

(7.4) *Intraoperative EEG monitoring* is performed using continuous routine EEG visual inspection alone or in combination with quantitative EEG monitoring. The most common application of intraoperative EEG monitoring is for carotid endarterectomy surgery. Thresholds for EEG changes at different levels of cerebral blood flow are used to alert the surgeon to the need to either shunt the patient or increase blood pressure.

(7.5) *Continuous EEG and video monitoring* is used to verify the presence of a seizure disorder, classify seizure type in patients with epilepsy, and localize the epileptogenic zone (the area of the brain that must be removed in order to control seizures). The EEG signal can be acquired by *radiotelemetry* (using a radio transmitter worn by the patient) or by *cable telemetry* (via a lightweight cable directly attached to the patient). Systems that record the video in a digital format provide much faster access for review of events than those using videotape. In general, all patients with medically intractable epilepsy and those being considered for surgical procedures to treat epilepsy (e.g., vagus nerve stimulator implantation or brain surgery) should undergo epilepsy monitoring.

(7.6) *Ambulatory monitoring* provides continuous 24 h (or longer) EEG recording using a small device that records and stores at least 16 channels of EEG. The EEG storage devices vary but the goal in most cases is to document the presence of electrographic seizure activity. The EEG recording is reviewed on an oscilloscope (if the EEG is stored as an analog signal) or computer monitor (if the EEG is stored digitally) using direct visual inspection. Automated seizure detection software can also be used to scan large segments of recording for possible seizures.

7.1 QUANTITATIVE EEG ANALYSIS

Quantitative EEG analysis refers to the transformation of a particular EEG feature into a numerical value. A method of signal analysis commonly used to perform quantitative EEG analysis is spectral analysis. An example of a feature typically calculated is the numerical value that represents the amount of all alpha (8–13 Hz) frequency activity recorded over a certain period of time. Quantitative EEG measures can be used for comparison with routine visual inspection, statistical comparisons, or for other forms of EEG display, such as topographic mapping. Although most methods of quantitative EEG analysis give very precise and reproducible results, it is important to recognize that virtually all are approximations and therefore contain a certain degree of error. *Automated event detection* or feature extraction refers to the use of the computer to recognize or isolate a selected EEG activity. An example is the automated detection of electrographic seizure activity. Quantitative analysis is most often used to: (1) quantitate EEG features for statistical analysis; (2) create topographic displays of EEG activity; (3) detect epileptiform activity; or (4) monitor selected EEG features in the ICU and OR.

Quantitative EEG analysis continues to be investigated as a method for detecting clinically relevant changes that are not revealed by routine visual inspection. Despite a number of reports suggesting that computer analysis is helpful for differential diagnosis, convincing verification of such findings by independent investigators has not been forthcoming. Currently, quantitative EEG analysis is best viewed as an extension of the routine EEG in clinical practice and as an important research tool. It cannot be overemphasized that clinicians attempting to apply these techniques in clinical practice should be experienced electroencephalographers who have a thorough understanding of the signal analysis methods being applied. Statistical quantitative EEG analysis is not reliable as an independent measure of abnormal brain function and should not be used as such for medical or legal purposes.

In order to quantitate the frequency components of the EEG signal, methods have been devised which transfer the EEG signal from the *time domain* into *the frequency domain*. The *time domain* refers to signals described in terms of *amplitude vs. time,* as displayed in the routine EEG. The *frequency domain* refers to signals described in terms of *amplitude* (or phase) vs. *frequency*. In Fig. 7.1, the original EEG signals displayed in la and 2a (i.e., in the time domain), have been transformed into the frequency domain (lb and 2b). Thus, lb and 2b show the relative intensities of different frequencies present in signals la and 2a. In the example in Fig. 7.1 the frequencies analyzed were from 0 to 20 Hz.

It is important to recognize that analyzing a signal in the frequency domain (Fig. 7.1) means that its original waveform morphology can no longer be seen. The advantages of this critical sacrifice of data are that: (1) a great deal of data can be summarized by a few descriptors; (2) selected features in the signal can be examined quantitatively; and (3) the relation-

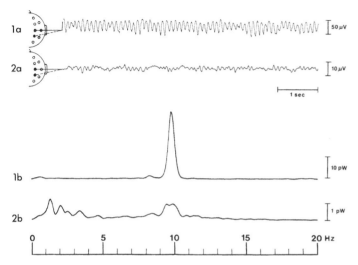

Fig. 7.1. Power spectra of normal (1) and abnormal (2) EEGs. The top two tracings (a) show strips of the paper tracing recorded between the right central and parietal electrode in a normal subject (1a) and a patient (2a). The bottom section shows power spectra (b) computed from about 13 s of the same recordings. The power spectrum of the normal subject (1b) shows activity mainly at 10 Hz, representing the 10 Hz waves seen in 1a; the power spectrum from the patient in 2b shows activity at about 1–4 Hz and at 10 Hz, reflecting the combination of slow waves and 10 Hz waves in 2a. Vertical calibration is in picowatts (pW).

ships between signals can be revealed more precisely than by visual inspection (see also 7.4.7).

The mathematical manipulation commonly used to make the conversion from the time to the frequency domain, and the one used in Fig. 7.1, is known as *the fast Fourier transform* (FFT). The FFT function is based on the fact that any signal can be described as a combination of sine and cosine waves of various phases, frequencies and amplitudes. Accordingly, the FFT generates a number of numerical coefficients that represent the sine and cosine waves present in the original signal in terms of frequency, amplitude, and phase. By using all of the Fourier sine and cosine values (coefficients), the signal can be reconstructed from the frequency domain back into its original form in the time domain.

A common approach to analyzing the FFT so that the signal can be viewed in terms of frequency vs. intensity consists of squaring the Fourier coefficients to create what is referred to as the *power spectrum* (as shown in Fig. 7.1, 1b and 2b). The power spectrum contains far less data than the original EEG. This makes the storage of spectral information much more efficient than raw EEG data storage. Unfortunately, the original EEG signal cannot be reconstructed from the power spectrum (it does not contain phase information). In addition, the squaring of coefficients changes the amplitude relationships of the various frequency components. For example, if the distances of two lines measuring 2 and 4 m are squared, then both become longer, but their relative difference in length becomes twice as great as it was originally. The amplitude relationships of the various frequency components of the EEG are similarly altered by power spectral analysis. This effect can be overcome by deriving the equivalent of the square root of the power spectrum, thereby creating an *amplitude spectrum*. Not surprisingly, the amplitude relationships displayed in the amplitude spectrum compare more directly with routine visual EEG analysis than do power spectrum amplitude measures.

Certain spectral features of the EEG signal may be examined once the amplitude or power spectrum has been derived. These commonly include: (1) *absolute band amplitude, or power;* (2) *relative band amplitude, or power;* (3) *the spectral edge frequency;* (4) *mean peak frequency;* and (5) *the absolute peak frequency.* Each of these values may, in turn, be statistically analyzed or plotted on a topographic display according to electrode position.

The *absolute band* value corresponds approximately to the area under the curve of the spectrum between the two frequencies that define the bandwidth. The *relative band* value refers to one absolute band value divided by another. In the example of a topographic map of relative bands shown in Fig. 7.2, the 0–4 Hz band is divided by the 0–20 Hz band and the corresponding value at each electrode site is plotted according to a gray scale that is displayed to the right of the map. As with absolute band values, the upper and lower limits of each band must be stated. Relative band values are often used because: (1) errors created by differences in amplifier gain between channels are minimized; and (2) the effects of amplitude differences of noncerebral origin (such as those due to varying skull thickness or asymmetrical interelectrode distances) are theoretically minimized.

The *spectral edge frequency* refers to the frequency below which a pre-selected percentage of the total frequency range absolute band value lies. For example, if the spectral edge frequency is set at 90%, then the computer will determine the frequency below which 90% of the area under the entire spectral curve is contained. The spectral edge frequency has been used as a gross indicator showing trends in the EEG over time. The median peak frequency can be determined by simply calculating the spectral edge frequency at 50%. Alternatively, a mean peak frequency (also referred to as the *centroid)* equivalent to the center of gravity of the area under the spectral plot may be used.

The *absolute peak frequency* refers to the peak value in a selected band of the frequency spectrum. A frequency band is selected at the keyboard and the computer calculates the highest spectral peak in that frequency band. Absolute peak frequency measures have been used to compare the alpha frequency between homotopic derivations, between individuals, and within individuals over time or in response to medications. These studies suggest that differences of as little as 0.3 or 0.4 Hz may be abnormal when comparing left and right occipital derivations with certain montages. In contrast, using routine visual analysis a peak alpha rhythm frequency asymmetry of less than 1 Hz is difficult to appreciate and differences of less than 0.5 Hz cannot be accurately assessed. However, clearly dominant spectral peak frequencies in the alpha frequency band may be poorly defined in both normal and abnormal individuals (particularly when increasingly longer EEG epoch lengths are analyzed), making the uniform appli-

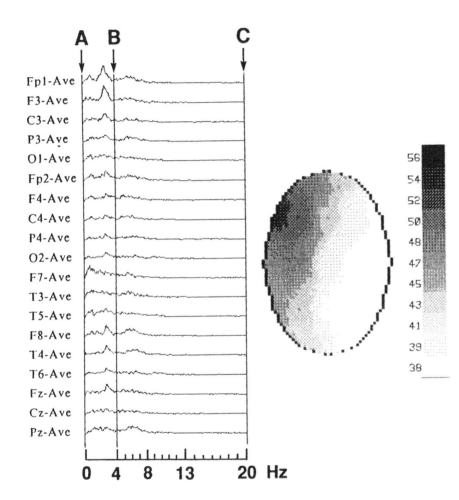

Fig. 7.2. The amplitude spectrum and topographic map of relative delta activity during light sleep. The EEG was recorded using a linked ear reference montage and subsequently reconstructed into a common average reference montage (7.4.5). Four 8 s epochs of apparently artifact-free EEG were selected using a monitor screen and the spectrum of each epoch was computed in each channel. The four spectra from each of the 8 s EEG epochs in each channel were then averaged to yield the final spectral plots for each channel as shown on the left side of the figure. The absolute band value (the approximate area under the spectral plot) between 0 and 4 Hz (A and B) was divided by the absolute band value between 0 and 20 Hz (A and C) and multiplied times 100 to yield the final relative percentage 0–4 Hz frequency band. The relative band percentage values on the topographic map are shown on the gray scale at the far right. The routine recording demonstrated left anterior temporal background slowing and occasional epileptiform spikes that could be seen on the topographic map as increased activity in the 0–4 Hz relative band.

cation of absolute peak frequency measures in clinical practice difficult.

As noted above, a major limitation of spectral analysis is the loss of the waveform morphology once the EEG has been transformed into the frequency domain. A particular band value gives no indication of waveform morphology, nor does it give any indication of how many times a specific frequency waveform has occurred. Thus, the same spectral band value could result from either continuous, identical, low amplitude waveforms or from intermittent high amplitude waveforms in the same frequency range. Because the morphology and repetition of waveforms cannot be appreciated in the frequency domain, it is important that the unprocessed EEG be viewed and interpreted by an experienced electroencephalographer. Otherwise, clinically useful information (such as the presence of epileptiform spikes) contained in the EEG may be lost. It is also important that an experienced electroencephalographer selects the segments of EEG for quantitative analysis. This is done to avoid artifact contamination and to facilitate the interpretation of the results. A computer monitor display is used to select EEG segments for processing.

Short EEG epoch FFT analysis (less than 2.5 s in duration) is often used to increase the likelihood that there will be artifact-free data available for analysis. In this way some segments of artifact-free EEG can usually be obtained, even in poorly cooperative patients. Once the individual EEG epochs have been transformed to the frequency domain, their separate frequency spectra can be averaged together to form a final spectrum more representative of a longer time span; a process known as *spectral averaging*. Spectral averaging decreases the influence of any infrequent activity (cerebral or artifactual) and may reduce variability when comparisons are made with subsequent recordings. However, spectral averaging also has inherent limitations. It is based on the assumption that, as in evoked potential recording, there is some feature of the signal that persists with little or no change from epoch to epoch. Unfortunately, the EEG is relatively stationary over only short periods of time (typically 20–40 s with behavioral control) and this variability depends largely on maintaining the behavioral state of the individual being recorded. Therefore, if spectral averaging is to be performed, it is preferable to try to average spectral EEG epochs in which the patient is in approximately the same state. This can be accomplished in a variety of ways. One approach is to ask the subject to quietly count the number of tones presented during a recording session lasting several minutes. At the end of the session the subject is asked how many tones were presented to verify that relative wakefulness was maintained during the recording.

It is also noteworthy that averaging short FFT epochs of EEG is a compromise solution to the problem of artifact contamination because shorter EEG epochs produce poorer frequency resolution. This occurs because the frequency resolution of an FFT is directly related to EEG epoch length. Integer multiples of the slowest waveform that can be fully described by the epoch length determine spectral frequency resolution. For example, if a 2 s epoch is selected, the slowest complete waveform that can be fitted into a 2 s period of time is 0.5 Hz (i.e., a 2 s wavelength). For this epoch length only frequency differences within the EEG of 0.5 Hz or greater can be resolved using FFT analysis. In such a case, a difference between 0.5 Hz and 0.62 Hz activity cannot be detected. But if a 4 s epoch is selected, then differences of as little as 0.25 Hz can be resolved. If one is interested in distinguishing between absolute peak frequencies that differ by 0.1 Hz, then epoch lengths of at least 10 s (to resolve 0.1 Hz differences) are needed. Other approaches to signal analysis besides the FFT, such as the autoregressive model, are better suited for assessing peak frequency using extremely short epoch lengths.

Methods that compare signal similarities in frequency, amplitude and phase have long been applied to EEG. These methods have been used for a variety of purposes such as localizing the mu rhythm, investigating inter- and intrahemispheric cortical relationships, elucidating the role of the thalamus in the generation of the alpha rhythm, and determining the anatomic pathways of spreading electrographic seizure activity. Most of these applications are based on, or derived from, the *cross-correlation* and *coherence functions*.

Cross-correlation evaluates the relationship between two signals recorded simultaneously. Similarities of both amplitude and shape are measured as the covariance of the signals; similarities of shape regardless of amplitude are expressed by the correlation coefficient which varies between +1, indicating that the signals have identical shape and polarity, and −1, indicating that they have identical shape but opposite polarity.

If the two sources generate signals that have similar shape but different timing, the correlation coefficient will vary; the dependence of the correlation coefficient on the time interval is represented by the correlation function. The correlation coefficient also varies with the frequency of the EEG components; the dependence of the correlation coefficient on the EEG frequency is the coherence function. Two signals that are identical are said to be completely coherent.

7.2 TOPOGRAPHIC MAPPING

Special displays of EEG and evoked potential activity have been developed to emphasize either the trends in EEG activity over time (Figs. 7.3 and 7.4) or the distribution of activity over the scalp (Fig. 7.2). The display of the distribution of scalp recorded activity is referred to as *topographic mapping* (TM).

TM may be used for the display of: (1) EEG voltage distributions at a particular point in time *(time domain mapping);* (2) EEG background features derived from frequency analysis *(frequency domain mapping);* and (3) statistical comparisons *(statistical mapping).* Examples from the first category include evoked potentials (EP) and averaged epileptiform spikes. Spike averaging may reveal the presence of widespread field distributions that cannot otherwise be appreciated. Whether spike averaging will contribute substantially to the anatomical localization of epileptogenic foci awaits further investigation. As with spike averaging, EP mapping has been used mainly to illustrate, rather than elucidate, field distributions. Although absolute EP amplitude measures are clinically less useful than peak latencies, EP spatial distributions have not been studied as extensively.

Amplitude measurements for time domain TM are determined according to deviations from the electrical zero baseline set by the analog to digital converter. In actual practice the baseline for the data point being mapped is almost always different from the electrical zero baseline used by the computer. Often the waveform is superimposed on a slower waveform arising from cerebral or non-cerebral activity. This effect can be reduced by digitally filtering out waveforms above and below the frequency of the waveform of interest. In the case of evoked potentials, the signal baseline may also be altered by stimulus artifact. Even more difficult to identify are baseline distortions that arise from amplifier drift (amplifier offset) and changes in resting potentials generated at the scalp–electrode interface. These effects can all lead to TM displays with misleadingly high or low amplitude values that vary in degree from channel to channel.

Frequency domain TM of background activity is accomplished by plotting one of several features derived from a spectral average. Fig. 7.2 shows a typical example of a topographic map of the relative band value of the 0–4 Hz (0–4 Hz absolute band value divided by the 1–20 Hz absolute band value). Four 8 s EEG segments were selected during light sleep. Only those epochs without apparent artifact were chosen for analysis. The spectra from all four 8 s epochs were averaged together to form the final averaged spectra for each of the channels, as shown on the left of the figure. Each band value is plotted at each electrode site according to the percentage scale to the right of the map.

It is important to recognize that the only 'real' values on topographic maps are those that represent the actual channel values. In the example shown in Fig. 7.2 there are only 19 points (pixels) on the entire map that are real values. All the rest are estimated or interpolated between the real values to make the map more visually pleasing. This is, however, analogous to a situation in which only the location of one point near the top of a mountain and three or four points near the base are known. It cannot be assumed that connecting those points with straight lines correctly demonstrates the shape of the mountain or even the highest peak. The only way to improve the spatial resolution of maps is to increase the number of recording electrodes (i.e., actual data points) and vary the montage design. A second important feature of maps that must be kept in mind is that, as in routine EEG recording, there is no such thing as an inactive reference, and the best approximation of one, a non-cephalic reference montage, is difficult to implement in spectral analysis because of ECG artifact. Thus, the activity displayed never reveals the true topography of the EEG. It is therefore probably best to analyze TM, as in routine practice, with more than one montage. Unfortunately, published topographic studies have rarely been performed with more than one montage.

Until reliable statistical methods and usable normal limits

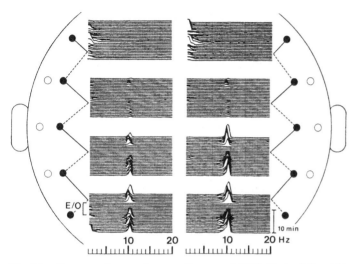

Fig. 7.3. Compressed spectral array of a normal EEG. Each of the eight blocks of tracings represents power spectra computed from simultaneous EEG recordings derived between the electrodes indicated on the head diagrams at the sides of the illustration. Each line in the blocks represents one power spectrum plotted for a recording period of about 35 s; successive spectra are stacked vertically. The posterior head regions show power mainly at about 10 Hz which disappears with eye opening (E/O) midway in the recording and reappears after the eyes are closed. The power in the low frequency range in the frontal regions is due to eye movement artifacts.

for mapped values are established, routine clinical applications for frequency domain TM are limited to the role of in-

forming the electroencephalographer that reinspection of the routine EEG may be necessary. Electrographic evidence for a cerebral dysfunction should not be based on frequency domain TM in the absence of abnormal routine EEG findings.

7.3   AUTOMATED EVENT DETECTION

Automated event detection is used clinically in epilepsy monitoring. The computer is programmed to 'recognize' either interictal epileptiform activity or electrographic seizures and then to store these events in a separate file for subsequent printing or display. Several approaches to seizure detection have been developed and refined. They all detect changes in rhythmicity or background activity using a variety of signal processing methods including artificial neural networks. At present, programs that have been developed for this purpose lack specificity, particularly those used to detect interictal epileptiform activity. However, they are sensitive, i.e., there are many false positives but rare few false negatives. The main advantage of automated seizure detection is that it provides the electroencephalographer with a powerful tool for reducing the amount of EEG recording that needs to be reviewed or stored for further analysis. Automated artifact detection is currently used in evoked potential recording to remove signals that: (1) contain excessive 60 cycle contamination; (2) exceed a preset voltage range; or (3) present as a flat line.

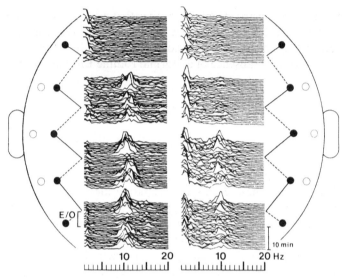

Fig. 7.4. Compressed spectral array of an abnormal EEG. Power spectra are plotted with the same method as used in Fig. 7.2. The spectra from the right posterior head regions differ from those from the left side in that they show a considerable amount of power below 8 Hz with a maximum at 1–3 Hz. Power at 10 Hz is reduced on the right side as compared to the left, especially in the frontocentral region. Eye opening (E/O) reduces power at 10 Hz noticeably on the left side but hardly at all on the right.

7.4 INTRAOPERATIVE AND INTENSIVE CARE UNIT MONITORING

Quantitative EEG analysis is being used increasingly to moni-

tor cerebral function in the operating room and intensive care unit. In the OR the scalp recorded EEG is useful for monitoring the level of general anesthesia and for detecting ischemia during *carotid endarterectomy*. Although this kind of monitoring can also be accomplished easily and reliably by routine visual EEG inspection, different methods of computerized analysis have been implemented. One well-known method consists of stacking successive power or amplitude spectral plots. This is referred to as a *compressed spectral array*. As shown in Figs. 7.3 and 7.4, gross changes which occur over time can be readily detected. Alternatively, a more precise evaluation of individual spectral features, such as the spectral edge frequency, can be plotted as a function of frequency (y-axis) vs. time (x-axis).

Intraoperative monitoring during carotid endarterectomy is performed with a relatively light level of general anesthesia. This allows the EEG to be more sensitive to ischemic changes. At a relatively light depth of anesthesia the EEG shows anterior dominant activity in the alpha frequency range with intermixed theta and delta waveforms. A critical time for monitoring is at the time of carotid artery clamping. If the EEG shows no change from a 10 min baseline prior to clamping the carotid artery, then placement of a shunt can be avoided. The majority of ischemic induced changes occur in the first 20 s after clamping and severe or major changes occur earlier than moderate or mild changes. Major changes are those which should be used to immediately alert the surgeon that severe ischemia may be occurring. Major changes include any of the following:

(1)   a 75% alteration of all activity
(2)   a >100% increase in delta activity ≤1 Hz
(3)   a >50% loss of all activity
(4)   a >50% loss of 8–15 Hz activity

The most severe change is a loss of amplitude. Abnormal EEG changes beginning with an attenuation of faster frequencies and an increase in slowing >1 Hz begin at cerebral blood flow (rCBF) levels of 18–23 ml/100 g/min. Below 18 ml/100 g/min major EEG changes occur. EEG slowing increases at 15 ml/100 g/min, and the EEG becomes isoelectric (inactive) at 12 ml/100 g/min. The threshold for cerebral infarction in man is thought to be 10 ml/100 g/min. Generalized changes may be due to anesthetic effects (excessive anesthesia) or relative hypotension, both of which should be immediately corrected by the anesthesiologist. The recording should be continued throughout the operative procedure and during recovery from anesthesia in order to provide the surgeon with the correct information about the onset of any ischemic changes. The choice of montage varies somewhat between centers but most use a longitudinal bipolar montage. The 'paper speed' should be 15 mm/s to enhance the visualization of slower waveforms. A sensitivity of 3–5 μV/mm is recommended.

In comparison to OR monitoring, the application of quantitative EEG analysis in the ICU setting has been limited by: (1) the difficulties of maintaining the integrity of an EEG recording system over long periods of time; and (2) the detection and elimination of artifacts. Unlike the OR, EEG monitoring in the ICU is usually performed over long periods of time without an EEG technologist in attendance. Quantitative EEG analysis in such a situation is ideal because the EEG can be compressed into displays of selected spectral features plotted over long durations of time for quick review. However, without the original EEG, or an on-site technologist, the correct interpretation of artifacts is problematic. ICU EEG monitoring has been used successfully for the early detection of vasospasm following aneurysm rupture. In some cases spectral trending (e.g., compressed spectral array) has been used to identify the presence of subclinical seizures; however, automated seizure detection algorithms are more effective.

7.5   AMBULATORY EEG RECORDING

Ambulatory EEG cassette or digital recording is routinely performed with 16- to 32-channel systems. Each channel has a preamplifier (made from a solid state amplifier chip) that may be located inside the cassette recording unit or digital computer worn by the patient or attached to a separate portable unit near the patient's head. Additional channels may be used to encode the time, to record other physiological signals (e.g., ECG) or document clinical events each time the patient presses a button. Each system typically records for at least

24 h. After recording, the analog tape or digitally stored EEG is scanned using a monitor to search for the occurrence of electrographic seizure activity. During scanning the EEG signal can also be played through a speaker allowing for the detection of electrographic events by changes in sound pattern. In addition, automated seizure detection software is used to select epochs of interest for review.

Ambulatory recording has clearly been shown to be an efficient method for confirming the diagnosis of epilepsy. It is also sometimes helpful for seizure localization. Prolonged monitoring appears to add little to the initial detection of seizures in neonates beyond that gained by performing a routine neonatal EEG recording because neonatal seizures usually occur at frequent intervals. The main disadvantages of ambulatory recording are: (1) the lack of simultaneous visual information, and (2) the frequent occurrence of artifacts.

The main clinical indications for ambulatory monitoring are: (1) to determine whether or not abnormal behavioral events are epileptic, (2) to quantify the frequency of epileptic seizures, and (3) to classify the patient's seizure disorder (e.g., partial vs. generalized, absence vs. complex partial). It is important to remember that the absence of an electrographic seizure pattern during a patient's behavioral attack is not necessarily proof that the attack is not epileptic in nature, particularly without the benefit of a recording of the patient's behavior. Similarly, pre-surgical evaluations for epilepsy surgery should be performed with video monitoring.

7.6 EEG RECORDING WITH SIMULTANEOUS VIDEO MONITORING

Prolonged monitoring with continuous video and EEG recording (V/EEG) allows the electroencephalographer to combine both EEG and clinical information in the classification of seizure disorders. Indeed, the classification of seizures (see Appendix III) is now based on information obtained from V/EEG monitoring.

V/EEG monitoring is also essential for localizing the anatomical site of seizure onset in patients being evaluated for possible surgical intervention. If behavioral events follow electrographic events, then the site of onset of the ictal activity is more likely to have accurate localizing value. However, if behavioral events precede the electrographic changes, then anatomical localization of ictal onset is less certain. In most cases of non-invasive epilepsy monitoring using scalp electrodes clear, localized ictal onset follows the behavioral onset and the electrographic seizure only becomes apparent as the *symptomatogenic zone* (that area of the brain that yields the first behavioral changes) is invaded by the seizure. That area of the brain may be at a considerable anatomical distance from the *ictal onset zone* (that area of the brain from which the seizure initially arises). Patients undergoing V/EEG usually require 3–5 days of recording, although this may vary greatly in individual cases. To reduce monitoring time to a minimum, anticonvulsants are usually partially withdrawn the day prior to admission to the epilepsy monitoring unit.

Ideally, the epilepsy monitoring unit is isolated from a regular patient ward and has a dedicated nursing staff, large single patient rooms, and a dayroom equipped with video cameras to provide some environmental variety for the patient during monitoring. When a seizure occurs a button is pressed by the patient or nurse that triggers an alarm. Behavioral testing is then performed to examine memory, language and motor functions that may help to classify the seizure and localize the area of brain involvement.

Current monitoring systems typically consist of the following components: (1) EEG amplifier/encoders, (2) a lightweight, flexible electrode cable to carry the signal from the electrodes to the amplifiers, (3) a decoder, (4) a special effects generator (splitter-inserter), (5) a reformatter, (6) digital video storage and processing, (7) an audio system, (8) a titler/time-code generator, (9) a monitor, and (10) video camera(s). The most recent advance in V/EEG monitoring is digital video processing. Digital video is a major time saving advantage because it allows the electroencephalographer to immediately view behavioral events after they have occurred instead of having to access them from videotape.

The encoder combines the signals from all channels into a single signal according to one of a variety of methods of signal multiplexing. The multiplexed signal is reconstructed into the original EEG signal by the decoder. The reformatter transforms the recorded EEG signal into a video display on the monitor and the special effects generator is used to combine the EEG and picture of the patient on the same monitor screen. The titler/time code generator prints the time on the monitor screen and alphanumerics can be entered onto the picture from a keyboard. Systems that use digital video do not require a reformatter because videotape is not necessary. Using more than one video camera is helpful, since one camera can be focused on the patient's face (or other area of special interest) while the other provides a wider view of the entire body. The latter view also reduces the likelihood that the patient will move out of the view of the camera entirely.

The storage of the EEG and video signal on video cassette tape and on digital hard drives obviates the need for an EEG machine during the actual recording. EEG events for interpretation performed with digital technology (i.e., retrospective filter, amplitude, 'paper speed,' and montage formatting) are analyzed using a high resolution monitor (or monitors). The system should allow the user to print out the same recorded segment with montage reformatting so that the same electrographic events can be seen using a variety of montages. During review a precise correlation in time can be made between behavioral and EEG events.

Since monitoring typically produces several days worth of data it is important to have efficient methods for reducing the amount of data to be reviewed. This is accomplished in two ways. First, the patient, the epilepsy monitoring nurse, or someone with the patient, presses a button which triggers the storage of a time code whenever a seizure occurs. A list showing the times at which the button was triggered is displayed on a computer monitor screen so that the EEG events can be viewed using digital EEG and the behavioral events can be reviewed using digital video or videotape. Second, electrographic seizure activity is automatically detected by computerized signal analysis.

In some systems, instead of a direct lightweight electrode cable connection between the patient and the monitoring equipment (i.e., *cable telemetry)*, the EEG electrodes are plugged into a radiotransmitter worn by the patient which transmits the multiplexed EEG signal to a receiver and then to a decoding unit. The potential disadvantages of radiotelemetry are that: (1) the signal may be interrupted if the patient wanders beyond the range of the radiotransmitter, and (2) most patients are more likely to remain in view of the camera if a direct cable is used.

REFERENCES

American EEG Society Statement on the Clinical Use of Quantitative EEG (1987) J. Clin. Neurophysiol. 4: 75.

Barlow, J.S. (1985) Methods of analysis of nonstationary EEGs, with emphasis on segmentation techniques: a comparative review. J. Clin. Neurophysiol. 2: 267–304.

Binnie, C.D., Batchelor, B.G., Bowring, P.A., Darby, C.E., Herbert, L., Lloyd, D.S.L., Smith, D.M., Smith, G.F. and Smith, M. (1978) Computer-assisted interpretation of clinical EEGs. Electroenceph. Clin. Neurophysiol. 44: 575–585.

Blume, W.T. and Sharbrough, F.W. (1993) EEG monitoring during carotid endarterectomy and open heart surgery. In: E. Niedermeyer and F. Lopes da Silva (Eds.), Electroencephalography: Basic Principles, Clinical Applications, and Related Fields, 3rd Edn. Williams and Wilkins, Baltimore, pp. 747–756.

Cooper, R., Osselton, J.W. and Shaw, J.C. (1981) EEG Technology, 3rd Edn. Butterworth, London.

Duffey, F.H., Bartels, P.H. and Burchfiel, J.L. (1981) Significance probability mapping: an aid in the topographic analysis of brain electrical activity. Electroenceph. Clin. Neurophysiol. 51: 455–462.

Ebersole, J.S. (1989) Ambulatory Monitoring. Raven Press, New York.

Ebersole, J.S. and Wade, P.B. (1991) Spike voltage topography identifies two types of fronto-temporal epileptic foci. Neurology 41: 1425–1433.

Epstein, C.M. (1994) Computerized EEG in the courtroom. Neurology 44: 1566–1569.

Faught, E. (1993) Current role of electroencephalography in cerebral ischemia. Stroke 24: 609–613.

Fisch, B.J. and Pedley, T.A. (1989) The role of quantitative topographic mapping or 'neurometrics' in the diagnosis of psychiatric and neurological disorders: the cons. Electroenceph. Clin. Neurophysiol. 73: 5–9.

Fisch, B.J., Pedley, T.A. and Keller, D.L. (1988) A topographic background symmetry display for comparison with routine EEG. Electroenceph. Clin. Neurophysiol. 69: 491–494.

Gabor, A.J. and Seyal, M. (1992) Automated interictal EEG spike detection using artifical neural networks. Electroenceph. Clin. Neurophysiol. 83: 271–280.

Gasser, T., Bacher, P. and Mocks, J. (1982) Transformations towards the normal distribution of broad band spectral parameters of the EEG. Electroenceph. Clin. Neurophysiol. 53: 119–124.

Gevins, A.S. and Rémond, A. (1987) Methods of Analysis of Brain Electrical and Magnetic Signals. Handbook of Electroencephalography and Clinical Neurophysiology (revised series), Vol. 1. Elsevier, Amsterdam, 31–38.

Gevins, A.S., Le, J., Martin, N.K. et al. (1994) High resolution EEG: 124-channel recording, spatial deblurring and MRI integration methods. Electroenceph. Clin. Neurophysiol. 90: 337–358.

Gotman, J. (1985) Practical use of computer-assisted EEG interpretation in Epilepsy. J. Clin. Neurophysiol. 2: 251–266.

Gotman, J., Ives, J.R. and Gloor, P. (1985) Long-term monitoring in epilepsy. Electroenceph. Clin. Neurophysiol. Suppl. 37: 444.

Gregory, D.L. and Wong, P.K. (1984) Topographical analysis of the centro-temporal discharges in benign Rolandic epilepsy of childhood. Epilepsia 25: 705–711.

Gumnit, R.J. (Ed.) (1987) Intensive Diagnostic Monitoring. Advances in Neurology, Vol. 46. Raven Press, New York.

Isley, M.R., Cohen, M.J., Wadsworth, S. et al. (1998) Multimodality neuro-monitoring for carotid endarterectomy surgery: determination of critical cerebral ischemic thresholds. Am. J. EEG Technol. 38: 65–122.

Jordan, K.G. (1993) Continuous EEG and evoked potential monitoring in the neuroscience intensive care unit. J. Clin. Neurophysiol. 10: 445–475.

Kahn, E.M., Weiner, R.D., Brenner, R.P. et al. (1988) Topographic maps of brain electrical activity – pitfalls and precautions. Biol. Psychiatr. 23: 628–636.

Kamp, A. and Lopes da Silva, F.H. (1987) Special techniques of recording and transmission. In: E. Niedermeyer and F.H. Lopes da Silva (Eds.), Electro-encephalography: Basic Principles, Clinical Applications and Related Fields. Urban and Schwarzenberg, Baltimore, pp. 619–694.

Lemos, M.S. and Fisch, B.J. (1991) The weighted average montage. Electro-enceph. Clin. Neurophysiol. 79: 361–370.

Lopes da Silva, F.H. (1987) Computerized EEG analysis: a tutorial overview. In: A.M. Halliday, S.R. Butler and R. Paul (Eds.), A Textbook of Clinical Neurophysiology. Wiley, New York, pp. 61–104.

Lopes da Silva, F.H. and Storm van Leeuwen, W.S. (1986) Clinical applications of computer analysis of EEG and other neurophysiological signals. In: Handbook of Electroencephalography and Clinical Neurophysiology, revised series, Vol. 2. Elsevier, Amsterdam.

Mocks, J. and Gasser, T. (1984) How to select epochs of the EEG at rest for quantitative analysis. Electroenceph. Clin. Neurophysiol. 58: 89–92.

Nunez, P.L. (1981) Electric Fields of the Brain. Oxford University Press, London, pp. 176–213.

Nunez, P.L. and Pilgreen, K.L. (1991) The spline-Laplacian in clinical neuro-physiology: a method to improve EEG spatial resolution. J. Clin. Neuro-physiol. 8: 397–413.

Nuwer, M.R. (1988) Quantitative EEG: 1. Techniques and problems of fre-quency analysis and topographic mapping. J. Clin. Neurophysiol. 5: 1–44.

Nuwer, M.R. (1997) Assessment of digital EEG, quantitative EEG, and EEG brain mapping. Report of the American Academy of Neurology and the American Clinical Neurophysiology Society. Neurology 49: 277–292.

Nuwer, M.R. and Hauser, H.H. (1994) Erroneous diagnosis using EEG dis-criminant analysis. Neurology 44: 1998–2000.

Nuwer, M.R., Lehmann, D., Lopes da Silva, F. et al. (1994) IFCN guidelines for topographic and frequency analysis of EEGs and EPs. Report of an IFCN committee. Electroenceph. Clin. Neurophysiol. 91: 1–5.

O'Brien, P. (1994) A primer on the discrete Fourier transform. Am. J. EEG Technol. 34: 190–223.

Oken, B.S. and Chiappa, K.H. (1986) Statistical issues concerning computer-ized analysis of brain wave topography. Ann. Neurol. 19: 493–494.

Pfurtscheller, G., Maresch, H. and Schuy, S. (1977) Inter- and intrahemi-spheric differences in the peak frequency of rhythmic activity within the alpha band. Electroenceph. Clin. Neurophysiol. 42: 77–83.

Picton, T.W. (Ed.) (1988) Human Event-Related Potentials. Handbook of EEG (revised series), Vol. 3. Elsevier, Amsterdam.

Porter, R.J. and Sato, S. (1987) Prolonged EEG and video monitoring in the diagnosis of seizure disorders. In: E. Niedermeyer and F.H. Lopes da Silva (Eds.), Electroencephalography: Basic Principles, Clinical Appli-cations and Related Fields. Urban and Schwarzenberg, Baltimore, pp. 634–644.

Qu, H. and Gotman, J. (1993) Improvement in seizure detection performance by automatic adaptation to the EEG of each patient. Electroenceph. Clin. Neurophysiol. 86: 79–87.

Roy, O.Z (1976) Section III. Biotelemetry and telephone transmission. In: A. Rémond (Ed.), Handbook of Electroenceph. Clin. Neurophysiol., Vol. 3A. Elsevier, Amsterdam, pp. 46–66.

Soong, A.C.K., Lind, J.C., Shaw, G.R. et al. (1993) Systematic comparisons of interpolation techniques in topographic brain mapping. Electroenceph. Clin. Neurophysiol. 87: 185–195.

Van Hufflen, A.C., Poortvliet, D.C.J. and Van der Wulp, C.J.M. (1984) Quantitative electroencephalography in cerebral ischemia. Detection of abnormalities in 'normal' EEGs. In: G. Pfurscheller, E.J. Jonkman and F.H. Lopes da Silva (Eds.), Brain Ischemia: Quantitative EEG and Imaging Techniques. Elsevier, Amsterdam, pp. 3–28.

Walter, D.O. (Ed.) (1972) Part B. Digital processing of bioelectric phenomena. In: A. Rémond (Ed.), Handbook of Electroenceph. Clin. Neurophysiol., Vol. 4B. Elsevier, Amsterdam.

Webber, W.R., Litt, B., Wilson, K. and Lesser, R.P. (1994) Practical detection of epileptiform discharges (EDs) in the EEG using an artificial neural network: a comparison of raw and parameterized EEG data. Electroenceph. Clin. Neurophysiol. 91: 194–204.

Yingling, C.D., Galin, D., Fein, G. et al. (1986) Neurometrics does not detect 'pure' dyslexics. Electroenceph. Clin. Neurophysiol. 63: 426–430.

Yvert, B., Bertrand, O., Echallier, J.F. et al. (1996) Improved dipole localization using local mesh refinement of realistic head geometries: an EEG simulation study. Electroenceph. Clin. Neurophysiol. 99: 79–89.

Part B

The normal EEG

8 Definition of the normal EEG, relation to brain function

SUMMARY

(8.1) An EEG is called normal because it lacks abnormal patterns known to be associated with clinical disorders. A statistically rare EEG pattern is not necessarily a clinically relevant finding.

(8.2) A normal EEG does not guarantee the absence of cerebral pathology because not all abnormalities of brain structure and function produce abnormalities of the EEG.

(8.3) An abnormal EEG does not always indicate a clinically significant cerebral abnormality. A few specific mild EEG abnormalities can be seen in some instances in persons without any apparent or clinically significant cerebral disorder.

8.1 DEFINITION OF THE NORMAL EEG

A wide variety of normal EEG patterns can be seen in different persons of the same age, and an even greater variety of normal patterns can occur in different age groups; recordings during wakefulness and drowsiness generally show more variability between subjects than recordings performed during sleep. It cannot be overemphasized that *statistically unusual or rare findings are not necessarily abnormal*. For example, many of the benign pseudoepileptiform patterns occur infrequently or rarely but rarity of occurrence is not the same thing as clinical significance. It is therefore not practical to define the normal EEG by listing all normal patterns and their variations; such a list would be too long. Nor can the normal EEG usually be defined by requiring that specific normal components be present; in this regard, the EEG differs somewhat from other tests such as the electrocardiogram. The problem of defining the normal EEG is therefore better approached in a different way. In contrast to the great variety of normal patterns, there are only a few EEG components, such as spikes and sharp waves, certain slow waves and amplitude changes, which have been proven to be definitely abnormal in each age group. The normal EEG can therefore be defined more effectively by the absence of abnormal components than by the presence of normal patterns. Conversely, an EEG is considered abnormal if it contains abnormal components regardless of whether or not it also contains normal components. The EEG reader therefore has to know the major features of the normal EEG at different ages and to distinguish from them abnormal components by using a set of precise descriptors (Chapter 9).

8.1.1 *The normal EEG up to the age of 19 years.* The normal EEG undergoes striking changes from the early premature period to about the age of 19 years. Characteristic patterns appear at fairly predictable ages and later disappear or change into more mature patterns. The variety of normal patterns is greater during this period than during adulthood. Even abnormalities such as spikes and slow waves in the neonate have different clinical implications than when seen later in life. Little is known about the clinical significance of the failure of normal patterns to appear and disappear at expected ages; less than severe failure of electrographic maturation is suggestive but not indicative of behavioral retardation.

8.1.2 *The normal EEG of adults.* Between the ages of 20 and 60 years, the typical normal EEG shows only few changes. The limits between normal and abnormal patterns are more easily identified in this age group than in younger persons and abnormal patterns correspond fairly well with basic types of brain lesions.

8.1.3 *The normal EEG above the age of 60 years.* The normal EEG at this age is similar to that of younger adults except that a few specific patterns which would be considered abnormal in younger adults become acceptable as normal.

8.2   A NORMAL EEG DOES NOT ALWAYS MEAN NORMAL BRAIN FUNCTION

Although acute, severe and anatomically large abnormalities of the brain are likely to cause EEG abnormalities, normal EEGs may be seen in some cases with small lesions or in others with long-standing, mild and limited cerebral abnormalities. For instance, a small infarct in the internal capsule far from the recording electrodes may cause a catastrophic hemiplegia but little or no EEG abnormality. A large infarction near the recording electrodes may cause EEG changes that last for a few weeks or months but then disappear even though some neurological deficit persists. The EEG may remain normal for a long period in slowly progressive, widespread brain diseases, such as Alzheimer's dementia, which cause cerebral atrophy and mental changes. An epileptogenic focus may escape detection if it does not fire during the recording or if its orientation or distance from the convexity of the brain interferes with volume conduction to the recording electrodes.

8.3   AN ABNORMAL EEG DOES NOT NECESSARILY MEAN CLINICALLY ABNORMAL BRAIN FUNCTION

Most abnormal EEG patterns indicate abnormal brain function. However, abnormal patterns occur occasionally in persons not showing evidence of brain disease. The type and incidence of these patterns are fairly well known in adults. A slight excess of a certain kind of slow waves (21.1.2) and an EEG of unusually low amplitude (24.2.2) occur in about 5–

15% of clinically normal persons after the age of 20 years. One might be inclined to call these patterns normal, especially since they occur most commonly in apparently normal persons; however, the same patterns can be seen to develop in patients with mild forms of diseases which, in their more severe stages, are associated with more pronounced expressions of the same EEG patterns. This suggests that in at least some persons, mild manifestations of these patterns indicate mild neurophysiological abnormalities. In order not to overlook the possibility of such cerebral abnormalities, one should therefore categorize even the mild forms of these patterns as EEG abnormalities. This attitude finds some support in studies showing that the incidence of these mild EEG abnormalities decreases in groups of healthy persons, such as airline pilots, who have passed rigorous examinations.

REFERENCES

Goldensohn, E.S., Legatt, A.D., Koszer, S. and Wolf, S.M. (1998) EEG Interpretation: Problems of Overreading and Underreading. Second revised and updated edition. Futura, Armonk, New York.

Hawkes, C.H. and Prescott, R.J. (1973) EEG variation in heatlhy subjects. Electroenceph. Clin. Neurophysiol. 34: 197–199.

Hughes, J.R. (1987) Normal limits in the EEG. In: A.M. Halliday, S.R. Butler and R. Paul (Eds.), A Textbook of Clinical Neurophysiology. Wiley, Chichester, pp. 105–154.

Kellaway, P. (1979) An orderly approach to visual analysis: the parameters of the normal EEG in adults and children. In: Current Practice of Clinical Neurophysiology. Raven Press, New York, pp. 69–148.

Klass, D.W. (1987) Identifying the abnormal EEG. In: A.M. Halliday, S.R. Butler and R. Paul (Eds.), A Textbook of Clinical Neurophysiology. Wiley, Chichester, pp. 189–200.

Maulsby, R.L. (1979) EEG patterns of uncertain diagnostic significance. In: D.W. Klass and D.D. Daly (1979) Current Practice of Clinical EEG. Raven Press, New York, pp. 411–420.

Maulsby, R.L., Kellaway, P., Graham, M., Forst, J., Proler, M.L., Low, M.D. and North, R.R. (1968) The Normative Electroencephalographic Data Reference Library. Final Report, Contract NAS 9–1200, National Aeronautics and Space Administration, 172 pp.

Van Dis, H., Corner, M., Dapper, R., Hanewald, G. and Hok, H. (1979) Individual differences in the human electroencephalogram during quiet wakefulness. Electroenceph. Clin. Neurophysiol. 47: 87–94.

Westmoreland, B.F. (1982) Normal and benign EEG patterns. Am. J. EEG Technol. 22: 3–31.

9 Descriptors of EEG activity

SUMMARY

To properly describe and analyze the EEG, the reader needs to understand the following terms: (1) *morphology*; (2) *repetition*; (3) *frequency*; (4) *amplitude*; (5) *distribution*; (6) *phase relation*; (7) *timing*; (8) *persistence*; and (9) *reactivity*. Digital signal analysis can be used to more precisely examine waveform features such as peak-to-peak amplitude, precise frequency content (e.g., using spectral analysis), similarities between signals (timing and waveforms) and their topography (distribution) over the head.

9.1 WAVEFORM

Waveform is a term used to describe the shape of a wave. Other synonyms used include *waveform morphology* or *configuration*. Any change in the difference of the electrical potential between two recording electrodes is called a *wave*, regardless of its form. Any wave or sequence of waves is simply referred to as EEG *activity*. Many waves repeat themselves in a series with an essentially unchanging morphology. A rhythmic run of waveforms of similar shape is referred to as *regular* or *monomorphic* (Fig. 9.1, Part 1). When regular waves are similar to sine waves they are described as *sinusoidal* (Fig. 9.1, Part 2) while other regular waves may be arch-shaped (wicket-shaped) or saw-toothed (asymmetrical triangular-shaped). Waveforms that do not have a sinusoidal or simple geometric shape are referred to as *irregular*. *Irregular activity* consists of waveforms with constantly changing shape and duration (Fig. 9.1, Part 4).

A *monophasic* wave has a single deflection either up or down from the baseline. A *diphasic* wave has two components on opposite sides of the baseline while a *triphasic* wave has three components alternating about the baseline. A *polyphasic* or *multiphasic* wave has two or more components of different direction. These terms do not indicate whether a wave has relatively positive or negative electrical polarity (3.4.1) or whether it was recorded with a bipolar or referential electrode montage (4.1).

A *transient* is an event that clearly stands out against the background. It consists of either a single wave or a *complex,* i.e., a sequence of two or more waves that have a characteristic form or recur with a fairly consistent shape (Fig. 9.1, Part 5).

A *sharp transient* is a wave of any duration that has a pointed peak at conventional EEG recording speed. Sharply contoured waveforms that are not judged to be abnormal epileptiform waveforms are often referred to as *sharp transients*. *Epileptiform* is a term used to describe EEG patterns that are identical to those that have been specifically associated with seizures or epilepsy. Epileptiform patterns usually consist of apiculate (i.e., sharply contoured) waveforms referred to as

spikes or *sharp waves*. A *spike* is a sharply contoured waveform with a duration of 20–70 ms (Fig. 9.1, Part 7). A *sharp wave* has a duration of 70–200 ms and may not be as sharply contoured as a spike (Fig. 9.1, Part 6).

The duration of an epileptiform spike or sharp wave is a reflection of the size of the anatomical area of activity and synchrony of the participating neuronal population: the longer duration sharp wave is associated with less synchronous

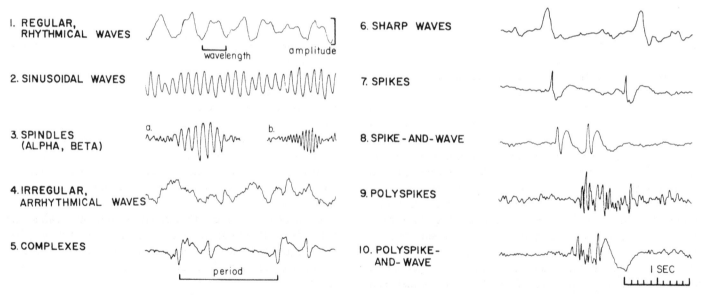

1. REGULAR, RHYTHMICAL WAVES

wavelength   amplitude

2. SINUSOIDAL WAVES

3. SPINDLES (ALPHA, BETA)

4. IRREGULAR, ARRHYTHMICAL WAVES

5. COMPLEXES

period

6. SHARP WAVES

7. SPIKES

8. SPIKE-AND-WAVE

9. POLYSPIKES

10. POLYSPIKE-AND-WAVE

I SEC

Fig. 9.1. Characteristic waveforms.

146

neuronal cell population discharge. The actual clinical importance of distinguishing between spikes and sharp waves is uncertain. Therefore, although spikes and sharp waves are clearly defined, most electroencephalographers use these terms interchangeably, in particular substituting the term spike(s) for sharp wave(s). Sharply contoured waveforms that: (1) appear as part of the background rhythm (e.g., the mu rhythm), (2) appear at different times either in isolation or as part of the background rhythm (e.g., wicket spikes; 19.4.5), (3) demonstrate a varying morphology, or (4) only occur once in the entire record usually, cannot be identified as epileptiform abnormalities and are therefore referred to as *sharp transients* or *non-specific sharp transients* (see also 17.1.1).

A spike may be followed by a slow wave and form a *spike-and-wave complex* (Fig. 9.1, Part 8) which may occur in isolation or repeat at regular intervals. Rhythmic runs of spike-and-wave complexes occurring at rates below 3 Hz are called *slow spike-and-wave complexes*. A sharp wave may also be followed by a slow wave and form a *sharp-and-slow-wave complex;* complexes of this kind usually last longer than a third of a second and therefore do not repeat at rates over 3 Hz. In some cases, two or more spikes occur in sequence, forming *multiple spike complexes (*formerly referred to as *polyspike complexes,* Fig. 9.1, Part 9). These complexes may be followed by a slow wave and thus form part of a *multiple spike-and-slow-wave complex,* also referred to as a *polyspike-and-slow-wave complex* (Fig. 9.1, Part 10). Spikes recorded in the EEG are not the same as action potentials or other brief electrophy-

siological events recorded directly from single nerve cells through microelectrodes. Although they are also often referred to as spikes they are never observed in the surface EEG.

Single spikes and sharp waves, and complexes that contain spikes and sharp waves and last for less than a few seconds are referred to as *interictal epileptiform activity;* longer lasting activity of this type of epileptiform activity that shows an evolving pattern in terms of amplitude and frequency is referred to as an *electrographic seizure pattern* or *ictal pattern* (17.1). Although seizure patterns are often associated with clinical seizure manifestations, they may occur without such correlates and are then called *subclinical electrographic seizure patterns.* Both interictal and ictal patterns are commonly called *epileptiform* despite the definition in the glossary of the International Federation of Societies for Electroencephalography and Clinical Neurophysiology which uses the term 'epileptiform' only for interictal patterns.

A *paroxysm* or a *paroxysmal discharge* consists of one or more waves that begin abruptly, stand out from the ongoing EEG activity, reach maximum amplitude rapidly, and disappear suddenly. Paroxysms often consist of complexes (Fig. 9.1, Part 5), whereas not all complexes begin and end abruptly, and not all paroxysms recur with a similar shape. *Paroxysms* or *paroxysmal discharges* may be normal (as in sudden onset patterns of drowsiness or benign pseudoepileptiform patterns) or they may be abnormal (as in epileptiform ictal or interictal patterns). Unfortunately, these terms have been used interchangeably by some electroencephalographers with the terms *epileptiform* and *electrographic seizure pattern* causing some confusion. Therefore it is best to always qualify these terms as being abnormal or normal and as being epileptiform or not and to not use them interchangeably with more precise terms. Similarly, the terms spike(s) and sharp wave(s) have been used by some electroencephalographers to describe epileptiform patterns, but they are not synonymous with abnormal epileptiform activity. Thus, *if epileptiform activity is considered to be present, then the term epileptiform should be added to any other descriptive term used.* For example, if an epileptiform abnormality is present it would be incorrect to simply state: The EEG is abnormal due to the presence of spikes that are maximal over the left anterior temporal area. Instead it should be rephrased as: The EEG is abnormal due to the presence of epileptiform spikes maximal over the left anterior temporal area.

9.2   REPETITION

Repetition of waves in a particular frequency range may be referred to as *rhythmic, semirhythmic,* or *irregular. Rhythmical* repetitive waves have similar intervals between individual waves; the waveforms are usually regular and often sinusoidal in shape (Fig. 9.1, Parts 1–3). *Spindles* are groups of rhythmical repetitive waves that gradually increase and then decrease in amplitude (Fig. 9.1, Part 3). Rhythmical repetitive waves are also referred to as *monorhythmic* or *monomorphic. Semi-*

rhythmic repetitive waves contain some recurring similar morphology waveforms as well as some intermixed irregular waveforms. *Irregular* repetitive waves are characterized by variable, irregular intervals between individual waveforms that vary in their shape (Fig. 9.1, Part 4). Thus they appear as a sequence of waves of different morphology that usually have an asymmetric, non-sinusoidal shape. Irregular repetitive waves are also referred to as polyrhythmic or polymorphic.

9.3   FREQUENCY

Frequency refers to the number of times a repetitive wave recurs in 1 s. A wave that can complete three cycles in 1 s is called a 3 Hz or 3/s waveform. The frequency of single or repetitive waves can be determined by measuring the duration of an individual wave, the *wavelength* (Fig. 9.1, Part 1), and calculating the reciprocal. For instance, a wave lasting 250 ms or 0.25 s is said to have a frequency of 4 Hz, regardless of whether or not it repeats. Single waves and complexes may repeat at intervals longer than the wavelength and are then called periodic, the *period* being the time interval between them (Fig. 9.1, Part 5).

The frequency of EEG waves is divided into 4 groups or *frequency bands,* namely:
– delta frequency band: under 4 Hz;
– theta frequency band: from 4 to under 8 Hz;

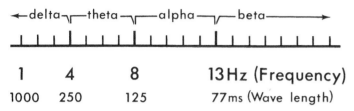

Fig. 9.2. Frequency bands. Delta, theta, alpha and beta frequency bands, defined by wave frequency and length.

– alpha frequency band: from 8 to 13 Hz;
– beta frequency band: over 13 Hz (Fig. 9.2).

Notice, these band definitions leave *no gaps* between individual frequency bands. These divisions are somewhat arbitrary in the sense that many EEGs contain waves of frequencies extending across the boundaries of the bands, for instance waves of 3–5 Hz. Nonetheless, they help the electroencephalographer to describe the most important normal and abnormal waves in the EEG, and frequency is one of the most important criteria for assessing abnormality in clinical EEG. Although waves under 8 Hz are commonly called *slow waves* and waves over 13 Hz are commonly called *fast waves,* it is more accurate and therefore preferable to either state the frequency of the activity (e.g., 3–5 Hz) or describe it according to the frequency band(s) it occupies (e.g., delta and theta activity). Activity that is either less than 0.5 Hz or greater than 20 Hz is of limited clinical utility in routine scalp recordings because it is often unclear if such activity is of cerebral origin

(6.1–3). Frequencies and frequency ranges are usually stated in divisions no smaller than 0.5 Hz. For example the alpha rhythm given by routine visual inspection may be stated as 9–9.5 Hz, not 9–9.25 Hz because it is usually not possible to make 0.25 Hz distinctions by routine visual inspection alone. Using digital EEG signal analysis more precise frequency measures may be determined.

9.4 AMPLITUDE

Amplitude of EEG waves is measured in microvolts (μV). It is determined by measuring and comparing the total vertical distance of a wave (Fig. 9.1, Part 1) to the height of a calibration signal recorded at the same gain and filter settings (3.3.1). Thus, if the height of an EEG wave measures 14 mm and a calibration signal of 50 μV measures 7 mm, the amplitude of the wave is 100 μV. If the sensitivity of an amplifier is known to be 7 μV/mm (3.4.2), a wave of 7 mm can be inferred to have an amplitude of 50 μV without direct comparison with a calibration pulse. Amplitude should not be expressed in terms of the height of the pen deflection in millimeters because this varies with the amplifier settings.

In clinical EEG, amplitude is often not reported in terms of microvolts but described loosely as *low* (under 20 μV), *medium* (20–50 μV), or *high* (over 50 μV). However, these terms often are used to describe amplitude of certain waves relative to that of other waves in the same record. For instance, a wave of 60

μV is not referred to as high amplitude if it occurs on a background of 40–50 μV activity. Moreover, it is meaningless to state the μV value without naming the montage because changing the montage changes the voltage. *Longer interelectrode distances produce increasing amplitudes up to an interelectrode distance of about 8 cm.*

Amplitude asymmetry is defined as the difference in amplitude of activity that is recorded simultaneously from corresponding mirror image parts of the two sides of the head. As stated in Chapter 4, an asymmetry seen in one bipolar montage should be verified using another montage oriented at 90° to the first (e.g., longitudinal vs. transverse bipolar) or a reference montage. Even slight differences of amplitude may be of clinical importance (23.2) if they persist; this is true especially of the adult EEG, with the exception of the alpha rhythm (11.1) and posterior occipital sharp transients (POSTs) of sleep.

Differences of amplitude are sometimes caused by factors outside the brain, especially by unequal spacing and impedance of the recording electrodes; the technologist should therefore verify correct electrode placements (2.3) and impedances (2.2) before accepting that an abnormal amplitude difference is genuine.

9.5   DISTRIBUTION

Distribution refers to the occurrence of electrical activity recorded by electrodes positioned over different parts of the head. EEG patterns may appear over large areas on both sides of the head, over one side only, or in a restricted, small area.

9.5.1   *Widespread, diffuse* or *generalized* distribution refers to activity which occurs at the same time over most or all of the head. Generalized activity may have a clear maximum within its field of distribution, recognized by the highest amplitude in referential recordings and by phase reversal in bipolar recordings from that area (4.1).

9.5.2   *Lateralized* distribution refers to activity which appears only or mostly on one side of the head. Lateralized activity is abnormal and suggests a cerebral abnormality either on the side where abnormal activity is present or on the side where normal activity is absent. Normal patterns (such as vertex waves or sleep spindles) may demonstrate *shifting lateralization*; that is, they appear on one side of the head at one time and then occur on the other side a few seconds or minutes later (9.7).

9.5.3   *Focal* or *localized* activity is restricted to one or a few electrodes over an area of the head. Some of the neighboring electrodes may pick up the same activity with lower amplitude. This restricted distribution must be distinguished from a wide or generalized distribution that may have a maximum in one area. This distinction is important especially with regard to abnormal slow waves and to sharp waves. Criteria that sometimes help in making this distinction are that *focal slow waves* often have a lower frequency and fewer intermixed alpha and beta waveforms at the area of maximum amplitude, whereas generalized slow waves do not. *Focal sharp waves* with a tendency to spread can often be distinguished from generalized sharp waves with a local maximum of amplitude by their greater persistence at the focus.

Activity arising from a single unilateral focus is almost always abnormal. Activity from a midline focus or from two foci located symmetrically in the two hemispheres may be part of a normal pattern.

Multifocal epileptiform pattern is a term only applied to recordings in which there are three or more anatomically distinct areas generating epileptiform spikes or sharp waves.

In describing the location of focal or localized patterns in the descriptive part of the EEG report, *electrode names should be used, not head regions or brain areas*. In contrast, in the impression or clinical correlation portion of the report head or brain regions should be stated to convey meaningful information to the referring physician.

9.6 PHASE RELATION

Phase refers to the timing and polarity of components of waves in one or more channels. Waves of different frequency may occur in different channels so that the troughs and peaks occur at the same time; these waves are said to be *in phase*. If they do not coincide in this manner, they are said to be *out of phase*. The phase difference may be expressed in terms of phase angle. For instance, peaks pointing in opposite directions are said to be 180° out of phase. Such a *'phase reversal'* is the major indicator of the origin of EEG potentials in bipolar recordings (4.1.1). In a single channel, phase refers to the time relationship between different components of a rhythm; for instance, the peak of a sine wave is said to 'lead' the preceding crossing of the zero line by 90° and to 'lag' behind the next following peak by 360°.

9.7 TIMING

Timing of waves in different areas of the head may be similar or different. The terms *'simultaneous'* and *'synchronous'* are used to indicate that two events occurred at the same time. These terms are usually used with the same meaning, but 'synchronous' is more often used to denote precise phase coincidence of waveforms appearing simultaneously over both hemispheres.

Using analog systems the eye can hardly distinguish a horizontal difference of less than 1 mm between corresponding points on two waves even in neighboring channels. A horizontal distance of only 1 mm corresponds to a time difference of 33 ms at the conventional EEG recording speed. The resolution of time relations deteriorates if more distant channels are compared and if the writing units are not perfectly aligned;

because of the curvilinear movement of the pens, synchronous excursions of different amplitude seem to have occurred at different times (3.6.1). In contrast, very precise timing distinctions can be made using digital instruments. A 1 s time epoch can be spread across the entire monitor screen so that 5 ms or less timing differences can be appreciated. If any difference in timing between two signals is seen using such precise measurement, it is assumed that it is the result of propagated or transsynaptic transmission. If no timing difference can be seen then it is likely that the spread of a given waveform has taken place by volume conduction.

Waves which occur at the same time on both sides of the head are called 'bilaterally synchronous' or 'bisynchronous'. These terms consider mainly the relationship between the two sides but not necessarily that on the same side; thus, bilaterally synchronous waves may be out of phase in the same hemisphere. In some instances, waves are delayed against each other by the same amount in successive channels which record activity from electrodes placed from the front to the back of the head, giving the impression that these waves spread from front to back. For instance, this type of gradual phase delay from the front to the back of the head can be seen in triphasic waves of metabolic encephalopathies (19.2.6).

Waveforms that occur in different channels without constant time relation to each other are called 'asynchronous'. This usually implies that the waveforms are present in different areas at the same time even though they do not fall in phase with each or do not have the same frequency. If waves occur in one area at one time and in other areas at another time, they are said to be *independent;* for instance, spikes in both temporal lobes may occur bisynchronously or independently; each case has different implications regarding a possible triggering mechanism.

9.8 PERSISTENCE

Persistence describes how often a wave or pattern occurs during a recording. Some waveforms occur only occasionally or intermittently, either in the form of a single wave or trains of waves; other waves are present through most or all of the recording. The persistence of waves can be estimated by measuring the proportion of time during which these waves appear. This is called the *index.* For instance, a delta index of 20% means that delta activity was present 20% of the recording time. In polysomnography a delta index measure is to determine the presence or absence of stages III and IV sleep in each 30 s epoch of recording. Stage III sleep is present if 20–50% of an epoch contains 2 Hz or slower waveforms with amplitudes of 75 μV or greater in C3 to A2. Stage IV sleep is present if greater than 50% of an epoch contains 2 Hz or slower waveforms with amplitudes of 75 μV or greater in C3 to A2. Because the clinical importance of EEG patterns often depends not only on their persistence but also on their amplitude, the persistence and amplitude are often described together in terms of their *quantity, amount* or *prominence.* The term 'abundance', previously used to describe this combination of persistence and amplitude, is no longer used.

Single waves and complexes may occur with a high, moderate or low persistence or incidence; the persistence of these events can be expressed as an interval index, i.e., their average number in 1 s or 1 min. They may occur periodically or at irregular intervals. Irregular and infrequent occurrence is also often referred to as *'sporadic'*. (The terms 'random' and 'diffuse' should not be used to describe persistence of EEG patterns.) Hemispheric differences in rhythmic background patterns (such as the alpha rhythm) may not consist of amplitude differences but of differences in how consistently the pattern is present over one hemisphere compared to the other. If a background rhythm is less *persistent* over one hemisphere it may also be described as *poorly sustained,* whereas the background pattern over the opposite hemisphere is described as *well sustained.*

9.9   REACTIVITY

Reactivity refers to changes that can be produced in some normal and abnormal patterns by various maneuvers. Some patterns are induced or increased, diminished or blocked by opening or closing the eyes, hyperventilation, photic or sensory stimuli, changes in levels of alertness, movements or other maneuvers. Abnormal slow waves in toxic and metabolic encephalopathies are often diminished by alerting and enhanced by hyperventilation and drowsiness whereas abnormal slow waves seen in cases of structural lesions usually show less attenuation or blocking during alerting maneuvers.

A recording should not be considered complete unless at least simple alerting maneuvers have been performed to demonstrate the effects of arousal on the EEG. These maneuvers include eye opening and closing (this may be passively performed for infants or other individuals who cannot respond to verbal commands) and questions requiring greater vigilance such as those testing memory and simple calculations. If the patient is unable to respond to verbal commands then vigorous auditory and vigorous or painful tactile stimulation should be applied. These maneuvers will also help clarify if background slowing is actually present or if the patient was merely excessively drowsy during the recording. In patients in coma not due to general anesthesia, hypothermia, or hypotension, an invariant pattern (a pattern lacking spontaneous variability) and a complete absence of EEG reactivity are almost always indicative of a poor prognosis for survival.

REFERENCES

Binnie, C.D. (1987) Electroencephalography and epilepsy. In: A. Hopkins (Ed.), Epilepsy. Demos, New York, pp. 169–200.
Blume, W.T. and Lemieux, J.F. (1988) Morphology of spikes in spike-and-wave complexes. Electroenceph. Clin. Neurophysiol. 69: 508–515.
Daube, J.R. (1996) Waveform parameter classification. In: J. Daube (Ed.), Clinical Neurophysiology. F.A. Davis, Philadelphia, pp. 60–64.

Chatrian, G.E., Bergamini, L., Dondey, M., Klass, D.W., Lennox-Buchthal, M. and Petersén, I. (1974) A glossary of terms most commonly used by clinical electroencephalographers. Electroenceph. Clin. Neurophysiol. 37: 538–548.

Gastaut, H. (1975) Section 1. The significance of the EEG and of ictal and interictal discharges with respect to epilepsy. In: A. Rémond (Ed.), Handbook of Electroenceph. Clin. Neurophysiol., Vol. 13A. Elsevier, Amsterdam, pp. 3–6.

Niedermeyer, E. (1993) Abnormal EEG patterns: Epileptic and paroxysmal. In: E. Niedermeyer and F. Lopes da Silva (Eds.), Electroencephalography: Basic Principles, Clinical Applications and Related Fields. Urban and Schwarzenberg, Baltimore, pp. 217–240.

Pedley, T.A. (1980) Interictal epileptiform discharges: Discriminating characteristics and clinical correlations. Am. J. EEG Technol. 20: 101–109.

Westmoreland, B.F. (1996) Epileptiform electroencephalographic patterns. Mayo Clin. Proc. 71: 501–511.

10 The normal EEG from premature age to the age of 19 years

SUMMARY

The maturation of EEG patterns parallels the anatomical and physiological development of the brain. As with brain development, the most dramatic EEG changes occur between the early premature age and the first 3 months of life.

The EEG patterns expressed during the first 6 months following birth are closely correlated with the infant's conceptional age (CA), i.e. the gestational age plus the legal age (time since birth), or actual physiological age. The premature baby develops new EEG patterns and modifies the acquired ones within fairly narrow ranges of conceptional age. Different periods of premature and mature neonatal life can be distinguished according to EEG and behavioral patterns that appear at various conceptional ages.

(10.1.1) *Less than 29 weeks,* the EEG is continuously discontinuous and bilaterally synchronous (a pattern referred to as *tracé discontinu*). The *delta brush* pattern emerges at 26 weeks CA.

(10.1.2) *29 to 31 weeks,* greater periods of continuous activity emerge, periods of suppression rarely exceed 30 s, delta brushes appear frequently. Interhemispheric synchrony during tracé discontinu is at its lowest and the *temporal theta burst* pattern, a distinctive finding at this age, is seen.

(10.1.3) *32 to 34 weeks,* EEG reactivity to vigorous stimulation is established, periods of diffuse attenuation usually last less than 15 s, and *multifocal sharp transients* and *delta brushes* are abundant.

(10.1.4) *34 to 37 weeks,* EEG reactivity to stimulation is present in all states, *delta brushes* begin to appear less often and are more frequent in quiet than active sleep, *multifocal sharp transients* are less frequent and well formed medium to high amplitude *frontal sharp transients* appear. The *tracé discontinu* pattern is replaced by the less strikingly discontinuous pattern of *tracé alternant*.

(10.1.5) *At the conceptional age of 38 weeks* the premature infant has developed EEG patterns similar to those of the full-term (40 weeks CA) newborn. Wakefulness, active sleep, and quiet sleep are clearly differentiated and the 4 basic EEG neonatal patterns are established:

(a) *low voltage irregular* (LVI, seen in wakefulness and active sleep),

(b) *mixed voltage* pattern (MV, seen in wakefulness, transitional sleep and active sleep),

(c) *high voltage slow* (HVS, seen in quiet sleep), and

(d) *tracé alternant* (TA, seen in quiet sleep).

(10.2) *After 46 weeks conceptional age,* the neonatal patterns are replaced by patterns which show different rhythms in different areas. This differentiation, and the frequency of the rhythms, increases rapidly during the first year of life.

(10.3) *During the first 3 months after birth in a full-term infant* there is a gradual loss of neonatal patterns and a posterior dominant amplitude gradient is prominent during wakefulness and quiet sleep. Five to 6 Hz rhythms are present over the central head regions that increase to 5–8 Hz by 4–6 months of age. Between 3 and 4 months of age approximately three-fourths of normal infants demonstrate a 3–4 Hz occipital rhythm during wakefulness that is activated by passive eye closure and attenuated by passive eye opening or alerting. This reactive occipital rhythm is the precursor of the alpha rhythm. Between 2 and 3 months of age sleep spindles appear over the central head regions with varying interhemispheric synchrony and symmetry.

(10.4) *During childhood and late adolescence,* several age-specific patterns appear transiently, but frequency of background waveforms during wakefulness continues to shift higher into the alpha (8–13 Hz) and beta (>13 Hz) range.

10.1 NEONATAL EEG

Neonatal EEG recording places special demands on both the electroencephalographer and the technologist. First, there are a number of age specific normal electrographic features that are prominent for only several weeks at a time. Second, many of the patterns occurring in the neonatal period have very different clinical implications than when seen at later ages (such as multifocal sharp transients or discontinuous patterns). Finally, special polygraphic recording techniques are necessary for measuring a variety of physiological functions in the routine neonatal EEG recording (eye movements, muscle tone, respiratory effort, and airflow) so that the main behavioral states of the newborn (wakefulness, transitional or indeterminate sleep, active sleep and quiet sleep) can be recorded (5.2).

With few exceptions, the EEG of the neonate is a function of the actual age of the brain. The actual age of the neonate from the time of conception is referred to as the *conceptional age* (CA). Knowledge of the conceptional age is essential for accurate EEG interpretation and should always be noted on the record by the technologist. The conceptional age is determined by adding the estimated *gestational age* (the number of weeks and days of intrauterine life since the last menstrual period) to the *legal age* (the number of days and weeks since the time of birth). Thus, the EEG of a normal 4-week-old neonate who was born at 30 weeks gestation will show the same kinds of EEG patterns as a l-week-old born at 33 weeks of gestation since they both have the same conceptional age (34 weeks). Under abnormal circumstances a pattern that is appropriate at one conceptional age may appear at a later age. This persistence or reappearance of patterns with immature features is referred to as *dysmaturity* or *anachronism*. Dysmaturity may be transient and associated with reversible cerebral disorders (such as electrolyte disturbances or mild anoxia due to pulmonary disease), or may be present on repeated recordings and associated with more enduring disorders of cerebral function (e.g., ischemic-hypoxic encephalopathy or intraventricular hemorrhage). When a more mature EEG pattern than expected is seen it is usually because the conceptional age has been underestimated. The term dysmaturity is also used to describe records in which there is a combination of patterns that are both appropriate and inappropriate for age.

The EEG and other physiological findings that define the behavioral state of the neonate develop together in an organized and predictable fashion. Behavioral states are assessed from the EEG and polygraphic electrographic recordings of body movements, eye movements, respiratory pattern and EMG. Frequent notations by the technologist are extremely important for verifying the accuracy of the electrographic monitors and providing a final source of information about specific movements, behavioral changes, artifacts and the activities of other individuals in the recording environment. Body movements in the neonate can usually be characterized as phasic (rapid) or tonic (slow and sustained muscle contractions). Respiration can be described as regular (appearing as monorhythmic fluctuations in recordings from nasal thermistor or thoracic strain gauge monitors) or irregular (in repetition rate and amplitude).

Each neonatal recording should ideally include the following monitors (as described in Chapter 4):

(1) eye movement monitors (2 channels),
(2) a submental EMG activity monitor,
(3) an electrocardiogram monitor recorded in one channel using electrodes placed on either arm (this channel can then also be used for detecting body movements), and
(4) two respiratory monitors: a thoracic strain gauge or motion transducer to detect chest wall movements in one channel, and a nasal and oral thermistor to detect airflow in the other channel.

As in adults, *central apnea* (an absence of breathing due to a complete interruption of both diaphragmatic and chest wall movement) will appear as the cessation of activity in both monitors, whereas *obstructive apnea* (a block in air flow due to intermittent upper airway obstruction) will appear as continuing chest wall movement without evidence of airflow.

Neonatal EEG recordings may be performed with electrodes placed either at all the standard 10–20 positions or with a reduced array. There are several reasons why most laboratories use a reduced number of electrode positions (see Table 4.4 and Section 5.2):

(1) the relatively small head size of the neonate allows for an adequate sampling of EEG activity with fewer electrodes;
(2) the crowding together of a full set of electrodes increases the likelihood of inadvertently connecting adjacent electrodes with salt bridges; and
(3) the use of fewer electrodes simplifies the recording procedure which is often performed in very fragile or unstable patients and under difficult circumstances.

However, *the newborn EEG can contain focal patterns with remarkably high amplitude compared to the EEG in later life*. For example, the omission of a Cz electrode has been shown to result in a complete failure to record electrographic seizure patterns that were not apparent at adjacent electrodes. Therefore, the electrode array should sample all major head regions.

Although premature and full-term neonatal EEG recordings are often run at routine paper recording speeds of 3 cm/s, many laboratories perform part or all of the recording at a slower speed of 1.5 cm/s. Slower recording speeds make it easier for the technologist to appreciate discontinuous background changes, transitions between continuous and discon-

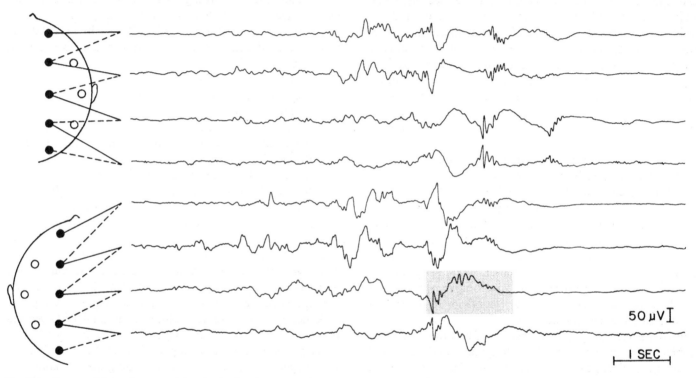

50 μV

1 SEC

Fig. 10.1. Pattern of discontinuous activity of quiet sleep in a normal premature baby of a conceptional age of 34 weeks, recorded 5 days after birth. Delta brush is marked by shading.

158

tinuous backgrounds, certain seizure patterns and the symmetry and rhythmicity of slower waveforms. During subsequent analysis with digital EEG recording speed is less of an issue because a variety of 'paper speeds' can be selected retrospectively. The duration of the routine neonatal record should be approximately 45–60 min. This usually allows for a sampling of all of the neonate's typical behavioral states. In the full-term infant sleep cycles usually last 45–60 min and consist of about 25 min of *active sleep*, 20 min of *quiet sleep*, and 10–15 min of *indeterminate sleep* (also referred to as *transitional sleep*). Wakefulness often makes recording impractical due to excessive movement artifact, but quiet wakefulness usually occurs soon after feeding and is more likely to produce an interpretable record. Therefore, it is advisable to *always try to record normal active newborns immediately following feeding*.

10.1.1 *Premature infants of less than 29 weeks conceptional age.* At approximately 28 weeks of life the major sulci of the brain are just beginning to appear. At this time there is relatively little variation in behavior except for occasional fluctuations in body motility. Open eye movements are rare but can occur spontaneously or only in response to vigorous stimulation. Respiration is continuously irregular. When body movements occur they are mostly tonic. Single or repetitive clonic jaw jerks are sometimes mistaken for seizure activity, but are normal at this age and throughout prematurity. Rarely clonic jaw jerks are also seen in full-term newborns.

EEG background activity this early in life is predominantly discontinuous (a finding which is universal among mammalian species in early prematurity) and consists of bursts of medium to high amplitude waveforms that are usually maximal over the posterior head regions. This activity interrupts an otherwise nearly flat background. Periods of EEG activity are typically brief, lasting less than 15 s. The intervals between the bursts have an average duration of 8–12 s but may occasionally last up to 25–30 s. This pattern is referred to as *tracé discontinu*. The duration of the relative flattening becomes shorter during periods of increased motor activity and with increasing age. Under abnormal circumstances, such as cerebral hypoxia, the interburst interval becomes longer in duration. As the newborn matures the tracé discontinu pattern eventually gives way to a less strikingly discontinuous pattern called *tracé alternant* in which the inter-burst periods have more activity and are shorter in duration. The tracé alternant pattern is well established between 34 and 36 weeks conceptional age (10.1.4) and rarely may be seen as late as 46 weeks conceptional age.

Interhemispheric synchrony, defined as a *less than 1.5 s difference in the time of onset of EEG burst activity between hemispheres during tracé alternant or tracé discontinu*, is well developed at this age. Indeed, approximately 90–100% of bursts begin within 1.5 s of each other until the neonate reaches 29–30 weeks CA. After that interhemispheric synchrony begins to decline and then in the last 6 weeks prior to birth reverses course increasing to almost 100% by term. The relationship

159

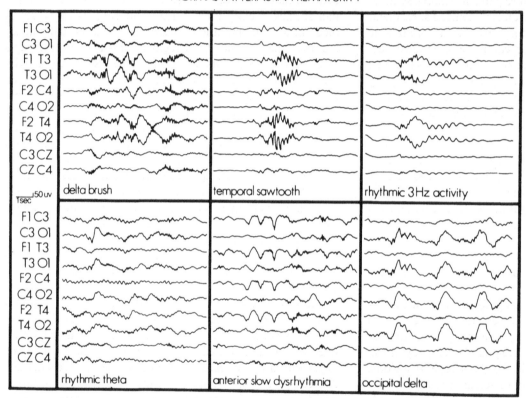

Fig. 10.2. These normal patterns seen in premature infants are sometimes mistaken for abnormalities. They were recorded at (from left to right, above to below): 33 weeks, 30 weeks, 28 weeks, 29 weeks, 35 weeks and 28 weeks conceptional age. (Courtesy S.S. Werner, J.E. Stockard and R.G. Bickford, Atlas of Neonatal EEG, Raven Press, New York, 1977.)

160

of interhemispheric synchrony to conceptional age summarized by Lombroso (1993) is as follows:

Conceptional age (weeks)	Indeterminate sleep (%)	Quiet sleep (%)	Active sleep (%)
26–28	90–100		
29–30	80–100		
31–32		50– 70	70–90
33–34		60– 80	
35–36		70– 85	
37–39		80–100	
40–42		100	

Thus, interhemispheric synchrony declines rapidly at 31–32 weeks CA and then gradually increases to nearly 100% at term.

The characteristic EEG feature seen at this age is the *delta brush pattern*. It first appears at about 26 weeks CA located over the central head region. Delta brushes consist of medium to high voltage (25–200 μV) 0.3–1.5 Hz delta waves with superimposed 10–150 μV rhythmic fast activity. The 'brush', or fast activity, is typically in the 8–22 Hz range, although somewhat slower, 4–6 Hz activity, may be also seen, particularly at this age. The abundance of delta brushes gradually declines throughout prematurity. The approximate frequency of occurrence of delta brushes at different ages can be summarized as follows (Lombroso, 1979):

Conceptional age (weeks)	Active sleep	Quiet sleep
31–32	6–11 min	4–10 min (tracé discontinu)
33–34	2–6 min	3– 8 min (tracé discontinu)
35–36	1.5 min	3– 7 min (tracé alternant)
37–38	Rare	1– 3 min (tracé alternant)

At less than 28 weeks CA delta activity may appear in rhythmic runs over the central head regions, or for shorter periods of time (less than 3 s) over the occipital area. Occipital theta or alpha activity lasting up to 10 s may also be present.

10.1.2 *Premature infants of 29–31 weeks of age.* Behavior at this age is characterized by more prominent variations between quiescence and body motility, rare periods of regular respiration, and irregular rapid eye movements (REM). Thus, differentiation of behavioral states begins to emerge at this stage of life. At the same time, the intensity of stimulation required to produce eye opening begins to decrease.

Active sleep, characterized by the appearance of continuous EEG activity in association with REM, irregular respiration and increased body motility occurs rarely. Well defined *quiet sleep,* characterized by discontinuous EEG activity, reduced eye and body movements and regular respiration is also infrequent. Thus, in the majority of routine recordings quiet and active sleep still cannot be clearly differentiated.

Interhemispheric synchrony is lowest between 31 and 32 weeks of conceptional age with approximately 30–50% of the onset of bursts between the left and right hemispheres occurring more than 1.5 s apart.

Delta brushes occur more frequently, particularly over the central, occipital and temporal head regions, and occur most often during periods of active sleep. In contrast, after 33–34 weeks conceptional age delta brushes are more often seen during quiet sleep. After 32 weeks CA the number of delta brushes begins to decline.

Theta bursts (also referred to as *temporal sawtooth waves* or *temporal theta rhythm*) with amplitudes up to 200 μV occur frequently over the temporal head regions in short runs (less than 1 s) of rhythmic, theta (4 to <8 Hz) frequency sharp wave complexes that occasionally resemble delta brushes (Fig. 10.2). They may appear in a unilateral or bisynchronous fashion. They are seen so rarely prior to 29 weeks or after 32 weeks that they are considered highly useful for estimating conceptional age.

10.1.3 *Premature infants of 32–34 weeks of age.* Motor activity is now more often phasic than tonic. Eye movements tend to occur in clusters and periods of regular respiration are more frequent.

Although activity typical of active and quiet sleep (as described in 10.1.2) is more likely to be seen than previously, much of the recording still contains *transitional (indeterminate) sleep* (sleep states which are not identifiable as either quiet or active sleep). Continuous EEG activity is seen more frequently and is associated with eye movements, active sleep and quiet wakefulness. *Tracé discontinu* contains shorter duration periods of relative inactivity. However, by 32 weeks CA these periods normally rarely exceed 15 s. Intermittent amplitude gradients appear with greater amplitude activity in the delta frequency range over the posterior head regions. Delta brushes are present in both active and quiet sleep predominantly over the central, temporal and occipital head regions.

Two other distinctive changes also occur at this age. The first is an increase in the number of *multifocal sharp transients* (Fig. 10.3) in all states. The second is the appearance of *EEG reactivity*: stimulation of the neonate now produces clear changes in the EEG.

10.1.4 *Premature infants of 34–37 weeks of age.* EEG reactivity is now present in all states and appears as either a widespread attenuation of activity or, less often, as an augmentation of activity. Active sleep is further defined by: (1) the appearance of more active eye movements during REM periods (including more vertical eye movements than seen previously) and (2) a decrease in tonic EMG activity (revealed by an attenuation of activity in the submental EMG monitor). Quiet sleep is seen more often in association with longer periods of regular respiration.

During periods of continuous EEG activity a spatial amplitude gradient appears intermittently with predominantly lower amplitude faster activity maximally over the anterior head

NORMAL TRANSIENTS IN PREMATURITY

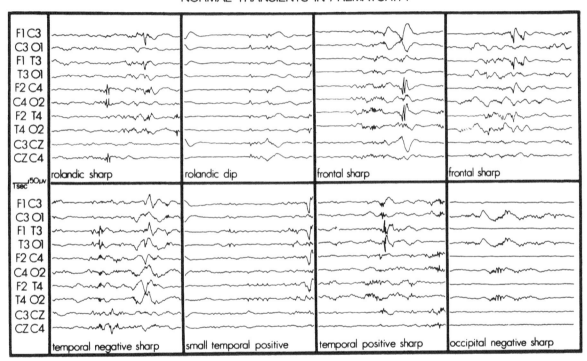

Fig. 10.3. These records illustrate the variability in location, amplitude, and duration of transients recorded in normal prematures at (from left to right, above to below): 33 weeks, 30 weeks, 28 weeks, 28 weeks, 33 weeks, 30 weeks, 33 weeks and 30 weeks. (Courtesy S.S. Werner, J.E. Stockard and R.G. Bickford, Atlas of Neonatal EEG. Raven Press, New York, 1977.)

regions and predominantly higher amplitude delta activity appearing maximally over the posterior head regions. *Delta brushes* are now more frequent during quiet sleep than during active sleep. It is also during this stage of life that the overall abundance of delta brushes begins to decline. This trend continues until they disappear at approximately 40 weeks CA, lastly appearing over the temporal or occipital head regions. With the appearance of clearly defined active and quiet sleep states the *tracé alternant* pattern (10.1.1) gradually replaces the *tracé discontinu* pattern. The onset of 60–80% of all bursts between hemispheres (interhemisphere synchrony) differs by no more than 1.5 s at 33–34 weeks of age. This degree of interhemispheric synchrony increases to 70–85% at 35–36 weeks CA and >90% at 38 weeks CA.

Multifocal sharp transients are less abundant, but well developed *frontal sharp waves* (also referred to as *frontal sharp transients* or *encoches frontales)* are first seen at this age (Fig. 10.4). Frontal sharp waves are biphasic, sharply contoured waveforms that may be unilateral, asymmetric, or bilateral and synchronous. They are maximal in amplitude over the frontal and mid-frontal head regions. They occur most often during sleep and are rarely seen after 46 weeks CA.

Monorhythmic frontal slowing (also referred to as *anterior slow dysrhythmia)* occurs frequently at this age and persists into the perinatal period. It consists of short runs of bilateral, monomorphic or rhythmic, 2–4 Hz, 50–150 μV activity (Fig. 10.2). It should not be confused with abnormal patterns, particularly neonatal epileptiform patterns.

Prior to this age wakefulness is difficult to record because it occurs infrequently and is often associated with movement-related artifacts. However, when quiet wakefulness appears it is usually associated with activity similar to that seen during active sleep. It is relatively low in amplitude with little evidence of an antero-posterior amplitude gradient; a pattern sometimes referred to as *activité moyenne* (Fig. 10.5).

10.1.5 *Infants of 38–42 weeks of age.* Wakefulness, active sleep, and quiet sleep are now clearly differentiated. Four main EEG patterns are seen. The first consists of continuous widespread 25–50 μV theta activity with intermixed lower amplitude delta activity and is present during quiet wakefulness and active sleep. This pattern is referred to as the low *voltage irregular pattern* (Fig. 10.5), although the voltage is low only in relation to other activity present at this age. The second type of pattern contains similar features but also has intermixed intermittent higher amplitude 2–4 Hz delta waveforms. Because it combines low and high amplitude components it has been referred to as the *mixed pattern* (Fig. 10.6). It is also seen during wakefulness and active sleep. The other two patterns occur during quiet sleep. In one there is continuous 25–150 μV slow delta activity, referred to as either the *high voltage slow (HVS)* pattern or *continuous slow wave pattern* (CSWP; Fig. 10.7). The HVS pattern represents the first appearance of continuous activity in quiet sleep and is first seen at 38 weeks CA. However, at term quiet sleep is dominated by the fourth pattern: *tracé alternant* (Fig. 10.8). Nearly 100% of the bursts of activity occurring in the tracé alternant pattern are synchronous by 40 weeks CA. Brushes are very infrequent and, if present, occur almost exclusively during quiet sleep.

Frontal sharp waves (also referred to as *frontal sharp transients*) and *monorhythmic frontal delta (slow anterior dysrhyth-mia)* occur frequently, particularly during indeterminate (transitional) sleep. Sharp transients are also regularly seen over the central and temporal head regions. Because multifocal sharp transients in the neonate are sometimes misinterpreted as being suggestive of a seizure disorder, the following

DEVELOPMENT OF FRONTAL SHARP TRANSIENTS

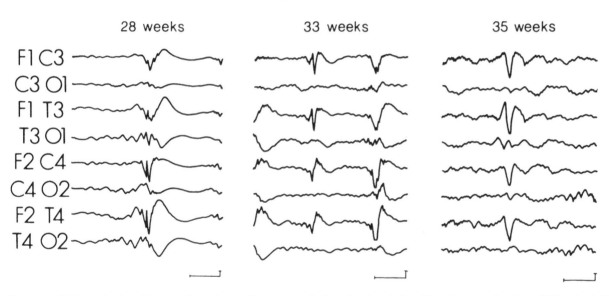

Fig. 10.4. High amplitude 'spikey' or polyphasic transients are seen in frontal regions before 36 weeks conceptional age. Calibration is 50 μV and 1 s. (Courtesy S.S. Werner, J.E. Stockard and R.G. Bickford, Atlas of Neonatal EEG. Raven Press, New York, 1977.)

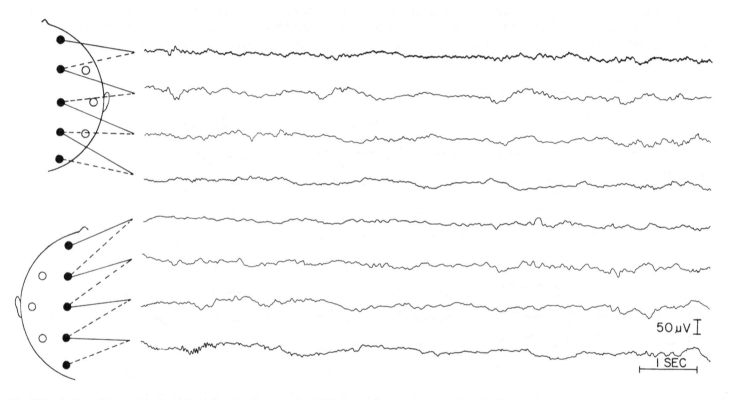

50 μV

1 SEC

Fig. 10.5.   Pattern of low voltage irregular theta and delta waves ('activité moyenne') in a wakeful normal full-term infant, 10 days old.

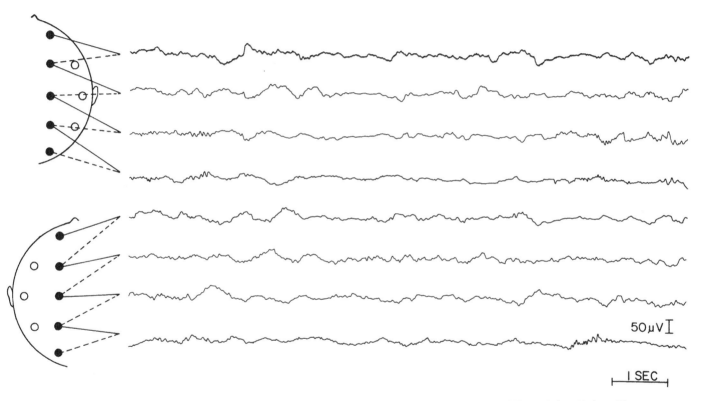

50μV

1 SEC

Fig. 10.6.　Pattern of low voltage irregular slow waves, including larger delta waves, during active sleep in a normal full-term infant, 10 days old.

167

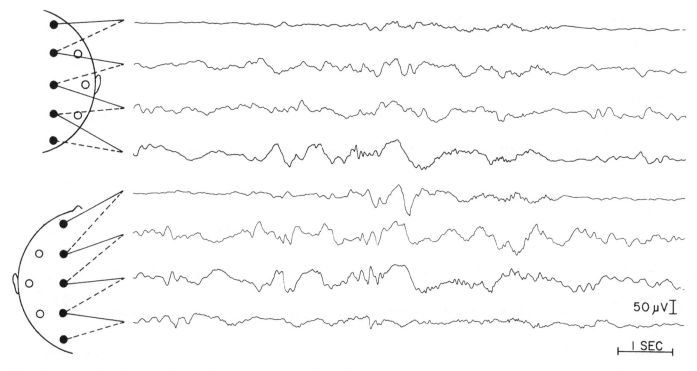

Fig. 10.7.   Pattern of continuous high amplitude slow waves of quiet sleep in a normal full-term infant, 4 days old.

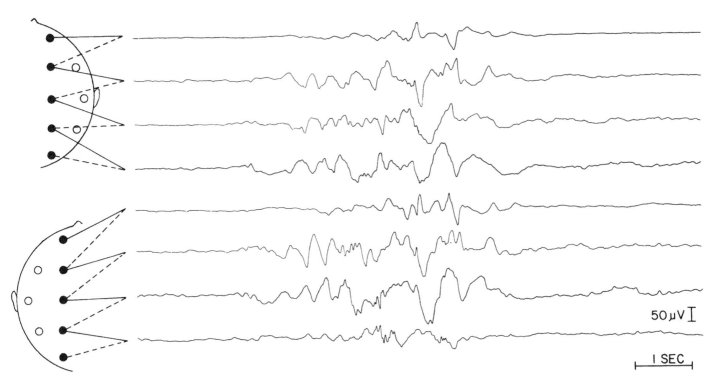

50μV

1 SEC

Fig. 10.8.   Pattern of quiet sleep ('tracé alternant') in a normal full-term infant, 4 days old.

points warrant emphasis. Sporadic multifocal sharp transients in either wakefulness or sleep in a 28–42 week CA infant are a normal finding. Moreover, although they decrease in occurrence after 40 weeks CA, rare (2–3/h) multifocal spikes in any state are considered normal up to 46 weeks CA. In addition to frontal sharp waves, sharp transients commonly occur as part of the burst phase of the tracé alternant pattern and may occur sporadically over the rolandic head regions during quiet sleep. An abnormal increase in the abundance of multifocal sharp transients represents a non-specific response to any encephalopathic process and does not specifically suggest the presence of a seizure disorder. If it is the only abnormal finding, then the EEG is interpreted as mildly abnormal. Frequent sharp transients occurring in any one particular location during wakefulness or active sleep after 42 weeks CA are abnormal (see also 19.1).

10.2 INFANTS FROM FULL TERM TO 3 MONTHS OF AGE

Between term and the end of the first 3 months of life precursors of adult patterns appear and neonatal patterns gradually disappear. The tracé alternant pattern occurs less and less frequently until it disappears completely at 46 weeks CA. At term, and thereafter, interhemispheric synchrony during tracé alternant is present nearly 100% of the time. As noted in 10.1.5, frontal sharp waves and monorhythmic frontal delta

(slow anterior dysrhythmia) are associated with sleep, particularly transitions between active and quiet sleep, and are commonly seen up to 41 weeks CA. However, it has not been determined beyond what CA their presence constitutes a significant abnormality and frontal sharp transients may occur very rarely up to 48 weeks CA. Multifocal sharp transients, which are most commonly seen in all states between 32 and 34 weeks CA, decline in frequency and retreat into quiet sleep, become rare by 42 weeks CA and finally disappear at 44 weeks CA.

Wakefulness in the first 3 months of life is characterized by an admixture of predominantly delta and theta activity. Five to 6 Hz rhythmic activity is present over the central head regions and may represent the earliest manifestations of the mu rhythm.

Drowsiness between full term and 5 months of life is usually characterized by gradual generalized background slowing which increases in amplitude and progresses smoothly into sleep. This often occurs when the infant appears to be awake and resting with the eyes partially or fully open. Because of the frequent lack of obvious EEG and behavioral changes during drowsiness, the reliable detection of the onset of drowsiness by clinical observation is difficult in the first 5 months of life.

At term approximately 80% of episodes of sleep onset consist of active sleep. But by 46 weeks CA the majority of sleep onset episodes begin with quiet sleep. This shift in sleep state at sleep onset is roughly paralleled by a shift in the relative time occupied by active and quiet sleep; from 40 to 48 weeks

CA active sleep decreases from approximately 50 to 40% of total sleep time. Background activity during quiet sleep shifts from the tracé alternant pattern (which occupies most of quiet sleep at term) to the high voltage slow (continuous slow wave) pattern which predominates by 45–46 weeks CA. At 40 weeks CA this activity is often maximal over the posterior head regions and by 3 months of age an amplitude gradient with greater amplitude activity over the posterior than the anterior head regions is well established and persists until approximately 10 years of age.

Sleep spindles may be present in rudimentary form at 40 weeks CA, but they are not consistently seen until 2–3 months of age. They appear as 12–14 Hz runs of low to medium amplitude rhythmic activity with maximal amplitude over the central and parasagittal head regions that usually last 3–5 s. In the first 3 years of life sleep spindles have a characteristic rectified morphology (the negative phase is sharply contoured and the positive phase is arched or rounded) that differentiates them from the more sinusoidal appearing sleep spindles in older individuals (Fig. 10.9, Part 3). Until approximately 8 months of life they are frequently asynchronous over the 2 hemispheres and at other times appear to shift from one side to the other. After this time asynchronous sleep spindles gradually occur less often and after 2 years of age asynchronous sleep spindles are considered abnormal. Sleep spindles should also be considered abnormal at any age if they only appear unilaterally or demonstrate a consistent amplitude asymmetry of more than 50%.

Tactile or auditory stimulation during sleep can produce one of several non-specific reactions in the EEG: (a) a negative vertex spike (up to 100 μV); (b) generalized flattening; (c) bursts of generalized slow waves; (d) bursts followed by flattening; and (e) change in state, especially from tracé alternant to diffusely slow or low voltage patterns. In addition, more specific responses may be elicited during wakefulness and sleep in the form of visual evoked potentials in response to single flashes (5.2; 7.6.1; 14.3.1) in approximately 60% of newborns. This response is typically a high amplitude (75–200 μV), sharply contoured triphasic waveform that has a much longer latency of onset following the flash (up to 200 ms) than that seen in adults. It fatigues rapidly and occurs only with single flashes or at slow rates of stimulation (1/s or less). It may be elicited at the onset or cessation of more rapid rates of stimulation (sometimes referred to as the *on* and *off* response). Rarely, *lambda waves* (occipital waveforms evoked by looking at complex patterns; 11.4) appear when the infant is looking around the room. When present (as in childhood and adulthood) lambda waves are usually associated with a prominent flash evoked response.

10.3 INFANTS FROM 3 MONTHS TO 12 MONTHS OF AGE

10.3.1 *Wakefulness* is characterized by patterns that begin to show regional differences and to react to stimulation. *Back-*

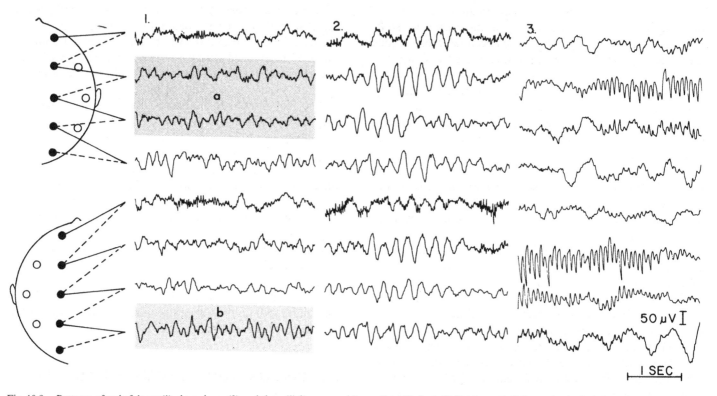

Fig. 10.9.   Patterns of wakefulness (1), drowsiness (2) and sleep (3) in a normal 8-month-old infant. (1) During wakefulness, rhythmical theta waves of 4–5 Hz in the central regions (a) can be distinguished from a rhythm of 6 Hz in the occipital areas (b). (2) Drowsiness is associated with high amplitude bisynchronous waves of 3–4 Hz. (3) During sleep, prominent spindles appear in the central regions, slightly asynchronous on the two sides; they are superimposed on generalized slow waves of under 2 Hz.

ground activity consists of rhythmical and arrhythmical slow waves in the delta and theta frequency range. These waves are generalized, and often more prominent over the occipital areas. By 4–6 months of age intermittent background activity in the 5–8 Hz frequency range appears over the central head region. Delta waves diminish considerably during the first year. Before the age of 5 months, rhythmical occipital activity develops (Fig. 10.9, Part 1). The relative contributions of different frequency background activity over different head regions at different ages are summarized in Fig. 10.12.

Occipital rhythms that can be clearly distinguished from the background first appear at 3 months of age. These rhythms have frequencies of 3–4 Hz and are reduced in amplitude by eye opening. They become more regular and increase in frequency to about 5 Hz at 5 months of age and to 6–8 Hz at the end of the first year of life (Fig. 10.9, Part 1). The amplitude decreases somewhat from 50–100 μV to 50–75 μV at 12 months. The trend of the development of the reactive occipital dominant frequency in relation to age in a group of normal individuals is shown in Fig. 10.10.

10.3.2 *Drowsiness up* to the age of 6–8 months is associated with a smooth transition from patterns of wakefulness to those of sleep; characterized by a generalized and progressive increase of amplitude and a decrease of frequency to 2–3 Hz. At 3 months of age approximately 30% of infants show a specific pattern of drowsiness referred to as *hypnogogic hypersynchrony* which consists of rhythmical and bisynchronous 3–5

Hz waves of high amplitude (75–200 μV; Fig. 10.9, Part 2). These waves begin rather abruptly and are widely distributed. They sometimes have an anterior, temporal or posterior predominance and occur intermittently or continuously for up to several minutes at the beginning (hypnogogic) and at the end (hypnopompic) of sleep. Nearly all normal infants between 6 and 8 months of age show this pattern and it is present in the majority of infants and children between 4 months and 2 years of age. Hypnogogic hypersynchrony vanishes gradually and is rarely seen by 12 years of age. The rhythmical slow waves lose amplitude and become asynchronous and are thus transformed into the adult pattern of drowsiness. A few infants do not show this pattern of drowsiness but instead show occipital or widespread rhythmical and asynchronous 4–5 Hz waves of low to medium amplitude; this pattern more closely resembles the adult patterns of drowsiness.

10.3.3 *Sleep* activity shows several major changes during the first year of life. Active sleep develops into REM sleep in which the two infantile EEG patterns previously seen during active sleep (low voltage irregular and mixed voltage) are transformed into electrical patterns which gradually come to resemble the low amplitude patterns of the adult REM stage of sleep (12.2.6). REM sleep, at first occupying about one-half of the total sleep time, decreases to about 40% of total sleep time at the age of 3–5 months, and to about 30% in the second half of the first year. The tracé alternant and high voltage slow patterns of quiet sleep disappear 4–6 weeks after term and are

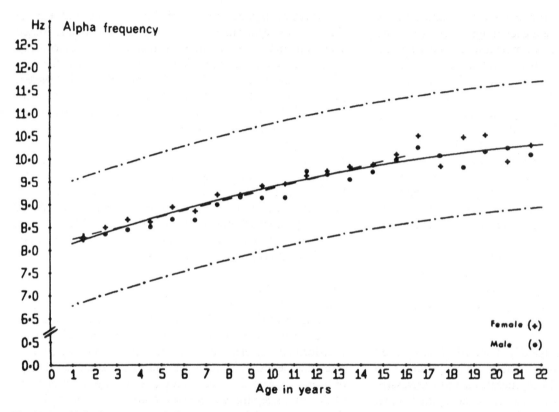

Fig. 10.10. Alpha frequency in relation to age in highly selected normals (continuous line). The diagram is based on a second degree polynomial (parabolic function). The dot-dash lines indicate 95% confidence limits. (Courtesy P. Kellaway, Current Practice of Clinical EEG. Raven Press, New York, 1979.)

replaced by sleep patterns which contain elements resembling those of adults. At the age of about 6 months, the EEG begins to show features similar to those which distinguish the adult non-REM sleep stages I–IV (12.2). After the age of 3 months, sleep no longer begins with the active phase, infants now fall directly into non-REM sleep and go into REM sleep 40–50 min later. During non-REM sleep there is generalized, posterior dominant, delta activity with occasional intermixed moderate to high amplitude bi- or triphasic delta waveforms that appear over the occipital head regions. These intermixed occipital waveforms have a prominent negative phase and are referred to as *cone waves,* or 'O' waves. They are most prominent during stages II and III sleep and are commonly observed up to 5 years of age.

REM sleep can generally be distinguished from non-REM sleep by EEG patterns, by the occurrence of rapid eye (phasic) and limb movements, decreased muscle tone, and by irregular breathing. However, in infants and young children the behavioral manifestations of REM sleep are not always correlated with the EEG pattern of REM sleep. For example, irregular breathing, characteristic of REM sleep in adults, occurs also in non-REM sleep in infants. Furthermore, the EEG patterns of REM sleep in infants consist of delta and theta waves which gradually change towards the pattern of low amplitude diffuse asynchronous waves characteristic of the adult EEG during REM sleep. In contrast to adults, normal infants may have sharp waves in the occipital regions during REM sleep.

Non-REM sleep is usually associated with regular breathing, absence of movements and presence of tonic neck muscle activity. Non-REM sleep can be divided into 4 stages characterized by EEG patterns similar to those of adults (12.2). These patterns begin to become distinguishable in the second half of the first year.

The most important elements of sleep activity acquired during the first year of life are sleep spindles, vertex sharp transients and K complexes.

Sleep spindles continue to increase in distribution and abundance up to 3–6 months of age to the point where they typically occur in prolonged runs lasting 8 s or longer separated by intervals of less than 10 s. After that time, the duration of spindle bursts decreases. An absence of sleep spindles between the ages of 5 and 12 months may be considered abnormal, but only if the duration of uninterrupted recorded sleep exceeds approximately 30 min (i.e., a reasonable sample of non-REM sleep states is obtained). Spindles are commonly asynchronous over the two hemispheres until the age of 8 months in normal infants; continuously asynchronous spindles after 2 years of age are abnormal. Spindle bursts are fairly asymmetrical in normal infants, but a marked and persistent reduction on one side raises the suspicion of an ipsilateral cerebral dysfunction.

Vertex sharp transients (V waves) and *K complexes* can be distinguished in rudimentary form in some infants during the neonatal period. They appear in well developed form for the first time at the age of 5–6 months. V *waves* have negative polarity, an amplitude of up to 250 μV, a wide distribution about the vertex, and a duration of usually less than 200 ms. V waves in the first 3 months of life tend to be difficult to identify; they are smaller, longer lasting and more asymmetrical than later. In infants and young children, vertex waves often appear in short bursts (Fig. 10.11, Part 3a) or repetitive runs and tend to have a sharper configuration compared to those seen in adolescents and adults. K complexes consist of a sharp, negative, high amplitude wave (often over 200 μV in ear reference recordings) followed by a moderate to high amplitude longer duration positive wave. Their topography is similar to that of vertex waves, but they are readily distinguished by their longer duration (greater than 0.5 s). They occur spontaneously during non-REM sleep and can be elicited during sleep by sensory stimulation (particularly auditory). The positive component usually occurs approximately 0.75 s after the stimulus. They may or may not be followed by a 1–2 s run of sleep spindles.

10.4   CHILDREN AND ADOLESCENTS FROM 1 TO 19 YEARS OF AGE

The EEG during resting wakefulness can now be recorded more reliably and shows differentiation of patterns similar to those seen in adults. The waking and drowsy record becomes the major indicator of structural lesions and metabolic abnormalities of the brain; the sleep EEG becomes useful for the activation of epileptiform activity. Hyperventilation and photic stimulation during wakefulness can be used as test conditions which may add information to that of the spontaneous EEG.

Resting wakefulness in children and adolescents is often associated with a mixture of an alpha rhythm and more widespread alpha and theta waveforms. In general, there is more variability in the relative amounts of delta and theta activity between normal children of the same age during the first 10 years of life than in older individuals. The relative amounts of activity in various frequency ranges is shown from birth to age 20 in Fig. 10.12. Note that some admixture of activity below 7 Hz is normal throughout childhood and adolescence.

The alpha rhythm, defined as a posterior dominant alpha frequency activity that attenuates with alerting maneuvers or eye opening and is enhanced by eye closure or relaxed wakefulness, develops from the rhythmical background activity in the occipital regions (Fig. 10.11, Part 1). Fully developed, it consists of sinusoidal waves of 8–13 Hz which are greatest in amplitude over the posterior head regions and may extend forward to the central regions and beyond. The alpha rhythm appears during relaxed wakefulness, usually while the eyes are closed. It is blocked or clearly attenuated by eye opening, attention, and by mental effort. The alpha rhythm slows in frequency and then disappears in drowsiness. The frequency of the alpha rhythm increases gradually with age (Fig. 10.10) and reaches 8 Hz in over 80% of children by 3 years of age. Be-

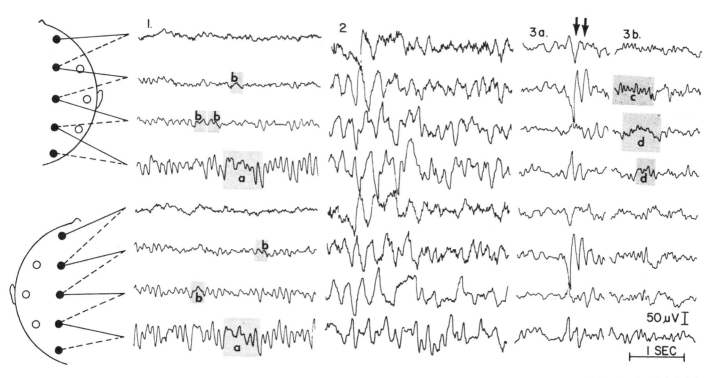

Fig. 10.11.   Patterns of wakefulness (1), drowsiness (2) and sleep (3) in a normal boy of 12 years. (1) Wakefulness is associated with well developed occipital alpha rhythm of 9–10 Hz superimposed on bilaterally synchronous intermittent slow waves of 1–2 Hz (a), and with central theta waves (b). (2) Drowsiness is characterized by generalized bilaterally synchronous slow waves of 2–4 Hz of high amplitude. (3) Sleep is associated with repetitive V waves (arrows) in 3a, and with sleep spindles (c) and slow waves (d) in 3b.

177

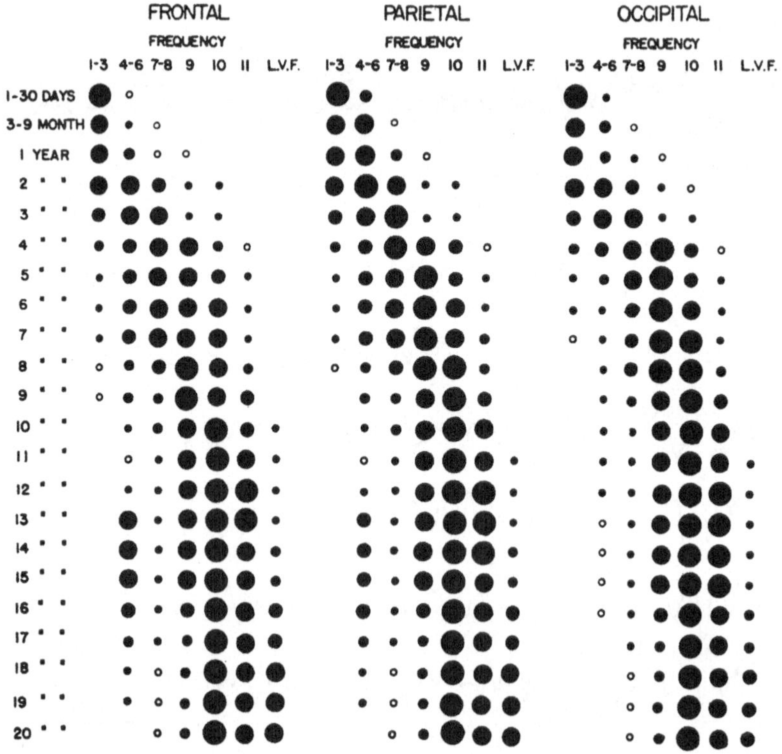

Fig. 10.12. The relative contributions of different frequency waveforms to the normal waking EEG during development. The relative amounts of a particular frequency of activity are indicated by the size of the circles. The activity was measured by spectral analysis and therefore gives no indication of waveform shape. It does, however, provide a rough estimation of the relative contributions of activities over different head regions. Note that slower waveforms make a significant contribution to the overall frequency content of the EEG even in adolescents (Gibbs and Knott, 1949).

tween childhood and adolescence it reaches the 9–11 Hz range.

The amplitude of the alpha rhythm also increases up to the age of 10 years and averages 50–60 μV (measured in T5-O1) between the ages of 3 and 15. In some children (particularly those between 6 and 9 years of age) the amplitude may exceed 100 μV. Children rarely show low amplitude (less than 20 μV in T5-O1) alpha rhythms and, in contrast to adults, either absent or very low amplitude alpha rhythms (less than 15 μV in T5-O1) are abnormal between 3 and 12 years of age. The alpha rhythm is frequently asymmetric, usually with greater amplitude on the right. However, the hemisphere with greater alpha amplitude should not exceed the amplitude of the opposite hemisphere by more than 1.5 times.

Slow waves decrease in prominence with age. Theta waves are more prominent than alpha waves up to the age of 4 years. Between 5 and 6 years, the amounts of alpha and theta activity are about equal. After this age, alpha waves are normally more prominent than theta waves. Rhythmical theta waves during wakefulness in the teenage years are usually most prominent over the temporal and posterior head regions (Fig. 10.11, Part 1). They also appear over the frontocentral head regions in approximately 15–20% of normal individuals between 8 and 16 years of age. Frontocentral theta may even occur in early adulthood. Therefore, the presence of 5–7 Hz frontal or frontocentral theta in runs lasting several seconds are a normal finding in young individuals. Anterior theta activity should only be considered abnormal if it occurs during wakefulness with amplitudes of 100 μV or greater in bipolar montages or when the amplitude clearly exceeds that of the alpha rhythm. Random frontal delta activity diminishes rapidly after 5 years of age and is rarely seen after 9 years of age.

Intermixed theta and delta waveforms are commonly seen over the posterior head regions during childhood and adolescence. They occur less often thereafter but may still be seen in over 5% of normal individuals up to 30 years of age. These waveforms, like frontocentral theta, are commonly misinterpreted as an abnormal finding. Rhythmic, 1–3 s runs of 2.5–4.5 Hz activity of less than 100 μV make up less than 2% of the waking record in up to 25% of children between the ages 1 and 15 years. This activity is most likely to be seen between 5 and 7 years of age. It is occasionally accentuated by hyperventilation.

Between the ages of 6 months and 2 years moderate to high amplitude, diphasic, approximately 0.75 s duration, waveforms appear over the occipital head regions immediately following the onset of eye blinks in a minority of individuals. They may have a sharp component but should not be mistaken for abnormal background slowing or abnormal epileptiform waves. They have been referred to as *shut eye waves.*

After 8 years of age prominent occipital slow waves normally occurring during wakefulness often fall into the categories of either the *slow alpha variant* (Fig. 11.1, Part 4) or *posterior slow waves of youth* (Fig. 10.11, Part 1a). The *slow alpha variant* occurs rarely and consists of a series of waves with approximately half the frequency of the surrounding alpha rhythm. Because of its morphology, distribution, and frequency, and because it demonstrates the same reactivity as the alpha rhythm, it is thought be a subharmonic of the alpha rhythm.

Posterior slow waves of youth are also considered to be formed from the alpha rhythm and therefore share the same distribution and reactivity to eye opening. They are most likely to be seen between the ages of 8 and 14 years, but occur commonly between 2 and 21 years of age. Although they occur infrequently after 21 years of age, if clearly identifiable, they should be considered a normal variant at any age. Each waveform has the duration of 3–6 combined waveforms from the surrounding alpha rhythm. They may occur in rapid succession or be separated from each other by one to several seconds. They often have a characteristic fused alpha wave morphology in which individual alpha waves appear with increasing definition during the second half of the waveform.

The precise point at which posterior slowing becomes abnormal, particularly in children, is poorly defined. As noted above, a substantial portion of normal slow waves that occur over the posterior head regions do not fall into the categories of either posterior slow waves of youth or the slow alpha variant. The correct interpretation of posterior slow waves in individuals less than 9 years of age is also made difficult by the fact that posterior dominant slowing frequently occurs as a non-specific response to a variety of diffuse cerebral dysfunctions such as head injury, CNS infection and toxic or metabolic encephalopathies. After 9 years of age, anterior dominant or generalized slowing is more commonly seen with a diffuse cerebral dysfunction. There are, however, several useful guidelines for assessing posterior slowing during wakefulness:

(1) a monorhythmic occipital rhythm that attenuates with eye opening (performed passively by the technologist when necessary) that has an appropriate frequency for the age of the child is normal;

(2) normal slower waveforms rarely exceed the amplitude of the alpha rhythm by more than 1.5 times;

(3) asymmetries of slower waveforms that are normal should conform to a similar asymmetry in the ongoing alpha rhythm, i.e., normal slow waves usually have approximately the same topographic distribution as the alpha rhythm; and

(4) normal posterior slow waves should attenuate with the alpha rhythm during alerting.

As in adults, rhythmical, bisynchronous, occipital slow waves of about half the frequency of alpha rhythm may alternate or mix with the alpha rhythm to form slow alpha variants (11.1.7). Unlike adults, some normal teenagers show intermittent or briefly repetitive posterior slow waves of medium or high amplitude which transiently replace alpha rhythm.

Beta activity occurs only rarely in children and adolescents during wakefulness. At any age beyond the neonatal period the voltage of beta activity recorded during wakefulness between adjacent electrodes (e.g., F3-C3) should not exceed 25 μV. Excessive beta activity, particularly in the 18–25 Hz band, is almost always seen as a medication effect. It is reliably produced in most individuals by benzodiazepines and barbiturates, even at non-sedating levels. For this reason, *chloral hydrate*, which rarely produces excessive beta activity at the minimal doses required for sedation, has been commonly used for sedation in the EEG laboratory. However, higher doses of chloral hydrate (e.g., several grams) will also produce beta activity. Aside from drug-induced beta activity, the clinical significance of excessive, symmetric beta activity during wakefulness is uncertain. A more important clinical finding is an asymmetry of beta activity. In general, *for beta activity the difference in amplitude between homologous hemispheric head regions should be less than approximately 35% of the amplitude of the side with the greater amplitude.* If an abnormal asymmetry is present, then in contrast to activity that is below the beta frequency range, it is almost always the case that the abnormal side is the side with lower amplitude. Very rarely a localized increase in beta activity has been associated with brain tumors. Almost always a localized increase in beta activity is due to a skull defect (developmental, traumatic or surgical, with or without an associated underlying lesion). The skull defect results in an ipsilateral increase in beta amplitude and is commonly referred to as a *breach rhythm*. The breach rhythm is usually, but not always, located directly over the skull defect.

Mu rhythm is defined as a 7–11 Hz rhythm that appears maximally over the central or centroparietal regions during wakefulness. It is blocked (suppressed) by contralateral limb movement or sensory stimulation. In some cases it can also be blocked by ipsilateral limb movement or the thought of contralateral limb movement. It begins in childhood or adolescence and is similar in appearance to that seen in the adult (11.3). It has a frequency that is usually within 1 Hz of the alpha rhythm.

Drowsiness may be associated with the following patterns:

(1) Between the ages of 6 months and 2 years the majority of children demonstrate *hypnogogic hypersynchrony;* it is rarely seen after 12 years of age. This pattern may at times appear abruptly on an otherwise quiescent background with intermixed low amplitude spike-like waves that give it an abnormal epileptiform appearance (Figs. 19.17 and 19.18), sometimes referred to as *paroxysmal hypnogogic hypersynchrony*.

(2) Between 6 months and 2 years an increase in beta activity in the predominantly 20–25 Hz range often appears maximally over the central and posterior head regions during drowsiness and stages 1 and 2 sleep. In older children and adults beta activity may also be activated by drowsiness, but it usually appears more anteriorly, over the frontocentral head regions.

(3) At approximately 10 years of age adult patterns of drowsiness become more common. The earliest sign of drowsiness, when present, is *slow lateral eye movements.* These movements produce waveforms of 1 Hz or less that have maximal amplitude and opposite polarity at the F7 and F8 electrodes. They frequently occur at a time when the alpha rhythm is still present or waxing and waning. With continued drowsi-

ness the alpha rhythm may slow by 1–2 Hz. If the frequency of the alpha rhythm is inadvertently assessed during drowsiness it may appear to be abnormally slow. *Therefore, it is extremely important that the frequency of the alpha rhythm be determined during wakefulness, and that wakefulness is clearly established by performing alerting maneuvers* (e.g., ask the patient to respond to verbal commands or answer questions about orientation to place, time, or person, or to perform mental calculations). These maneuvers should be followed or preceded by eye opening and closing on command (see also Bancaud's phenomenon).

(4) Between 10 and 20 years of age prominent frontal rhythmic theta activity occurs commonly during drowsiness.

Sleep activity shows maturation of stages and the development of new patterns.

The sleep stages I–IV of non-REM sleep and the *stage of REM sleep* become more similar to those of adults (12.2) and can be distinguished more easily from each other. Sleep cycles also mature. The proportion of time spent in REM sleep gradually drops from about 30% of the total sleep time at 1–2 years to the adult fraction of about 25%.

Positive occipital sharp transients (POSTs) of sleep similar to those of adults (12.1.2) begin to appear in light sleep during childhood.

Fourteen and 6 Hz positive bursts (a benign pseudoepileptiform pattern) are frequently seen during drowsiness and sleep in children and adolescents and are more common at these ages than in adults.

Vertex waves in children, particularly between the ages of 3 and 5, often have a very sharply contoured morphology and may occur in repetitive runs. Because of these features they are sometimes misinterpreted as abnormal central epileptiform spikes.

Cone waves or *'O' (for occipital) waves* (10.3) are often present during non-REM sleep from infancy until 5 years of age. They appear as isolated, medium to high amplitude, predominantly monophasic, triangular shaped, delta waves over the occipital head region.

REFERENCES

Andersen, C.M. and Torres, F. (1985) The EEG of the early premature. Electroenceph. Clin. Neurophysiol. 60: 95–105.

Aso, K., Scher, M.S. and Barmada, M.A. (1989) Neonatal electroencephalography and neuropathology. J. Clin. Neurophysiol. 6: 103–124.

Blume, W.T. (1982) Atlas of Pediatric EEG. Raven Press, New York.

Blume, W.T. and Kaibara, M. (1995) Atlas of Adult Electroencephalography. Raven Press, New York.

Clancy, R.R., Chung, H.J. and Temple, J.P. (1993) Neonatal electroencephalography. In: M.R. Sperling and R.R. Clancy (Eds.), Atlas of Electroencephalography, Vol. 1. Elsevier, Amsterdam.

Dreyfus-Brisac, C. and Curzi-Dascalova, L. (1975) Section II. The EEG during the first year of life. In: A. Rémond (Ed.), Handbook of Electroenceph. Clin. Neurophysiol., Vol. 6B. Elsevier, Amsterdam, pp. 24–30.

Dreyfus-Brisac, C. and Monod, N. (1975) Section I. The electroencephalogram of full-term newborns and premature infants. In: A. Rémond, (Ed.), Handbook of Electroenceph. Clin. Neurophysiol., Vol. 6B. Elsevier, Amsterdam, pp. 6–23.

Eeg-Olofsson, O. (1971) The development of the electroencephalogram in normal adolescents from the age of 16 through 21 years. Neuropaediatrie 3: 11–45.

Ellingson, R.J. (1979) The EEGs of premature and full-term newborns. In: D.W. Klass and D.D. Daly (Eds.), Current Practice of Clinical Electroencephalography. Raven Press, New York, pp. 149–169.

Ellingson, R.J. and Peters, J.F. (1980) Development of EEG and daytime sleep patterns in normal full-term infants during the first 3 months of life: longitudinal observations. Electroenceph. Clin. Neurophysiol. 49: 112–124.

Gibbs, F.A. and Knott, J.R. (1949) Growth of the electrical activity of the cortex. Electroenceph. Clin. Neurophysiol. 1: 223–229.

Hahn, J.S., Monyer, H. and Tharp, B.R. (1989) Interburst interval measurements in the EEGs of premature infants with normal neurological outcome. Electroenceph. Clin. Neurophysiol. 73: 410–418.

Hanley, J.W. (1981) A step-by-step approach to neonatal EEG. Am. J. EEG Technol. 21: 1–13.

Holmes, G.L. (1986) Morphological and physiological maturation of the brain in the neonate and young child. J. Clin. Neurophysiol. 3: 209–238.

Hrachovy, R.A., Mizrahi, E.M. and Kellaway, P. (1990) Neonatal EEG. In: D.D. Daly and T.A. Pedley (Eds.), Current Practice of EEG, 2nd Edition. Raven Press, New York.

Hughes, J.R. (1987) Normal limits in the EEG. In: A.M. Halliday, S.R. Butler and R. Paul (Eds.), A Textbook of Clinical Neurophysiology. Wiley, Chichester, pp. 105–154.

Jankel, W.R. and Niedermeyer, E. (1985) Sleep spindles. J. Clin. Neurophysiol. 2: 1–36.

Kellaway, P. (1979) An orderly approach to visual analysis: parameters of the normal EEG in adults and children. In: D.W. Klass and D.D. Daly (Eds.), Current Practice of Clinical Electroencephalography. Raven Press, New York, pp. 69–147.

Kellaway, P. (1990) An orderly approach to visual analysis: characteristics of the normal EEG of adults and children. In: D.D. Daly and T.A. Pedley (Eds.), Current Practice of Clinical Neurophysiology: Electroencephalography, 2nd Edition. Raven Press, New York, pp. 139–200.

Kellaway, P. and Mizrahi, E.M. (1989) Clinical electroencephalographic, therapeutic, and pathophysiological studies of neonatal seizures. In: C.B. Wasterlain and P. Vert (Eds.), Neonatal Seizures: Pathophysiology and Pharmacologic Management. Raven Press, New York.

Lombroso, C.T. (1979) Quantified electrographic scales on 10 pre-term healthy newborns followed up to 40–43 weeks of conceptional age by serial polygraphic recordings. Electroenceph. Clin. Neurophysiol. 46: 460–474.

Lombroso, C.T. (1993) Neonatal EEG polygraphy in normal and abnormal newborns. In: E. Niedermeyer and F. Lopes da Silva (Eds.), Electroencephalography: Basic Principles, Clinical Applications and Related Fields, Third Edition. Williams and Wilkins, Baltimore, pp. 803–876.

Monod, N., Pajot, N. and Guidasci, S. (1972) The neonatal EEG: Statistical studies and prognostic value in full-term and pre-term babies. Electroenceph. Clin. Neurophysiol. 32: 529–544.

Niedermeyer, E. (1993) Maturation of the EEG: Development of waking and sleep patterns. In: E. Niedermeyer and F. Lopes da Silva (Eds.), Electroencephalography: Basic Principles, Clinical Applications and Related Fields. Williams and Wilkins, Baltimore, pp. 167–191.

Pampiglione, G. (1977) Development of rhythmic EEG activities in infancy. (waking state). Rev. Electroencephalogr. Neurophysiol. 7: 327–333.

Petersén, I. and Eeg-Olofsson, O. (1970) The development of the electroencephalogram in normal children from the age of 1 through 15 years. Nonparoxysmal activity. Neuropaediatrie 2: 247–304.

Petersén, I. and Eeg-Olofsson, O. (1971) The development of the electroencephalogram in normal children from the age of 1 through 15 years nonparoxysmal activity. Neuropaediatrie 2: 247–304.

Petersén, I., Eeg-Olofsson, O. and Sellden, U. (1968) Paroxysmal activity of normal children. In: P. Kellaway and I. Petersén (Eds.), Clinical Electroencephalography of Children. Almqvist and Wiksell, Stockholm, pp. 167–187.

Petersén, I., Sellden, U. and Eeg-Olofsson, O. (1975) Section III. The evolution of the EEG in normal children and adolescents from 1 to 21 years. In: A. Rémond (Ed.), Handbook of Electroenceph. Clin. Neurophysiol., Vol. 6B. Elsevier, Amsterdam, pp. 31–68.

Pope, S.S., Werner, S.S. and Bickford, R.G. (1992) Atlas of Neonatal Electro-encephalography. Raven Press, New York.

Slater, G.E. and Torres, F. (1979) Frequency-amplitude gradient. A new parameter for interpreting pediatric sleep EEGs. Arch. Neurol. 36: 465–470.

Stockard-Pope, J.E., Werner, S.S. and Bickford, R.G. (1992) Atlas of Neonatal Electroencephalography. 2nd Edn. Raven Press, New York.

Tharp, B.R. (1986) Neonatal and pediatric electroencephalography. In: M.J. Aminoff (Ed.), Electrodiagnosis in Clinical Neurology. Churchill Livingstone, New York, pp. 77–124.

Tharp, B.R. (1990) Electrophysiological brain maturation in premature infants: a historical perspective. J. Clin. Neurophysiol. 7: 302–314.

Tharp, B.R., Cukier, F. and Monod, N. (1981) The prognostic value of the electroencephalogram in premature infants. Electroenceph. Clin. Neurophysiol. 51: 219–236.

Werner, S.S., Stockard, J.E. and Bickford, R.G. (1977) Atlas of Neonatal EEG. Raven Press, New York.

Westmoreland, B.F. and Klass, D.W. (1996) Electroencephalography: Electroencephalograms of neonates, infants, and children. In: J. Daube (Ed.), Clinical Neurophysiology. F.A. Davis, Philadelphia, pp. 104–113.

Westmoreland, B.F. and Sharbrough, F.W. (1975) Posterior slow wave transients associated with eye blinks in children. Am. J. EEG Technol. 15: 14–19.

11 The normal EEG of wakeful resting adults of 20–60 years of age

SUMMARY

The normal EEG of the wakeful adult at rest may show various types of activity alone or in combination:

(11.1) *The alpha rhythm* consists of sinusoidal waveforms ≥8 Hz and ≤13 Hz maximal over the posterior head region that are blocked by eye opening (and other alerting maneuvers) and disappear in drowsiness and sleep. The alpha rhythm is >8.0 Hz in normal adults.

(11.2) *Beta rhythms* are less common and consist of waves over 13 Hz that appear either in a wide distribution, or limited to the frontal or posterior head regions.

(11.3) *Mu rhythm.*

(11.4) *Lambda waves.*

(11.5) *Vertex sharp transients.*

(11.6) *Kappa rhythm.*

(11.7) *Intermittent posterior theta rhythms* are rarer than alpha and beta rhythms.

(11.8) *Low voltage activity* may be the only pattern of the EEG in some normal adults.

(11.9) *Abnormalities* commonly include epileptiform spikes and sharp waves, more than a minimum of slow waves, asymmetrical or very low amplitude activity, or deviations from normal patterns.

11.1 THE ALPHA RHYTHM

The alpha rhythm is defined by its frequency, its distribution and its reactivity (Fig. 11.1, Parts 1–5). Thus, the terms *alpha rhythm* and *alpha frequency* or *activity* are not synonymous.

11.1.1 The *alpha rhythm* consists of regular (monomorphic) *waveforms* that have sharp points at the top or bottom or are sinusoidal. Single alpha waves with sharp peaks may be distinguished from abnormal sharp waves by their similarity to other, repetitive alpha waves in the same recording.

11.1.2 The *frequency* ranges from >8 to ≤13 Hz in different normal subjects. An alpha rhythm frequency that never exceeds 8.0 Hz in an awake adult is abnormal. It is fairly constant in a given subject but may decrease by 1 Hz or more with drowsiness and increase momentarily after eye closure. This brief increase in frequency after eye closure followed by rapid deceleration to the individual's normal baseline frequency is referred to as the *squeak phenomenon.* Because the alpha rhythm frequency is variable depending on the behavioral state of the individual, it should only be measured when it is clear the subject is awake and not drowsy. This is accomplished by assessing the frequency during periods of eye opening and closure in association with mental activation. The alpha rhythm frequency is one of the few quantitative meas-

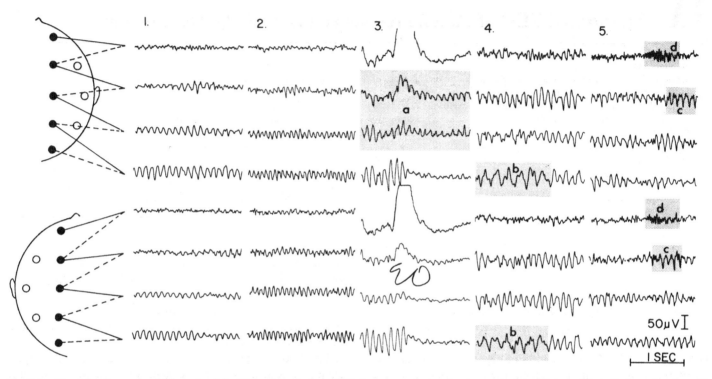

Fig. 11.1. Normal patterns of wakefulness in adults. (1) An alpha rhythm of 9 Hz in the posterior head regions and minimal beta activity in the frontal regions. (2) An alpha rhythm of 12–13 Hz extending from the posterior to the central regions. (3) An alpha rhythm of 9–10 Hz in the posterior head regions is present at the beginning and is then blocked by eye opening (EO); a central mu rhythm on the right side persists after eye opening (a). (4) Slow alpha variant of 4–5 Hz, maximal in the occipital regions (b), alternates with an alpha rhythm of about 9 Hz in a wider posterior distribution; a beta rhythm is present in the frontal regions. (5) An alpha rhythm of 8–9 Hz posteriorly, mu rhythm of similar frequency frontocentrally (c), and beta rhythm frontally (d).

ures that can be assessed on every recording in which an alpha rhythm is present. It should always be included in the descriptive portion of the EEG report for comparison with subsequent recordings. Because the alpha rhythm frequency in a given individual remains nearly constant throughout their adult life, a decline of 1 or more Hz is abnormal even if their absolute frequency remains in a normal range above 8 Hz.

The frequency of the alpha rhythm in the two hemispheres should be the same at any moment; even a slight difference is suspicious of abnormality if it persists, and a difference of over 1 Hz at any time is definitely abnormal. Using digital EEG spectral analysis the finding of a 0.5 Hz or greater peak frequency difference is abnormal. The hemisphere with the lower frequency is abnormal.

11.1.3 The *phase relation* of the alpha rhythm over different parts of the brain may vary. Individual alpha waves are often not in phase in different areas in normal EEGs, even though the alpha rhythm normally appears and disappears simultaneously in the two hemispheres.

11.1.4 The *distribution* of the alpha rhythm is posterior: the alpha rhythm has the greatest amplitude and is most persistent in the occipital posterior temporal and parietal areas. It often extends into the temporal areas and sometimes into the central areas, especially in young subjects. The alpha rhythm may appear in recordings from a frontal electrode referred to an electrode on the ear, the mastoid or other posterior placements because these reference electrodes pick up the alpha rhythm in posterior locations (4.1.2; Fig. 11.2). Cerebral rhythms of alpha frequency that appear only or mainly in the frontal regions in an adult are abnormal (25.3.1). *Alpha frequency activity that is restricted to the frontopolar (Fp1 and Fp2) electrodes is eye movement artifact until proven otherwise.* During the early stages of drowsiness, activity in the alpha frequency range may become more prominent over the frontocentral head regions when recorded using a neck/chest, average, or ear reference montage. This shift in the topography of alpha activity during drowsiness occurs somewhat more often in older individuals. It may not be apparent if longitudinal bipolar montages are used.

11.1.5 The *amplitude* of the alpha rhythm often waxes and wanes. While the amplitude may differ between the two hemispheres at different times, an estimate of the average amplitude of the alpha rhythm during a recording may show it to be symmetrical on the two sides. However, even persistent asymmetries of the alpha rhythm are not necessarily abnormal. A higher amplitude of the alpha rhythm on the right side is common, but even so the amplitude on the left side should be at least 50% of that seen on the right side (Fig. 11.1). Occasionally normal subjects have an alpha rhythm with slightly higher amplitude on the left side. The normal asymmetry of the alpha rhythm in some cases may be due to an asymmetry of occipital bone thickness. It does not depend on whether a subject is right-handed or left-handed. Abnormal asymmetries can be seen in many conditions (23.7.1).

The amplitude and persistence of the alpha rhythm decrease with age from its maximum in childhood (10.7.1). Because of the wide variation of the alpha rhythm between normal adults, low amplitude, rare occurrence, or even complete absence of the alpha rhythm in adults (11.8) is not necessarily abnormal. Therefore, no clinical significance can be attached to distinctions which have been made between dominant and rare alpha rhythms, or between 'plus' or persistent ('P-type'), reactive ('R-type') and 'minus' or minimal ('M-type') alpha rhythms. Only if the alpha rhythm changes significantly between sequential recordings from the same subject (24.1.2; 24.1.4) can one suspect the development of an abnormality (24.7).

11.1.6 The *reactivity* of the alpha rhythm can be tested with various maneuvers. The alpha rhythm is blocked by eye opening (Fig. 11.1, Part 3), sudden alerting, attention to visual and other stimuli, and mental concentration. The degree of reactivity varies in different subjects and in the same subject at different times. The alpha rhythm may be blocked completely for many seconds or its amplitude may be attenuated only briefly. However, the complete absence of any reduction is abnormal (25.2.2). Unilateral blocking of the alpha rhythm always indicates the presence of an abnormality of the non-reactive hemisphere (Bancaud's phenomenon). Recently, it has been demonstrated that this is not an all-or-none process. That is, a clearly recognizable, reproducible, *partial failure* of

alpha reactivity over one hemisphere also indicates an abnormality of that hemisphere.

The alpha rhythm also attenuates when alertness decreases to the level of drowsiness (12.2.2). This attenuation may be associated with a decrease of frequency and is often gradual and intermittent. Drowsiness can also produce a normal variation of alpha blocking, namely a *paradoxical alpha rhythm* which appears on eye opening as the result of partial alerting. This alpha rhythm will disappear with eye closure if drowsiness returns (Fig. 11.2, top). A normal alpha rhythm can be demonstrated in individuals who have a paradoxical alpha rhythm (Fig. 11.2, bottom).

The effect of eye opening should be studied in every routine clinical EEG recording to: (a) study the reactivity and symmetry of alpha blocking; (b) demonstrate the artifacts produced by eye opening, eye closing and eye movements to distinguish them from frontal slow waves; (c) bring out rhythms hidden by the alpha rhythm; (d) test the reactivity of other EEG activity; and (e) precipitate abnormal reactions to eye opening and eye closing, for instance epileptiform discharges. In addition, *testing alpha reactivity with mental calculation during eye closure may demonstrate unilateral failure of alpha blocking that is not apparent with eye opening alone.*

11.1.7 *Alpha variants* are normal rhythms that resemble the alpha rhythm in distribution and reactivity but differ from it by having slower or faster frequency.

Slow alpha variants are rhythms of 3.5–6.5 Hz; half the fre-

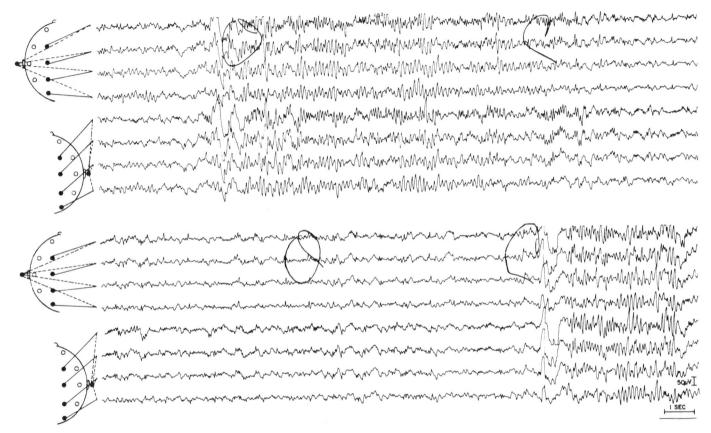

Fig. 11.2. Paradoxical alpha rhythm (top) and normal return of the alpha rhythm (bottom) in a normal drowsy teenager. *Top:* The alpha rhythm appears on eye opening (O) and disappears soon after eye closure (C); activity characteristic of drowsiness is present before and after the period of eye opening. *Bottom:* The alpha rhythm appears after eye closure (C); activity before eye opening (O) and until shortly before eye closing is characteristic of drowsiness; the bottom section was recorded about 1 min after the top section.

quency of the alpha rhythm that appears elsewhere in the same record (Fig. 11.1, Part 4). Because it consists of an admixture of normal alpha activity it appears over the posterior head, usually alternates with the alpha rhythm of the usual frequency, and blocks like the alpha rhythm. Slow alpha variants are rare but normal and should not be confused with the intermittent occipital slow waves seen in children (10.4) and adults (11.7.2).

Fast alpha variants are described with beta rhythms (11.2).

11.1.8 The *physiological purpose* of the alpha rhythm remains unknown. The posterior distribution, blocking with eye opening, and other characteristics of the alpha rhythm indicate that it is integrated with visual system function and possibly represents activity which appears in the absence of specific input to that system. Like other rhythmic cortical activities it is modulated by thalamic and cortical interactions.

11.2   BETA RHYTHMS

Unlike the alpha rhythm, beta rhythms are defined only by frequency, although they can be further subdivided according to distribution and reactivity.

11.2.1 The *frequency* of beta rhythms is over 13 Hz. Although any rhythmical activity above that frequency is called beta rhythm, beta rhythms of over 30 Hz have usually very low amplitude and are difficult to record with conventional EEG techniques (3.5.2). The upper beta range has sometimes been referred to as the gamma range.

11.2.2 The *distribution* and reactivity of beta rhythms vary. Three main types can be distinguished. All of them disappear in sleep, but the first two usually persist longer during drowsiness than does the alpha rhythm.

Frontal beta rhythm is the most common type. It often extends into the central regions (Fig. 11.1, Part 5). In some instances, this type of beta rhythm is blocked by movement, the intention to move, and tactile stimulation. The blocking effect is greater in the hemisphere contralateral to the moved or stimulated side.

Widespread beta rhythm can be recorded over most areas of the head, usually at the same time (Fig. 11.3, Part 1). It is not blocked by any stimulus.

Posterior beta rhythm or *fast alpha variant* has a frequency of about twice that of the alpha rhythm (usually 16–20 Hz) and either intermixes or alternates with the alpha rhythm or replaces it (Fig. 11.3, Part 2). This beta rhythm is blocked by the same maneuvers that block the alpha rhythm.

In addition to these beta patterns, it is common to see an accentuation of beta activity during drowsiness. Beta activation by stage I sleep (drowsiness) is usually maximal over the frontocentral head regions, although it is sometimes maximal over the posterior head regions in early childhood.

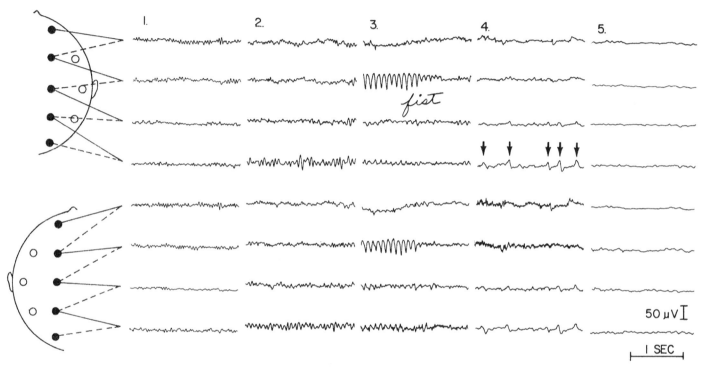

Fig. 11.3. Normal patterns of wakefulness in adults. (1) Generalized beta rhythm of a low amplitude or 'low voltage fast activity'. (2) Fast alpha variant of about 15 Hz in the posterior head regions and faster beta rhythm elsewhere. (3) Frontocentral mu rhythm, blocked by making a fist; posterior alpha rhythm is blocked by eye opening during this recording. (4) Lambda waves (arrows) in the occipital areas, triggered by visual scanning of a picture. (5) Low voltage pattern; subject was alert and had eyes closed during the recording.

11.2.3 The *amplitude* of beta activity is usually lower than that of alpha activity in the same record, but amplitude and persistence of beta rhythm may be abnormally high (24.8). Amplitude and distribution of all normal beta rhythms are symmetrical; amplitude in homologous head regions should not differ by more than 35%. A significant (35%) asymmetry or unilateral or focal appearance of beta rhythm is abnormal (19.3.6; 23.7.2). In the absence of a skull defect the hemisphere with the lower amplitude is abnormal. A skull defect (e.g., fracture or burr hole) creates a low resistance pathway for EEG currents. This can result in a localized increase in beta activity nearby or at a distance from the skull defect referred to as *breach rhythm*.

11.2.4 Since alpha activity tends to decrease during adult life (11.1.5), the ratio of beta to alpha activity increases with age (13.2). However, the absence of these age-dependent changes is not a clinically significant finding. Only in a general manner does the presence of beta activity in an older person signal better cerebral function than does its absence.

Excessive prominent beta activity in wakefulness and drowsiness is almost always the result of a medication effect, most reliably produced by benzodiazepines or barbiturates. Otherwise excessive generalized beta activity is of little diagnostic significance.

11.2.5 The *physiological significance* of beta activity is not clear. The blocking mechanism of frontal beta suggests a relationship between this type of beta rhythm and sensorimotor functions of the underlying cortex; a similar relationship may be postulated for the mu rhythm (11.3). The presence of beta activity is highly dependent on normal cortical function. *Therefore beta activity is almost always a good prognostic sign.* For example, patients in coma with prominent or exclusive beta activity usually make a full recovery with adequate medical support. Posterior beta rhythm probably has the same significance as the alpha rhythm (11.1.8); it is of no known clinical importance.

11.3 MU RHYTHM

Older names for this rhythm which are no longer used are 'wicket', 'comb' or 'arceau' rhythm. The mu rhythm, seen prominently in less than 5% of EEGs and most commonly in younger adults, consists of arch-shaped waves at 7–11 Hz which appear in trains of usually up to a few seconds over the central or centroparietal regions (Fig. 11.3, Part 3). These trains often appear at different times on the two sides of the head. Because they are a local activity they are better seen in bipolar montages (that filter out more widespread waveforms) than in referential recordings. Mu waves intermix or alternate with beta activity (Fig. 11.1, Part 5) and then often have half the frequency of the beta waves. Because the mu rhythm has a frequency similar to that of the alpha rhythm, it usually is best recognized when the alpha rhythm is blocked by eye opening

(Fig. 11.1, Part 3). The appearance of the mu rhythm is said to be facilitated while a subject scans visual images.

Like the frontal beta rhythm, the mu rhythm is often blocked by voluntary, reflex or passive movement, by the intention to move, or by tactile stimuli (Fig. 11.3, Part 3). The effect is greatest over the hemisphere opposite the side of the movement or stimulation. If the alpha rhythm is present while the mu reactivity is tested, the alpha rhythm may be blocked along with the mu rhythm if the test alerts the subject. A paradoxical mu rhythm is a mu rhythm that is induced by contralateral movement or touch after the mu rhythm has dropped out in drowsy subjects. The same events that induce a paradoxical mu rhythm may also alert the subject, and a paradoxical alpha rhythm may be induced at the same time.

Because the mu rhythm is normally intermittent and asynchronous, an EEG is not abnormal if it shows only a few trains of mu rhythm on one side, or only a moderate difference in the incidence of mu rhythm on the two sides. However, frequent trains of mu rhythm appearing only on one side, or a consistent asymmetry of amplitude or frequency of mu rhythm, suggest an abnormality on the side of the lower amplitude or frequency. Mu rhythms can be detected in more than 10% of individuals if bipolar, or Laplacian montages are used and the frequency spectra of the at rest vs. during movement periods of EEG are averaged and subtracted from each other. The physiological significance of mu rhythm may be related to somatosensory processes associated with movement. This is suggested by the distribution of mu rhythm, by

the blocking effect of sensory stimuli and of passive movement, and by the onset of the mu blocking before actual and intended movement. The mu rhythm, like the alpha rhythm, may represent the idling of a sensory system not processing specific input from thalamic nuclei.

11.4   LAMBDA WAVES

Sharp transients of sawtooth shape and of positive polarity occur in the occipital regions of some subjects when they look at images containing visual detail (Fig. 11.3, Part 4). The duration of lambda waves is roughly 100–250 ms. They are usually diphasic with the highest amplitude component positive and less than 50 μV in amplitude in bipolar or referential montages. Lambda waves resemble positive occipital sharp transients (POSTs) of sleep. Indeed, subjects with prominent lambda waves almost always also have prominent POSTs and photic driving responses. Unlike POSTs that occur during drowsiness and sleep, lambda waves are accompanied by eye movement and eye blink artifact. Lambda waves are infrequently encountered in routine clinical EEGs, in part because visual scanning of complex images is not part of the routine recording procedure.

Neither the presence nor the absence of lambda waves is abnormal, but a marked asymmetry suggests an abnormality on the side of lower amplitude. Lambda waves resemble visual evoked potentials elicited by intermittent flash stimuli in terms of distribution, waveform and latent period between the change of visual input and the wave peak. Each lambda wave is preceded by a scanning eye movement, usually recognizable as an eye movement artifact in frontal derivations. It is therefore likely that lambda waves partly represent visual evoked potentials, but not necessarily in response to light. They persist to some extent in association with eye movements in the dark and probably also reflect other events, perhaps processes related to eye movement or to the blocking of visual input during changes of gaze.

11.5   VERTEX SHARP TRANSIENTS (V WAVES)

Sharp transients of negative polarity at the vertex are a common element of normal sleep activity (12.1.3). They occur very rarely in wakeful adults following a sudden loud noise or other unexpected stimuli, but are more easily evoked in children, for example by percussing the hands or feet. The amplitude of V waves during wakefulness is much lower than that of V waves occurring during sleep. V waves may form part of a generalized response to startling stimuli; such a response may also include eye blinks and scalp movements.

V waves probably represent a late component of evoked potentials which is non-specific insofar as it does not depend on the modality of the sensory stimulus and appears in a larger region of the cortex than the relatively small specific sensory area. Because of its wider distribution, evoked vertex waves are more likely to be recorded in the EEG than the earlier parts of sensory responses which are restricted to the specific sensory pathways and cortical receiving areas and usually need enhancement by computer averaging to be seen clearly. V waves tend to be more sharply contoured in younger individuals. They are also more likely to appear at times with a maximum amplitude over the midparietal head region (Pz) in children. Also, during childhood V waves are more likely to occur in bursts or rhythmic trains that can be confused with epileptiform abnormalities.

11.6   KAPPA RHYTHM

This rhythm consists of bursts of very low amplitude waves of alpha or theta frequency which have been recorded in a few instances in the temporal regions of subjects engaged in mental activity and are rarely seen in routine clinical recordings. It is not clear whether these waves represent electrocerebral activity in the temporal lobes generated by mental effort or whether they are due to fine rhythmical eye movements associated with eyelid flutter.

11.7   NORMAL POSTERIOR THETA RHYTHMS

Two very rare patterns of rhythmical theta activity can be distinguished in some normal EEGs. Their distribution and reactivity resembles that of alpha rhythms. They are the only exceptions to the rule that synchronous and repetitive theta waves in the EEG of wakeful resting adults are abnormal (11.9.2).

11.7.1 *Slow alpha variant* has been described (11.1.7).

11.7.2 *Rhythmical slow waves of about 4–5 Hz* appear intermittently in the occipital and temporal areas in probably less than 1% of normal adults. Even though the distribution of these rhythms differs slightly from that of alpha waves, they are blocked by eye opening and alerting and disappear in drowsiness and sleep. The incidence of this pattern decreases during adult life.

11.8   THE LOW VOLTAGE EEG

Some EEGs show no activity over 20 μV in recordings from any part of the head (Fig. 11.3, Part 5). At a high gain, a wide range of frequencies can be distinguished, including beta, theta and some delta waves, and sometimes posterior alpha waves (Fig. 11.4). The term 'low voltage fast EEG', which has sometimes been used to describe this pattern, is therefore not entirely accurate. Waves of higher amplitude can sometimes be induced by hyperventilation, photic stimulation and sleep.

Low voltage EEGs are not seen in normal children, but they become more common with advancing age. They are sometimes seen in tense subjects who show normal amplitude when relaxed. However, low voltage EEGs may be abnormal reflecting bilateral reduction of amplitude which can be recognized if a prior record from the same subject shows higher amplitude. Very low voltage, i.e., no activity over 10 μV, is more likely to be abnormal (24.2.2).

EEGs with no activity more than 2 μV in amplitude are considered to be evidence of electrocerebral inactivity and are highly correlated with the presence of brain death or a severe suppression of brain function.

11.9   MAJOR ABNORMALITIES

11.9.1 *Spikes and sharp waves* are abnormal except for (a) vertex sharp transients (11.5); (b) lambda waves which can easily be recognized by their shape and distribution and by the specific precipitating mechanisms (11.4); (c) most 6 Hz spike-and-slow-wave complexes (19.5.1); and other normal variants described in 19.5.

11.9.2 *Slow waves* of ≤8 Hz during wakefulness should be absent or very rare. They can be considered normal only if they are single, of theta frequency, without focal, regional or lateral predominance, asynchronous and not much higher in amplitude than the background. Theta rhythms that appear to be harmonic combinations of other frequency waveforms (such as RMTD or psychomotor variant) are also normal.

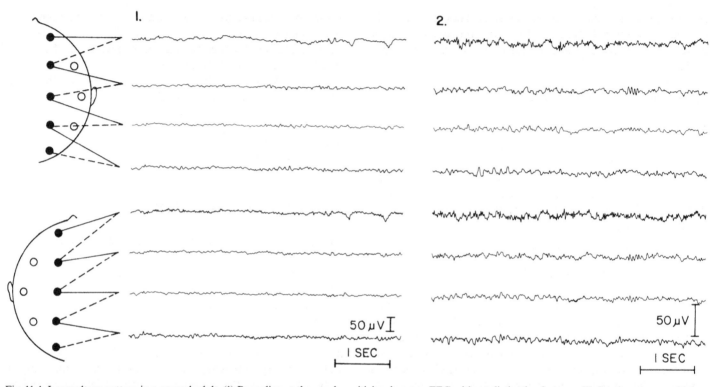

Fig. 11.4. Low voltage pattern in a normal adult. (1) Recording at the usual sensitivity shows an EEG without distinctive features. (2) Continuation at a higher sensitivity shows a mixture of a wide range of frequencies.

Slow waves are abnormal if they are repetitive or frequent, of delta frequency, of focal, regional or lateral distribution, bilaterally synchronous or of clearly higher amplitude than the background. A rare exception are the bilaterally synchronous theta rhythms in the posterior head regions of a few adults (11.7).

11.9.3 *Low amplitude* generally can best be diagnosed as being abnormal if the amplitude can be shown to be decreased in comparison with a preceding or subsequent record from the same subject. Low amplitude (<10 μV) observed in a single recording, although strictly an abnormal EEG feature, may not be associated with clinical abnormalities (24.2.2). However, a single recording of very low amplitude (<5 μV) usually indicates a clinical abnormality.

11.9.4 *Deviations from normal patterns* such as changes of the frequency or reactivity of alpha rhythm and the occurrence of alpha frequency patterns in coma are important abnormalities (25).

REFERENCES

Adrian, E.D. and Matthews, B.H.C. (1934) The Berger rhythm: potential changes from the occipital lobes in man. Brain 57: 355–385.

Aird, R.B. and Gastaut, Y. (1959) Occipital and posterior electroencephalographic rhythms. Electroenceph. Clin. Neurophysiol. 11: 637–656.

Barlow, J.S. and Cigánek, L. (1969) Lambda responses in relation to visual evoked responses in man. Electroenceph. Clin. Neurophysiol. 26: 183–192.

Blume, W.T. and Kaibara, M. (1995) Atlas of Adult Electroencephalography. Raven Press, New York.

Chapman, R.M., Armington, J.C. and Bragdon, H.R. (1962) A quantitative survey of kappa and alpha EEG activity. Electroenceph. Clin. Neurophysiol. 14: 858–868.

Chatrian, G.E. and Lairy, G.C. (Eds.) (1976) Part A. The EEG of the waking adult. In: A. Rémond (Ed.), Handbook of Electroenceph. Clin. Neurophysiol., Vol. 6A. Elsevier, Amsterdam.

Cobb, W.A., Guiloff, R.J. and Cast, J. (1979) Breach rhythm: the EEG related to skull defects. Electroenceph. Clin. Neurophysiol. 47: 251–271.

Fourment, A., Calvet, J. and Bancaud, J. (1976) Electrocorticography of waves associated with eye movements in man during wakefulness. Electroenceph. Clin. Neurophysiol. 40: 457–469.

Gibbs, F.A. and Gibbs, E.L. (1951) Atlas of Electroencephalography, Vol. 1: Methodology and Controls, 2nd Edn. Addison-Wesley Publishing Co., Reading.

Gloor, P. (Ed.) (1969) Hans Berger on the Electroencephalogram of Man. The Fourteen Original Reports on the Human Electroencephalogram. Electroenceph. Clin. Neurophysiol. Suppl. 28. Elsevier, Amsterdam.

Goldensohn, E.S., Legatt, A.D., Koszer, S. and Wolf, S.M. (1999) Goldensohn's EEG Interpretation: Problems of Overreading and Underreading. 2nd Edition. Futura Publishing Company, Armonk, New York.

Hoovey, Z.B., Heinemann, U. and Creutzfeldt, O.D. (1972) Inter-hemispheric 'synchrony' of alpha waves. Electroenceph. Clin. Neurophysiol. 32: 337–347.

Hughes, J.R. (1987) Normal limits in the EEG. In: A.M. Halliday, S.R. Butler and R. Paul (Eds.), A Textbook of Clinical Neurophysiology. Wiley, Chichester, pp. 105–154.

Hughes, J.R. and Cayaffa, J.J. (1977) The EEG in patients at different ages without organic cerebral disease. Electroenceph. Clin. Neurophysiol. 42: 776–784.

Kellaway, P. (1979) An orderly approach to visual analysis: the parameters of the normal EEG in adults and children. In: D.W. Klass and D.D. Daly (Eds.), Current Practice of Clinical Electroencephalography. Raven Press, New York, pp. 69–148.

Kellaway, P. (1990) An orderly approach to visual analysis: characteristics of the normal EEG of adults and children. In: D.D. Daly and T.A. Pedley (Eds.), Current Practice of Clinical Neurophysiology: Electroencephalography. 2nd Edition. Raven Press, New York, pp. 139–200.

Klass, D. and Westmoreland, B. (1996) Electroencephalography: general principles and adult electroencephalograms. In: J. Daube (Ed.), Clinical Neurophysiology. F.A. Davis, Philadelphia, pp. 73–103.

Kozelka, J.W. and Pedley, T.A. (1990) Beta and mu rhythms. J. Clin. Neurophysiol. 7: 191–208.

Kuhlman, W.N. (1978) Functional topography of the human mu rhythm. Electroenceph. Clin. Neurophysiol. 44: 83–93.

Lehmann, D. (1971) Multichannel topography of human alpha EEG fields. Electroenceph. Clin. Neurophysiol. 31: 439–449.

Leissner, P., Lindholm, L.E. and Petersén, I. (1970) Alpha amplitude dependence on skull thickness as measured by ultrasound technique. Electroenceph. Clin. Neurophysiol. 29: 392–399.

Liske, E., Hughes, H.M. and Stowe, D.E. (1967) Cross-correlation of human alpha activity: normative data. Electroenceph. Clin. Neurophysiol. 22: 429–436.

Markand, O. (1990) Alpha rhythms. J. Clin. Neurophysiol. 7: 163–190.

Niedermeyer, E. and Lopes da Silva, F. (Eds.) (1993) Electroencephalography: Basic Principles, Clinical Applications and Related Fields. Urban and Schwarzenberg, Baltimore.

Perez-Borja, C., Chatrian, G.E., Tyce, F.A. and Rivers, M.H. (1962) Electrographic patterns of the occipital lobe in man: a topographic study based on use of implanted electrodes. Electroenceph. Clin. Neurophysiol. 14: 171–182.

Pfurtscheller, G., Maresch, H. and Schuy, S. (1977) Inter- and intrahemispheric differences in the peak frequency of rhythmic activity within the alpha band. Electroenceph. Clin. Neurophysiol. 42: 77–83.

Santamaria, J. and Chiappa, K.H. (1987) The EEG of Drowsiness. Demos, New York.

Schoppenhorst, M., Brauer, F., Freund, G. and Kubicki, S. (1980) The significance of coherence estimates in determining central alpha and mu activities. Electroenceph. Clin. Neurophysiol. 48: 25–33.

Sperling, M.R. and Morrell, M.J. (1993) Pediatric and adult electroencephalography. In: M.R. Sperling and R.R. Clancy (Eds.), Atlas of Electroencephalography. Elsevier, Amsterdam.

Westmoreland, B.F. (1982) Normal and benign EEG patterns. Am. J. EEG Technol. 22: 3–31.

12 The normal sleep EEG of adults over 20 years

SUMMARY

The sleep EEG of adults shows less variation of patterns between individuals than does the waking EEG.

(12.1) The elements of the sleep EEG differ completely from those of the waking EEG and consist of slow waves, sleep spindles, positive occipital sharp transients (POSTs) of sleep, vertex sharp waves, K complexes, medium to high amplitude delta activity, and sawtooth waves. Eye movements and muscle activity may be picked up incidentally from routine EEG electrode placements but are recorded intentionally with special electrode placements for scoring sleep stages.

(12.2) *Sleep stages* are distinguished by EEG patterns consisting of different combinations of electrographic elements. These patterns serve to distinguish *stages I–IV of slow wave sleep,* representing progressively deeper levels of essentially dreamless sleep, and the *stage of rapid eye movement (REM) sleep,* which has some EEG characteristics of very light sleep and is associated with dreaming.

(12.3) *Sleep cycles* are characteristic sequences of sleep stages. Cycles can only be studied in all-night sleep recordings. REM sleep does usually not begin until 90–120 min after sleep onset. Stages III and IV sleep (also referred to as *slow wave sleep* or *delta sleep*) are concentrated in the first two-thirds of the night and REM in the last two-thirds of the night. Slow wave sleep is specifically associated with the secretion of growth hormone. Sleep stages are recognized by monitoring EEG, eye movement and submental muscle tone. Polysomnograms usually also include ECG, thoracic and abdominal wall movement, tibialis anterior muscle and nasal/oral air flow monitoring to allow for the detection of sleep disordered breathing (e.g., sleep apnea), periodic leg movements, and cardiac arrhythmias.

(12.4) Deviations from normal sleep include the absence of normal sleep features, REM periods at the onset of sleep (i.e., sleep within 20 min of sleep onset, so-called 'sleep onset REM periods'), and sleep disorders characterized by disturbances of sleep timing (circadian rhythm disturbances), abnormal respiration (e.g., sleep apnea), and unusual behaviors in sleep referred to as *parasomnias,* such as sleep walking, night terrors, nocturnal seizures, or REM behavior disorder. The multiple sleep latency test (12.4.5) is used to detect REM onset sleep in patients with suspected narcolepsy and to document excessive daytime sleepiness.

12.1 ELEMENTS OF NORMAL SLEEP ACTIVITY

12.1.1 *Slow waves* occur in a wide distribution and are often more prominent posteriorly than anteriorly. In lighter stages of non-REM sleep they are generally less persistent, more asynchronous, of lower amplitude and faster frequency (Fig. 12.1, Parts 2 and 3) than in deeper stages (Fig. 12.2, Parts 1 and 2).

12.1.2 *Positive occipital sharp transients* (POSTs) are mono- or biphasic, triangular waves in the occipital regions (Fig. 12.1, Parts 2 and 3; Fig. 12.2, Part 1). Because they have posi-

199

tive electrical polarity, they produce upgoing pen deflections in channels connected to the occipital electrodes through input 2, such as P3-O1 (3.4.1). POSTs occur intermittently and spontaneously, either simultaneously or independently, on the two sides of the head. They usually recur irregularly at intervals of over 1 s, but they may repeat up to 4–6 times/s. Intermittent independent POSTs of high amplitude may resemble focal epileptiform discharges but should not be confused with them.

POSTs have also been called 'lambdoid waves' because they resemble lambda waves in shape and distribution (11.4); like lambda waves, they depend on normal central visual acuity. However, because the mechanisms responsible for generating the two types of waves are not known, the term 'lambdoid' should not be used.

Individuals with prominent lambda waves are more likely to demonstrate both POSTs and prominent photic driving. Awareness of this relationship is sometimes helpful in distinguishing high amplitude asymmetric POSTs from epileptiform activity.

12.1.3 *Vertex sharp transients (V waves)* are bilaterally synchronous waves which have a maximum amplitude at the vertex and often extend into frontal, temporal and parietal areas (Fig. 12.1, Part 3). Children are most likely to show parietal dominant vertex waves. V waves have negative polarity and therefore cause upgoing pen deflections in channels connected to an electrode close to the vertex placed in amplifier input 1

and to a more distant electrode in amplifier input 2 (3.4.1; 4.1). V waves are symmetrical on average even though their amplitude on either side may fluctuate transiently and sometimes dramatically. They are single and often recur at irregular intervals, rarely more often than 2 times/s. They may appear in response to a sensory stimulus, such as tapping on the foot or hands in asleep or awake individuals, particularly children (11.5). When they occur in runs they are sometimes mistaken for abnormal epileptiform activity.

12.1.4 *Sleep spindles* have a frequency range of 11–15 Hz, but are usually defined as 12–14 Hz waveforms with a duration of >0.5 s that may last up to a few seconds (Fig. 12.1, Part 3, Fig. 12.2, Part 1). They have a wide distribution, with a maximum over the central regions. After 2 years of age they always appear simultaneously over both hemispheres and are approximately symmetric.

12.1.5 *K complexes* resemble V waves in distribution, reaction to sensory stimuli and polarity of the major component, but they are significantly longer in duration (≥0.5 s) and less sharply contoured (Fig. 12.2, Part 1). A more detailed description is given in 10.3.

12.2 SLEEP STAGES

12.2.1 *Stage W* or wakefulness at the transition to drowsiness may show some slowing and greater prominence of alpha rhythm (Fig. 12.2, Part 1). Beta rhythms may be present and continue into stage I of sleep; they are especially prominent when sleep is induced by sedatives. Movement and muscle artifacts may obscure the EEG at the transition to sleep.

Slow lateral eye movements (SEMs), typically less than 0.5 Hz, are often the first obvious electrographic sign of drowsiness and often occur at a time when the alpha rhythm is still present. According to Santamaria and Chiappa (1987) earlier stages of drowsiness can be detected using a sensitive movement transducer taped over the outer aspect of the upper eyelid. By this technique wakefulness during eye closure is accompanied by the presence of *mini-blinks* (rapid eye deflections; predominantly vertical) that occur 5–10 times/10 s, each with a duration of less than 400 ms. They correspond to low amplitude deflections in the eye lead monitors. The earliest stage of drowsiness occurs when mini-blinks disappear. In approximately one-third of normal individuals with further drowsiness the mini-blinks are replaced by small fast irregular eye movements. The latter have a faster repetition rate (5–30/ s) and are lower in amplitude than mini-blinks. Finally, SEMs appear. In approximately one-third of normal individuals SEMs are accompanied by small fast rhythmic (3–8 Hz) eye movements, visible with movement transducer monitoring.

12.2.2 *Sleep stage I* begins with the disappearance of the alpha rhythm and the appearance of slow waves of 2–7 Hz (Fig. 12.1, Part 2). *In polysomnography, a 30 s epoch is scored as sleep (vs. waking) if less than 50% of the epoch contains the waking alpha background activity.* At the early part of this stage, most persons show low amplitude activity of mixed frequencies, but some have medium to high amplitude slow wave bursts immediately after the disappearance of the alpha rhythm. Alpha waves may recur briefly; this is the time when the *paradoxical alpha* rhythm (produced by alerting instead of eye closure and relaxation) appears on slight alerting (11.1.6). Muscle activity diminishes. Slow eye movements may occur and last for several seconds.

A variety of sudden or paroxysmal medium to high amplitude patterns consisting of various admixtures of delta, theta, and alpha activity can occur during the transition from wakefulness to stage I and II sleep. It is important to be aware that these somewhat unusual or striking patterns can occur during drowsiness so that they are not misinterpreted as paroxysmal abnormalities or, more specifically, epileptiform abnormalities.

Slow waves and paroxysmal slowing during drowsiness and stage I sleep may at times be difficult to distinguish from pathological slowing, particularly since many abnormal changes appear predominantly during eye closure at rest or early drowsiness. Normal slowing during drowsiness is most likely to occur in patients who have either been sedated in order to obtain a sleep recording or who spontaneously achieve stages I and II sleep during the recording. Other findings consistent with drowsiness are the presence of SEM and a reduction in muscle artifact. Finally, alerting maneuvers

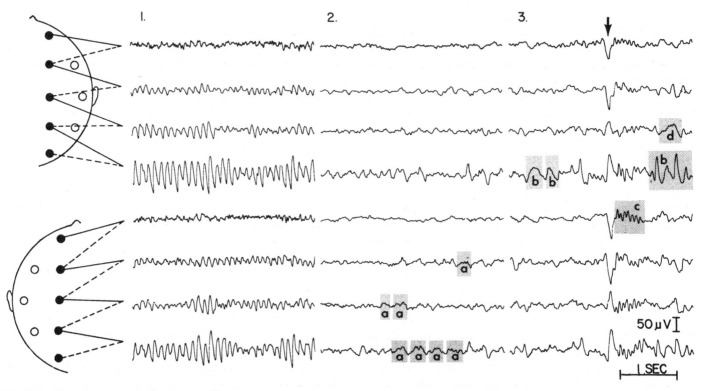

Fig. 12.1.   Normal patterns of wakefulness and light sleep in an adult. (1) Stage W (wakefulness) with alpha rhythm and frontal beta rhythm. (2) Stage I (drowsiness) with irregular slow waves at 3–7 Hz (a). (3) Stage II (light sleep) with a V wave (arrow), POSTs (b), sleep spindles (c), and slow waves of 2–7 Hz (d).

should be performed at some point in *every* recording to produce a state of clear wakefulness. To reiterate, *it is best to assess the frequency of the alpha rhythm during alerting maneuvers since during drowsiness it may slow by 1–2 Hz.* Alerting maneuvers should *always* include more than the simple commands to open and close the eyes (such as mental calculation, orientation to time, or other questions appropriate to age and clinical condition), otherwise sustained wakefulness may not occur. In addition, mental calculations performed during eye closure may reveal an abnormal asymmetry of posterior alpha reactivity (failure of attenuation over the abnormal hemisphere) that does not appear with eye opening.

In deeper parts of stage I, slow waves are of medium amplitude and may form irregularly spaced bursts. Vertex waves may occur in response to alerting stimuli or apparently spontaneously in this stage and in stage II. At the end of stage I, POSTs appear in many subjects.

12.2.3 *Stage II is characterized by the presence of either sleep spindles of at least 0.5 s in duration or K complexes or both* (Fig. 12.1, Part 3). Slow waves of 2–7 Hz continue to be seen and are often bilaterally synchronous; slow waves of less than 2 Hz are absent or not prominent. POSTs often persist in stage II.

12.2.4 *Stage III is* characterized by the presence of a moderate amount of very slow waves of high amplitude: *in sleep scoring stage III sleep is considered present if 20–50% of an epoch (i.e., 30 s of recording) is occupied by waves of 2 Hz or less of over 75 μV* (Fig. 12.2, Part 1) recorded in C3-A1 or C4-A2. K complexes are often present. Sleep spindles may be present or absent. POSTs can usually be distinguished.

12.2.5 *Stage IV is* characterized by more slow wave activity than is present in stage III. In sleep scoring *stage IV sleep is considered present if over 50% of the 30 s epoch is occupied by waves of 2 Hz or less that are over 75 μV in amplitude recorded in C3-A1 or C4-A2.* K complexes blend with slow waves. Spindles and POSTs may be seen but are rare (Fig. 12.2, Part 2). After 55 years of age stage III and IV sleep become rare if only the amplitude criteria for sleep scoring are applied. Therefore, most polysomnographers assess the presence of slow wave sleep (i.e., stages III or IV) according to frequency content rather than amplitude.

12.2.6 *REM* sleep is characterized by low voltage EEG patterns, rapid eye movements, and reduced muscle activity (atonia); it is associated with dreaming. In sleep scoring *REM sleep is considered to be present when more than 50% of a 30 s epoch contains low voltage EEG activity with prominent theta activity preceded by rapid eye movements* and accompanied by reduced muscle tone as measured from submental electrodes. Although the EEG and some behavioral changes suggest that sleep is lighter during this stage, the threshold for arousal by auditory stimuli is increased, suggesting a deeper stage of sleep. Brain metabolic activity during REM sleep as measured by positron emission tomography is as great or greater than

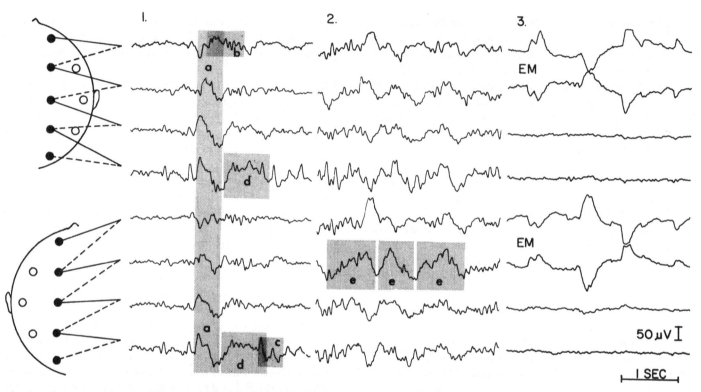

Fig. 12.2.   Normal patterns of deep sleep and REM sleep in an adult. (1) Stage III (deep sleep) with a K complex (a), sleep spindle (b), POSTs (c), and slow waves of less than 2 Hz (d). (2) Stage IV (very deep sleep) with slow waves of less than 2 Hz and over 75 μV during over 50% of the recording (e). (3) Stage REM (rapid eye movement sleep) with eye movements indicated by eye movement monitors (EM) used during this part of the recording.

that seen during wakefulness. These conflicting findings (sleep with atonia and high cerebral metabolic activity) have led various authors to refer to REM as *'paradoxical sleep'*.

The EEG during REM sleep shows asynchronous low voltage waves of mixed frequency (Fig. 12.2, Part 3). It may resemble the pattern of stage I sleep except that it contains no V waves. REM sleep usually produces a specific EEG pattern of brief runs of medium amplitude sawtooth shaped theta waves over the central and frontal head regions (*sawtooth waves*). It is a common misconception that REM sleep looks like the waking EEG. Although alpha frequency waveforms may be present, they are always 1–2 Hz less than the frequency of the alpha rhythm during wakefulness and theta activity is abundant.

Rapid eye movements are often picked up with routine prefrontal electrode placements but are more reliably monitored with recording electrodes placed near the eyes (4.3.1). Such recordings show irregular deflections with extremely fast initial components due to rapid lateral changes of eye position (Fig. 12.2, Part 3).

Changes of muscle tone and other activity are recorded with EEG electrodes placed on neck muscles below the chin (4.3.4). Muscle tone reaches its lowest level during the REM stage of sleep. However, paroxysms of muscle activity may appear in such recordings and often are associated with vigorous bursts of REM and brief twitches of face and limb muscles. This is referred to as *phasic* REM activity as opposed to *tonic* REM. Blood pressure and heart rate increase, breathing becomes faster and irregular, and gastrointestinal movement ceases; males have erections during almost every REM period.

REM sleep is rarely encountered during routine recordings in children, adolescents, and adults because the latency of REM sleep exceeds routine recording times. Therefore, the appearance of REM sleep in a routine recording raises the question of a sleep disorder such as narcolepsy, sleep apnea, sleep deprivation, or a circadian rhythm disorder.

12.3 SLEEP CYCLES

Normal nightly sleep is organized in characteristic sequences of sleep stages (Fig. 12.3). The first cycle begins with stage I and proceeds through increasingly deeper stages of non-REM sleep to REM sleep. This is followed by another cycle of gradual descent through non-REM sleep to REM sleep. Normally, there are about 4–7 such cycles during a night. The first cycle is the shortest, but later cycles do not vary much in length and last about 80–120 min. REM sleep normally occurs only at the end of each cycle and thus first appears 70–90 min after the onset of sleep. REM is almost always entered through stage II sleep. The highest serum levels of growth hormone in a 24 h period occur during the first cycle of stage III and IV sleep (slow wave sleep; delta sleep) of the night.

Several features of sleep vary with age. Although total sleep time is fairly constant through adulthood, the number and duration of the individual sleep stages change. A normal

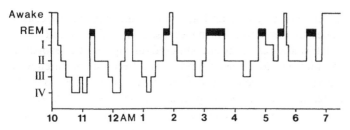

Fig. 12.3. Diagram of sleep cycles during an all-night sleep recording in a normal young adult. Sleep stages are plotted against time of the night.

young adult spends about 30–50% of sleep time in stage II, 20–40% in stages III and IV, and 5–10% in stage I. The percentage of stages III and IV decreases with age so that greater amounts of sleep time are spent in lighter stages. The proportion of REM sleep decreases slightly from about 25% in young adults to about 20% in the fifth decade, but overall remains stable throughout life.

To chart sleep stages, an all-night sleep recording is scored during successive periods of 30 s. The sleep stage prevailing during these periods is plotted as a function of time from the onset of sleep forming a hypnogram (Fig. 12.3). To identify the sleep stages accurately, eye movements and muscle activity are recorded in addition to the EEG (5.3). A thorough study of sleep cycles for research purposes requires that recordings be made during more than 1 night to overcome the distorting 'first night effect' which is due to the subject's unfamiliarity with the environment of the sleep laboratory and the recording procedures.

12.4   DEVIATIONS FROM NORMAL SLEEP

With the exceptions of epileptiform activity, non-epileptiform abnormalities present in the waking record, or the absence of normal sleep activity (e.g., unilateral loss of sleep spindle activity due to an ipsilateral thalamic lesion), sleep disorders are detected either by multiple sleep latency testing (MSLT) or overnight polysomnography.

12.4.1   *Spikes and sharp waves* appear during sleep in many patients with convulsive disorders. Therefore sleep is often used as an activation procedure in the diagnosis of epilepsy, particularly partial seizure disorders (14.2.1). Spikes and sharp waves must be carefully distinguished from positive occipital sharp transients (12.1.2) and vertex sharp transients (12.1.3).

12.4.2   *Short latency to sleep onset* of an average of less than 5 min on the MSLT across all daytime naps can be found in patients with narcolepsy and other disorders (25.4.3).

12.4.3   *Sleep onset REM periods* are characteristically seen in patients with narcolepsy and may occur rarely in patients with sleep apnea (25.4.3). Single daytime naps are not reliable indicators of this disorganization of the first sleep cycle because naps occasionally begin with REM sleep in persons without sleep disorders, and may begin without REM periods in some patients with narcolepsy. However, REM sleep occurring on a routine EEG recording always raises the question of a sleep disorder, particularly narcolepsy. *REM sleep during two or more naps of the MSLT is virtually pathognomonic of narcolepsy if other disorders that cause daytime somnolence have been ruled out by polysomnography.*

12.4.4 *Disorders of sleep cycles* such as excessive arousals from sleep or the absence of REM sleep occur in various conditions (25.4.5). To diagnose these conditions, it is necessary to perform overnight polysomnography using extracerebral physiological monitoring in addition to the EEG (4.3). An arousal index, defined as the number of arousals per hour of sleep, in excess of 15 from any cause is almost always associated with pathological daytime sleepiness. Respiratory body movement and air flow must be monitored to study sleep apnea, characterized by frequent and long periods without breathing (>10 s is scored as an apnea) that can cause severe daytime sleepiness or dangerous arrhythmia producing hypoxemia ($< 65\%$ S_aO_2). Electrodes are placed over the tibialis anterior muscle on each leg to detect periodic leg movements (PLMs) that resemble spontaneous Babinski responses. Almost all patients with restless leg syndrome also have excessive PLMs. Video recording during polysomnography is essential for the study of parasomnias (abnormal behaviors) that disrupt sleep: sleep walking, night terrors, and confu-

sional arousals occur during stage III and IV sleep and nightmares and REM behavior disorder during REM sleep.

12.4.5 The multiple sleep latency test (MSLT) is used: (1) to detect the presence of REM onset sleep in patients with suspected narcolepsy, and (2) to evaluate complaints of excessive daytime drowsiness. Since REM onset sleep and excessive drowsiness may both be caused by sleep deprivation, the MSLT is most revealing when performed in a controlled inpatient setting that allows for polysomnographic monitoring of the patient's sleep pattern the night before testing.

The MSLT is performed by giving the patient 5 opportunities to fall asleep during the day. The first nap should begin at approximately 9:00 or 10:00 a.m. and the remaining are performed at 2 h intervals. For each nap the patient is given 20 min to fall asleep. *Sleep onset is* defined as either (1) 3 consecutive 30 s epochs of stage I sleep, or (2) any single epoch of stage II, III, or REM sleep. Each nap is terminated if the patient is not asleep at 20 min after the onset of testing or if the patient sleeps for 15 consecutive minutes. The nap is also terminated if the patient awakens at any time beyond 20 min from the onset of the test. Wakefulness is defined as 2 consecutive 30 s epochs of wakefulness.

The *mean sleep latency* (i.e., the time between the beginning of the nap period and the beginning of *sleep onset)* is calculated for each of the 5 naps. A mean sleep latency of less than 5 min is considered highly abnormal and suggests the presence of excessive drowsiness. The number of nap periods with

REM sleep is also calculated. If two or more nap periods contain REM sleep, then a diagnosis of narcolepsy is highly likely. However, it is important to be aware that the MSLT results are extremely difficult to interpret in individuals who are either sleep deprived or taking medications that may alter sleep (e.g., amphetamines or antidepressant medications).

REFERENCES

American Electroencephalographic Society (1994) Guideline fifteen: Guidelines of polygraphic assessment of sleep-related disorders. J. Clin. Neurophysiol. 11: 116–124.

ASDA Atlas Task Force (1993) Recording and scoring leg movements. Sleep 16: 749–759.

Association of Sleep Disorders Centers and the Association for the Psychophysiological Study of Sleep (1979) Glossary of terms used in the sleep disorders classification. Sleep 2: 123–129.

Bartel, P., Robinson, E. and Duim, W. (1995) Burst patterns occurring during drowsiness in clinical EEG. Am. J. EEG Technol. 35: 283–295.

Broughton, R. (1993) Polysomnography: principles and applications in sleep and arousal disorders. In: E. Niedermeyer and F. Lopes da Silva (Eds.), Electroencephalography: Basic Principles, Clinical Applications and Related Fields. Urban and Schwarzenberg, Baltimore, pp. 765–802.

Browman, C.P., Krishnareddy, S.G., Yolles, S.F. and Mitler, M. (1986) Forty-eight hour polysomnographic evaluation of narcolepsy. Sleep 9: 183–188.

Daly, D.D. and Yoss, R.E. (1957) Electroencephalogram in narcolepsy. Electroenceph. Clin. Neurophysiol. 9: 109–120.

Decoster, R. and Foret, J. (1979) Sleep onset and first cycle of sleep in human subjects: change with time of day. Electroenceph. Clin. Neurophysiol. 46: 531–537.

Dement, W.C. (1976) Daytime sleepiness and sleep 'attacks'. In: C. Guilleminault, W.C. Dement and P. Passouant (Eds.), Narcolepsy. Spectrum, New York, pp. 17–42.

Dement, W.C. (1990) A personal history of sleep disorders medicine. J. Clin. Neurophysiol. 7: 17–47.

Dement, W. and Kleitman, N. (1957) Cyclic variations in EEG during sleep and their relation to eye movements, body mobility, and dreaming. Electroenceph. Clin. Neurophysiol. 9: 673–690.

Erwin, C.W., Somerville, E.R. and Radtke, R.A. (1984) A review of electroencephalographic features of normal sleep. J. Clin. Neurophysiol. 1: 253–274.

Fisch, B.J. (1994) Neurological aspects of sleep. In: M.J. Aminoff (Ed.), Neurology and General Medicine, 2nd Edition. Churchill Livingstone, New York.

Guilleminault, C. and Baker, T.L. (1984) Sleep and electroencephalography: points of interest and points of controversy. J. Clin. Neurophysiol. 1: 275–291.

Guilleminault, C., Stoohs, R., Clerk, A. et al. (1993) A cause of excessive daytime sleepiness. The upper airway resistance syndrome. Chest 104: 781–787.

Hauri, P. and Olmstead, E.M. (1973) Alpha-delta sleep. Electroenceph. Clin. Neurophysiol. 34: 233–237.

Hauri, P. and Olmstead, E.M. (1989) Reverse first night effect in insomnia. Sleep 12: 97–105.

Hughes, J.R. (1985) Sleep spindles revisited. J. Clin. Neurophysiol. 2: 37–44.

Jankel, W.R. and Niedermeyer, E. (1985) Sleep spindles. J. Clin. Neurophysiol. 2: 1–36.

Kales, A. and Kales, J.D. (1974) Sleep disorders. Recent findings in the diagnosis and treatment of disturbed sleep. New Engl. J. Med. 290: 487–499.

Kryger, M.H., Roth, T. and Dement, W.C. (1994) Principles and Practice of Sleep Medicine. W.B. Saunders, Philadelphia.

Lavie, P., Gadoth, N., Gordon, C.R., Goldhammer, G. and Bechar, M. (1979) Sleep patterns in Kleine–Levin syndrome. Electroenceph. Clin. Neurophysiol. 47: 369–371.

Mahowald, M.W. and Schenck, C.H. (1989) REM sleep behavior disorder. In: M.H. Kryger, T. Roth and W.C. Dement (Eds.), Principles and Practice of Sleep Medicine. W.B. Saunders, Philadelphia, pp. 389–401.

Mitler, M. (1984) The multiple sleep latency test as an evaluation for excessive somnolence. In: C. Guilleminault (Ed.), Sleeping and Waking Disorders, Indications and Techniques. Addison-Wesley, Reading, pp. 145–153.

Mitler, M.M., Van den Hoed, J., Carskadon, M.A., Richardson, G., Park, R., Guilleminault, C. and Dement, W.C. (1979) REM sleep episodes during the multiple sleep latency test in narcoleptic patients. Electroenceph. Clin. Neurophysiol. 46: 479–481.

Numminen, J., Mäkelä, J.P. and Hari, R. (1996) Distributions and sources of magnetoencephalographic K-complexes. Electroenceph. Clin. Neurophysiol. 99: 544–555.

Parkes, J.D. (1985) Sleep and Its Disorders. Saunders, Philadelphia.

Passouant, P. (1975) EEG and sleep. In: E.K. Killam and K. Killam (Eds.), Handbook of EEG and Clinical Neurophysiology, Vol. 7A. Elsevier, Amsterdam, pp. 5–25.

Rechtschaffen, A. and Kales, A. (1968) A Manual of Standardized Terminology, Techniques and Scoring System for Sleep Stages of Human Subjects. PHS, U.S. Government Printing Office, Washington, DC.

Richardson, G.S., Carskadon, M.A., Flagg, W., Van den Hoed, J., Dement, W.C. and Mitler, M.M. (1978) Excessive daytime sleepiness in man: multiple sleep latency measurement in narcoleptic and control subjects. Electroenceph. Clin. Neurophysiol. 45: 621–627.

Roth, M., Shaw, J. and Green, J. (1956) The form, voltage distribution and physiological significance of the K-complex. Electroenceph. Clin. Neurophysiol. 8: 385–402.

Santamaria, J. and Chiappa, K.H. (1987) The EEG of Drowsiness. Demos, New York.

Shepard, Jr., J.W. (1991) Atlas of Sleep Medicine. Futura Publishing Company, Mount Kisco, NY.

Sleep Disorders Atlas Task Force of the American Sleep Disorders Association (1992) EEG arousals: scoring rules and examples. Sleep 15: 174–184.

Therapeutics and Technology Assessment Subcommittee of the American Academy of Neurology (1992) Assessment: techniques associated with the diagnosis and management of sleep disorders. Neurology 42: 269–275.

Vignaendra, V., Matthews, R.L. and Chatrian, G.E. (1974) Positive occipital sharp transients of sleep: relationships to nocturnal sleep cycle in man. Electroenceph. Clin. Neurophysiol. 37: 239–246.

Williams, R.L., Karacan, I. and Hursch, C.J. (1974) Electroencephalography (EEG) of Human Sleep. Wiley, New York.

13 The normal EEG of adults over 60 years of age

SUMMARY

The normal EEG of adults over 60 years of age is similar to that of younger adults with a few exceptions.

(13.1) The alpha rhythm may be slower, less persistent and less reactive.

(13.2) *Beta activity* is often more prominent.

(13.3) *Sporadic generalized slow waves* may be slightly more common than in younger adults.

(13.4) *Intermittent temporal slow waves* appear in some apparently normal subjects, especially on the left side.

(13.5) *Sleep* is less deep and more often interrupted by wakefulness.

(13.6) *Major abnormalities* at this age are similar to those of younger adults except that a wider range of slow waves is acceptable as normal in old age.

13.1 ALPHA RHYTHM

Alpha rhythm decreases in frequency, prominence and reactivity.

13.1.1 The frequency of alpha rhythm drops from mean values of about 10–11 Hz in groups of young adults to means of about 9 Hz in persons over 60 years and of 8–9 Hz in centenarians. This progression to slower rates can be seen in recordings from the same individual made at different ages.

The frequency of the alpha rhythm may fall below 8 Hz in adults; although such rhythms are abnormal and outside the alpha frequency range, they are commonly, however imprecisely, called 'alpha rhythm' as long as they retain the distribution and reactivity of the alpha rhythm. It was previously thought that a frequency as low as 7.0 Hz was not abnormal in persons between 60 and 70 years of age and that frequencies of 6–7 Hz could be normal in some persons over 70 years. But an alpha rhythm of 8.0 Hz or less is now generally considered abnormal, even in elderly persons (Fig. 13.1). The frequency of the alpha rhythm becomes a more sensitive indicator of cerebral dysfunction if a previous baseline recording is available for comparison. For example, provided that the alpha rhythm is assessed during definite wakefulness (e.g., with alerting maneuvers), even a well sustained alpha rhythm of 9.0 Hz is an abnormal finding if the individual's baseline alpha rhythm is 11.0 Hz.

13.1.2 The *voltage and persistence* of alpha rhythm decrease with age. Low voltage patterns (11.8) become more common after age 60.

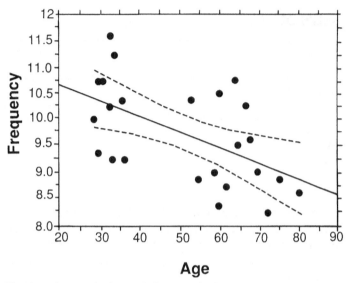

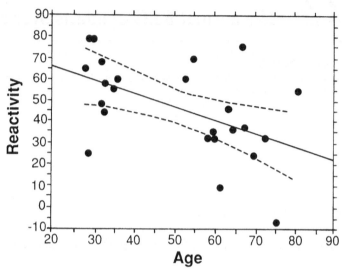

Fig. 13.1. Age vs. absolute peak frequency in the 8–13 Hz range in a group of carefully screened (medication-free) normal individuals. The spectral peak frequency of activity recorded in Ol-A1A2 derivation was determined by computer analysis. The amplitude spectra analyzed were obtained from an average of four 8 s epochs (yielding a frequency resolution of 0.125 Hz).

Fig. 13.2. Age vs. alpha reactivity recorded in T5-O1 in a group of carefully selected (medication-free) normal individuals. Alpha reactivity was calculated by subtracting the 8–13 Hz amplitude spectral band value during eye opening from the 8–13 Hz band value during eye closure and then dividing the difference by the 8–13 Hz band value during eye closure. The final value multiplied by 100 yields the percentage of change in the eyes closed 8–13 Hz band caused by eye opening. The spectra used for these calculations were obtained by averaging four 8 s epochs in each condition (eyes opened and eyes closed). During the recording the subjects were instructed to hold their eyes open or closed every 10 s.

13.1.3 The *reactivity* of the alpha rhythm is decreased. The percentage of attenuation of the alpha rhythm in response to eye opening decreases with age. This has been demonstrated by computerized quantitative EEG analysis (as shown in Fig. 13.2). It is also thought that the onset of attenuation following eye closure is delayed and the degree of sustained attenuation is of shorter duration.

212

13.1.4 The *topography* of activity in the alpha frequency range when recorded with non-cephalic, common average, or ear reference montages is often shifted from a posterior to a more frontocentral dominant location during eye closure at rest. This occurs somewhat more often in elderly individuals than in young adults, particularly during drowsiness.

13.2 BETA RHYTHM

The incidence and amplitude of beta rhythms increase during middle life (11.2.4). Beta activity is found in at least half of the elderly, more commonly in women than in men. Fast activity tends to disappear in very old age. Its disappearance is probably not a normal phenomenon but generally correlates with the development of cerebral atrophy.

13.3 SPORADIC GENERALIZED SLOW WAVES

Sporadic generalized slow waves are not much more prominent between 60 and 75 years than in younger adults. After age 75, a slight increase of slow waves mainly in the theta range may represent normal, age-dependent EEG changes, but more continuous theta activity or the appearance of generalized delta waves represents an EEG abnormality. Abnormal generalized slow waves correlate more strongly than other age-related EEG changes with dementia of Alzheimer's

type. However, senile dementia may progress to considerable severity before the EEG shows any deviation from the normal range.

13.4 INTERMITTENT TEMPORAL SLOW WAVES

Intermittent temporal slow waves of elderly persons have several characteristic features. They appear in the form of either single waves or of brief bursts of theta or delta activity (Fig. 13.1). Although these bursts have medium or high amplitude, they occur infrequently and remain separated from each other by normal background activity. Approximately two-thirds arise from the left temporal area. Similar slow waves of lower amplitude sometimes appear simultaneously or independently in the right temporal regions. Since such slow waves usually are distributed either evenly over the left and right temporal areas or more frequently on the left, the finding of a right-sided predominance should raise the question of an underlying right temporal abnormality.

Although these slow waves are probably not the result of normal aging but of degenerative and perhaps vascular cerebral changes, they are often found in apparently normal elderly individuals. They are best seen in bipolar or Cz reference montages and least well seen in ipsilateral ear reference montages. They can usually be distinguished from an abnormal slow wave focus by their clearly intermittent occurrence between long periods of normal background activity and by their restricted distribution. According to Arenas at al. (1986), 'normal' temporal slowing in the delta frequency range should occupy less than 1% of the waking record. 'Normal' temporal slowing in the theta frequency range should occupy less than 10% of the waking record. In contrast, abnormal focal slow waves of comparable amplitude occur more frequently, may extend into neighboring areas, especially the frontal regions, and are often associated with generalized slow waves. Sharp transients may occur with some temporal slow wave bursts that occasionally resemble focal epileptiform sharp waves (17.1.2), but their configuration usually shows greater variability. As in younger individuals, temporal intermittent rhythmic delta activity has a higher association with seizure disorders than other non-specific abnormal patterns.

13.5 SLEEP

13.5.1 *Sleep onset* may be associated with fairly prominent slow waves beginning abruptly as soon as alpha activity has dropped out. Some normal old persons show trains of bilaterally synchronous delta waves in drowsiness. Sudden transitions to stage II sleep, sometimes referred to as telescoping sleep onset, also occur in normal individuals.

13.5.2 *Sleep depth and sleep consolidation is reduced.* The proportion of time spent in stages III and IV decreases through adult life and reaches less than 10% in old age. How-

ever, if the amplitude criteria (>75 μV in C3-A2) for scoring stages III and IV sleep are ignored and the frequency criteria (activity 2 Hz or less occupying more than 20% of a 30 s epoch for stage III or more than 50% for stage IV) is used, then slow wave sleep occupies more time. The loss of amplitude is thought to be due in part to the reduction in the number of cortical synapses that occurs with aging. Although the total time spent sleeping in a 24 h period changes little with aging, the consolidation of sleep into the major nocturnal sleep period declines with age resulting in more fragmentation of sleep and increased daytime napping.

13.5.3 *REM sleep* decreases to less than 20% of total sleep time at the ages of 70–80 years.

13.6 MAJOR ABNORMALITIES

13.6.1 *Slow waves* in excess of those acceptable as normal at this age (13.3) are usually associated with clinical abnormalities.

13.6.2 *Extremely low amplitude* and *asymmetry of amplitude* are abnormal; the standards are the same as for younger adults (11.9.3).

13.6.3 *Spikes and sharp waves* are abnormal with the same

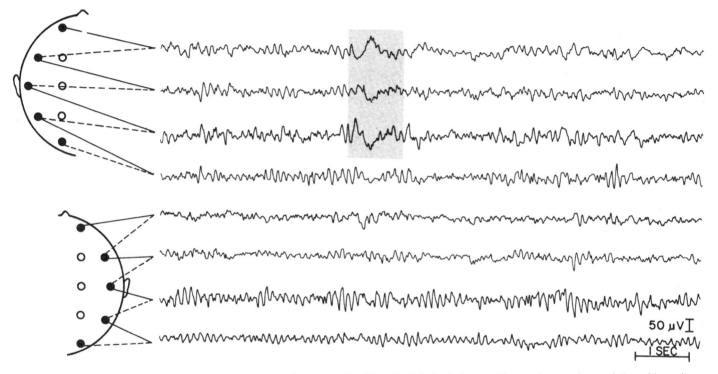

Fig. 13.3. Sporadic left temporal slow waves with sharp contours in 61-year-old subject (shaded) that is abnormal because it occurs in association with continuous irregular higher amplitude activity compared to the right hemisphere.

exceptions as for younger adults during wakefulness (11.9.1) and sleep (12.4.1).

REFERENCES

Arenas, A.M., Brenner, R.P. and Reynolds, C.F. (1986) Temporal slowing in the elderly revisited. Am. J. EEG Technol. 26: 105–114.

Bennet, D.R. (1981) Electroencephalographic and evoked potential changes with aging. Sem. Neurol. 1: 47–51.

Celesia, G. (1986) EEG and event related potentials in aging and dementia. J. Clin. Neurophysiol. 3: 99–112.

Ehlers, C.L. and Kupfer, D.J. (1989) Effects of age on delta and REM sleep parameters. Electroenceph. Clin. Neurophysiol. 72: 118–125.

Erwin, C.W., Somerville, E.R. and Radtke, R.A. (1984) A review of electroencephalographic features of normal sleep. J. Clin. Neurophysiol. 1: 253–274.

Hubbard, O., Sunde, D. and Goldensohn, E.S. (1976) The EEG in centenarians. Electroenceph. Clin. Neurophysiol. 40: 407–417.

Ingvar, D.H., Sjölund, B. and Ardo, A. (1976) Correlation between dominant EEG frequency, cerebral oxygen uptake and blood flow. Electroenceph. Clin. Neurophysiol. 41: 268–276.

Katz, R.I. and Horowitz, G.R. (1982) Electroencephalogram in the septuagenarian: studies in a normal geriatric population. J. Am. Geriat. Soc. 30: 273–275.

Kellaway, P. (1979) An orderly approach to visual analysis: the parameters of the normal EEG in adults and children. In: D.W. Klass and D.D. Daly (Eds.), Current Practice of Clinical Electroencephalography. Raven Press, New York, pp. 69–148.

Klass, D.W. and Brenner, R.P. (1995) Electroencephalography of the elderly. J. Clin. Neurophysiol. 27: 43–47.

Marsh, G.R. and Thompson, L.V. (1977) Psychophysiology of aging. In: J.E. Birren and K.W. Schaie (Eds.), Handbook of the Psychology of Aging. Reinhold van Nostrand, New York, pp. 219–248.

Mundy-Castle, A.C., Hurst, L.A., Beerstecher, D.M. and Prinsloo, T. (1954) The electroencephalogram in the senile psychoses. Electroenceph. Clin. Neurophysiol. 6: 245–252.

Obrist, W.D. (1976) Section V. Problems of aging. In: A. Rémond (Ed.), Handbook of Electroenceph. Clin. Neurophysiol., Vol. 6A. Elsevier, Amsterdam, pp. 275–292.

Obrist, W.D., Sokoloff, L., Lassen, N.A., Lane, M.H., Butler, R.N. and Feinberg, I. (1963) Relation of EEG to cerebral blood flow and metabolism in old age. Electroenceph. Clin. Neurophysiol. 15: 610–619.

Otomo, E. and Tsubaki, T. (1966) Electroencephalography in subjects sixty years and over. Electroenceph. Clin. Neurophysiol. 20: 77–82.

Pedley, T.A. and Miller, J.A. (1983) Clinical neurophysiology of aging and dementia. In: R. Mayeux and W.G. Rosen (Eds.), The Dementias. Raven Press, New York, pp. 31–49.

Prinz, P.N., Peskind, E.R., Vitaliano, P.P., Raskind, M.A., Eisdorfer, C., Zemcuznikov, N. and Gerber, C.V. (1982) Changes in the sleep and waking EEGs of nondemented and demented elderly subjects. J. Am. Geriat. Soc. 30: 86–93.

Soininen, H., Partanen, V.J., Helkala, E.L. and Riekkinen, P.J. (1982) EEG findings in senile dementia and normal aging. Acta Neurol. Scand. 65: 59–70.

Torres, F., Faoro, A., Loewenson, R. and Johnson, E. (1983) The electroencephalogram of elderly subjects revisited. Electroenceph. Clin. Neurophysiol. 56: 391–398.

Van Sweden, B., Wauquier, A. and Niedermeyer, E. (1993) Normal aging and transient cognitive disorders in the elderly. In: E. Niedermeyer and F. Lopes da Silva (Eds.), Electroencephalography: Basic Principles, Clinical Applications and Related Fields. Urban and Schwarzenberg, Baltimore, pp. 329–338.

Visser, S.L., Hooijer, C., Jonker, C., Van Tilburg, W. and De Rijke, W. (1987) Anterior temporal focal abnormalities in EEG in normal aged subjects;

correlations with psychopathological and CT brain scan findings. Electroenceph. Clin. Neurophysiol. 66: 1–7.

Williamson, P.C., Merskey, H., Morrison, S. et. al. (1990) Quantitative electroencephalographic correlates of cognitive decline in normal elderly subjects. Arch. Neurol. 47: 1185–1188.

14 Activation procedures

SUMMARY

Activation procedures are used to induce or enhance abnormal EEG patterns. These procedures also may induce normal patterns that are not seen in the spontaneous EEG.

(14.1) *Hyperventilation* is used routinely in most laboratories. The normal response consists of a buildup of generalized slow waves; this response is seen especially in persons who are young or in those who are hypoglycemic. Abnormal responses include electrographic seizures, spike-and-wave discharges, spikes, sharp waves, focal slow waves, enhancement of abnormal slow waves and enhancement of asymmetries.

(14.2) *Sleep* recordings are made after routine daytime waking records in many laboratories and are indicated especially in patients who are suspected of having epilepsy but show no epileptiform activity in the waking record. Recordings after a period of overnight *sleep deprivation* should be used in patients who give a history of having seizures, particularly after insufficient sleep.

(14.3) *Photic stimulation* using a stroboscopic diffuse light stimulus is performed routinely in most laboratories. The occipital dominant visual evoked potentials are referred to as *photic driving* when they occur in a rhythmic run time-locked to a train of repetitive flashes. Photomyogenic (photomyoclonic) responses are unusual; photoparoxysmal (photoconvulsive) responses are abnormal. Prominent photic driving at very slow flash rates is seen in early infancy and later in life in individuals with dementia.

(14.4) *Other stimuli* such as patterned light, a startling noise, or musical sounds should be used during EEG recordings in those patients who are known to react to these stimuli with behavioral changes suggestive of seizures.

(14.5) *Pentylenetetrazol* and other convulsant drugs are used only rarely and for very narrowly defined reasons.

14.1 HYPERVENTILATION

Hyperventilation should be performed for 3–5 min in all routine recordings with the few exceptions described in 5.1.

14.1.1 *Normal responses* consist of generalized slow waves that may begin soon after the onset of hyperventilation (Fig. 14.1). Initially, the slow waves are intermittent and may appear in the form of bilaterally synchronous bursts containing waves with sharp contours. The slow waves sometimes start as, or often develop into, long trains of rhythmical, bisynchronous, generalized delta waves of high amplitude that may become continuous. Normal slow waves of hyperventilation are not focal or lateralized in distribution even though they may have a maximum in the anterior or posterior head regions. In children the response to hyperventilation usually begins or re-

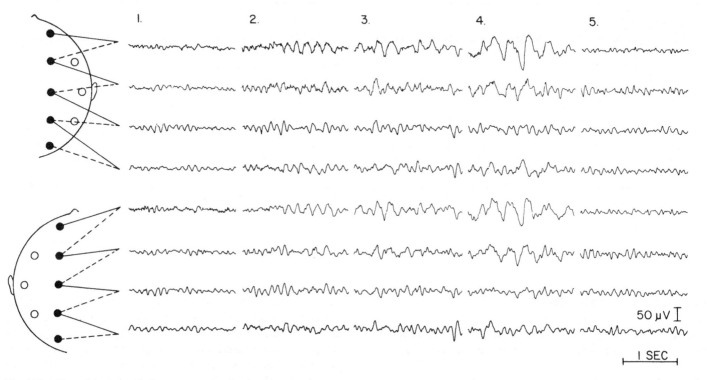

Fig. 14.1. Normal hyperventilation response in 45-year-old subject, 4–5 h after the last meal. (1) Before hyperventilation: normal EEG. (2) After 1 min of hyperventilation: rhythmical theta waves with frontal maximum. (3) After 2 min of hyperventilation: theta and delta waves with frontal maximum. (4) After 3 min of hyperventilation: fairly rhythmical delta waves, maximal frontally. (5) 1 min after the end of hyperventilation: return to initial EEG pattern.

mains maximal over the posterior head regions. In contrast, in teenagers and adults the response is almost always maximal over the anterior head regions. The normal response ends within 1 min after the patient stops hyperventilating. Children or older individuals who cry or sob during the recording may induce the hyperventilation response. Notations by the technologist are usually sufficient to prevent the electroencephalographer from misinterpreting the hyperventilation of sobbing or crying as abnormal slowing.

14.1.2 *The incidence and intensity* of the hyperventilation response in normal individuals depends on age, blood sugar level and cerebral responsiveness to hypocarbia. Hyperventilation responses are most pronounced in children and teenagers. They diminish in young adults and are rare in old persons, presumably because of reduced respiratory effort, reduced gas exchange across alveolar membranes, reduced cerebral vascular reactivity and reduced reactivity of neuronal structures to blood gas changes. Hyperventilation responses are more prominent in persons with low serum glucose or cerebral ischemia at the time of hyperventilation. The EEG changes produced by hyperventilation are generally thought to arise from constriction of cerebral blood vessels which leads to reduced cerebral blood flow and decreased delivery of oxygen and glucose to the brain. However, this mechanism of action has not been established conclusively, and other explanations, such as a brainstem mediated response to hypocarbia, have also been proposed.

14.1.3 *Abnormal responses* to hyperventilation can occur at any age. Subjective symptoms in a patient's history such as dizziness, numbness, tingling, transient blurring of vision, episodic changes of consciousness or awareness, or ringing in the ears often raise the clinician's suspicion of a convulsive disorder and prompt an EEG examination. However, all these symptoms may be reproduced during hyperventilation. If the EEG at that time shows no epileptiform abnormalities, it is very unlikely that the symptoms are due to a seizure disorder. This is one of the most useful pieces of information that can be obtained from hyperventilation. On the other hand, it is a common pitfall of interpretation to assume that the patient who does not respond during hyperventilation is having a seizure. In particular, *normal children frequently have brief lapses in responsiveness and awareness during intense hyperventilation that can be easily misinterpreted as behavioral evidence of a seizure disorder.* The activation of a complex partial or absence seizure during hyperventilation can usually be ruled out if: (1) the EEG contains approximately symmetrical activity, and (2) there are no clear epileptiform patterns. Because hyperventilation is very useful for diagnosing patients with hyperventilation attacks the technologist should document any symptoms that arise during hyperventilation (5.1). The electroencephalographer can then report the symptoms produced and state whether or not they were associated with EEG abnormalities (26.1.3).

An extremely intense or abnormally prolonged hyperventilation response, especially if occurring in a person after adolescence, raises the suspicion of low blood sugar or cerebral anoxia. However, it is also difficult to tell by bedside observation at what point an individual actually stops hyperventilating, even after being instructed to breathe normally. For this reason in routine recordings the point at which a response can be considered abnormally prolonged is uncertain.

A prominent asymmetric response, or *a response which reappears after hyperventilation has stopped* and the background has returned to baseline, suggests the presence of cerebrovascular insufficiency. In children and young adults the latter finding in particular should always raise the question of moyamoya disease.

Epileptiform discharges may be induced or enhanced by hyperventilation in some cases. Spike-and-wave discharges of 3 Hz are particularly sensitive to hyperventilation and in many cases appear only during this procedure during wakefulness in a single recording. Slow spike-and-wave discharges seen in patients with Lennox–Gastaut syndrome may also be activated in about 50% of patients by hyperventilation. Less often, generalized atypical spike-and-wave patterns, and least often focal epileptiform patterns are activated.

Slow waves in a wide distribution, if present in the spontaneous recording, may be enhanced during hyperventilation. They may also merge with the generalized slow waves of a normal hyperventilation response and are then difficult to recognize as abnormal. Hyperventilation is more likely to enhance rhythmical and generalized slow waves than arrhythmical and focal slow waves.

Asymmetries of background activity may be enhanced and become clearly significant during hyperventilation, or they may become less prominent and reduce the suspicion of an abnormality. Persistent asymmetries of the hyperventilation response itself are abnormal. Usually the abnormality is on the side of the higher amplitude response.

14.2 SLEEP

14.2.1 *Sleep recordings* (those which clearly contain stage II sleep) can help in the diagnosis of epilepsy (12.4.1) and in the assessment of non-specific EEG abnormalities. Although most epileptiform abnormalities can be found in waking records, recordings which contain a period of sleep can help to (1) detect these abnormalities in some patients who do not show them during wakefulness and (2) discover or delimit an epileptogenic focus in patients showing epileptiform activity without clear focal origin during wakefulness. Foci in the temporal lobes are especially likely to appear in sleep. An attempt should therefore be made to obtain a sleep recording, either spontaneous or drug-induced (5.1) in all patients who are suspected of having a convulsive disorder but do not show epileptiform discharges in the waking EEG or whose waking EEG contains only non-epileptiform localized abnormalities. Epileptiform activity may occur in any non-REM stage of sleep. It is less likely to appear during REM sleep and more likely to appear in deeper stages of non-REM sleep.

Non-specific lateralized or focal EEG abnormalities such as background slowing, background asymmetry or focal slowing are often most apparent during stage I sleep and least apparent during alert wakefulness.

14.2.2 *Sleep deprivation* is frequently used as a method for inducing epileptiform activity in susceptible individuals. Contrary to current opinion, its use has certain practical limitations.

It is difficult to keep most individuals awake for more than 20 h without behavioral monitoring. It is therefore always difficult to know the extent of sleep deprivation. Although it is likely, it has been difficult to clearly establish that sleep deprivation offers significant advantages over the activating effect of spontaneous or drug-induced sleep in most individuals with epilepsy. However, sleep deprivation should still be considered as a method of activation in patients who have a history of seizures, particularly after insufficient sleep, and those who do not show epileptiform activity in routine waking and sleep recording.

The most practical approach is to use a sedative such as chloral hydrate in those individuals who fail to sleep despite self-reported sleep deprivation at the time of testing. Adults undergoing sedation or complete sleep deprivation should ideally be accompanied by an adult who can assist them in traveling to and from the laboratory. Although many hospitals require a nurse or anesthetist to be present at the time of sedation with chloral hydrate, this is medically unnecessary.

14.3 PHOTIC STIMULATION

14.3.1 *Normal cerebral responses* to stimulation with flashes of diffuse light (5.1) consist of occipital visual evoked potentials produced by each flash of light. When the light stimulus is administered in a repetitive train a string of evoked potentials occurs referred to as *photic driving*. These responses appear mainly in the occipital areas but may extend into the parietal and posterior temporal areas and occasionally even more anteriorly.

Visual evoked potentials recorded in the EEG usually consist of a monophasic wave of positive polarity with a peak appearing 80–150 ms after the flash. When extracted from the ongoing EEG by computer averaging techniques, the potential shows additional smaller components.

Photic driving usually occurs at flash rates over 3 Hz (Fig. 14.2). At these rates, individual components of the visual evoked potential often merge into rhythms that consist of an admixture of components that have the frequency of the stimulus as well as other harmonic or subharmonic frequencies that are multiples of the flash frequency. The response may develop gradually and change in amplitude and configuration as the repetitive stimulation continues. The response on one side may differ from that on the other, both in waveform and in amplitude; these differences may vary with the stimulus rate. The largest responses are often obtained with stimulus frequencies at or near the frequency of the subject's alpha rhythm.

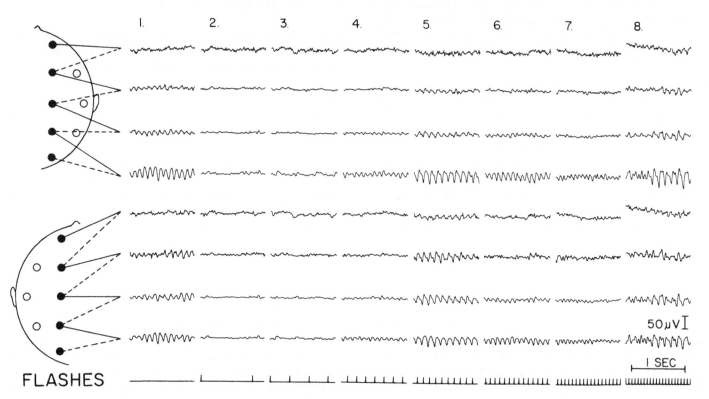

FLASHES

Fig. 14.2. Normal responses to photic stimulation in a 58-year-old subject with closed eyes. Flashes are indicated on the bottom line. (1) Before stimulation: normal EEG with posterior alpha rhythm. (2–8) During photic stimulation at rates of 1, 3, 6, 9, 12, 15 and 18 Hz. Note that the posterior responses have the highest amplitude at a rate near that of the alpha rhythm (part 5) and at twice that rate (part 8).

While the amplitude of photic driving, like that of alpha rhythm, is often higher on the right side, even a 2-fold difference of amplitude of photic driving on either side is not definitely abnormal in the absence of other EEG abnormalities. High frequency components of the response may be so prominent as to form spikes time-locked to the flash frequency as part of a normal photic driving response.

The incidence and prominence of photic responses depend on the frequency, intensity, color and pattern of the stimulus, and on the alertness and attention of the subject. Flashes given while the eyes are closed often elicit a response of higher amplitude and different configuration than flashes given while the eyes are open. Responses may appear, change and disappear during continued stimulation. Many subjects show photic driving only at some stimulus frequencies, usually in the range of 8–15 Hz. Driving at high rates is rare in young infants and old persons. Driving cannot be elicited in newborns. Photic responses may be entirely absent in normal subjects even though they can be demonstrated in virtually all subjects of any age by computer averaging of diffuse light evoked potentials.

14.3.2 *Photomyogenic* (formerly called *photomyoclonic) responses* consist of brief muscle contractions triggered in a few susceptible subjects by flashes given while the eyes are closed. The contractions involve mainly the eyelids but may extend into other muscles of the head, neck and body and lead to rather violent twitching (Fig. 14.3). Photomyogenic responses are statistically significant in that they occur rarely, but they have no known clinical significance. Rarely, individuals with photomyogenic responses may show gradual recruitment with evolution into a generalized convulsion, particularly during barbiturate withdrawal.

14.3.3 *Abnormalities of photic responses* consist of extreme variations in amplitude or of *photoparoxysmal* (epileptiform) responses.

As an isolated finding, an asymmetric driving response is not considered clinically significant. If it is associated with other abnormal findings in a consistent fashion, then it is appropriate to consider it as an additional abnormality (Fig. 14.4). The question of whether the higher or the lower amplitude indicates the abnormal side can often be answered if the recording also contains other lateralized abnormal findings such as slow waves or spikes and sharp waves.

A marked bilateral increase or decrease of amplitude, established by comparison with a control recording obtained from the same subject under the same recording and stimulating conditions, raises the suspicion of an abnormality. However, a single recording showing either very high amplitude or a complete absence of responses is not abnormal.

Photoparoxysmal (photoepileptiform, photoconvulsive) responses consist of spikes and other epileptiform activity. While normal photic responses may contain sharp waves and spikes which repeat at the stimulus rate, remain maximal in the posterior head regions and end with the cessation of stimulation,

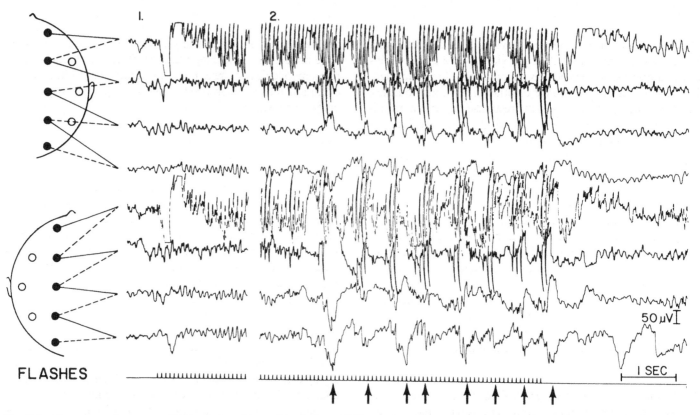

Fig. 14.3.   Photomyogenic response. (1) Stimulation with repetitive flashes at 13 Hz, monitored at the bottom, causes muscle artifact in the frontal regions at the rate of the flashes. The posterior head regions show the beginning of photic driving. (2) Five seconds after part 1, the muscle artifact is spreading to the posterior head regions and repetitive movement artifacts at 1–2 Hz (arrows) develop, corresponding with jerking of the head and neck. Muscle and movement artifacts end promptly at the end of the flash stimuli. This 37-year-old woman has a history of syncope, headaches and high blood pressure; the neurological examination was normal.

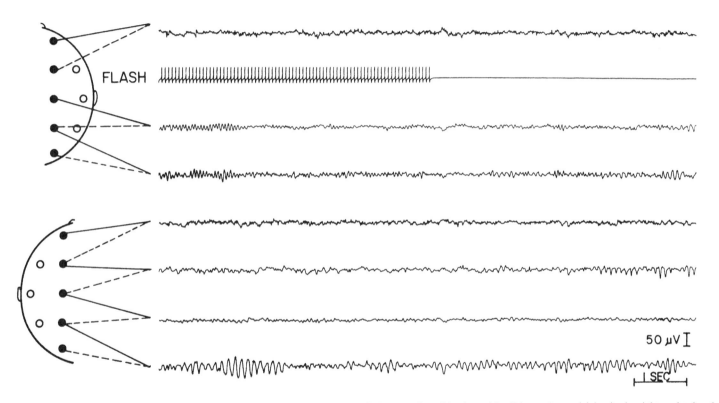

FLASH

50 μV

1 SEC

Fig. 14.4. Significant asymmetry of photic driving. Stimulation with repetitive flashes, monitored in channel 2, elicits moderate driving in the right parietal and occipital areas; there is no response on the left where alpha waves continue. This is a part of a recording also used in Fig. 25.1 to illustrate unilateral failure of alpha blocking on eye opening.

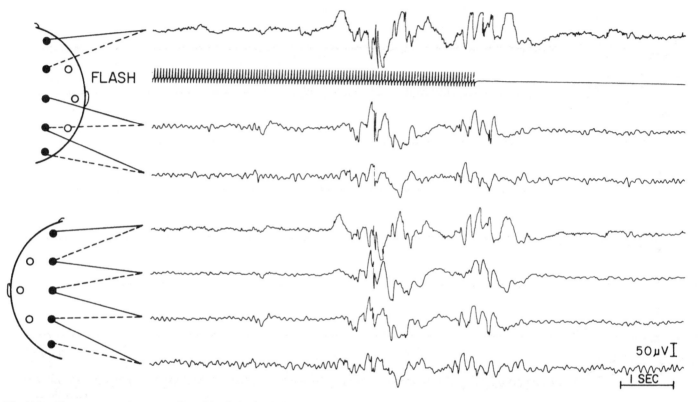

FLASH

50μV

1 SEC

Fig. 14.5.   Photoparoxysmal response. Repetitive flash stimulation, monitored in channel 2, elicits no driving; rather, a paroxysm of irregular spikes, sharp and slow waves appears suddenly and in a wide distribution. The generalized epileptiform activity outlasts the end of photic stimulation. Similar paroxysms were elicited repeatedly with similar stimuli in other parts of the same recording. This 23-year-old woman had a generalized tonic-clonic seizure 1 day before the EEG recording. The seizure began while the patient looked at a television screen showing horizontal bars which turned over vertically.

228

photoparoxysmal (photoepileptiform) responses usually show no clear relationship to the stimulus frequency, often involve the frontal head regions or the entire head and may outlast the end of stimulation.

Photoparoxysmal responses that are maximal over the frontal and central head regions and outlast the duration of the photic stimulus are most often associated with seizure disorders (Fig. 14.5). Photic stimulation rarely evokes a focal epileptiform response and is therefore most useful when a primarily generalized seizure disorder is suspected. Indeed, *the presence of a generalized (symmetric) photoparoxysmal response in an EEG argues strongly for primary generalized epilepsy and against epilepsy with partial seizures.* Juvenile myoclonic epilepsy is the most common form of primary generalized epilepsy associated with photoparoxysmal responses. Patients with photoparoxysmal responses whose epilepsy disappears with aging often show *degraded photoparoxysmal responses* consisting of bursts of irregular mixed waveforms rather than clearly epileptiform patterns in response to photic stimulation.

EEG technologists all need the expertise necessary to rapidly identify a photoparoxysmal response. In some cases prolonged stimulation after the onset of a response will trigger a generalized convulsion. Once a response has been clearly identified it is generally good policy to cease stimulation. However, *to demonstrate that the epileptiform pattern is actually due to the stimulus (rather than a chance occurrence), stimulation at that flash frequency must be repeated.*

Photoparoxysmal responses were initially reported to occur in nearly half of all patients in acute alcohol withdrawal. However, Fisch et al. (1989) did not find any instances of photoparoxysmal responses in response to either diffuse light or patterned light stimulation in the only other study thus far of untreated patients in alcohol withdrawal. Thus, it is now generally accepted that *acute alcohol withdrawal does not cause a photoparoxysmal response.* The presence of a photoparoxysmal response in individuals in alcohol withdrawal therefore usually indicates a genetic tendency to photosensitivity, the co-existence of primary generalized epilepsy, or non-alcoholic sedative drug withdrawal.

14.4   OTHER STIMULI

Other activation procedures may be used in cases where episodic symptoms or signs suggest a convulsive disorder triggered by known stimuli and where a diagnosis is wanting. These procedures should be used with caution and with the intention of inducing EEG abnormalities while avoiding precipitation of a seizure. The benefits of the diagnostic information obtainable by activation of EEG discharges must be weighed against the minor risk of inducing a seizure. Great care should be taken to precisely reproduce the triggering conditions that are suspected to bring on seizures in the patient under study. Many of these triggering conditions consist of very specific visual, auditory or other sensory stimuli.

14.4.1 *Pattern or video game sensitivity* is characterized by generalized epileptiform discharges, similar to photoparoxysmal responses, that can be induced in the EEG while a patient looks at an image containing visual detail. The triggering mechanism can be further analyzed in terms of visual content and manner of looking. For example, a patient may be sensitive to a parallel line pattern in which sensitivity depends on the lines having a certain width, direction, brightness, contrast and color, and insensitive to other, slightly different, patterns. The pattern may be effective only when the patient keeps scanning it or switches from looking at the pattern to looking at a blank surface. While the effective stimulus condition remains constant in some patients, responsiveness varies in others. *Virtually all patients with pattern sensitivity also show sensitivity to photic stimulation. However, very few patients with sensitivity to photic stimulation also have pattern sensitivity.* An important advantage of identifying individuals with pattern sensitivity is that they can then be instructed to avoid clothes, pictures, wall paper designs, etc., containing certain patterns and to wear dark glasses as needed.

Some patients have seizures while watching television. This may be due to one or more mechanisms, including the appearance of effective patterns. Occasionally, the television becomes an effective stimulus when it malfunctions so as to produce a flickering stimulus. With the advent of video games and their widespread use among non-adults reports of video-induced seizures have become common. In one study of 40 patients with photoparoxysmal responses to stroboscopic photic stimulation, 30% of the patients also demonstrated sensitivity to video games (Hormes et al., 1995). Some patients may give a history of video game-induced seizures and not demonstrate sensitivity to photic stimulation. Rarely, the visual stimulus that evokes an epileptiform response or seizure can be quite specific. For example, the film archives of the Mayo Clinic contain a case of an infant who had a seizure evoked by looking at one of his hands that was then prevented by covering the hand with a glove (Donald Klass, M.D., personal communication).

14.4.2 *Auditory stimuli* of several different kinds may trigger epileptiform discharges in the EEG as well as clinical seizures. In some patients, a sudden loud noise may be more effective than other startling stimuli. In such cases the seizure usually begins with a series of myoclonic jerks. Other patients require more specific auditory stimuli such as a certain sound, a specific musical piece, or a musical piece played with certain instrumentation or by a certain orchestra ('musicogenic epilepsy'). Some stimuli may have an emotional impact on the patient, and this may be at least as important for the triggering as the sensory quality of the stimulus. This is probably true of some rare seizure triggering mechanisms such as the hearing of a particular word or sentence or the confrontation with the need to make a decision.

14.4.3 *Reading* may induce epileptiform activity and clinical seizures through one of two mechanisms.

Primary reading epilepsy, also called 'intrinsic' or 'perceptive', is characterized by paroxysmal abnormalities that appear only with reading. Epileptiform bursts occur after a period of reading, have a maximum in the parieto-occipital regions, and are often associated with jaw jerking or 'clicking' while reading. These facial movements may progress to a generalized seizure or a generalized seizure may be preceded by epileptiform activity.

Secondary reading epilepsy, also called 'extrinsic' or 'sensorial', is characterized by epileptiform discharges which appear not only with reading but also under other conditions. This form of reading epilepsy may be associated with pattern sensitivity and photoparoxysmal and photomyogenic responses, suggesting that the abnormal responses depend not on the deciphering of the written text but on the visual stimulation resulting from the scanning eye movements and visual patterns produced by alphanumeric figures.

14.4.4 *Eye opening and closing and mental concentration* are routinely used to attenuate and activate the alpha rhythm. Unilateral failure to attenuate with eye opening (Bancaud's phenomenon) indicates a serious abnormality of the hemisphere that fails to attenuate. A more sensitive test of alpha rhythm reactivity that has similar clinical implications as Bancaud's phenomenon is the failure of unilateral attenuation during mental calculation and eye closure. Rarely, mental concentration, such as mental arithmetic, will precipitate a seizure.

14.4.5 *Tactile stimulation* of certain parts of the body may induce or abolish epileptiform activity and seizures in some patients. So-called somatosensory epilepsy is characterized by interictal medium to high amplitude spikes over the perisylvian or central parasagittal head regions that can be evoked by tapping on the distal contralateral extremities.

14.5 PENTYLENETETRAZOL, BEMEGRIDE AND OTHER CONVULSANT DRUGS

When given in sufficient doses, these drugs induce generalized seizures. The addition of photic stimulation during administration of pentylenetetrazol ('photometrazol test') often brings out paroxysms and seizures at slightly lower drug doses. Because the effective doses for the production of seizures and epileptiform EEG discharges under either condition are not clearly different for persons with and without epilepsy, convulsant drugs cannot be used to establish the diagnosis of epilepsy.

In the past convulsant drugs were used only in patients with medically refractory seizures as part of the evaluation for epilepsy surgery. These agents were used to: (1) determine the precise location of the epileptogenic zone by triggering the patient's typical seizure during EEG recording, and (2) exclude the existence of additional epileptogenic foci which could continue to produce seizures after surgery. These agents are rarely used today since it is now known that they may evoke seizures from ectopic foci producing misleading localizing information in up to 10% of subjects. Instead seizure localization is accomplished by recording the patient's typical seizures during long-term monitoring and by obtaining indirect localizing evidence through neuroimaging procedures. However, convulsant drugs remain useful in studying seizures that must occur under controlled conditions such as the performance of positron emission tomography or magnetic resonance imaging.

REFERENCES

Achenbach-Ng, J., Siao, T.C.P., Mavroudakis, N., Chiappa, K.H. and Kiers, L. (1994) Effects of routine hyperventilation on pCO_2 and pO_2 in normal subjects: implications for EEG interpretations. J. Clin. Neurophysiol. 11: 220–225.

Ahuja, G.K., Mohandas, S. and Narayanaswamy, A.S. (1980) Eating epilepsy. Epilepsia 21: 85–89.

Anderson, N.E. and Wallis, W.E. (1986) Activation of epileptiform activity by mental arithmetic. Arch. Neurol. 43: 624–626.

Bancaud, J. (1976) EEG activation by metrazol and megimide in the diagnosis of epilepsy. In: A. Rémond (Ed.), Handbook of Electroencephalography and Clinical Neurophysiology. Elsevier, Amsterdam.

Bickford, R.G. (1979) Activation procedures and special electrodes.In: D.W. Klass and D.D. Daly (Eds.), Current Practice of Clinical Electroencephalography. Raven Press, New York, pp. 269–306.

Bickford, R.G., Whelan, J.L., Klass, D.W. and Corbin, K.B. (1956) Reading epilepsy: clinical and electroencephalographic studies of a new syndrome. Trans. Am. Neurol. Ass. 81: 100–102.

Binnie, C.D., Coles, P.A. and Margerison, J.H. (1969) The influence of end-tidal carbon dioxide tension on EEG changes during routine hyperventilation in different age groups. Electroenceph. Clin. Neurophysiol. 27: 304–306.

Binnie, C.D., Rowan, A.J. and Gutter, T. (1982) A Manual of Electroencephalographic Technology. Cambridge University Press, Cambridge.

Blume, W.T. and Kaibara, M. (1995) Atlas of Adult Electroencephalography. Raven Press, New York.

Bostem, F. (1976) Section II. Hyperventilation. In: A. Rémond (Ed.), Handbook of Electroenceph. Clin. Neurophysiol., Vol. 3D. Elsevier, Amsterdam, pp. 74–88.

Chatrian, G.E. and Perez-Borja, C. (1964) Depth electrographic observations in two cases of photooculoclonic responses. Electroenceph. Clin. Neurophysiol. 17: 71–75.

Coull, B.M. and Pedley, T.A. (1978) Intermittent photic stimulation. Clinical usefulness of nonconvulsive responses. Electroenceph. Clin. Neurophysiol. 44: 353–363.

DeMarco, P. and Tassinari, C.A. (1981) Extreme somatosensory evoked potentials (EPSEP): an EEG sign forecasting the possible occurrence of seizures in children. Epilepsia 22: 569–575.

Drury, I. (1997) Activation procedures. In: E. Wyllie (Ed.), The Treatment of Epilepsy. Principles and Practice, 2nd Edition. Williams and Wilkins, Baltimore, pp. 251–263.

Ellingson, R.J., Wilken, K. and Bennett, D.R. (1984) Efficacy of sleep deprivation as an activation procedure in epilepsy patients. J. Clin. Neurophysiol. 1: 83–102.

Engel, J. (1974) Selective photoconvulsive responses to intermittent diffuse and patterned photic stimulation. Electroenceph. Clin. Neurophysiol. 37: 283–292.

Epstein, M.A., Duchowny, M., Jayakar, P., Resnick, T.J. and Alvarez, L.A. (1994) Altered responsiveness during hyperventilation-induced EEG slowing: a non-epileptic phenomenon in normal children. Epilepsia 35: 1204–1207.

Ferrie, C.D., De Marco, P., Grunewald, R.A., Giannakodimos, S. and Panayiotopoulos, C.P. (1994) Video game induced seizures. J. Neurol. Neurosurg. Psychiatr. 57: 925–931.

Fisch, B.J., Hauser, W.A., Brust, J.C.M., Gupta, G.S., Lubin, R., Tawfik, G. and Hyacinthe, J.C. (1989) The EEG response to diffuse and patterned photic stimulation during acute untreated alcohol withdrawal. Neurology 39: 434–436.

Forster, F.M. (1977) Reflex Epilepsy, Behavioral Therapy and Conditional Reflexes. C.C. Thomas, Springfield.

Fountain, N.B., Kim, J.S. and Lee, S.I. (1998) Sleep deprivation activates epileptiform discharges independent of the activating effects of sleep. J. Clin. Neurophysiol. 15: 69–75.

Gabor, A.J. and Seyal, M. (1986) Effect of sleep on the electroencephalographic manifestations of epilepsy. J. Clin. Neurophysiol. 3: 23–38.

Gloor, P. (1976) Section V. Intracarotid amobarbital and pentylenetetrazol activation. In: A. Rémond (Ed.), Handbook of Electroenceph. Clin. Neurophysiol., Vol. 3D. Elsevier, Amsterdam, pp. 121–151.

Harden, A., Pampiglione, G. and Picton-Robinson, N. (1973) Electroretinogram and visual evoked response in a form of 'neuronal lipidosis' with diagnostic EEG features. J. Neurol. Neurosurg. Psychiat. 36: 61.

Hiraga, H., Aoki, Y. and Kodama, N. (1980) Electroencephalographic findings in moyamoya disease: its diagnostic value and classification. Clin. EEG (Okasaka) 22: 513–526.

Holmes, G.L., Blair, S., Eisenberg, E., Scheebaum, R., Margraf, J. and Zimmerman, A.W. (1982) Tooth-brushing induced epilepsy. Epilepsia 23: 657–661.

Hormes, J.T., Mellinger, J.F. and Klass, D.W. (1995) Testing for electroencephalographic activation with video games in patients with light sensitivity. Am. J. EEG Technol. 35: 37–45.

Jeavons, P.M. and Harding, G.F.A. (1975) Photosensitive Epilepsy. A Review of the Literature and a Study of 460 Patients. Heinemann, London.

Klass, D.W. and Fischer-Williams, M. (1976) Section 1. Sensory stimulation, sleep and sleep deprivation. In: A. Rémond (Ed.), Handbook of Electroenceph. Clin. Neurophysiol., Vol. 3D. Elsevier, Amsterdam, pp. 5–73.

Lesser, R.P. (1985) Psychogenic seizures. In: T.A. Pedley and B.S. Meldrum (Eds.), Recent Advances in Epilepsy, Vol. 2. Churchill/Livingstone, Edinburgh, pp. 273–296.

Matsuoka, H., Takahashi, T., Hasegawa, T. and Okuma, T. (1983) The role of psychic tension in the precipitation of epileptic seizures, with special reference to the findings obtained from neuropsychological EEG activation. J. Jpn. Epil. Soc. 1: 128–138.

Meier-Ewert, K. and Broughton, R.J. (1967) Photomyoclonic response of epileptic and non-epileptic subjects during wakefulness, sleep and arousal. Electroenceph. Clin. Neurophysiol. 23: 142–151.

Mesri, J.C. and Pagano, M.A. (1987) Reading epilepsy. Epilepsia 28: 301–304.

Newmark, M.E. and Penry, J.K. (1979) Photosensitivity and Epilepsy. A Review. Raven Press, New York.

Panayiotopoulos, C.P. (1974) Effectiveness of photic stimulation on various eye-states in photosensitive epilepsy. J. Neurol. Sci. 23: 165–173.

Patel, V.M. and Maulsby, R.L. (1987) How hyperventilation alters the electroencephalogram: a review of controversial viewpoints emphasizing neurophysiological mechanisms. J. Clin. Neurophysiol. 4: 101–120.

Paulson, O.B. and Sharbrough, F.W. (1974) Physiologic and pathophysiologic relationship between the electroencephalogram and the regional cerebral blood flow. Acta Neurol. Scand. 50: 194–220.

Puglia, J.F., Brenner, R.P. and Soso, M.J. (1992) Relationship between prolonged and self-limited photoparoxysmal responses and seizure incidence: study and review. J. Clin. Neurophysiol. 9: 137–144.

Reilly, E.L. and Peters, J.F. (1973) Relationship of some varieties of electroencephalographic photosensitivity to clinical convulsive disorders. Neurology 23: 1050–1057.

So, E.L. and Fisch, B.J. (1998) Drug withdrawal and other activating techniques. In: J. Engel, Jr. and T.A. Pedley (Eds.), Epilepsy. A Comprehensive Textbook. Volume 2. Lippincott-Raven, Philadelphia, pp. 1021–1028.

So, E.L., Ruggles, K.H., Ahmann, P.A. and Olson, K.A. (1993) Prognosis of photoparoxysmal response in nonepileptic patients. Neurology 43: 1719–1722.

Sperling, M.R. (1984) Hypoglycemic activation of focal abnormalities in the EEG of patients considered for temporal lobectomy. Electroenceph. Clin. Neurophysiol. 58: 506–512.

Sunder, T.R., Erwin, C.W. and Dubois, P.J. (1980) Hyperventilation induced abnormalities in the electroencephalogram of children with moyamoya disease. Electroenceph. Clin. Neurophysiol. 49: 414–420.

Sutherling, W.W., Hershman, L.M., Miller, J.Q. and Lee, S.I. (1980) Seizures induced by playing music. Neurology 30: 1001–1004.

Takahashi, T. (1993) Activation methods. In: E. Niedermeyer and F. Lopes da Silva (Eds.), Electroencephalography: Basic Principles, Clinical Applications, and Related Fields. Urban and Schwarzenberg, Baltimore, pp. 241–262.

Thorensen, M., Henriksen, O., Wannag, E. and Laegreid, L. (1997) Does a sedative dose of chloral hydrate modify the EEG of children with epilepsy? Electroenceph. Clin. Neurophysiol. 102: 152–157.

Tyner, F.S., Knott, J.R. and Mayer, Jr., W.B. (1983) Fundamentals of EEG Technology. Vol. 1: Basic Concepts and Methods. Raven Press, New York, pp. 267–279.

Vignaendra, V., Thian Ghee, L., Chong Lee, L. and Siew Tin, C. (1976) Epileptic discharges triggered by blinking and eye closure. Electroenceph. Clin. Neurophysiol. 40: 491–498.

Wiebers, D.O., Westmoreland, B.F. and Klass, D.W. (1979) EEG activation and mathematical calculation. Neurology 29: 1499–1503.

Wilkins, A. and Lindsay, J. (1985) Common forms of reflex epilepsy: physiological mechanisms and techniques for treatment. In: T.A. Pedley and B.S. Meldrum (Eds.), Recent Advances in Epilepsy, Vol. 2. Churchill/Livingstone, Edinburgh, pp. 239–272.

Wilkins, A.J., Darby, C.E., Binnie, C.D., Stefansson, S.B., Jeavons, P.M. and Harding, G.F.A. (1979) Television epilepsy. The role of pattern. Electroenceph. Clin. Neurophysiol. 47: 163–171.

Wyler, A.R., Richey, E.T., Atkinson, R.A. and Hermann, B.P. (1987) Methohexital activation of epileptogenic foci during acute electrocorticography. Epilepsia 28: 490–494.

Part C

The abnormal EEG

15 Abnormal EEG patterns, correlation with underlying cerebral lesions and neurological diseases

SUMMARY

(15.1) An EEG is usually called abnormal not because it lacks normal patterns but because it contains: (A) epileptiform activity, (B) slow waves, (C) abnormalities of amplitude, or (D) specific deviations from normal patterns. These abnormalities can be subdivided into a few basic abnormal EEG patterns.

(15.2) The basic abnormal EEG patterns correspond fairly well with a few anatomical and pathophysiological kinds of cerebral lesions.

(15.3) The basic abnormal EEG patterns do not correlate directly with specific neurological diseases because similar cerebral lesions, and thus similar EEG patterns, may be produced by a great variety of neurological diseases. Moreover, many diseases may produce more than one abnormal pattern. Although there are a few specific patterns that help to narrow the differential diagnosis considerably, the EEG alone cannot be used to make an etiological diagnosis. The EEG is used to help to establish the presence, severity, and cerebral distribution of neurological disorders and to aid the physician in selecting one of several possible diagnoses.

15.1 DEFINITION OF THE ABNORMAL EEG

An EEG is abnormal if it contains (A) epileptiform activity, (B) slow waves, (C) amplitude abnormalities, or (D) certain patterns resembling normal activity but deviating from it in frequency, reactivity, distribution or other features. In most abnormal EEGs, the abnormal patterns do not entirely replace normal activity: they appear only intermittently, only in certain head regions, or only superimposed on a normal background.

The most important EEG abnormalities can be divided into the following basic abnormal EEG patterns that are discussed in the subsequent chapters.

(A) Epileptiform activity
  (1) Localized epileptiform activity
  (2) Generalized epileptiform activity
  (3) Special epileptiform patterns
(B) Slow waves
  (1) Localized slow waves
  (2) Generalized asynchronous slow waves
  (3) Bilaterally synchronous slow waves
(C) Amplitude abnormalities
  (1) Localized amplitude changes: asymmetries
  (2) Generalized amplitude changes
(D) Deviations from normal patterns

15.2 CORRELATION BETWEEN ABNORMAL EEG PATTERNS, GENERAL CEREBRAL PATHOLOGY AND SPECIFIC NEUROLOGICAL DISEASES

Each of the basic abnormal EEG patterns listed above can be caused by one or a few types of intracranial abnormalities characterized by their unstable or destructive character and by their cortical, subcortical and epicortical locations. The correlation between EEG patterns, cerebral pathology and specific diseases is summarized in a series of tables and discussed in the subsequent chapters. The four major categories of abnormal EEG patterns are the subject of Table 15.1 – Basic epileptiform patterns, 15.2 – Basic patterns of slow wave abnormalities, 15.3 – Basic patterns of abnormal amplitude and 25.1 – Deviations from normal patterns. The epileptiform patterns listed in Table 15.1 are further detailed in Tables 17.1, 18.1, 19.1, 19.2, 19.3 and 19.4; the patterns of abnormal amplitude listed in Table 15.3 are shown in more detail in Tables 23.1 and 24.1

15.2.1 *Epileptiform activity is* outlined in Table 15.1. Local epileptiform activity is usually due to a focal irritative lesion of the cerebral cortex; in infants, such activity may be the result of widespread lesions or of toxic, metabolic or electrolytic abnormalities. Generalized epileptiform activity is either not associated with demonstrable lesions or associated with a variety of conditions which increase the excitability of subcortical centers, of wide parts of the cerebral cortex, or of both.

Special epileptiform patterns have a large variety of pathological correlates.

15.2.2 *Slow wave abnormalities* and their correlates are shown in Table 15.2.

Local slow waves are often due to circumscribed damage of the white matter of the hemispheres with or without involvement of the cortex. Generalized asynchronous slow waves suggest a widespread disturbance of cerebral function, often due to greater involvement of subcortical white matter than of the cerebral cortex. Bisynchronous slow waves are often due to widespread involvement of subcortical and cortical grey matter or to local involvement of deep midline structures; this may be due to structural damage or to metabolic or toxic disorders.

15.2.3 *Amplitude changes* are described in Table 15.3. Local reductions of amplitude are often due either to superficial lesions which reduce the electrical potentials generated in the cortex or to matter that is interposed between cortex and recording electrodes and interferes with the electrical conduction of cortical potentials to the recording electrodes; a local increase of amplitude often results from skull defects. Generalized reductions of amplitude are due either to a widespread decrease of the production of electrocortical potentials or to a generalized increase of the conducting media between cortex and recording electrodes.

TABLE 15.1

Basic epileptiform patterns: pathological and clinical correlates

Basic patterns	General pathological correlates	Examples of specific diseases
1. *Local epileptiform activity* (Table 17.1)	(1) Chronic local cortical lesions	Cortical scars after strokes and injuries, tumors; with or without recurring partial seizures: symptomatic epilepsy
	(2) Acute local cortical lesions	Acute strokes, head injuries; with or without acute partial seizures
	(3) In young infants (a) Widespread structural damage	Perinatal injury, anoxia, ischemia; with or without partial, uni- or bilateral seizures
	(b) Toxic, metabolic, electrolytic abnormalities	Hypoglycemia, pyridoxine deficiency, phenylketonuria; with or without seizures as above
	(4) Children without detectable lesion	Benign epilepsy of childhood with partial seizures
2. *Generalized epileptiform activity* (Table 18.1)	(1) No detectable abnormality	Idiopathic epilepsy with primary generalized seizures
	(2) Diffuse cortical and subcortical disorders: (a) Structural (aa) Acute damage	Acute anoxia, head injury, encephalitis; with or without primary generalized seizures
	(bb) Chronic diseases	Postanoxic and posttraumatic generalized cerebral damage, myoclonus epilepsy; with or without primary generalized seizures
	(b) Toxic, metabolic, endocrine, electrolytic disorders	Hypoglycemia, renal encephalopathy, alcohol withdrawal; with or without primary generalized seizures during the disorder
3. *Special epileptiform patterns* 3.1 Infantile and juvenile patterns of multifocal and generalized spikes (Table 19.1)	Widespread structural or metabolic cerebral disease; patterns are more specific for age than for cause	Pre-, peri- and postnatal injury, cerebromacular degeneration, tuberous sclerosis, phenylketonuria, leukodystrophies; with or without partial or generalized seizures
3.2 Periodic complexes (Table 19.2)	Acute or subacute, fairly widespread cerebral damage or metabolic derangements	Acute cerebral infarcts, Jakob-Creutzfeldt disease, subacute sclerosing panencephalitis, barbiturate intoxication, herpes simplex encephalitis, metabolic encephalopathies; with or without myoclonus
3.3 Ictal patterns without spikes and sharp waves (Table 19.3)	No common pathological correlate	Certain partial complex seizures, tonic seizures, neonatal seizures, absence seizures, epilepsia partialis continua
3.4 Epileptiform patterns without known pathological correlates and without seizures (Table 19.4)	No detectable abnormality	No known diseases or seizures

TABLE 15.2

Basic patterns of slow wave abnormalities: pathological and clinical correlates

Basic patterns	General pathological correlates	Examples of specific diseases
1. Local slow waves	(1) Local structural damage of	
	(a) Subcortical white matter	Strokes, tumors, abscesses
	(b) Thalamus	As above
	(2) Local disorders of cerebral blood flow or metabolism	Transient ischemic attacks, migraine, postictal condition
2. Generalized asynchronous slow waves	(1) No detectable abnormality in some cases of mild or moderate slow waves	No known disease, in 10–15% of normal adults
	(2) Widespread structural damage including subcortical white matter	Widespread degenerative and cerebrovascular disease
	(3) Generalized disorders of cerebral function	Acute anoxia, syncope, coma, postictal condition
3. Bilaterally synchronous slow waves	Deep midline gray matter involvement by	
	(1) Diffuse diseases damaging subcortical and cortical gray matter more than white matter	Presenile dementia, progressive supranuclear palsy
	(2) Local structural lesions which directly involve or compress, distort or render ischemic deep midline structures of the mesencephalon, diencephalon, mesial and orbital parts of frontal lobe	Tumors, strokes at or near the bottom of the anterior, middle or posterior fossa
	(3) Metabolic, toxic, and endocrine encephalopathies	Hepatic, renal, hypoparathyroid encephalopathies

15.2.4 *Deviations from normal patterns* are listed in Table 25.1. These patterns have some features seen in normal patterns but deviate from them in specific ways, for instance in frequency, reactivity or distribution; some of them correlate with particular cerebral abnormalities.

15.3   THE DIAGNOSTIC VALUE OF THE EEG

Most cerebral lesions and EEG patterns can be caused by a wide variety of different neurological diseases (examples are listed in the right columns of the tables). The correlation between patterns and diseases is complicated by the observation

TABLE 15.3

Basic patterns of abnormal amplitude: pathological and clinical correlates

Basic patterns	General pathological correlates	Examples of specific diseases
1. Local differences of amplitude (asymmetries) (Table 23.1)	(1) Locally decreased EEG production	
	(a) Structural cortical damage	Cortical infarct, contusion
	(b) Disorder of cortical function	Cortical transient ischemia, migraine
	(2) Local change of media between cortex and recording electrode	
	(a) Increase	Subdural hematoma, subgaleal hematoma
	(b) Decrease	Surgical skull defect
2. Generalized changes of amplitude (Table 24.1)	(1) Generally decreased EEG production	
	(a) No detectable abnormality in some cases of mild or moderate reduction	No known disease, in 5–10% of normal adults
	(b) Structural diseases of cerebral cortex	Huntington's chorea, postanoxic encephalopathy
	(c) Disorders of cortical function	Hypothyroidism, acute anoxia, hypothermia, intoxications, anxiety, postictal
	(2) Bilateral increase of media between cortex and recording electrodes	Subdural hematoma

that many diseases cause more than one type of cerebral lesion and, therefore, more than one pattern. Moreover, not all cases of certain neurological diseases cause an EEG abnormality; for instance the EEG may be normal especially if the cerebral lesion is small, chronic or located deeply in the brain. A disease may also produce EEG abnormalities that are intermittent and so infrequent that they do not appear during the period of a routine EEG recording. Finally, the EEG may be abnormal in some persons who show no other evidence for a disease; for instance, an EEG abnormality may precede or outlast all other signs of a disease.

Because each abnormal EEG pattern can be caused by more than one disease and because some diseases cause more than one abnormal EEG pattern, the EEG alone cannot be used to make a specific clinical diagnosis. Even so, the EEG becomes a powerful diagnostic tool when it is used in combination with the clinical history, physical examination and other laboratory information. For example, in an alcoholic

241

patient in coma who is suspected of having either anoxia, non-convulsive status epilepticus, or hepatic encephalopathy, a suppression-burst pattern would suggest anoxia, an epileptiform pattern would indicate a seizure disorder, and a triphasic wave pattern with all intermixed waveforms <5 Hz would favor hepatic encephalopathy.

Even in cases where the clinical options are wider, the EEG may select some as being more likely. For instance, in an elderly patient with increasing episodes of confusion spikes in the temporal lobe suggest that he may suffer from complex partial seizures; focal slow waves over a frontal area would suggest a structural lesion such as a frontal lobe tumor; triphasic waves or diffuse background slowing would suggest a metabolic/toxic encephalopathy or a nearly normal EEG raising the question of the early stages of Alzheimer's disease.

Obviously, the EEG is essential in the diagnostic evaluation of epilepsy, status epilepticus and in differentiating an acute reactive seizure disorder from a chronic seizure disorder (i.e., epilepsy).

In general, the EEG reflects changes of cerebral function more directly and reliably than it detects structural lesions, especially if the structural lesions are not discrete and localized near the surface of the hemispheres. As a result, the EEG has been found to be more useful in the differential diagnosis of some disorders than in that of others. The indication for ordering an EEG therefore depends on the diagnoses entertained in each case. The diagnostic value of an EEG is likely to be:

(a) *High* in sudden and rapidly progressive disorders of the hemispheres and midline diencephalic and mesencephalic structures, for instance in: (1) seizure disorders; (2) toxic-metabolic encephalopathies; (3) coma of undetermined cause; (4) suspected cerebral death; (5) reduction of cerebral blood flow during carotid endarterectomy; (6) encephalitis; (7) Jakob-Creutzfeldt disease, and (8) stroke.

(b) *Moderate* in recent or progressive focal mass lesions of the hemispheres or of midline diencephalic and mesencephalic structures; although these lesions are more precisely localized by MRI or computerized tomographic brain scans, in some cases they may be recognized earlier by EEG. Examples are: (1) brain tumor; (2) strokes; (3) head injury; (4) chronic subdural hematoma; and (5) cerebral abscess.

(c) *Low* in lesions below the hemispheres and not impinging upon midline diencephalic and mesencephalic structures, and in mild, old, stationary or slowly progressive generalized disorders of the hemispheres, namely in: (1) cerebellar diseases and lesions; (2) brainstem lesions involving cranial nerves and long tracts but not the reticular core; (3) non-organic psychiatric diseases; (4) early Alzheimer's disease, Parkinson's disease, Wilson's disease, spinocerebellar degenerations; and (5) chronic headaches of undetermined cause.

Even though the diagnostic value of the EEG is generally low in certain diseases, it may be of value by excluding other diagnostic possibilities; for instance, although the EEG in Alzheimer's disease may show only mild generalized slow waves, the finding of such slow waves may help to rule out other possible causes of dementia such as a metabolic or toxic encephalopathy, pseudodementia, or depression. The EEG is also useful for monitoring the progress of a patient's disease or the effect of treatment. This is true for a wide variety of acute and subacute disorders of cerebral structure and function. For instance, the EEG may help to demonstrate recovery from postanoxic coma, intoxications, metabolic encephalopathy or status epilepticus. To maximize the value of the EEG it is important to obtain a baseline recording early in the course of these disorders and before the beginning of any treatment.

REFERENCES

Goldensohn, E.S., Legatt, A.D., Koszer, S. and Wolf, S.M. (1999) Goldensohn's EEG Interpretation: Problems of Overreading and Underreading, 2nd Edition. Futura Publishing Company, Armonk, NY.

Kiloh, L.G., McComas, A.J., Osselton, J.W. and Upton, A.R.M. (1981) Clinical Electroencephalography. Appleton-Century-Crofts, New York.

Klass, D.W. (1987) Identifying the abnormal EEG. In: A.M. Halliday, S.R. Butler and R. Paul (Eds.), A Textbook of Clinical Neurophysiology. Wiley, Chichester, pp. 189–200.

Klass, D. and Westmoreland, B. (1996) Electroencephalography: general principles and adult electroencephalograms. In: J. Daube (Ed.), Clinical Neurophysiology. F.A. Davis, Philadelphia, pp. 73–103.

Kooi, K.A., Tucker, R.P. and Marshall, R.E. (1978) Fundamentals of Electroencephalography. Harper and Row, Hagerstown.

Maulsby, R.L. (1979) EEG patterns of uncertain diagnostic significance. In: D.W. Klass and D.D. Daly (Eds.), Current Practice of Clinical Electroencephalography. Raven Press, New York, pp. 411–420.

Petty, G.W., Labar, D.R., Fisch, B.J., Pedley, T.A., Mohr, J.P. and Khandji, A. (1995) Electroencephalography in lacunar infarction. J. Neurol. Sci. 134: 47–50.

Rémond, A. (Ed.) (1971–1978) Handbook of Electroencephalography and Clinical Neurophysiology, Vols. 1–16. Elsevier, Amsterdam.

Rowan, A.J. and French, J.A. (1988) The role of the electroencephalogram in the diagnosis and management of epilepsy. In: T.A. Pedley and B.S. Meldrum (Eds.), Recent Advances in Epilepsy. Churchill/Livingstone, London, pp. 63–92.

Salinsky, M., Kanter, R. and Dasheiff, R.M. (1987) Effectiveness of multiple EEGs in supporting the diagnosis of epilepsy: an operational curve. Epilepsia 28: 331–334.

Schaul, N., Gloor, P. and Gotman, J. (1981) The EEG in deep midline lesions. Neurology 31: 157–167

Schaul, N., Green, L., Peyster, R. and Gotman, J. (1986) Structural determinants of electroencephalographic findings in acute hemispheric lesions. Arch. Neurol. 20: 703–711.

Sharbrough, F.W. (1993) Nonspecific abnormal EEG patterns. In: E. Niedermeyer and F. Lopes da Silva (Eds.), Electroencephalography: Basic Principles, Clinical Applications and Related Fields. 3rd Edition. Williams and Wilkins, Baltimore, pp. 197–215.

Werner, S., Stockard, J.E. and Bickford, R.G. (1977) Atlas of Neonatal Electroencephalography. Raven Press, New York.

Williams, G.W., Lüders, H.O., Brickner, A., Goormastic, M. and Klass, D.W. (1985) Interobserver variability in EEG interpretation. Neurology 35: 1714–1719.

Zifkin, B.G. and Cracco, R.Q. (1990) An orderly approach to the abnormal EEG. In: D.D. Daly and T.A. Pedley (Eds.), Current Practice of Clinical Neurophysiology: Electroencephalography. 2nd Edition. Raven Press, New York, pp. 253–268.

16 Classification of seizures

SUMMARY

This chapter differs from those that follow in that it deals more with the clinical and behavioral aspects of seizures and epilepsy than with EEG patterns. This is essential for preparing the reader for the clinical correlates of epileptiform EEG patterns.

(16.1) *Definitions: Seizures* are episodes of sudden relatively brief disturbances of mental, motor, sensory or autonomic activity caused by an abnormal paroxysmal cerebral activity. *Convulsions* are seizures consisting of violent involuntary contractions of somatic muscles. *Seizure disorder* and *convulsive disorder* are terms describing the condition of patients who have had one or more seizures or convulsions. *Epilepsy* is defined clinically as a state of chronic recurrent seizures; the cause may be known ('symptomatic epilepsy') or unknown ('idiopathic epilepsy' or 'cryptogenic epilepsy'). *Status epilepticus* is the recurrence of seizure episodes at intervals too short to allow recovery to the pre-seizure condition. *Epilepsia partialis continua* consists of repetitive seizure manifestations, usually rhythmical twitching of a distal limb or lower face, persisting for several days, weeks, or years and not forming discrete seizure episodes.

(16.2) *The international classification of epileptic seizures* divides seizures by their clinical manifestations as shown in Table 16.1. The goal of seizure classification is to incorporate it into an epilepsy syndrome diagnosis that facilitates proper counseling and selection of therapeutic alternatives. Although there are many epilepsy syndromes the initial diagnostic step is to determine whether the patient's seizures are partial or generalized and whether the seizure disorder is idiopathic (cryptogenic or genetic) or symptomatic (acquired or secondary to a neurological disease).

16.1 DEFINITIONS

16.1.1 *Seizures,* in neurological terms, are episodes of sudden disturbances of consciousness, mental functions, motor, sensory and/or autonomic activity. Seizures invariably involve a paroxysmal malfunction of cortical neurons that produce an excessive discharge of synaptic and action potentials. Seizures are discrete episodes lasting only one or a few minutes and involving either part or all of the brain. Most seizures show varying manifestations during their course. They may progressively involve different parts of the body or they may produce more than one manifestation, for instance a sustained tonic contraction, before another motor manifestation, for instance rhythmical, clonic contractions. Seizures are often followed by a transient paralysis of that function which had been most involved during the seizure ('Todd's paralysis'). Seizures occurring in the same person usually resemble each other closely. These characteristics in most instances clearly distinguish seizures from other conditions producing an episodic loss of consciousness or changes in behavior (such as syncope, transient ischemic attacks or psychiatric disturbances).

16.1.2 *Convulsions* are violent involuntary contractions of the body musculature. In neurology, this term is usually limited to contractions produced by cerebral seizure activity.

16.1.3 *Seizure disorder* and *convulsive disorder* are terms used to describe the condition of patients who have had one or more seizures or convulsions.

16.1.4 *Epilepsy* describes the condition of patients who have recurring seizures due to some lasting cerebral abnormality. Patients who have had only one seizure or who have recurrent seizures due to transient cerebral abnormalities or to abnormalities primarily outside the brain such as alcohol withdrawal, hypoglycemia or fever are considered to have reactive seizures rather than epilepsy. Approximately 5% of the population will experience isolated seizures whereas slightly less than 1% have epilepsy.

16.1.5 *Status epilepticus* describes the recurrence of seizures separated by intervals too short to allow recovery of the condition that existed before the onset of the seizures. Usually more than two or three seizures occur and form cycles of discrete seizure episodes separated from each other by only brief pauses. The seizure episodes consist of constant or progressively changing manifestations, each episode usually resembling the others.

16.1.6 *Epilepsia partialis continua is* a continuous and rather stereotyped repetition of one, fairly constant, type of epileptic activity, usually rhythmical jerking of a limb or of part of a limb or lower face; alertness may be mildly reduced. This activity may last for weeks, months or years. Sometimes, it may be interrupted by discrete partial or generalized seizures or may become less violent or more restricted and even disappear intermittently.

16.1.7 *Reflex epilepsy* denotes seizures triggered by sensory stimuli and other mechanisms specific for each patient (14.4; 25.5.2). Many patients with reflex epilepsy also have seizures which are not triggered by these mechanisms.

16.2 CLASSIFICATION OF SEIZURES – GENERAL

The most widely used and generally accepted classification of epileptic seizures is that proposed by the Commission on Classification and Terminology of the International League Against Epilepsy. Unlike other classifications, it defines seizure types only in terms of clinical manifestations and EEG findings. It also differs from previous classifications because it is based on the study of videotape recordings of simultaneously recorded EEG and clinical epileptic seizures. The classification is divided into four major categories as shown in Table 16.1. *Partial seizures,* the first major category, are those in which the first clinical and electrographic changes indicate the initial involvement of a group of neurons limited to part of one cerebral hemisphere. If consciousness is not impaired during the attack, as evidenced by amnesia for some or all of the events during the attack, then the seizure is classified as a *simple partial seizure.* If consciousness is impaired, then the seizure is classified as a *complex partial seizure. Simple partial seizures* often involve only one hemisphere electrographically, whereas complex partial seizures frequently involve both hemispheres in routine recordings. *Simple partial seizures may not show any electrographic changes, whereas complex partial seizures virtually always produce some change, however nonspecific, in routine scalp recordings. Simple partial seizures* can be further categorized according to accompanying symptoms and signs as listed in Table 16.1. *Generalized seizures,* the second major category, are those in which the first clinical and electrographic changes indicate initial involvement of both hemispheres. They usually produce loss of consciousness, bilateral motor activity, or both.

The third category, *unclassified epileptic seizures,* is included because certain kinds of seizures cannot yet be properly characterized due to either a lack of data or a consensus of opinion among investigators. This category includes certain forms of neonatal seizures. The fourth category emphasizes circumstances that influence the occurrence of seizures, such as the sleep-waking cycle or specific triggering stimuli associated with certain forms of reflex epilepsy, and includes definitions of the terms *status epilepticus* and *epilepsia partialis continua.*

Each of the terms used in the classification has been defined by the Commission on Classification and Terminology of the International League Against Epilepsy and can be found in Appendix III. The reader is strongly encouraged to carefully review Table 16.1 and Appendix III. The electroencephalographic ictal and interictal patterns associated with specific types of seizures will be presented in subsequent chapters.

It is important to recognize that efforts are continually under way to revise the current classification of seizures according to new clinical and laboratory data. One aspect of this continuing revision will concern the way in which a given seizure may evolve. The current classification already recognizes that a *simple partial seizure* may progress to a *complex partial seizure* or to a *generalized tonic-clonic seizure,* or that a *complex partial seizure* may evolve into a *generalized tonic-clonic seizure.* However, other known patterns of seizure evolution, such as absence seizures that evolve to tonic-clonic seizures or tonic-clonic seizures that begin with myoclonic or clonic activity (so-called clonic-tonic-clonic seizures) have also been well documented.

In addition to the International Classification of Epileptic Seizures, there is also an International Classification of the Epilepsies. The classification of the epilepsies attempts to classify chronic, recurrent seizure disorders into specific syndromes or clinical categories. The categories are organized according to: (1) whether the seizures are partial or general-

TABLE 16.1

Proposal for revised seizure classification*

I. Partial (focal, local) seizures

Partial seizures can be classified into one of the following three fundamental groups:

A. Simple partial seizures
B. Complex partial seizures
    1. With impairment of consciousness at onset
    2. Simple partial onset followed by impairment of consciousness
C. Partial seizures evolving to generalized tonic-clonic convulsions (GTC)
    1. Simple evolving to GTC
    2. Complex evolving to GTC (including those with simple partial onset)

Clinical seizure type	EEG seizure type	EEG interictal expression
A. *Simple partial seizures* (consciousness not impaired)	Local contralateral discharge starting over the corresponding area of cortical representation (not always recorded on the scalp)	Local contralateral discharge

1. With motor signs
    (a) Focal motor without march
    (b) Focal motor with march (Jacksonian)
    (c) Versive
    (d) Postural
    (e) Phonatory (vocalization or arrest of speech)		

2. With somatosensory or special-sensory symptoms (simple hallucinations, e.g., tingling, light flashes, buzzing)
    (a) Somatosensory
    (b) Visual
    (c) Auditory
    (d) Olfactory
    (e) Gustatory
    (f) Vertiginous		

* Adapted from Epilepsia, 22: 498–501, 1981.

TABLE 16.1 *(continued)*

Clinical seizure type	EEG seizure type	EEG interictal expression
3. With autonomic symptoms or signs (including epigastric sensation, pallor, sweating, flushing, piloerection and pupillary dilatation)		
4. With psychic symptoms (disturbance of higher cerebral function). These symptoms rarely occur without impairment of consciousness and are much more commonly experienced as complex partial seizures (a) Dysphasic (b) Dysmnesic (e.g., déjà vu) (c) Cognitive (e.g., dreamy states, distortions of time sense) (d) Affective (fear, anger, etc.) (e) Illusions (e.g., macropsia) (f) Structured hallucinations (e.g., music, scenes)		
B. *Complex partial seizures* (with impairment of consciousness; may sometimes begin with simple symptomatology) 1. Simple partial onset followed by impairment of consciousness (a) With simple partial features (A.1.–A.4.) followed by impaired consciousness (b) With automatisms 2. With impairment of consciousness at onset	Unilateral or frequently bilateral discharge, diffuse or focal in temporal or frontotemporal regions	Unilateral or bilateral generally asynchronous focus; usually in the temporal or frontal regions

249

TABLE 16.1 *(continued)*

Clinical seizure type	EEG seizure type	EEG interictal expression
(a) With impairment of consciousness only (b) With automatisms		
C. *Partial seizures evolving to secondarily generalized seizures* (This may be generalized tonic-clonic, tonic, or clonic) 1. Simple partial seizures (A) evolving to generalized seizures 2. Complex partial seizures (B) evolving to generalized seizures 3. Simple partial seizures evolving to complex partial seizures evolving to generalized seizures	Above discharges become secondarily and rapidly generalized	

II. Generalized seizures (convulsive or nonconvulsive)

Clinical seizure type	EEG seizure type	EEG interictal expression
A. 1. *Absence seizures*	Usually regular and symmetrical 3 Hz but may be 2–4 Hz spike-and-slow-wave complexes and may have multiple spike-and-slow-wave complexes. Abnormalities are bilateral	Background activity usually normal although paroxysmal activity (such as spikes or spike-and-slow-wave complexes) may occur. This activity is usually regular and symmetrical
(a) Impairment of consciousness only		

TABLE 16.1 *(continued)*

Clinical seizure type	EEG seizure type	EEG interictal expression
(b) With mild clonic components (c) With atonic components (d) With tonic components (e) With automatisms (f) With autonomic components (b through f may be used alone or in combination)		
2. *Atypical absence*	EEG more heterogeneous; may include irregular spike-and-slow-wave complexes, fast activity or other paroxysmal activity. Abnormalities are bilateral but often irregular and asymmetrical	Background usually abnormal; paroxysmal activity (such as spikes or spike-and-slow-wave complexes) frequently irregular and asymmetrical
May have: (a) Changes in tone that are more pronounced than in A.1 (b) Onset and/or cessation that is not abrupt		
B. *Myoclonic seizures* Myoclonic jerks (single or multiple)	Polyspike and wave, or sometimes spike and wave or sharp and slow waves	Same as ictal
C. *Clonic seizures*	Fast activity (10 c/s or more) and slow waves; occasional spike-and-wave patterns	Spike-and-wave or polyspike-and-wave discharges

TABLE 16.1 *(continued)*

Clinical seizure type	EEG seizure type	EEG interictal expression
D. *Tonic seizures*	Low voltage, fast activity or a fast rhythm of 9–10 c/s or more decreasing in frequency and increasing in amplitude	More or less rhythmic discharges of sharp and slow waves, sometimes asymmetrical. Background is often abnormal for age
E. *Tonic-clonic seizures*	Rhythm at 10 or more c/s decreasing in frequency and increasing in amplitude during tonic phase, interrupted by slow waves during clonic phase	Polyspike-and-wave or spike-and-wave, or, sometimes, sharp-and-slow-wave discharges
F. *Atonic seizures* (astatic) (combinations of the above may occur, e.g., B and F, B and D)	Polyspikes and wave or flattening or low-voltage fast activity	Polyspikes and slow wave

III. Unclassified epileptic seizures

Includes all seizures that cannot be classified because of inadequate or incomplete data and some that defy classification in hitherto described categories. This includes some neonatal seizures, e.g., rhythmic eye movements, chewing, and swimming movements.

IV. Addendum

Repeated epileptic seizures occur under a variety of circumstances:

(1) as fortuitous attacks, coming unexpectedly and without any apparent provocation; (2) as cyclic attacks, at more or less regular intervals (e.g., in relation to the menstrual cycle, or the sleep-waking cycle); (3) as attacks provoked by:(a)non-sensory factors (fatigue, alcohol, emotion, etc.), or (b) sensory factors, sometimes referred to as 'reflex seizures'.

Prolonged or repetitive seizures (status epilepticus). The term 'status epilepticus' is used whenever a seizure persists for a sufficient length of time or is repeated frequently enough that recovery between attacks does not occur. Status epilepticus may be divided into partial (e.g., Jacksonian), or generalized (e.g., absence status or tonic-clonic status). When very localized motor status occurs, it is referred to as epilepsia partialis continua.

ized, and (2) whether they are idiopathic or symptomatic of an identifiable underlying abnormality. The classification of the epilepsies will not be described in detail here since it is not essential for the correct identification of clinical seizures by behavioral or EEG criteria. Special, well established epileptic syndromes with characteristic EEG patterns will be described in the following chapters. Those readers interested in the classification of the epilepsies are referred to the bibliography referenced at the end of the chapter.

16.3   CLASSIFICATION OF SEIZURES – SPECIFIC

I.   *Partial seizures*

These seizures are restricted to part of the brain and produce symptoms involving those body parts or mental functions which are most affected by the area of seizure involvement.

A.   *Simple partial seizures*
These seizures produce focal motor, sensory, autonomic, mixed or psychic symptoms without change of consciousness.

1.   *Partial seizures with motor symptoms:*
(i) *Focal motor seizures* consist of sustained tonic contractions or intermittent clonic contractions, or of a sequence of tonic and clonic movements. They involve the face, one part of a limb, an entire limb or half of the body.

(ii) *Jacksonian seizures* are focal motor seizures which successively involve adjacent parts on one side of the body during a seizure. This march is due to the spread of the seizure activity over adjacent parts of the motor cortex.

(iii) *Versive seizures* cause turning of the body, usually in a direction away from the side of the seizure discharge. They are also called 'adversive' or 'contraversive' seizures.

(iv) *Postural seizures* consist of involuntary changes of body posture.

(v) *Inhibitory motor seizures* may cause a paroxysmal cessation of all muscle tone in a part of the body.

(vi) *Aphasic seizures* are characterized by expressive, receptive or global loss of language. They result from seizure activity in language areas.

(viii) *Phonatory seizures* consist of vocalization or of speech arrest.

2.   *Partial seizures with special sensory and somatosensory symptoms:*
(i) *Somatosensory seizures* produce sudden sensations such as tingling, heaviness, numbness or burning which, like motor symptoms, either remain in one part of the body or march over part, or all, of the side of the body opposite to the seizure discharge in the somatosensory area of the brain.

(ii) *Visual seizures* produce hallucinations of white or colored simple shapes, for instance stars and flashes or alterations of visual perception or highly structured visual images.

(iii) *Auditory seizures* cause hallucinations of simple sounds or structured, recognizable sounds.

(iv) *Olfactory seizures* produce hallucinations of odors; they often precede complex partial seizures.

(v) *Gustatory seizures* consist of hallucinations of taste.

(vi) *Vertiginous* seizures cause transient vertigo; unless associated with other seizure manifestations, these rare seizures may be difficult to distinguish from vertigo of other causes.

3. *Partial seizures with autonomic symptoms* are rarely seen in isolation, but autonomic symptoms are often part of other partial seizures. The seizure symptoms consist of salivation, perspiration, changes in pupillary size, heart beat, respiration or skin color, sexual symptoms, urination, epigastric discomfort or increased gastrointestinal activity. Abdominal epilepsy is a rare cause of periumbilical pain and may be associated with symptoms of complex partial seizures, but this diagnosis requires strict exclusion of local abdominal abnormalities as a cause of the paroxysmal pain. The autonomic symptoms seem to depend on seizure discharges in the insula, the depth of the Sylvian fissure or the mesial frontal areas.

4. *Partial seizures with psychic symptoms* include:

(i) *Partial seizures with cognitive symptoms* may lead to disturbances of memory. Some patients feel and act as though in a dream ('dreamy state'). Other patients become conscious of a lack of memory while some feel that they have seen, heard, or lived through the same situation before ('déjà vu', 'déjà entendu') or that they are strangely unfamiliar with their situation ('jamais vu,' 'jamais entendu'). Ideational symptoms include the appearance and persistence of an idea or a thought that is out of context and seems to be forced upon the mind ('forced thinking') during the seizure. A careful history often reveals partial seizures with cognitive symptoms that aids in diagnosing other events in the same patient as seizures.

(ii) *Partial seizures with affective symptoms* may cause sudden, unprompted and seemingly inappropriate changes of affect. Most common is a display of fear. Less common are laughing and crying. Rage is not usually a primary seizure manifestation but may be induced as a reaction to restraining environmental factors. Patients with partial complex seizures are not capable of volitionally directed violent behavior; they may commit violent acts by accident or if another individual engages them physically during a seizure, not by intention.

B. *Complex partial seizures*

These seizures have often been called 'temporal lobe seizures' because they usually arise from foci in the mesial and inferior part of the temporal lobe or adjacent parts of the frontal lobe. The complex symptoms consist primarily of changes of the content of consciousness which reduce the ability of patients to interact with their surroundings; complete loss of consciousness is not a primary symptom. A variety of other mental symptoms may also occur. Patients have no recollection or only incomplete memory of events that occur during the seizure although they may remember simple symptoms at the onset of the seizure such as an awareness of a bad odor. Such olfactory hallucinations presumably arise from the uncus of the temporal lobe and are called 'uncinate fits'. In the overwhelming majority of cases olfactory auras arise in temporal lobe tumors.

1. *Partial seizures with impaired consciousness only* are associated with a reduction of awareness that is manifested by confusion.

2. *Partial seizures with automatisms* consist of repetitive movements which seem purposeful in themselves although they serve no obvious purpose in the actual situation; these movements may seem automatic ('automatism'). Simple movements may consist of scratching, patting, chewing, swallowing, mumbling and lip smacking. More highly organized symptoms include facial, gestural and verbal expressions.

C. *Partial seizures secondarily generalized*

These seizures begin like other partial seizures. They then evolve into a generalized seizure either suddenly or after gradually spreading to larger areas of the brain. Secondarily generalized seizures are usually symmetrical and tonic-clonic, but may be asymmetrical tonic-clonic movements with asynchronous movements of the left and right side of the body. The partial onset of the generalized seizure may be remembered by the patient or observed by witnesses; it may, however, be too short to produce any clinical manifestations. A focal onset may be suggested by the EEG in some cases of apparently primary generalized seizures, but it remains an open question whether some apparently primary generalized convulsive seizures are really secondary generalized and arise from clinically and electroencephalographically undetected cortical areas.

II. *Generalized seizures*

These seizures involve the entire brain and may produce bilateral and fairly symmetrical motor changes; autonomic manifestations may be pronounced. Most generalized seizures begin and remain associated with loss of consciousness. A variety of generalized seizure types are commonly seen in children; infants do not usually have bilaterally synchronous and symmetrical seizures, whereas adults rarely have non-convulsive generalized seizures.

1. *Absences ('petit mal' seizures)*

Absence attacks, formerly called 'petit mal' seizures, usually occur in childhood and rarely persist into adulthood. In most cases they are an idiopathic form of epilepsy and not associated with clinical or EEG abnormalities except during the attacks ('typical absences' or 'typical petit mal'). However, in some cases, absence attacks are associated with a disease acquired early in life and manifested by various EEG and clinical abnormalities which persist independent of attacks ('atypical absence' or 'petit mal variant').

(a) *Typical absence attacks* consist of impairment of consciousness without loss of muscle tone and posture. They often manifest as a momentary apparent inattentiveness, an empty stave, or an interruption of speech or motion. However, automatisms, myoclonic and clonic (3 Hz) activity also occur frequently. Usually the interrupted activity is promptly resumed after the attack and the patient has no memory of the lapse of awareness. Some patients retain awareness during the attacks but cannot respond with movement or speech. In some attacks simple repetitive movements begun just prior to the attacks continue during the attack. Attacks may go unnoticed unless they interrupt some motor activity or unless a lapse of awareness or memory can be demonstrated (5.1). Attacks are often triggered by hyperventilation and photic stimulation.

Absences may follow each other closely or continue without noticeable pause so that the patient remains confused or stuporous. This form of status epilepticus, sometimes called 'absence status', occurs usually in children. However, a similar behavioral attack with epileptiform activity may appear in adult patients who have not previously had absence attacks (Fig. 18.4). In those cases the epileptiform pattern is not a typical 3 Hz spike and wave.

(b) *Atypical absence attacks* are characterized by a combination of impaired consciousness and motor or autonomic changes, and usually pronounced changes in tone. Atypical absence seizures usually have more gradual onset and cessation than typical absence seizures. Examples of atypical absence seizures include:

(i) *retropulsive absences* are associated with a sudden increase of postural tone causing the patient to move backward;

(ii) *atonic absences* are combined with a decrease of postural tone producing drop attacks similar to those occurring in brief atonic seizures; and

(iii) *mixed forms* of absences may contain more than one of the components listed above.

2. *Bilateral massive epileptic myoclonus (myoclonic jerks)*

Bilateral massive epileptic myoclonus or myoclonic jerks are brief contractions which involve mainly flexor muscles on both sides of the body and may vary in distribution. The contractions may recur at irregular or regular intervals. In some cases, they are precipitated by photic stimulation. This type of generalized seizure is so brief that a loss of consciousness cannot usually be detected. Epileptic myoclonus, in contrast to non-epileptic myoclonic contraction, is associated with brief epileptiform activity in the EEG. Thus, epileptic myoclonus precipitated by photic stimuli differs from the more common photomyogenic (photomyoclonic) response (25.5.3).

3. *Infantile spasms*

Infantile spasms are brief sudden contractions mainly of flexor, or less often extensor, muscles of the limb girdle producing quick nodding or jack-knife movements of the body. The contractions may last for several seconds and they may recur irregularly for several minutes. Akinesia and reduced responsiveness follow the spasms in some instances and are the only seizure manifestation in others.

4. *Clonic seizures*

Clonic seizures consist of generalized rhythmical myoclonic movements which usually last for 1 min or more and are associated with loss of consciousness. These seizures commonly occur as febrile seizures in childhood.

5. *Tonic seizures*

Tonic seizures consist of contractions of the axial musculature of the entire body and produce flexor positions. They usually last up to 1 min and are associated with loss of consciousness.

6. *Tonic-clonic seizures ('grand mal' seizures)*

Tonic-clonic seizures, formerly called 'grand mal', are the most severe form of generalized seizures and are the most common type of generalized seizures in adults. They begin suddenly with loss of consciousness, sometimes preceded by a shrill cry. Few patients have vague premonitions up to a few hours or days before a seizure, but well-described symptoms preceding the loss of consciousness ('aura') raise the suspicion of a partial seizure with secondary generalization. During the initial tonic phase, most muscles of the body contract intensely, causing stiffening and occasional quivering of the entire body, respiratory arrest with cyanosis, increased heart rate and blood pressure, pupillary dilatation, and perspiration. After 10–20 s, the tonic muscle contraction gives way to rhythmic twitching which builds up to violent, generalized and bilaterally synchronous jerking movements of the entire body. This clonic phase may result in injury, tongue biting, irregular respiration and 'foaming at the mouth'. The clonic phase usually stops in about 30 s and leaves the patient in deep coma from which he gradually recovers after passing through the stages of sleep, somnolence and confusion. Urinary and fecal incontinence may occur in this stage.

7. *Atonic seizures*

Atonic seizures consist of sudden loss of muscle tone. They may be associated with myoclonic jerks to form myoclonic-atonic seizures.

(a) *Brief atonic seizures* or *epileptic drop attacks* lead to sudden falls; the attacks usually last 1 or 2 s.

(b) *Long atonic seizures* cause patients to suddenly lose consciousness, fall to the floor and remain completely flaccid for one or several minutes.

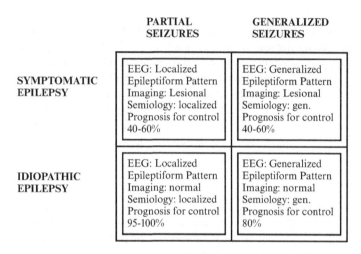

	PARTIAL SEIZURES	GENERALIZED SEIZURES
SYMPTOMATIC EPILEPSY	EEG: Localized Epileptiform Pattern Imaging: Lesional Semiology: localized Prognosis for control 40-60%	EEG: Generalized Epileptiform Pattern Imaging: Lesional Semiology: gen. Prognosis for control 40-60%
IDIOPATHIC EPILEPSY	EEG: Localized Epileptiform Pattern Imaging: normal Semiology: localized Prognosis for control 95-100%	EEG: Generalized Epileptiform Pattern Imaging: normal Semiology: gen. Prognosis for control 80%

Fig 16.1.   Diagnostic approach to epilepsy based on clinical and laboratory information. Initial diagnostic efforts are aimed at placing the patient into one of the four categories shown above. Imaging refers to brain MRI, semiology to ictal behavior and experience, and prognosis is described in terms of the percentage of all patients likely to have nearly complete control with medications alone. (Modified from Risinger, M., American Academy of Neurology, 1999.)

16.4   SEIZURE CLASSIFICATION AND EPILEPSY SYNDROME DIAGNOSIS

The purpose of seizure classification is to facilitate epilepsy syndrome diagnosis. Once the syndrome diagnosis is made, then the physician can move to the next step of counseling the patient and selecting the proper therapeutic regimen. Although there are many specific epilepsy syndromes the initial diagnostic step is aimed at placing the patient into one of four diagnostic categories as shown in Fig. 16.1. These categories are organized according to: (1) the classification of the patient's seizures as partial or generalized (based on ictal observation and EEG information), and (2) whether the seizure disorder is idiopathic (cryptogenic or genetic) or symptomatic (acquired or secondary to a neurological disease), as determined by the patient's history and neuroimaging information.

REFERENCES

Aicardi, J. (1988) Epileptic syndromes in childhood. Epilepsia 29 (Suppl. 3): Sl–5.
Aicardi, J. (1994) Classification of epileptic seizures and epilepsy. In: Epilepsy in Children, 2nd Edition. Raven Press, New York, pp. 9–17.
Blume, W.T., Berkovic, S.F. and Dulac, O. (1998) Search for a better classification of the epilepsies. In: J. Engel, Jr. and T.A. Pedley (Eds.), Epilepsy. A Comprehensive Textbook, Vol. 2. Lippincott-Raven, Philadelphia, pp. 779–790.
Commission on Classification and Terminology of the International League Against Epilepsy (1981) Proposal for revised clinical and electrographic classification of epileptic seizures. Epilepsia 22: 489–501.
Commission on Classification and Terminology of the International League Against Epilepsy (1985) Proposal for classification of epilepsies and epileptic syndromes. Epilepsia 26: 268–278.
Commission on Classification and Terminology of the International League Against Epilepsy (1989) Proposal for classification of epilepsies and epileptic syndromes. Epilepsia 26: 268–278.

Dreifuss, F.E. (1998) Classification of epileptic seizures. In: J. Engel, Jr. and T.A. Pedley (Eds.), Epilepsy. A Comprehensive Textbook, Vol. 2. Lippincott-Raven, Philadelphia, pp. 517–524.

Gastaut, H. and Broughton, R. (1972) Epileptic Seizures. Clinical and Electrographic Features, Diagnosis and Treatment. Thomas, Springfield, IL.

Holmes, G. (1987) Neonatal seizures. In: Diagnosis and Management of Seizures in Children. Saunders, Philadelphia, pp. 237–261.

Lüders, H.O., Burgess, R.C.B. and Noachtar, S. (1993) Expanding the international classification of seizures to provide localization information. Neurology 43: 1650–1655.

Masland, R.L. (1974) The classification of the epilepsies. A historical review. In: P.J. Vinken and G.W. Bruyn (Eds.), Handbook of Clinical Neurology. North-Holland, Amsterdam, pp. 1–29.

Mizrahi, E.M. (1987) Neonatal seizures: problems in diagnosis and classification. Epilepsia 28 (Suppl. 1): S46–55.

Mizrahi, E.M. and Kellaway, P. (1998) Diagnosis and Management of Neonatal Seizures. Lippincott-Raven, Philadelphia.

Mosewich, R.K. and So, E.L. (1996) A clinical approach to the classification of seizures and epileptic syndromes. Mayo Clin. Proc. 71: 405–414.

Porter, R.J. (1987) The classification of epileptic seizures and epileptic syndromes. In: H. Lüders and R. Lesser (Eds.), Epilepsy: Electroclinical Syndromes. Springer, New York, pp. 1–12.

Swartz, B.E. and Delgado-Escueta, A.V. (1987) Complex partial seizures of extratemporal origin: 'The evidence for'. In: H.G. Wieser, E.J. Speckman and J. Engel, Jr. (Eds.), The Epileptic Focus. Current Problems in Epilepsy. John Libbey, London, pp. 137–174.

Wolf, P. (1994) Epileptic seizures and syndromes: terms and concepts. In: P. Wolf (Ed.), Epileptic Seizures and Syndromes. John Libbey, London, pp. 3–7.

Wyllie, E. (1996) The Treatment of Epilepsy: Principles and Practice, 2nd Edition. Williams and Wilkins, Baltimore.

17 Localized epileptiform patterns

SUMMARY

(17.1) The *patterns* of localized epileptiform activity consist of single or multiple focal spikes or sharp waves often in combination with slow waves. Although the spikes and sharp waves may have multiple phases, the polarity of the highest voltage phase is usually electronegative. Epileptiform activity occurring between seizures is referred to as *interictal epileptiform activity*. Interictal epileptiform activity is usually brief in duration (typically lasting less than 1 s) and almost always exceeds the amplitude of the surrounding background activity. Localized *ictal epileptiform activity* (also referred to as *electrographic seizure activity)* usually persists for more than several seconds, begins abruptly, and consists of repetitive, rhythmic waveforms that tend to vary in form, frequency and topography throughout the seizure. Scalp recorded EEG changes during focal seizures may also be absent or so subtle that they appear as only a mild attenuation in amplitude or as other minor changes in the ongoing background activity. Subtle EEG alterations require correlation with simultaneous behavioral changes to be correctly identified as ictal events. More clearly identifiable ictal EEG patterns that occur in the absence of clinical seizure manifestations are referred to as *subclinical ictal* or *subclinical electrographic seizure activity*. Interictal localized activity is usually restricted to a few electrodes, while ictal activity often produces changes in a more widespread distribution or rapidly involves both hemispheres in an asymmetric fashion.

(17.2.1) *Clinical correlates* of localized epileptiform activity are partial seizures. The type of partial seizure depends on the location of the ictal discharge in the brain. Localized discharges in motor and sensory areas generally cause partial seizures with elementary motor and sensory symptoms. Localized discharges in the temporal areas are likely to cause partial seizures with psychic or special sensory symptoms. The correlation between the appearance of epileptiform discharges and clinical seizures is not perfect. Some patients suffer from seizures but show no epileptiform activity during the EEG recording, whereas few patients show epileptiform activity without ever having had a seizure.

(17.2.2) *Causes* of focal epileptiform activity in adults are acute or chronic lesions that produce partial damage in a circumscribed cortical area. It is not known why some lesions cause epileptiform activity while other, similar, lesions do not. In infants and children, single or multiple foci may be the result of fairly widespread cortical damage; such foci tend to shift in distribution and have little localizing value. In some patients with focal epileptiform activity, no underlying structural lesion can be demonstrated.

(17.3) *Other EEG abnormalities* associated with focal epileptiform activity may suggest specific clinical correlates and causes.

(17.4) *Mechanisms* underlying focal epileptiform activity include paroxysmal depolarizing shifts of the membrane potential of a group of cells synchronized by a few pacemaker neurons ('epileptic neurons', 'epileptic neuronal aggregate'). The depolarizing shifts are limited in time and space by hyperpolarizing mechanisms except during seizures when the depolarization becomes repetitive and may spread in distribution. The sustained depolarization shift is accompanied by a superimposed cluster of action potentials

(17.5) *Specific disorders* causing focal epileptiform activity are mainly cerebral injuries, tumors and strokes, but also include a wide variety of degenerative, developmental, metabolic, and infectious diseases.

17.1 DESCRIPTION OF PATTERNS

17.1.1 *Focal epileptiform activity* consists of spikes or sharp waves that appear at one or a few neighboring electrodes. Focal epileptiform activity is divided into interictal and ictal activity (9.1). Abnormal interictal focal (and generalized) epileptiform waveforms are distinguished from non-epileptiform sharp transients and other paroxysmal waveforms by the following criteria:

(1) Epileptiform spikes and sharp waves are usually asymmetric. The initial half of the wave (from the baseline to peak) often has a shorter duration than the second half of the wave (from the peak to baseline). In contrast, many non-epileptiform transients are often approximately symmetric (e.g., wicket spikes).

(2) Epileptiform spikes and sharp waves may be followed by a slow wave. The slow wave is not sharply contoured and it has a longer duration than the predominant background waveforms. The slow wave may range in frequency from the alpha to delta frequency ranges.

(3) Epileptiform spikes and sharp waves have more than one phase (usually 2 or 3), and the duration of each phase differs from the durations of the phases of the surrounding background waveforms.

(4) Epileptiform spikes and sharp waves do not appear as simply an abrupt increase in the amplitude of sharply contoured waveforms that are part of the ongoing background activity.

(5) Epileptiform activity often interrupts the ongoing background beyond the duration of the spike or sharp wave due to the presence of an aftergoing slow wave or surrounding irregular slower waveforms that may precede or follow the spike or sharp wave.

(6) Sharply contoured waveforms that are recorded from only one electrode may be non-cerebral in origin. Therefore, epileptiform activity should always be detected at more than one electrode site. When activity is only detected at one electrode, the impedance of that electrode should be tested and one or more additional recording electrodes should be placed near the active electrode.

In practice, interictal epileptiform activity often lacks some of the aforementioned features. Similarly, sharp transients and other pseudoepileptiform paroxysmal events may demonstrate some of these features (Fig. 17.1). Therefore, the correct identification of interictal epileptiform activity often depends largely on the experience and judgment of the electroencephalographer. However, the likelihood of correct interpretation increases according to the number of these criteria that are fulfilled.

Interictal and ictal activity differ in: (1) wave shape; (2) distribution; and (3) duration (Table 17.1).

(1) *The wave shape* of interictal activity consists of spikes or sharp waves that are sometimes followed by a slow wave; these discharges are usually intermittent but may repeat briefly with little or no variation of shape. In contrast, ictal

TABLE 17.1

Localized epileptiform activity

Interictal epileptiform pattern	Ictal epileptiform pattern	Clinical seizure type	Underlying brain lesion
Intermittent focal spikes, sharp waves, spike-and-waves, rarely repetitive	Episodes of repetitive epileptiform activity, usually different from interictal patterns	Partial seizures	
A. *Located usually outside of temporal and fronto-temporal areas, in:*	*Located usually in similar distribution as interictal patterns, but may occupy wider area*	*Simple partial seizures* ('focal seizures')	Often history or clinical findings consistent with a recent or old local cortical lesion
1. Motor cortex		1. With motor symptoms	
2. Sensory cortex		2. With sensory symptoms	
3. Insula, Sylvian fissure, mesial frontal cortex		3. With autonomic symptoms	
4. Cortex of more than one area		4. Compound forms	
	Patterns include: Fast waves of increasing amplitude and decreasing frequency; paroxysmal theta, delta or alpha activity; no EEG change		
B. *Located usually in temporal or fronto-temporal areas*	*Located usually in similar distribution as interictal patterns but may occupy wider and bilateral areas*	*Complex partial seizures and simple partial seizures with psychic symptoms*	Often no history or clinical evidence for a lesion
		1. With impaired consciousness	
		2. With cognitive symptoms	
		3. With affective symptoms	
		4. With illusions and halluci-nations	
		5. With automatisms ('psychomotor seizures')	
	Patterns include those in A above; 4–6 Hz unilateral or bisynchronous waves; bilateral 14–20 Hz waves; flattening of EEG	6. Compound forms	
C. *Followed by generalized epileptiform activity* As in A and B, occasionally followed by generalized epileptiform activity	*Ictal discharges begin as above in A and B,* then involve the entire brain	*Partial seizures secondarily generalized* Begin as above in A and B, followed by generalized seizure	As above in A and B

activity consists of rhythmical waves that continue to change in shape, frequency and amplitude during the discharge. Although the shapes of interictal and ictal patterns differ between patients, most adult patients have only one or a few interictal and ictal patterns; infants and children show a much greater variety of patterns and often have several interictal and ictal patterns. Both interictal and ictal activity may occur in the same recording, but interictal activity is seen much more commonly.

(2) *The distribution* of interictal discharges is usually limited to one or a few electrodes over an area which is variously referred to as the *irritative zone, spike focus,* or *sharp wave focus.* Occasionally, interictal spikes are widely distributed over one hemisphere with some lower amplitude components present over the opposite hemisphere. *The minimum area of cortical surface involved in the generation of an interictal spike visible at one scalp electrode site is approximately 6 cm^2, but most epileptiform spikes arise from a larger cortical area of at least 10–20 cm^2. Single high amplitude epileptiform spikes generated in depth electrodes in the hippocampus are never seen in scalp electrodes.* Ictal discharges often have a wider distribution; they may start at the focus of interictal activity and gradually extend to a larger area or they may initially appear in a large area that includes the focus of interictal activity. However, localized ictal discharges recorded from intracranial electrodes almost always persist for many seconds or even minutes before they are visible in scalp electrodes.

Usually interictal epileptiform spikes appear as radial dipoles with one distinct scalp area of maximal voltage. However, in some cases, such as rolandic epilepsy, the discharges are oriented at an angle that is more parallel than radial to the scalp surface. This produces a so-called horizontal dipole with simultaneous negativity and positivity in two adjacent scalp regions.

(3) *Duration.* It is important to recognize that the terms *ictal* and *interictal* epileptiform activity are electrographic descriptors, whose interpretation and clinical implications may be modified by clinical circumstances. For example, brief epileptiform activity most often occurs as an interictal phenomenon. Therefore, it is interpreted as interictal unless an associated behavioral change is observed. If an abnormal behavioral change or impairment of consciousness occurs at the time of the activity, then even if it has a brief duration and characteristic interictal appearance, it should be interpreted as an ictal event. Conversely, some discharges having a long duration and other EEG features usually associated with seizures may occur in the absence of apparent behavioral changes. If such activity occurs in individuals with abnormally impaired consciousness or those whose repertoire of behavioral responses limits behavioral testing (e.g., patients with severe encephalopathies or neonates), then the EEG pattern may be referred to as an *electrographic* or *subclinical* seizure discharge.

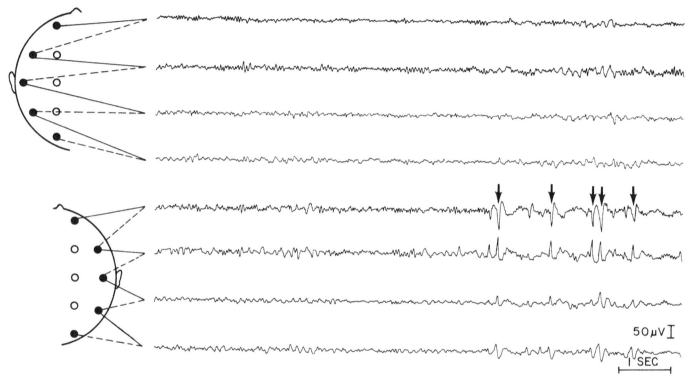

Fig. 17.1. Focal sharp waves in the right anterior temporal region (arrows). The patient is a 30-year-old man with a history of birth injury; for 15 years he has had partial seizures characterized by confusion and automatic behavior. Despite this history these waveforms recorded during wakefulness may represent wicket spikes.

17.1.2 *Specific interictal patterns* consist of spikes or sharp waves (Figs. 17.4 and 20.4) which may combine with slow waves to form spike-and-wave complexes or sharp-and-slow-wave complexes (Figs. 17.3 and 17.4). The major component of most spikes and sharp waves has negative electrical polarity and therefore causes upgoing pen deflections in channels in which the electrode near the focus is connected to input 1 of the amplifier, and downgoing pen deflections in channels connected to such an electrode through input 2 (4.1). Focal epileptiform activity is usually intermittent and rarely repeats to form polyspikes and repetitive spike-and-wave or polyspike-and-wave complexes; the repetition of these elements is often irregular in contrast to that of most generalized epileptiform activity. Some types of focal epileptiform activity that repeat periodically are described under 'special epileptiform patterns' (19.2). The location of foci remains fixed in many adults but often varies slightly from one moment to the next in some. More than one focus may occur in the same patient and the shape of the discharges from each focus may be different. Pairs of foci are often located in corresponding parts of the hemispheres, especially in the temporal areas, and are sometimes called 'mirror foci'. One focus may fire only when the other one occurs suggesting that it is triggered by the other, or both foci may occur independently of each other. Multiple foci that shift location from moment to moment are common in infants (18.2.3) and young children. Foci in older children are slightly more stable in location but may change location

between different recordings made at fairly short intervals (17.5.6).

17.1.3 *Specific ictal patterns* consist of repetitive waves which, in many instances, change configuration and/or distribution as the discharge progresses (Fig. 17.2). They often contain spikes or sharp waves mixed with slow waves and form a variety of patterns. Many ictal discharges begin with low amplitude rhythmical activity which increases in amplitude and decreases in frequency. Alternatively, the ictal pattern may evolve from a slower to a faster frequency discharge. Only some ictal discharges begin with spikes of the interictal type and only rarely do ictal discharges consist of a repetition of interictal discharges. Ictal discharges end abruptly or with a few intermittent bursts and may be followed first by a generalized depression of all activity and then by slow waves in the distribution of the discharge.

In routine scalp recordings in adults localized ictal discharges may occasionally be quite subtle compared to direct cortical or depth electrode recordings. Less often routine surface recordings may show no electrographic changes. In other cases the discharge may be clearly epileptiform but falsely localizing. These variations are largely due to: (1) the attenuation and dispersion of electrical activity caused by the skull and intervening tissues (particularly the dura and cerebrospinal fluid); (2) the orientation and location of the discharge in relation to the recording electrodes; and (3) the secondary

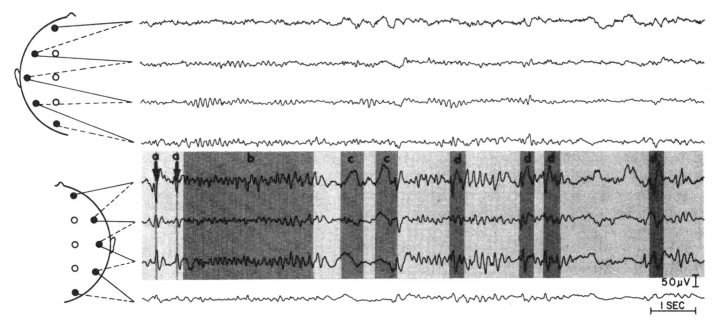

Fig. 17.2. Focal ictal discharge in the right anterior temporal region, consisting of initial intermittent spikes (a) followed by a rhythm of 10 Hz of increasing amplitude and decreasing frequency (b) which is interrupted by slow waves (c) and forms irregular spike-and-wave complexes (d). This short ictal discharge, occurring during light sleep, was not associated with any clinical manifestations. This 57-year-old man had a series of generalized convulsions 3 days before the EEG recording.

activation of cortical structures at a distance from the site where the discharge actually began. Ictal events in scalp recordings may therefore only appear as varying degrees of localized background attenuation, slowing or disorganization. Such non-specific patterns should not be considered as electrographic evidence for a possible seizure unless clearly correlated with typical ictal behavioral changes.

267

17.2 CLINICAL SIGNIFICANCE OF FOCAL EPILEPTIFORM ACTIVITY

17.2.1 *Association with seizures.* Many patients who show local epileptiform activity in their EEG have a history of partial or generalized seizures, and many patients with such a history show local epileptiform EEG activity. However, some patients showing epileptiform activity in their EEG never have a seizure, and a minority of patients with a history of seizures do not show epileptiform activity in an EEG recording. Focal interictal epileptiform activity located over the anterior temporal or frontal head region is most likely to be associated with a history of seizures.

(1) *Epileptiform activity in patients with seizure history.* In adults, the location of the epileptiform activity usually correlates with the seizure type. This correlation is fairly good for interictal discharges and very good for localized ictal discharges, especially those outside the temporal and frontotemporal areas. Focal discharges in the motor area are associated with partial seizures with motor symptoms, while focal discharges in sensory and other areas outside the temporal and frontotemporal regions are associated with partial seizures with the corresponding simple symptoms (16.2). Some patients with focal epileptiform activity have seizures that appear to be clinically generalized from the start. Although these seizures are usually due to the secondary generalization of a focal discharge, only a few of these patients show transi-

tions between focal and generalized discharges (17.3.2) in their EEG between seizures (Fig. 17.3). Patients with adult onset secondarily generalized seizures often present with a history of seizures that appear to be generalized from onset.

In a few patients, focal epileptiform discharges with or without seizure manifestations can be precipitated during the recording by activating procedures including special sensory stimuli (14.4).

Recurrent local ictal discharges are usually seen in status epilepticus but occasionally occur in patients not having clinical seizure manifestations; these patients are said to be in subclinical electrographic status epilepticus. Periodic discharges of focal epileptiform activity (19.2) or of slow waves (19.3.2) are seen in patients with epilepsia partialis continua or as an acute interictal pattern; in some cases, the periodic discharges are interrupted by episodes of focal seizure discharges.

The EEG can be of great value in the diagnosis of seizure disorders because clinical symptoms similar to those seen during some seizures can be caused by other conditions, namely syncope, hyperventilation, transient cerebral ischemia and psychiatric disorders. The EEG can make the diagnosis of a seizure disorder likely if it reveals epileptiform activity. The likelihood that a patient's symptoms are manifestations of seizures is further increased if the location of the focal epileptiform activity corresponds with the clinical manifestations of a patient's seizures. A positive identification of clinical symptoms as seizure manifestations can be made on those rare occasions when both an ictal discharge and the clinical manifestations of a seizure occur together during an EEG recording. Conversely, if the clinical symptoms occur during an EEG recording without being associated with epileptiform activity, unless they are very brief and unassociated with impaired consciousness, it is very unlikely that they are due to a convulsive disorder. Individuals with simple partial seizures occasionally do not demonstrate epileptiform activity or other definite EEG changes during the seizure (Table 16.1).

(2) *Epileptiform activity in persons without seizure history.* Focal interictal epileptiform activity similar to that seen in patients with epilepsy may rarely be found in the EEGs of individuals who have no history of seizures (less than 2%). In general, this is more likely if the epileptiform activity is localized to the parietal or occipital head regions than the anterior temporal, frontal or central head regions. Indeed, visual system defects are frequently associated with the development of occipital spikes in children who never develop seizures. In some cases interictal epileptiform activity may arise from epileptogenic lesions that have remained below a threshold for the production of clinical seizures. In infants and neonates in particular, focal epileptiform activity is the expression of a great variety of pathological conditions which do not produce seizures.

(3) *Patients with a history of seizures but without epileptiform*

EEG activity. Recordings between seizures may contain no epileptiform activity in approximately 20–40% of patients with a history of seizures even if the recordings include the activation procedures of hyperventilation, photic stimulation and sleep. Both longer recording periods and repeated sampling increase the likelihood of recording epileptiform activity. In separate studies it has been shown that approximately 50–60% of patients who will show interictal epileptiform do so on the first recording. Each subsequent recording yields approximately half as many new patients with interictal epileptiform activity as the previous one. Thus, there is usually little to be gained by performing additional routine recordings if 3 separate recordings with sleep, wakefulness, hyperventilation and photic stimulation have failed to show epileptiform changes. The likelihood of recording epileptiform activity does not directly depend on anticonvulsant medication (except in the case of valproate, clonazepam, or ethosuximide and typical generalized 3 Hz spike and wave activity) although it may decrease as anticonvulsants reduce the frequency of seizures. The incidence of interictal epileptiform activity varies little with the type of underlying lesion except that metastatic brain tumors are less likely to produce epileptiform activity between seizures than are other lesions producing seizures of similar frequency. Interictal focal epileptiform activity may fail to appear in the scalp EEG if the focus is small, is located deeply in the brain, or has an unusual spatial orientation with respect to the recording electrodes.

17.2.2 *Underlying cerebral abnormalities. Adults and adolescents* develop focal epileptiform activity often as the result of acute or chronic damage to a circumscribed area of the cerebral cortex. *Acute* damage causes epileptiform activity which usually lasts only for a few days. A common example is middle cerebral artery territory cortical infarction. *Chronic* epileptogenic lesions either are stationary, for instance scars resulting from head injuries or strokes, or are gradually progressive, as in cases of slowly growing tumors. In stationary lesions, epileptiform activity may not develop until after a period of several months or years, even in patients who have briefly shown epileptiform activity during the few days after an acute cerebral injury (e.g., stroke). Lesions in the temporal and frontal lobes are more likely than lesions in the parietal and occipital cortical areas to produce epileptogenic foci. Similarly, epileptiform spikes occurring in the frontal and temporal lobes are more likely to be associated with a seizure disorder than spikes occurring in the parietal and occipital lobes. In some patients with chronic recurrent epileptiform activity, no historical, clinical or laboratory evidence for a lesion can be found. It is, however, reasonable in view of the detection of smaller and more subtle epileptogenic anatomical abnormalities by MRI (e.g., cortical dysgenesis) to assume that in such cases microanatomical lesions are present.

Infants and children react to acute widespread damage with localized epileptiform discharges more often than do adults.

17.3 OTHER EEG ABNORMALITIES ASSOCIATED WITH FOCAL EPILEPTIFORM ACTIVITY

17.3.1 *Focal sharp transients,* which have less distinct and more variable shapes than do spikes and sharp waves (9.1), may be seen in recordings which also contain focal spikes and sharp waves in the same distribution. However, sharp transients unassociated with spikes and sharp waves, although perhaps suggesting some local hyperexcitability, are not suggestive of an epileptogenic focus.

17.3.2 *Generalized interictal epileptiform activity,* i.e., epileptiform activity that by routine visual inspection appears simultaneously on both sides of the head, is sometimes produced by a focal epileptogenic lesion. This may occur by a process referred to as *secondary bilateral synchrony* in which an epileptic focus is thought to either trigger a mirror image cortical area by transcallosal transmission or through a thalamic area that in turn produces a bilaterally synchronous epileptiform pattern (18.4.1). In such cases the interictal and ictal epileptiform patterns may be bisynchronous all or most of the time. Since *primary* and *secondary bilateral synchrony* have quite different clinical implications, it is important for the electroencephalographer to be familiar with those features that are sometimes helpful in distinguishing one from the other.

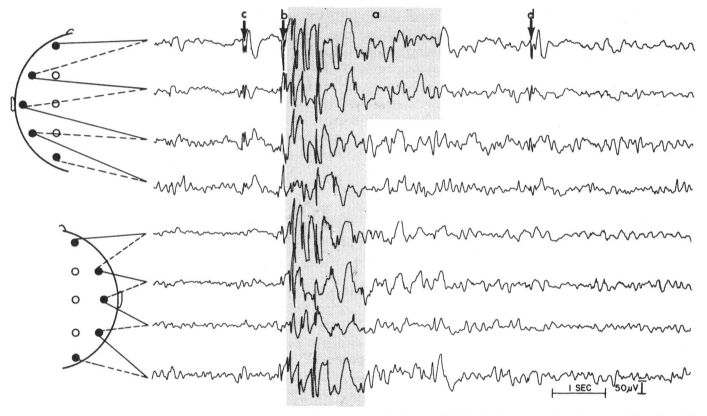

Fig. 17.3. Generalized spike-and-wave discharges (a) preceded by focal left temporal spike discharge (b). Focal left temporal spikes also appear before (c) and after (d) the generalized discharge. This 22-year-old man was hit on the head with a garbage can and passed out briefly 5 months before the recording; he began to have attacks of being dazed for 10–15 s 6 weeks before the recording and had a generalized seizure on the day of the recording.

Bilateral interictal discharges due to secondary bilateral synchrony are distinguished by the following features:

(1) they are most often less than 2.5 Hz when rhythmic;

(2) they may demonstrate considerable morphological variability from complex to complex;

(3) they usually contain a single site of phase reversal in transverse bipolar montages;

(4) they may be consistently asymmetrical; and

(5) consistently focal epileptiform spikes or sharp waves may be present (Fig. 17.3); EEG findings typically associated with cerebral lesions, particularly focal slowing or focal background attenuation, may be present.

In contrast, the discharges of primary bilateral synchrony are most often rhythmical with a repetition rate of 2.5 Hz or greater, show approximately the same morphology with each occurrence, often have more than one phase reversal in transverse bipolar montages, and are usually symmetrical. In general, when it is difficult to distinguish between primary and secondary bilateral synchrony, a prolonged recording often provides additional distinguishing features.

17.3.3 *Hemispheric epileptiform activity* may develop gradually or suddenly from focal interictal and ictal epileptiform activity. This unilateral form of generalization occurs practically only in infants and young children and is one of the EEG correlates of unilateral seizures.

17.3.4 *Local slow waves* may be the result of epileptogenic cerebral damage (Fig. 20.4) or of focal epileptiform activity itself. *Highly focal monorhythmic temporal intermittent rhythmic delta activity (TIRDA) is highly associated temporal lobe epilepsy and is considered by some to carry the same significance as epileptiform spikes and sharp waves.*

17.3.5 *Local reduction of amplitude* of the background in the area of the focal discharge has similar connotations as do focal slow waves except that postictal depression of amplitude usually persists for only a few seconds or minutes after the end of the ictal discharge.

17.3.6 *Generalized asynchronous and bisynchronous slow waves* may be due either to a recent secondarily generalized seizure, to a condition giving rise to both epileptiform and slow wave activity, or to unrelated causes.

17.4 MECHANISMS UNDERLYING FOCAL EPILEPTIFORM ACTIVITY

17.4.1 *Interictal focal epileptiform discharges* are the reflection of synchronized and abnormally intense fluctuations of membrane potentials of neurons in the epileptogenic focus. Microelectrode recordings from neurons within a focus suggest (a) that the abnormal synchronization is accomplished by a small group of neurons ('epileptic neurons' or 'epileptic neuronal aggregate') which send intermittent bursts of action potentials to many neurons in the focus, and (b) that the abnormally intense membrane fluctuation consists of a powerful paroxysmal depolarizing shift (which is probably triggered by an excitatory input) followed by a transient hyperpolarization. Frontal and temporal cortical neurons and hippocampal cells are more epileptogenic than parietal and occipital cortical cells in that they exhibit burst firing and are more readily 'kindled' into producing electrographic seizures with a series of subclinical electrical stimuli. The actual pathophysiological change responsible for the development of the epileptogenic zone is unclear. One current hypothesis is that neuronal excitability is increased through an accumulation of glutamate receptors (and perhaps sodium channels) combined with impaired glial cell removal of potassium from the extracellular space.

17.4.2 *Ictal focal epileptiform discharges* occur when, for reasons not yet understood, the hyperpolarization following each paroxysmal depolarizing shift weakens and is overwhelmed by depolarization. This leads to repetitive depolarizations manifested by rhythmical membrane fluctuations of neurons in the focus and by rhythmical ictal patterns in the EEG. Subcortical structures connected to the cortical focus may become involved in the seizure activity and probably serve to sustain it. Failure of surrounding inhibition can lead to the spread of focal ictal discharges to adjacent parts of the cortex.

17.4.3 *Acute focal epileptiform activity* is produced by various kinds of cerebral lesions. It can be explained by several mechanisms, all of which reduce the level of the neuronal membrane potential and thereby increase the tendency of the neuron to depolarize and to fire repetitively. Some of these mechanisms are: mechanical deformation of neuronal membrane, changes of membrane permeability resulting in abnormal ion exchanges; changes of ion concentrations, especially an increase in potassium and decrease in calcium in the extracellular space; ischemia, hypoxia and toxic products paralyzing the cellular metabolism needed to maintain the neuronal membrane potential.

17.4.4 *Chronic focal epileptiform activity* in adults is usually due to lasting structural change. Because spikes and ictal discharges in a chronic focus usually do not vary much in shape, it can be assumed that the sequence of the underlying neuronal events in the established focus is very stereotyped, i.e., that the epileptiform neuronal aggregate is rigidly organized. The long delay of several months or years between cerebral damage and the establishment of a discharging focus suggests that extensive reorganization of local circuitry takes place during this period. Following head trauma approximately 70% of patients who will develop epilepsy do so within 7 years of the trauma. Pathological studies of foci usually show scars of astrocytic gliosis at the site of the chronic epileptogenic focus. However, anatomical, histological, biochemical and other techniques have not so far been able to distinguish between lesions which produce epileptiform activity and those which do not.

The mechanisms immediately responsible for the production of epileptiform activity in the chronic focus include those listed for the acute focus. In addition, several other mechanisms have been considered important in the case of chronic focal activity. Partial deafferentation of cortical neurons may lead to altered sensitivity to synaptic transmitters. Reorganization of synaptic connections and collateral sprouting of axon terminals after injury may lead to increased excitation or decreased inhibition of neurons in the focus. Chronic foci unassociated with gross structural abnormalities may result from excessive afferent stimulation, for instance by repeated abnormal input from distant epileptogenic zones (17.1.2). The secondarily activated area is then referred to as a *secondary focus*. A contralateral homotopic secondary focus is referred to as a *mirror focus*. Currently, in humans there is only limited evidence to suggest that a secondary focus can actually generate seizures and sustain itself in the absence of a primary focus. That abnormal input alone can generate such a focus is suggested by the experimental phenomenon of *kindling* in animals: periodic electrical stimulation that is too low in intensity to actually trigger a seizure will eventually produce epileptiform activity and clinical seizures if applied repeatedly to certain susceptible parts of the brain (e.g., the amygdaloid nucleus). If the intermittent application of this initially subthreshold stimulus is continued, then in some cases even spontaneous seizures will occur without any stimulation. However, the more phylogenetically advanced the animal is, the more difficult it is to produce the kindling phenomenon. For this reason, and because it has not been unequivocally demonstrated in humans, the relevance of kindling to human epilepsy remains uncertain.

17.5 SPECIFIC DISORDERS CAUSING FOCAL EPILEPTIFORM ACTIVITY

17.5.1 *Degenerative, developmental and demyelinating diseases*

(1) *Senile and presenile dementia (Alzheimer's disease)* in some patients leads to sharp transients in the same distribution as the intermittent left temporal slow waves characteristically seen in normal older persons. The sharp transients often form complexes with the slow waves. Seizures occur slightly more often than in the general population in these patients.

(2) *Jakob–Creutzfeldt disease* is associated with periodic sharp wave complexes in many cases (Fig. 19.10). The sharp waves may be localized to one part of the brain (particularly the left or right parieto-occipital area) for several days or weeks before they become generalized. They are usually associated with myoclonic twitching.

(3) *Tuberous sclerosis* often presents with single or multiple spike foci in addition to single or multiple slow wave foci and generalized asynchronous slow waves, especially in children and adults with mental deficiency and epilepsy. Infants with tuberous sclerosis often show hypsarrhythmia (19.2.1) or multifocal independent spikes (19.2.3).

(4) *Sturge–Weber syndrome* is associated with epileptiform activity in about one-half of all cases. Local reductions of amplitude are very common. The epileptiform discharges may arise from one focus, from several foci near the involved area, or from the entire area. They may secondarily generalize or be generalized from the start.

(5) *Porencephaly, microgyria, pachygyria, agyria, holoprosencephaly and hydrocephaly of various causes* all can cause focal spikes although they more characteristically cause focal slow waves.

(6) *Bilateral optic neuritis* in children, if causing significant visual loss, may lead to occipital spikes unassociated with seizures (19.4.6).

(7) *Cortical dysplasia* characterized by abnormal migration and proliferation of neuronal cell aggregates is highly associated with focal epileptiform activity and clinical seizures.

17.5.2 *Metabolic and toxic encephalopathies*

(1) *Acute metabolic encephalopathies* such as those produced by hypoglycemia, hypoxia, hyperosmolar non-ketotic hyperglycemia, hypoparathyroidism and acute porphyria are most commonly characterized by generalized bisynchronous (22.6.2) and asynchronous (21.6.2) slow waves. Generalized epileptiform activity is common while focal spikes or sharp waves are less common and may be due to the activation of a chronic abnormality caused by earlier damage.

(2) *Cerebral lipidoses* may produce focal spikes, usually of the multifocal type (19.1). The late infantile form of ceroid lipofuscinosis (also referred to as the Bielschowsky–Jansky form) is specifically associated with excessively high amplitude occipital spikes that occur in a time-locked fashion in response to slow rates of photic stimulation.

17.5.3 *Cerebrovascular diseases*

(1) *Acute strokes* due to arterial thrombosis, embolism, intracerebral hemorrhage and subarachnoid hemorrhage extending into the brain may cause focal epileptiform discharges, usually associated with focal slow waves, generalized slow waves and amplitude asymmetries indicating recent structural damage. The focal epileptiform discharges are of the interictal and ictal types. Interictal epileptiform activity in the first week following ischemic stroke correlates highly with the occurrence of seizures. The predictive value of such activity for the occurrence of late seizures, months or years after the stroke, is uncertain. According to Fisch et al. (1986) periodic lateralized epileptiform discharges (19.3.1) occur acutely in 1–2% of individuals with non-hemorrhagic strokes involving cortical structures. Single or repetitive partial seizures, status epilepticus and epilepsia partialis continua may occur at the time of the acute infarction or hemorrhage.

(2) *Basilar artery migraine* has been noted to occur in association with posterior epileptiform activity or slow waves during or even between attacks.

(3) *Old strokes* can lead to the production of chronic epileptogenic foci several months or years after the acute event. This development is slightly more likely in patients who showed focal epileptiform activity at the time of the acute event. The background of the EEG and the clinical condition of the patient may show little or no residual evidence of the stroke when the chronic focus appears.

(4) *Chronic subdural hematoma* rarely causes focal epileptiform activity in the area of focal slow waves or amplitude reduction; such activity and partial seizures may, however, develop after surgical evacuation of the hematoma.

(5) *Arteriovenous malformations* and *venous angiomas* are commonly associated with epilepsy. This may be due in part to the epileptogenic effects of free iron deposited in the surrounding tissues.

17.5.4 *Cerebral trauma*

(1) *'Traumatic seizures'* or *'early posttraumatic seizures'* may occur during the first 1 or 2 weeks after head injuries of sufficient strength to produce cortical damage. The EEG may show focal spikes and sharp waves which are practically always associated with other EEG abnormalities. Similar abnormalities may occur after brain surgery. In children, early posttraumatic epileptiform activity is more common, more dramatic and more persistent than in adults; multiple shifting or stationary foci (19.1) are a common indicator of cerebral damage in infants and young children.

(2) *'Posttraumatic epilepsy'* or *'late traumatic epilepsy'* may develop several months or years after severe head injuries, primarily injuries which penetrate into the brain. The development of epilepsy as the result of head trauma without loss of consciousness is controversial. Spike foci develop not only in patients with this form of epilepsy but also in some patients with similar head injuries which do not lead to posttraumatic epilepsy. Focal epileptiform EEG discharges and epilepsy may also develop after brain surgery, especially after operations associated with major cortical damage; however, both abnormalities may occur after operations producing only minor cortical damage, for instance the insertion of a ventric-

ular shunt or of stereotaxic probes, although they occur more often after major cortical damage. Skull defects may enhance local sharp activity (23.4.2).

Posttraumatic, postoperative and other spike foci may require surgical excision if they generate a disabling seizure disorder which cannot be controlled medically. Before surgery, continuous non-invasive and invasive EEG and video monitoring, MRI studies, ictal SPECT, WADA testing and neuropsychological testing are often performed (14.5) to determine the extent of the *epileptogenic zone* (i.e., the area of the brain that is necessary to be removed to control seizures). During surgery, recordings from electrodes on the cortical surface can guide the excision of spike foci.

17.5.5 *Brain tumors. Supratentorial tumors* are most likely to produce an area of epileptiform activity if they grow slowly and near the cortex. Epileptogenic areas are therefore most common in oligodendrogliomas and angiomas, fairly common in astrocytomas and meningiomas, and least common in the faster growing glioblastomas and metastases. Epileptiform activity due to tumors is not always associated with clinical seizures; the association also depends on the type of tumor. While seizures are most common in oligodendrogliomas and angiomas, they are also fairly common in meningiomas and metastases and least common in astrocytomas and glioblastomas.

Although epileptiform activity caused by tumors is usually localized to the site of the tumor, it may also appear in a bilat-erally symmetric and synchronous or asynchronous fashion, or at a distance from the tumor. Thus, epileptiform activity caused by tumors, even when unilateral, does not have the same localizing value as continuous focal slowing or localized background attenuation.

17.5.6 *Focal epileptiform activity in seizure disorders without known underlying diseases and in normal persons*

(1) *Benign childhood epilepsy with centro-temporal spikes,* also referred to as 'rolandic epilepsy' is a fairly distinct and common convulsive disorder of childhood with onset between 2 and 12 years of age. It is benign in the majority of cases in that it typically disappears between the ages of 15 and 18 years. The history, clinical findings and laboratory tests give no evidence of a local brain lesion in spite of the clearly focal origin of the epileptiform activity and seizures. The EEG contains spikes which frequently have a characteristic morphology and are often followed by slow waves. *Unlike almost all other focal epilepsies, the spikes occur frequently, especially during drowsiness and sleep.* The spikes are sometimes grouped together in short runs with a repetition rate of 1.5–3 Hz (Fig. 17.4). They are located predominantly in the central or temporal areas and may demonstrate a slightly shifting distribution. They may also occur unilaterally (in approximately 70% of patients with a single recording) or bilaterally with varying degrees of interhemispheric synchrony. The individual spikes sometimes have the field distribution of horizontal dipoles

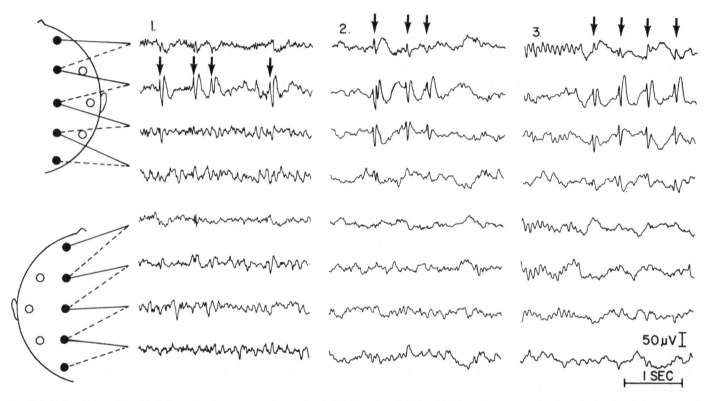

Fig. 17.4. Spikes (arrows), usually followed by slow waves and repeating in brief bursts at 1–2 Hz in the right fronto-central regions ('rolandic spikes'). (1) Awake: spikes limited to the area between frontal and central electrode. (2) Light sleep: slightly wider distribution and occasional polyphasic spikes. (3) Deeper sleep: widest distribution. This 6-year-old girl had her first seizure a few hours before the EEG recording. The seizure began in the left side of the face and then generalized. History, clinical examination and other test results were normal.

(also referred to as parallel generators) with a single spike showing a phase reversal in ear reference recordings and more than one phase reversal in longitudinal bipolar recordings. Drowsiness and light sleep activate the discharges, although occasionally they are abundant during wakefulness. The dramatic activation of spikes by drowsiness and sleep is a useful electrographic diagnostic feature. Generalized repetitive spike-and-wave patterns have recently been reported to occur in 5–20% of patients with rolandic epilepsy during all night recordings, but it is rarely encountered in routine EEG recordings. Apart from the background disturbance related to the epileptiform activity, the EEG is normal. Children with rolandic spikes most often have rare or no seizures. When seizures do occur they are usually simple partial seizures with motor symptoms. The motor activity may be tonic or clonic, limited to one side of the face, and associated with speech arrest or pharyngeal manifestations. Because the seizures typically occur at night they may go unnoticed. It is important to recognize, however, that only 50–70% of children with typical centro-temporal spikes actually have seizures. The seizure disorder as well as the electrographic findings are inherited in an autosomal dominant pattern with incomplete and age-dependent penetrance.

(2) *Childhood epilepsy with occipital paroxysms* is a more recently described syndrome of idiopathic epilepsy in which seizures begin in childhood and usually cease by adulthood. The seizures typically begin with visual symptoms and may be fol-

lowed by a postictal migrainous headache. The interictal EEG shows prominent occipital spikes or sharp waves that may occur in a semi-rhythmic pattern at 1–3 Hz. The discharges attenuate or disappear with eye opening and are not activated by photic stimulation. EEG background activity is usually normal. Onset between ages 2 and 8 and predominantly nocturnal seizures with deviation of the eyes and vomiting are thought to be favorable prognostic features.

Several factors combine to make this syndrome somewhat less well defined than the more common syndrome of rolandic epilepsy: (1) the prognosis is more variable, (2) a similar EEG pattern may be seen in individuals with underlying structural abnormalities, (3) headaches may precede or follow a variety of seizure types, and (4) there may be some overlap with rolandic epilepsy since it has been reported that some children with rolandic spikes may initially have epileptiform activity localized to the occipital head regions.

(3) *Landau–Kleffner syndrome of acquired epileptic aphasia* is a rare disorder that usually occurs in children and is characterized by seizures and a progressive disturbance of language function. The language disturbance may initially be limited to difficulty with comprehension and then progress to include speech. The seizures may precede or follow the onset of the language disturbance. Interictal epileptiform activity typically consists of moderate to high amplitude spikes or spike-and-wave complexes that are localized to the temporal head regions. The discharges may be strictly unilateral, but more often show either shifting lateralization or appear in a bilaterally independent fashion. They often become more abundant with the onset of sleep. Epileptic seizures in some cases are benign in that they are easily controlled with anticonvulsant medications and do not persist throughout life. A number of cases have also been described in which only epileptiform activity and language dysfunction are present without any evidence of clinical seizures. Although mild gliotic cortical changes have been described the etiology is unknown.

(4) *Normal individuals* may show certain EEG patterns that resemble epileptiform activity but have no clearly proven pathological significance. These so-called pseudoepileptiform patterns must therefore be distinguished from true epileptiform activity (19.5).

17.5.7. *Infectious diseases*

(1) *Meningitis and encephalitis* produce focal spikes only rarely in adults. Because infants are likely to react to widespread cerebral damage with focal spikes, such spikes may be seen in neonatal meningitis, syphilis and cytomegalic inclusion body disease; they may be associated with partial, unilateral or generalized seizures.

(2) *Cerebral abscesses* rarely produce interictal or ictal focal epileptiform abnormalities in adults.

(3) *Thrombophlebitis* of the cerebral venous sinus systems can produce focal or unilateral spikes in addition to decreased amplitude and slow waves. Septic phlebitis of the lateral or cavernous sinus may lead to the syndrome of hemiconvulsions, hemiplegia and epilepsy (HHE syndrome) in children. The acute phase of this syndrome is characterized by long-lasting and repetitive seizures of unilateral onset; this phase may be followed by epilepsy with partial complex seizures at a later age.

(4) *Herpes simplex encephalitis* often leads to periodic sharp waves in the temporal regions (19.3.1).

(5) *Subacute sclerosing panencephalitis* is usually associated with a high amplitude periodic sharp wave complexes which may begin locally (19.3.3).

17.5.8 *Psychiatric diseases.*
Behavior disorders and episodic psychotic or psychopathic behavior in children and adults have been found in association with focal spikes, especially in the temporal lobes. However, because the relationship between epileptiform activity and psychiatric abnormalities is unclear, focal cerebral lesions must be searched for in these patients. However, the relationship between epileptiform activity, epilepsy and psychiatric disorders is complex. Intracranial recordings reveal the presence of electrographic seizure activity without extracranial manifestations and episodic psychosis may occur in the setting of seizures.

REFERENCES

Aicardi, J. and Newton, R. (1987) Clinical findings in children with occipital spike wave complexes suppressed by eye opening. In: F. Andermann and E. Lugaresi (Eds.), Migraine and Epilepsy. Butterworth, Boston, pp. 111–124.

Ajmone Marsan, C. and Zivin, L.S. (1970) Factors related to the occurrence of typical paroxysmal abnormalities in the EEG records of epileptic patients. Epilepsia 11: 361–381.

Andermann, F. and Zifkin, B. (1998) The benign occipital epilepsies of childhood: an overview of the idiopathic syndromes and of the relationship to migraine. Epilepsia 39 (Suppl. 4): S9–S23.

Beaussart, M. (1972) Benign epilepsy of children with rolandic (centro-temporal) paroxysmal foci. A clinical entity. Study of 221 cases. Epilepsia 13: 795–811.

Binnie, C.D. (1987) Electroencephalography and epilepsy. In: A. Hopkins (Ed.), Epilepsy. Demos, New York, pp. 169–200.

Binnie, C.D., Batchelor, B.G., Gainsborough, A.J., Lloyd, D.S.L., Smith, D.M. and Smith, G.F. (1979) Visual and computer-assisted assessment of the EEG in epilepsy of late onset. Electroenceph. Clin. Neurophysiol. 47: 102–107.

Chabolla, D.R. and Cascino, G.D. (1996) Interpretation of extracranial EEG. In: E. Wyllie (Ed.), The Treatment of Epilepsy: Principles and Practice, 2nd Edition. Williams and Wilkins, Baltimore, pp. 264–279.

Cole, A.J., Gloor, P. and Kaplan, R. (1987) Transient global amnesia: the electroencephalogram at onset. Ann. Neurol. 22: 771–772.

Cole, A.J., Andermann, F., Taylor, L., Olivier, A., Rasmussen, T., Robitaille, Y. and Spire, J.P. (1988) The Landau–Kleffner syndrome of acquired epileptic aphasia: unusual clinical outcome, surgical experience, and absence of encephalitis. Neurology 38: 31–38.

Daly, D.D. and Pedley, T.A. (1990) Current Practice of Clinical Neurophysiology electroencephalography, 2nd Edition. Raven Press, New York.

Fisch, B.J., Rosenstein, R., Ramirez-Lassepas, M. and Hauser, W.A. (1986) The electroencephalogram as a predictor of epilepsy following occlusive cerebrovascular insult. Epilepsia 27: 615.

Frost, J.D., Hrachovy, R.A. and Glaze, D.G. (1992) Spike morphology in childhood focal epilepsy: relationship to syndromic classification. Epilepsia 33: 531–536.

Gastaut, H. and Zifkin, B.G. (1987) Benign epilepsy of childhood with occipital spike and wave complexes. In: F. Andermann and E. Lugaresi (Eds.), Migraine and Epilepsy. Butterworth, Boston, pp. 47–82.

Gastaut, H., Poirier, F., Payan, H., Salamon, G., Toga, M. and Vigouroux, M. (1960) H.H.E. syndrome: hemiconvulsions, hemiplegia, epilepsy. Epilepsia 1: 418–447.

Geier, S., Bancaud, J., Talairach, J., Bonis, A., Szikla, G. and Enjelvin, M. (1977) The seizures of frontal lobe epilepsy. A study of clinical manifestations. Neurology 27: 951–958.

Geiger, L.R. and Harner, R.N. (1978) EEG patterns at the time of focal seizure onset. Arch. Neurol. 35: 276–286.

Goldensohn, E.S., Legatt, A.D., Koszer, S. and Wolf, S.M. (1999) Goldensohn's EEG Interpretation: Problems of Overreading and Underreading. Second Edition. Futura Publishing Company, Armonk, NY.

Gotman, J. and Koffler, D.J. (1989) Interictal spiking increases after seizures but does not decrease after medication. Electroenceph. Clin. Neurophysiol. 72: 7–15.

Gotman, J. and Marciani, M.G. (1985) Electroencephalographic spiking activity, drug levels, and seizure occurrence in epileptic patients. Ann. Neurol. 17: 597–603.

Hughes, J.R. (1989) The significance of the interictal spike discharge: a review. J. Clin. Neurophysiol. 6: 207–226.

Hughes, J.R. and Zak, S.M. (1987) EEG and clinical changes in patients with chronic seizures associated with slowly growing brain tumors. Arch. Neurol. 44: 540–543.

Jennett, B. (1975) Epilepsy After Non-Missile Head Injuries. 2nd Ed. William Heinemann Medical Books, Chicago.

281

Jensen, I. and Klinken, L. (1976) Temporal lobe epilepsy and neuropathology. Acta Neurol. Scand. 54: 391–414.

Kellaway, P. (1981) The incidence, significance and natural history of spike foci in children. In: C.E. Henry (Ed.), Current Clinical Neurophysiology. Elsevier, Amsterdam, pp. 151–175.

King, D.W. and Ajmone Marsan, C. (1977) Clinical features and ictal patterns in epileptic patients with EEG temporal lobe foci. Ann. Neurol. 2: 138–147.

Klass, D.W. (1975) Electroencephalographic manifestations of complex partial seizures. In: J.K. Penry and D.D. Daly (Eds.), Advances in Neurology, Vol. 11. Raven Press, New York, pp. 113–140.

Klass, D. and Westmoreland, B. (1996) Electroencephalography: general principles and adult electroencephalograms. In: J. Daube (Ed.), Clinical Neurophysiology: Neurophysiology. F.A. Davis, Philadelphia, pp. 73–103.

Kuzniecky, R. and Rosenblatt, B. (1987) Benign occipital epilepsy: a family study. Epilepsia 28: 346–350.

Laskowitz, D.T., Sperling, M.R., French, J.A. and O'Connor, M.J. (1995) The syndrome of frontal lobe epilepsy: characteristics and surgical management. Neurology 45: 780–787.

Lerman, P. and Kivity, S. (1975) Benign focal epilepsy of childhood. Arch. Neurol. 32: 261–264.

Loiseau, P. and Duche, B. (1989) Benign childhood epilepsy with centromidtemporal spikes. Cleve. Clin. J. Med. 56 (Suppl. 1): S17–22.

Loiseau, P., Duche, B., Cordova, S., Dartigues, J.F. and Cohadon, S. (1988) Prognosis of benign childhood epilepsy with centrotemporal spikes: a follow-up study of 168 patients. Epilepsia 29: 229–235.

Lüders, H., Lesser, R.P., Dinner, D.S. and Morris, H.H. (1987) Benign focal epilepsy of childhood. In: H. Lüders and R.P. Lesser (Eds.), Epilepsy: Electroclinical Syndromes. Springer, New York, pp. 279–302.

Ludwig, B.I and Ajmone Marsan, C. (1975) Clinical ictal patterns in epileptic patients with occipital electroencephalographic foci. Neurology 25: 463–471.

Ludwig, B.I., Ajmone Marsan, C. and Van Buren, J. (1976) Depth and direct cortical recording in seizure disorders of extratemporal origin. Neurology 26: 1085–1099.

Markand, O.N., Wheeler, G.L. and Pollack, S.L. (1978) Complex partial status epilepticus (psychomotor status). Neurology 28: 189–196.

McLachlan, R.S. and Girvin, J.P. (1989) Electroencephalographic features of midline spikes in the cat penicillin focus and in human epilepsy. Electroenceph. Clin. Neurophysiol. 72: 140–146.

Michel, B., Gastaut, J.L. and Bianchi, L. (1979) Electroencephalographic cranial computerized tomographic correlates in brain abscess. Electroenceph. Clin. Neurophysiol. 46: 256–273.

Miller, J.W., Yanagihara, T., Peterwen, R.C. and Klass, D.W. (1987) Transient global amnesia and epilepsy. Arch. Neurol. 44: 629–633.

Niedermeyer, E. (1993) Abnormal EEG patterns: epileptic and paroxysmal. In: E. Niedermeyer and F. Lopes da Silva (Eds.), Electroencephalography: Basic Principles, Clinical Applications and Related Fields. Urban and Schwarzenberg, Baltimore, pp. 217–240.

Pampiglione, G. and Harden, A. (1977) So-called neuronal ceroid lipofuscinosis. Neurophysiological studies in 60 children. J. Neurol. Neurosurg. Psychiatr. 40: 323–330.

Panayiotopoulos, C.P. (1989) Benign childhood epilepsy with occipital paroxysms: a 15-year prospective study. Ann. Neurol. 26: 51–56.

Pedley, T.A. (1987) Epilepsy. In: A.M. Halliday, S.R. Butler and R. Paul (Eds.), A Textbook of Clinical Neurophysiology. Wiley, Chichester, pp. 231–267.

Pedley, T.A., Tharp, B.R. and Herman, K. (1981) Clinical and electroencephalographic characteristics of midline parasagittal foci. Ann. Neurol. 9: 142–149.

Quesney, L.F. (1986) Seizures of frontal lobe origin. In: T.A. Pedley and B.S. Meldrum (Eds.), Recent Advances in Epilepsy. Churchill/Livingstone, London, pp. 81–110.

Reiher, J., Beaudry, M. and Leduc, C.P. (1989) Temporal intermittent rhythmic delta activity (TIRDA) in the diagnosis of complex partial epilepsy: sensitivity, specificity, and predictive value. Can. J. Neurol. Sci. 16: 398–401.

Robertson, R., Langill, L., Wong, P.K.H. and Ho, H.H. (1988) Rett syndrome: EEG presentation. Electroenceph. Clin. Neurophysiol. 70: 388–395.

Salinsky, M., Kanter, R. and Dasheiff, R.M. (1987) Effectiveness of multiple EEGs in supporting the diagnosis of epilepsy: an operational curve. Epilepsia 28: 331–334.

Sammaritano, M., De Lothinière, A., Andermann, F., Olivier, A., Gloor, P. and Quesney, L.F. (1987) False lateralization by surface EEG of seizure onset in patients with temporal lobe epilepsy and gross focal cerebral lesions. Ann. Neurol. 21: 361–369.

Sammaritano, M., Gigli, G.L. and Gotman, J. (1991) Interictal spiking during wakefulness and sleep in the localization of foci in temporal lobe epilepsy. Neurology 41: 290–297.

Sawhney, I.M.S., Suresh, N., Dhand, U.K. and Chopra, J.S. (1988) Acquired aphasia with epilepsy – Landau–Kleffner syndrome. Epilepsia 29: 283–287.

Schwartzkroin, P.A. and Wyler, A.R. (1980) Mechanisms underlying epileptiform burst discharge. Ann. Neurol. 7: 95–107.

Sharbrough, F.W. (1987) Complex partial seizures. In: H. Lüders and R.P. Lesser (Eds.), Epilepsy: Electroclinical Syndromes. Springer, New York, pp. 279–302.

Shewmon, D.A. and Erwin, R.J. (1988a) The effect of focal interictal spikes on perception and reaction time. I. General considerations. Electroenceph. Clin. Neurophysiol. 69: 319–337.

Shewmon, D.A. and Erwin, R.J. (1988b) The effect of focal interictal spikes on perception and reaction time. II. Neuroanatomic specificity. Electroenceph. Clin. Neurophysiol. 69: 338–352.

Spencer, S.S., Williamson, P.D., Bridgers, S.L., Mattson, R.H., Cicchetti, D.V. and Spencer, D.D. (1985) Reliability and accuracy of localization by scalp ictal EEG. Neurology 35: 1567–1575.

Sperling, M.R. (1993) Intracranial electroencephalography. In: M.R. Sperling and R.R. Clancy (Eds.), Atlas of Electroencephalography. Elsevier, Amsterdam.

Sperling, M.R. and Clancy, R.R. (1998) Ictal EEG. In: J. Engel, Jr. and T.A. Pedley (Eds.), Epilepsy. A Comprehensive Textbook. Vol. 2. Lippincott-Raven, Philadelphia, pp. 849–886.

Sperling, M.R. and Morrell, M.J. (1993) Pediatric and adult electroencephalography. In: M.R. Sperling and R.R. Clancy (Eds.), Atlas of Electroencephalography. Elsevier, Amsterdam.

Swanson, J.W. and Vick, N.A. (1978) Basilar artery migraine. Neurology 28: 782–786.

Theodore, W.H., Sato, S. and Porter, R.J. (1984) Serial EEG in intractable epilepsy. Neurology 34: 863–867.

Thomas, J.E., Reagan, T.J. and Klass, D.W. (1977) Epilepsia partialis continua: a review of 32 cases. Arch. Neurol. 34: 266–275.

Trojaborg, W. (1968) Changes of spike foci in children. In: P. Kellaway and I. Petersén (Eds.), Clinical Electroencephalography of Children. Almqvist and Wiksell, Stockholm, pp. 213–225.

Walczak, T.S. and Jayakar, P. (1998) Interictal EEG. In: J. Engel, Jr. and T.A. Pedley (Eds.), Epilepsy. A Comprehensive Textbook. Vol. 1. Lippincott-Raven, Philadelphia, pp. 831–848.

Westmoreland, B.F. (1985) The electroencephalogram in patients with epilepsy. In: M.J. Aminoff (Ed.), Electrodiagnosis. Neurologic Clinics. W.B. Saunders, Philadelphia, pp. 599–614.

Westmoreland, B.F. (1996) Epileptiform electroencephalographic patterns. Mayo Clin. Proc. 71: 501–511.

Westmoreland, B.F. (1998) The EEG findings in extratemporal seizures. Epilepsia 39 (Suppl. 4): S1–S8.

Westmoreland, B.F. and Sharbrough, F.W. (1978) The EEG in cerebromacular degeneration. Electroenceph. Clin. Neurophysiol. 45: 28P–29P.

Zivin, L. and Ajmone Marsan, C. (1968) Incidence and prognostic significance of 'epileptiform' activity in the EEG of non-epileptic subjects. Brain 91: 751–778.

18 Generalized epileptiform patterns

SUMMARY

(18.1) *The patterns* of generalized epileptiform activity (Table 18.1) differ from those of focal epileptiform activity in that they appear over most or all parts of both hemispheres and usually have symmetrical shape, amplitude and timing in corresponding areas. Generalized discharges resemble focal ones in that they consist of sharp waves, spikes, multiple spikes and combinations with slow waves. Generalized interictal discharges, more commonly than local interictal discharges, consist of brief repetitive or rhythmical discharges, often spike-and-wave complexes that recur at regular intervals. Generalized ictal patterns consist either of longer repetitions of generalized interictal patterns, or patterns that contain different, progressively changing elements.

(18.2.1) *Clinical correlates* of generalized epileptiform activity (Table 18.1) are various kinds of generalized seizures. There is some correspondence between the type of seizure and the type of ictal discharge. *Typical 3/s spike-and-wave activity* is associated with non-convulsive absence seizures whereas *atypical spike-and-wave* is more likely to be associated with convulsive seizures. Multiple spike complexes increase the likelihood of myoclonus. *Slow-spike-and-wave activity* is likely to be associated with multiple seizure types and atypical absence seizures (e.g., Lennox–Gastaut syndrome). Infrequently, patients with a history of generalized seizures have normal EEGs whereas others may have generalized epileptiform activity in their EEG without having had any seizures.

(18.2.2) *Causes* of generalized epileptiform activity cannot be found in a large portion of patients. Those who have symmetrical and synchronous epileptiform activity and no other EEG and clinical abnormalities are said to have idiopathic epilepsy assumed to be due to an inherited or acquired genetic disorder. Other patients have epilepsy as a manifestation of widespread, lasting cerebral diseases that cause other clinical and EEG abnormalities as well. Another group of patients have generalized epileptiform discharges as a result of transient cerebral diseases or as the result of toxic, metabolic or other primary extracerebral disorders.

(18.3) *Other EEG abnormalities* do not usually occur in patients with idiopathic epilepsy. The appearance of other EEG abnormalities may therefore indicate underlying cerebral or extracerebral pathology.

(18.4) *Mechanisms* producing generalized interictal epileptiform discharges currently include *corticoreticular activation* for primarily generalized seizures and *secondary generalization* and *secondary bilateral synchrony* for partial or secondarily generalized seizures. An increased familial incidence of epilepsy in patients with primarily generalized seizures, genetic linkage studies, and no evidence of other cerebral or systemic abnormalities suggest a hereditary basis. The widespread and bilaterally synchronous appearance of epileptiform activity may be secondary to the interaction of a central, subcortical pacemaker with a diffusely and abnormally reactive cortex (the corticoreticular theory of primarily generalized seizures) or result from an extremely rapid spread of epileptiform activity via interhemispheric pathways from a focal epileptogenic cortical zone.

(18.5) *Specific disorders* causing generalized epileptiform activity include degenerative, metabolic, toxic, vascular and inflammatory disorders which involve large areas of the brain.

285

18.1 DESCRIPTION OF PATTERNS

18.1.1 *Generalized epileptiform activity* differs from focal epileptiform activity more in the distribution than morphology of the waveforms. It appears over corresponding parts of both hemispheres or the entire head. The waveforms usually have similar configuration, symmetrical amplitude, simultaneous onset and synchronous timing in corresponding parts of the two hemispheres, but may differ slightly in different parts of the same hemisphere. In many patients, the epileptiform discharges intermittently have a higher amplitude or are apparent only in one area of the brain, but discharges with local predominance are usually transient and may be followed by discharges having greater prominence in other areas. In other patients, generalized discharges begin consistently in the same area and often have higher amplitude and greater persistence in that area. These generalized discharges with focal emphasis suggest a focal origin of the generalized discharges, but this remains unproven unless focal discharges either consistently precede the generalized discharges and appear independent of the generalized discharges.

Like localized epileptiform activity, generalized discharges usually contain spikes and sharp waves, often in combination with slow waves, and can be divided into interictal activity lasting less than a few seconds and ictal activity which lasts longer (Table 18.1). Generalized interictal discharges, in contrast to localized interictal discharges, often consist of spike-and-wave and other complexes which repeat at regular rates.

Generalized ictal discharges, more often than focal ictal discharges, consist of long repetitions of interictal patterns. The shape of generalized ictal patterns is of greater clinical importance than that of localized ictal patterns because it often correlates with clinical seizure type (see also 17.1.1).

18.1.2 *Interictal patterns*

(1) *Three Hz spike-and-wave complexes,* also called *typical spike-and-wave complexes,* consist of a spike or spikes of high amplitude followed by a slow wave of similar or sometimes greater amplitude. The spike-and-wave complexes repeat at a frequency of about 3 Hz (Fig. 18.1). The slow wave immediately follows the spike, or the spike may appear to be superimposed on the beginning or end of the slow wave. The time relation between the spike-and-wave may differ in different derivations and may shift during the same discharge. In many instances 2 or 3 spikes appear with each slow wave. This is more likely to be observed if recording derivations with long interelectrode distances (e.g., ipsilateral ear reference montage) are employed. Although the frequency is often constant, some bursts begin at rates of 3–4 Hz and end at 2–3 Hz.

The typical spike-and-wave pattern usually has a frontal maximum, showing instrumental phase reversals in both longitudinal and transverse bipolar montages. At other times the background may contain bisynchronous slow wave bursts at 3 Hz resembling the 3 Hz spike-and-wave complexes without the spikes. There may also be brief runs of 3 Hz slow waves

TABLE 18.1

Generalized epileptiform activity

Interictal epileptiform pattern	Ictal epileptiform pattern	Clinical seizure type	Underlying brain lesion
Usually complexes of spike-and-waves or polyspike-and-waves, often repetitive; rarely single spikes and sharp waves	Episodes of prolonged activity of interictal type or of progressively changing activity	Generalized seizures	Unknown ('idiopathic') or widespread structural or metabolic diseases
1. Three Hz spike-and-waves or polyspike-and-waves, symmetrical and synchronous	Same as interictal pattern, but longer	*Absences* ('petit mal seizures')[a]	Unknown
2. Polyspike-and-waves, spike-and-waves, mono- and polyphasic sharp waves	Same as interictal, but repetitive	Bilateral massive epileptic myoclonus[a,c]	Unknown or widespread structural or metabolic diseases
3. Hypsarrhythmia and other patterns (Table 19.1)	(Table 19.1)	Infantile spasms[b]	As above
4. Spike-and-waves or polyspike-and-waves	Mixture of fast waves of over 10 Hz and slow waves with occasional spike-and-wave patterns	Clonic seizures[a]	As above
5. Slow spike-and-waves and other patterns (Table 19.1)	Rhythm of 10 Hz or more with increasing amplitude and decreasing frequency	Tonic seizures[b]	As above
6. Spike-and-waves or polyspike-and-waves	Rhythm of 10 Hz or more with increasing amplitude and decreasing frequency, later interrupted by slow waves	*Tonic-clonic seizures*[a] ('grand mal seizures')	As above
7a. Polyspike-and-waves or spike-and-waves	Polyspike-and-waves	Brief atonic seizures (epileptic drop attacks)	As above
7b. Polyspike-and-waves, spike-and-waves	Mixed fast and slow waves with occasional spike-and-wave patterns	Long atonic seizures[a] (incl. atonic absences)	As above
8. Polyspike-and-waves	Mixed fast and slow waves with occasional spike-and-wave patterns	Akinetic seizures[a]	As above

[a] Also occur with special infantile patterns (Table 19.1).
[b] Usually occur with special infantile patterns (Table 19.1).
[c] Also occur with periodic complexes (Table 19.2).

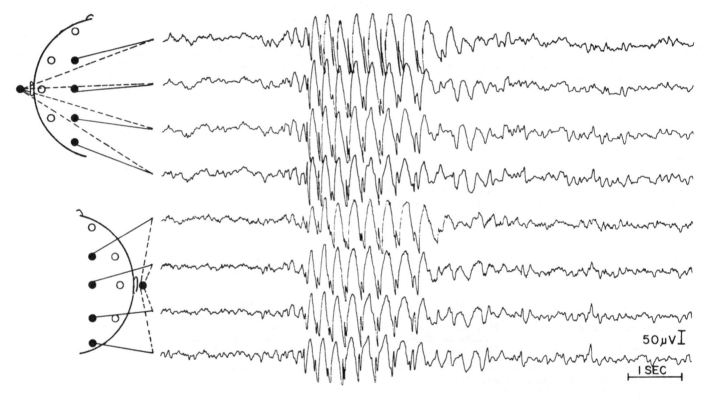

Fig. 18.1.　Interictal generalized 3 Hz spike-and-wave discharge, unassociated with clinical manifestations; the patient remembered a test word given during the discharge. This 22-year-old woman has a history of absence attacks since age 12 and of generalized tonic-clonic seizures since age 18.

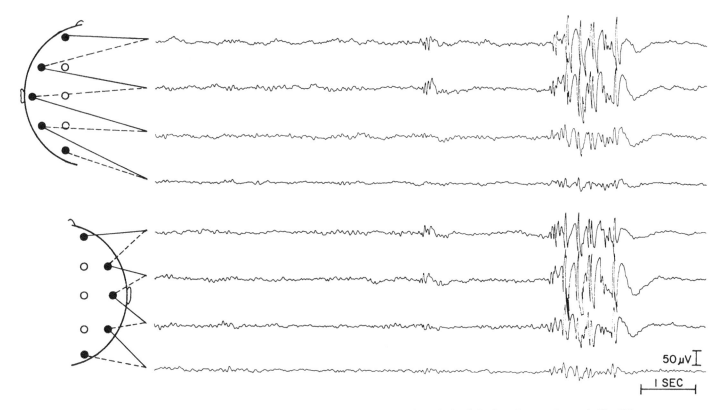

50 μV

1 SEC

Fig. 18.2.   Paroxysm of generalized 3–4 Hz spike-and-wave and polyspike-and-wave complexes during light sleep. Same patient as in Fig. 18.1.

that are maximal over the occipital head regions. This occipitally dominant pattern is not specifically related to epilepsy, but in approximately one-third of individuals in which it occurs, the typical 3 Hz spike-and-wave pattern may also be seen. The 3 Hz spike-and-wave pattern is readily detected in routine recordings (>98%) that include hyperventilation unless the patient is receiving anticonvulsant medication.

The sleep record regularly shows complexes of multiple spikes which are separated from each other by smaller slow waves than those in the waking epileptiform pattern (Fig. 18.2); these complexes may or may not repeat at 3 Hz. During wakefulness brief (less than 1 s) generalized or lateralized irregular epileptiform activity or bursts of theta and delta waves may also occasionally coexist with the typical 3 Hz spike-and-wave pattern. Other abnormalities of the background are very uncommon. Three Hz spike-and-wave discharges are usually activated by hyperventilation and associated with photoparoxysmal responses.

(2)   *Atypical spike-and-wave complexes* differ from the typical spike-and-wave pattern by either being less rhythmical or having a faster repetition rate. The frequency of spikes may vary in a burst or between bursts (Fig. 18.3). If the frequency reaches 6 Hz (Fig. 18.3, Part 2), these complexes must be distinguished from 6 Hz spike-and-slow-wave discharges (19.5.1) which are typically smaller, shorter lasting and usually not as widely distributed (Fig. 19.13). Generalized anterior dominant 4–6 Hz spike-and-wave patterns are basically associated with

juvenile myoclonic epilepsy (JME), although other generalized patterns, such as 3 Hz spike-and-wave, can also occur in patients with JME.

(3)   *Slow spike-and-wave discharges* (Fig. 19.6) are similar to the 3 Hz spike-and-wave complexes except that (a) they repeat at rates of less than 3 Hz, usually at 1.5–2.5 Hz; (b) the first component is more often a sharp wave than a spike; (c) the discharges may have focal preponderance or consistently focal onset in one area; (d) they are usually not facilitated by hyperventilation. The pattern of slow spike-and-wave discharges is discussed further in the next chapter (19.2).

(4)   *Hypsarrhythmia* is described in the next chapter (19.2).

(5)   *Intermittent spikes, polyspikes and sharp waves* occur either sporadically as rudiments of other interictal patterns or periodically as elements of periodic complexes (19.3). These elements are seen much less often as interictal generalized epileptiform activity than as interictal focal epileptiform activity.

(6)   *Generalized paroxysmal fast activity* is an infrequently encountered pattern that consists of runs of rapid spikes or sharply contoured waveforms in the beta frequency range (Fig. 19.7). It usually appears during sleep with maximal amplitude over the frontal or frontocentral head regions. The discharge typically lasts 2–4 s, but has been observed to last up to 18 s. Although it is occasionally seen in individuals with nor-

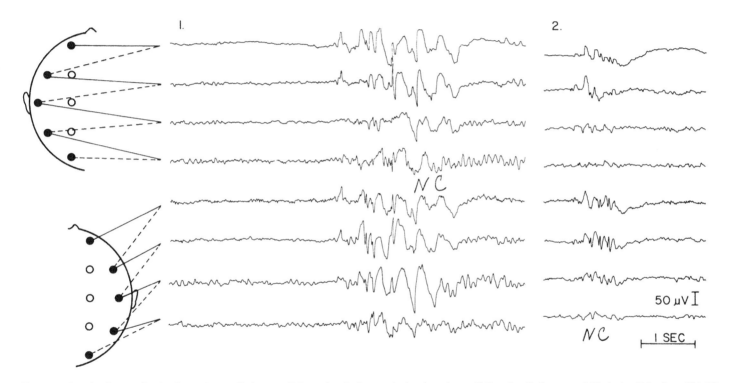

Fig. 18.3. Interictal generalized spike-and-wave discharges. (1) Irregular discharges during drowsiness. (2) Regular discharges at 6 Hz during light sleep. This 24-year-old woman has a history of generalized tonic-clonic seizures since the age of 4.

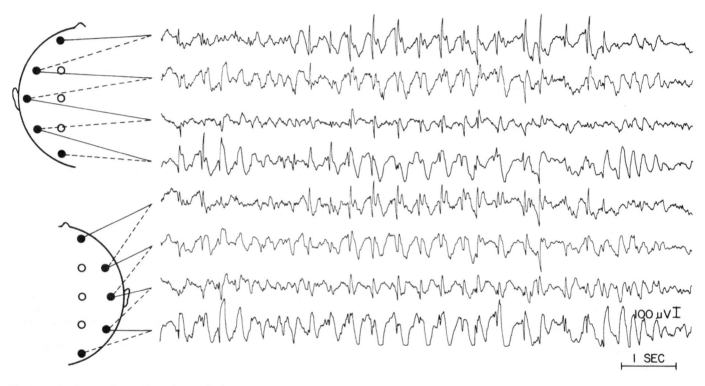

Fig. 18.4.   Ictal generalized spike-and-wave discharges at 2–3 Hz. This 60-year-old woman has a history of generalized tonic-clonic seizures since childhood with sudden onset of absence status 2 days before this recording.

mal intelligence, it is far more common in those with mental retardation. Most patients with this pattern have tonic-clonic and absence seizures, but other types of generalized seizures (e.g., tonic or clonic) may also occur.

18.1.3 *Ictal patterns* are of many different types (Table 18.1). Some of the more common patterns have fairly reliable associations with clinical seizure types. The most common ictal patterns are described below.

(1) *3 Hz spike-and-wave discharges* are repetitions of the interictal 3 Hz spike-and-wave pattern and last more than a few seconds. Most patients with this ictal pattern have the same interictal pattern, but not all patients with interictal 3 Hz spike-and-wave discharges show this ictal pattern. Patients with petit mat epilepsy (absence epilepsy) who are in absence status may show prolonged runs of typical 3 Hz spike-and-wave (so called petit mal status). In other patients with generalized non-convulsive status (also referred to as absence status) who have no history of typical absence seizures (petit mal seizures), less regular spike-and-wave complexes (e.g., multiple spike-and-wave complexes) are present continually with a variable repetition rate; this pattern is particularly common in adults and elderly individuals who may suddenly develop absence status with or without having had a history of prior seizures (Fig. 18.4).

(2) *Slow spike-and-wave discharges and sharp-and-slow-wave discharges* are repetitions of the corresponding interictal patterns. They are often associated with atypical absence attacks. They are related to infantile patterns and are further described in the next chapter (19.2).

(3) A *rhythm of 10 Hz or more* increases in amplitude and decreases in frequency to form repetitive spikes which are occasionally interrupted by slow waves before the discharge ends. A discharge of this kind forms the first of the two phases associated with generalized tonic-clonic seizures (Fig. 18.5). A similar discharge is often associated with tonic seizures (Fig. 19.7) and appears mainly in patients with interictal patterns described in the next chapter (19.2).

(4) *Multiple spike-and-wave discharges and spike-and-wave discharges* that are usually less regular than the 3 Hz spike-and-wave discharges appear in patients who often have interictal discharges of similar shape and suffer from a variety of different seizures. Similar discharges form the second phase of the diphasic discharge associated with generalized tonic-clonic seizures (Figs. 18.5–18.7).

(5) *An evolving discharge,* often associated with tonic-clonic seizures, consists of a sequence of the two last-described patterns (Figs. 18.5–18.7). A rhythm of 10 Hz or more which increases in amplitude and decreases in frequency corresponds with the tonic phase of the seizure; it lasts about 10–20 s. At the end, it may be interrupted by slow waves that appear at regular intervals and lead to a gradual development of the second phase. This clonic phase is characterized by high amplitude spike-and-wave or multiple spike-and-wave complexes that repeat at 1–4 Hz for about 30 s, having a faster rate initially. When they stop, the record usually shows no distinguishable activity for many seconds or a few minutes before slow waves of low amplitude begin to appear. The waves gradually increase amplitude and frequency until pre-ictal patterns eventually reappear. Postictal bilateral slow waves may very rarely remain as a residual EEG abnormality for up to several hours following a single generalized tonic-clonic seizure. Far more often the EEG returns to baseline within minutes. However, if more than one generalized convulsive seizure occurs, then postictal slowing may persist for hours or days.

Most patients with this ictal pattern have typical or atypical interictal spike-and-wave patterns although some patients show no interictal abnormalities at all.

(6) *A sudden transient decrease of amplitude* of all activity or a paroxysmal appearance of *generalized fast waves* are ictal patterns mainly seen in infants and very young children (19.2).

18.2 CLINICAL SIGNIFICANCE OF GENERALIZED EPILEPTIFORM ACTIVITY

18.2.1 *Association with seizures and epilepsy.* Most patients with generalized epileptiform EEG activity, similar to patients with focal epileptiform activity, have a history of seizures, and most patients with a history of chronic generalized seizures show generalized epileptiform activity in the EEG. Generalized electrographic seizures are almost always accompanied by obvious clinical seizure manifestations except in cases where the responses of the patient are limited (e.g., patients in coma or patients with severe, chronic encephalopathy). Rarely, generalized non-convulsive status (absence status) may be accompanied by a very mild impairment of mentation. In some patients, generalized epileptiform activity and seizure manifestations are precipitated by specific external sensory stimuli, mental tasks, or other factors. In contrast to patients with precipitated focal discharges and partial seizures, patients with precipitated generalized seizures are more susceptible to simple stimuli. The response often varies with stimulus intensity and has a short latency from the time of the stimulus presentation.

The occurrence of an interictal typical 3 Hz spike-and-wave pattern strongly suggests the presence of absence seizures. *In every recording in which this or any other generalized epileptiform pattern occurs, clinical response testing should be performed during the discharge to determine if there is an associated impairment of consciousness.* If an impairment is clearly documented, then the pattern is considered an ictal event, regardless of its duration. The presence of the typical spike-and-wave pattern does not necessarily mean that the patient with seizures has only absence seizures. Indeed, the majority of patients with typical absence seizures will even-

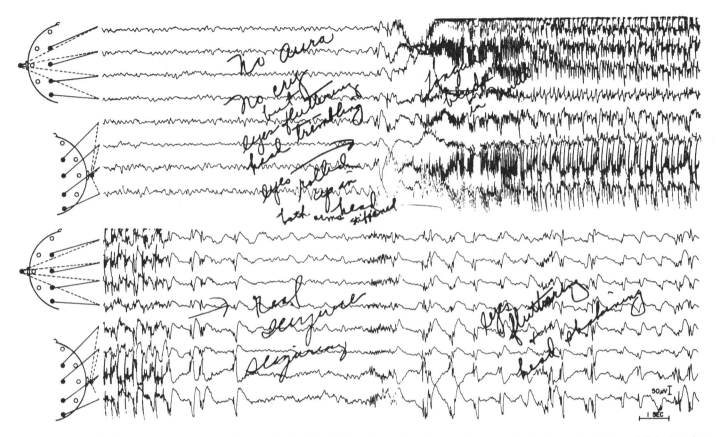

Fig. 18.5. Generalized tonic-clonic seizure in an 18-year-old girl with a life-long history of major and minor generalized seizures. *Top:* Pattern of slight drowsiness, suddenly interrupted by intermittent spikes and movement artifacts at the onset of a rhythm of generalized repetitive spikes of increasing amplitude and decreasing frequency which lasts about 10 s. Technician's comments read: 'No aura, no cry, but eyes fluttering, head trembling, eyes rolled up in head, both arms stiffened. Tongue blade in mouth'. This represents the tonic phase of the tonic-clonic seizure. *Bottom:* Spikes begin to be interrupted by slow waves. This signals the beginning of the clonic phase which starts with rhythmical high amplitude polyspike-and-wave and spike-and-wave complexes at about 1 Hz. Technician's notes read: 'Real seizure, seizuring. Eyes fluttering + head shaking'.

295

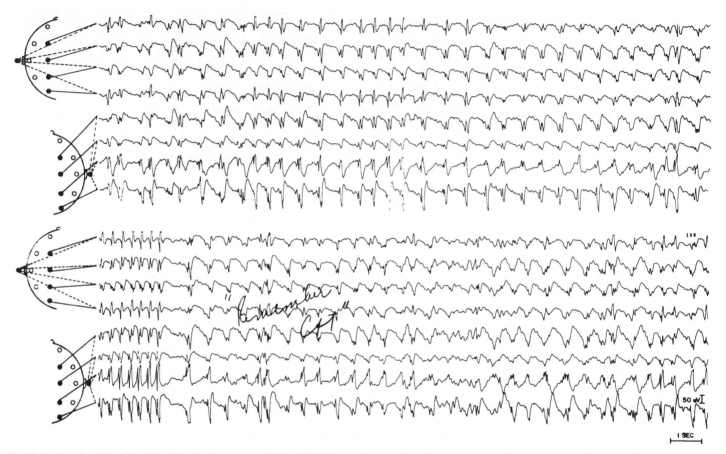

Fig. 18.6. Continuation of the generalized seizure shown in Fig. 18.5. High amplitude spike-and-wave discharges continue during the clonic phase. Top part is continuous with the bottom part of Fig. 18.5. Technician's note reads: 'Remember Cat', indicating that the technician was testing the patient's ability to remember a test word; the patient later did not recall anything.

296

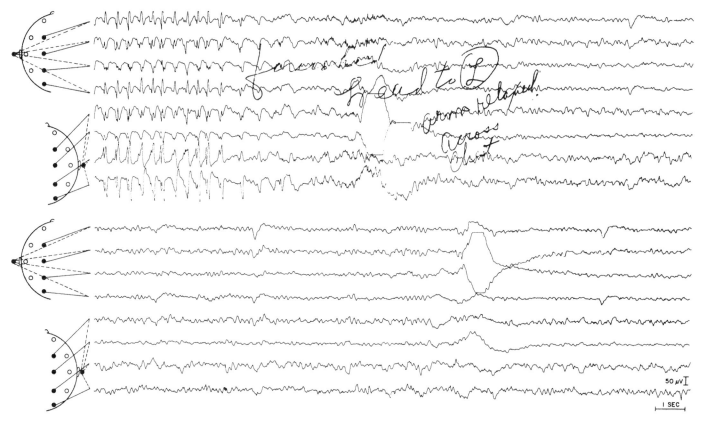

Fig. 18.7.   End of the generalized seizure shown in Figs. 18.5. and 18.6. Top part is continuous with bottom part of Fig. 18.6. The end of the high amplitude generalized bisynchronous spike-and-wave complexes represents the end of the clonic phase of the seizure. This is followed by slow waves, movement artifacts and gradual return of normal background activity. Technician's notes read: 'Head to left, arms relaxed across chest'. This was a mild generalized seizure. More violent seizures are usually followed by postictal depression of amplitude and longer lasting slow waves of lower frequency. Violent seizures can usually not be recorded completely because the recording electrodes become dislodged.

tually experience one or more tonic-clonic seizures. *To the extent that the interictal pattern deviates from the classical 3 Hz spike-and-wave pattern the likelihood of absence seizures becomes more uncertain and the likelihood of other kinds of generalized seizures becomes more likely.*

The presence or absence of the typical 3 Hz spike-and-wave interictal pattern in patients with idiopathic absence seizures can be used as a measure of the efficacy of therapeutic intervention. In this regard the typical spike-and-wave pattern differs from all other known focal or generalized interictal patterns. If anticonvulsant treatment is completely effective, then there is usually a dramatic, if not complete, suppression of 3 Hz spike-and-wave discharges at rest and during hyperventilation.

Like patients with localized epileptiform activity, some patients with generalized epileptiform activity have no evidence of seizures. This is commonly encountered in family members of patients with idiopathic primarily generalized seizures and occasionally in some patients with metabolic/toxic encephalopathies. The bilateral benign epileptiform (pseudo-epileptiform) patterns of 6 Hz phantom spike-and-wave, 14 and 6/s positive spikes, paroxysmal hypnogogic hypersynchrony, and subclinical rhythmic EEG discharges of adults (SREDA) also have no proven relation to seizures.

Epilepsy and seizures without obvious epileptiform activity may occur for several reasons. EEG recordings made between seizures may fail to show epileptiform activity for reasons discussed in connection with localized epileptiform activity. Patients with generalized seizures due to transient disorders such as drug withdrawal or toxic and metabolic encephalopathies are unlikely to show epileptiform activity after the disorder is resolved or at times other than during the periods of heightened susceptibility to seizures. Generalized seizures that produce an impairment of consciousness always show epileptiform activity (unless obscured by artifact) or prominent background changes with or without postictal slowing. Epileptiform activity during generalized convulsive ('tonic-clonic') seizures is often obscured by artifact, but postictal slowing always occurs and is easily discerned.

18.2.2 *Underlying cerebral abnormalities in adults and adolescents.* No demonstrable lesion is found in the majority of adults and adolescents with primary generalized epileptiform activity, especially in those who have bilaterally synchronous and symmetrical epileptiform patterns and no other EEG abnormalities. There is no historical, clinical or laboratory evidence of cerebral damage. These patients have idiopathic epilepsy.

Widespread lasting structural damage is present in some patients with generalized epileptiform activity. Most patients in this group have a history, clinical signs or laboratory findings pointing to the cause of the lesions; common etiologies include trauma, anoxia, meningoencephalitis, or encephalitis. The EEG may show other abnormalities in addition to generalized epileptiform discharges. The generalized epileptiform pattern is not typical spike-and-wave (3 Hz spike-and-wave).

Transient conditions that can cause seizures and generalized epileptiform activity are legion. Far more often these disorders occur without interictal generalized epileptiform activity. Some of the more common transient conditions associated with generalized epileptiform patterns and seizures include acute anoxia, recent severe head injury, hypoglycemia, withdrawal from barbiturates and other CNS depressant drugs and renal, hepatic or other metabolic encephalopathies. However, the EEG in these conditions more often shows other non-specific background abnormalities than epileptiform activity. If the underlying transient abnormality resolves without residual cerebral dysfunction, then the EEG returns to baseline.

18.3 OTHER EEG ABNORMALITIES ASSOCIATED WITH GENERALIZED EPILEPTIFORM ACTIVITY

18.3.1 *Focal epileptiform activity* in a record that also contains generalized epileptiform activity raises the question that the generalized epileptiform activity may be triggered by the focal discharge. *However, one of the most common pitfalls in EEG interpretation of generalized epileptiform patterns is to mistake a focal spike fragment of an otherwise generalized epileptiform pattern as evidence for focal onset. Such focal spikes should only be considered evidence for secondary generalization if they appear consistently and without any other contralateral*

focal spikes and without any evidence of photoparoxysmal responses (17.3.2).

18.3.2 *Focal slow waves* or a *local decrease of background amplitude* may suggest a focal brain lesion related to the generalized epileptiform discharges.

18.3.3 *Generalized asynchronous and bisynchronous slow waves and generalized decrease of amplitude* may indicate a generalized cerebral abnormality giving rise to generalized epileptiform discharges (e.g. metabolic encephalopathy, post-anoxic myoclonus, Jakob–Creutzfeldt disease). However, similar abnormalities may be the result of a generalized seizure discharge; mild postictal slow waves may rarely persist for hours after a seizure.

18.4 MECHANISMS UNDERLYING GENERALIZED EPILEPTIFORM ACTIVITY

18.4.1 *The involvement of intact cortex* by bilateral and approximately symmetrical and synchronous epileptiform activity distinguishes primarily generalized from secondarily generalized epileptiform activity. In secondarily generalized interictal epileptiform activity there is a focal cortical epileptogenic disturbance that gives rise to a generalized epileptiform pattern. One mechanism by which this occurs is commonly referred to as *secondary bilateral synchrony* and is discussed in Section 17.3.2. Cortical lesions giving rise to secondary bilateral synchrony are classically located in the mesial frontal cortex, but other cortical areas, including the temporal lobe, may be involved. Mesial frontal foci are best detected with transverse bipolar montages. Additional electrodes placed between the routine 10–20 electrode positions are often helpful since the critical finding is a single phase reversal that is lateralized to the left or right of the midline.

In 1954 Penfield and Jasper proposed the first modern theory of primarily generalized seizure propagation. They suggested that the epileptogenic discharge originated in a 'central integrating system of the higher brainstem'. Subsequently, such seizures were called *centrencephalic seizures* in accord with their postulated site of origin. Observations that supported the theory of centrencephalic seizures included the following:

(1) the apparently bisynchronous onset of epileptiform activity involving every area of the cortex simultaneously seemed to require a subcortical generator;

(2) Dempsey and Morison (1942) had demonstrated the existence of a diffuse non-specific projection system of thalamocortical connections by which medial and intralaminar thalamic nuclei could induce widespread cortical rhythmic activity; and

(3) an electrographic pattern approximating 3 Hz spike-and-slow-wave complexes could be produced in anesthetized or brainstem transected cats by electrical stimulation of the medial intralaminar region of the thalamus.

The centrencephalic theory has been considerably modified largely through the work of Gloor and colleagues who proposed that the cortex also plays a primary role in the propagation of primarily generalized seizures. This now generally accepted physiological explanation for primarily generalized seizures is referred to as the *corticoreticular* theory. Support for the corticoreticular theory includes the following experimental observations:

(1) high dose parenteral penicillin induces bilaterally synchronous bursts of 3–5 Hz spike-and-wave discharges that appear first in cortex, not in the thalamus or brainstem;

(2) generalized spike-and-wave activity can also be produced by the direct application of penicillin to the cortex, application to the thalamus is ineffective in producing epileptiform discharges;

(3) thalamic input appears to be the triggering event since thalamic stimulation which would normally induce sleep spindles or recruiting responses elicits spike-and-wave activity in the penicillin model;

(4) thalamic function and thalamocortical connections are prerequisites since depression of thalamic function by potassium chloride or thalamectomy abolishes spike-and-wave discharges; and

(5) the brainstem reticular formation appears to modulate spike-wave activity by altering the level of cortical excitability.

Hereditary predisposition also plays an important role in the genesis of epilepsy in individuals with primarily generalized seizures since: (1) the incidence of epilepsy in family members is significantly higher than in the general population, and (2) the incidence of epileptiform activity is also increased in unaffected family members. This familial tendency is most apparent among individuals with the least evidence of cerebral disease, as in those with petit mal epilepsy with typical absence seizures. Although it was initially thought that epilepsy with absence seizures was autosomal dominant, it is now known that the mode of inheritance is more complex.

18.5 SPECIFIC DISORDERS CAUSING GENERALIZED EPILEPTIFORM ACTIVITY

18.5.1 *Degenerative, developmental and demyelinating diseases*

(1) *Unverricht–Lundborg's myoclonus epilepsy* is associated with interictal multiple spikes or bursts of spikes and waves at 3–6 Hz which last for 1–2 s. The background contains theta and delta activity with superimposed beta waves. Photic stimulation may elicit multiple generalized spikes and waves with or without myoclonic jerks.

(2) *Lafora's inclusion body epilepsy* may show spikes, polyspikes and spike-and-wave complexes with focal or bilaterally synchronous distribution and with limited correlation to myoclonic jerks. The background may show diffuse asynchronous and bisynchronous delta waves of high amplitude.

(3) *Jakob–Creutzfeldt disease* often shows generalized periodic sharp waves (19.10).

(4) *Ramsey–Hunt's syndrome of dyssynergia cerebellaris myoclonica* may be associated with spikes, spikes and waves, multiple spikes and waves at 4–6 Hz, with an anterior maximum. Photic stimulation often elicits a paroxysmal response with jerks. Focal spikes may appear in sleep. Seizures are tonic-clonic or only clonic.

(5) *Sturge–Weber syndrome* may show bilateral spikes although it is often associated with local reduction of amplitude and local spikes.

(6) *Riley–Day's familial dysautonomia* may be associated with generalized epileptiform activity.

(a) Microgyria, agyria and holoprosencephaly may show generalized spikes, spikes and waves as well as focal slow waves, focal spikes, hypsarrhythmia and multifocal spikes (19.2).

(7) *Rett's syndrome* is a disorder of females that is associated with spikes that are often bisynchronous and diffusely distributed over the central and parasagittal head regions. The spikes may occur in runs with a repetition rate less than 3 Hz. In some cases the spikes can be suppressed with stimulation of the hand or elicited by tapping of the contralateral hand. Rett's syndrome is characterized clinically by a slow retrogression of motor and language skills beginning in late infancy or the second year of life. The patients also demonstrate a nearly diagnostic repetitive 'hand wringing' and hand washing movement. Most patients have either generalized convulsive, complex partial or simple motor seizures. By age 10 the epileptiform activity and seizures disappear and the EEG becomes dominated by delta activity.

18.5.2 *Metabolic and toxic encephalopathies.* Generalized spikes or sharp waves occur in many of these encephalopathies, usually on a background of widespread bisynchronous and asynchronous slow waves. Generalized epileptiform discharges occasionally repeat at regular intervals and may form complexes resembling spike-and-wave discharges. Regular, organized and sustained spike-and-wave patterns are rarely seen in adults except in some cases of dialysis encephalopathy. In infants and children, metabolic encephalopathies may be associated with multifocal or generalized epileptiform discharges of special types (19.1).

The following metabolic and endocrine encephalopathies may be associated with generalized epileptiform activity: Addison's disease, dialysis encephalopathy, hyperglycemia without ketoacidosis, hypoglycemia, hypocalcemia due to hypoparathyroidism or pseudohypoparathyroidism, hyponatremia, acute intermittent porphyria, pyridoxine deficiency and uremia (Table 22.1).

A very great number of toxic agents are capable of producing generalized epileptiform activity. Among the more common agents are high doses of therapeutic agents, such as phenothiazines, haloperidol, rauwolfia derivatives, INH, tricyclic antidepressants, environmental agents and organic solvents such as methyl bromide and chloride, pesticides, DDT, lead and mercury.

Withdrawal from chronic use of drugs depressing central nervous function can induce generalized epileptiform activity for a few days after withdrawal; photoparoxysmal responses are often seen in this condition. The most common agents are barbiturates.

Hyperthermia can induce or precipitate generalized epileptiform activity, especially in young children who tend to have seizures during febrile illnesses. These *febrile seizures* are usually tonic or clonic. Most of these children show no epileptiform EEG activity between seizures, but some of them develop such activity, and recurring generalized seizures, independent of fever.

18.5.3 *Cerebrovascular diseases*

(1) *Postanoxic encephalopathy* may produce generalized epileptiform activity in addition to many other EEG abnormalities. A special form of this activity consists of periodic sharp waves that are seen in cases of postanoxic myoclonus (19.3).

(2) *Cerebral infarction* rarely causes generalized epileptiform activity unless both hemispheres are affected, as for example in sickle cell disease or malaria. In such cases synchronous or asynchronous bilateral periodic lateralizing discharges (PLEDs) may occur (19.3). If epileptiform activity occurs as a result of cerebral infarction it is focal or lateralized.

18.5.4 *Cerebral trauma.* Severe head injuries can lead to secondarily generalized epileptiform activity and seizures. Like focal epileptiform abnormalities, the generalized abnormalities may appear soon after the injury or with a delay. The effects of cerebral injury on the EEG are especially pronounced in infants and young children who may react with special epileptiform patterns (19.1).

18.5.5 *Brain tumors.* The incidence of generalized epileptiform activity may be increased very slightly compared with that encountered in the general population.

18.5.6 *Generalized epileptiform activity in seizure disorders without known underlying diseases and in normal persons. Idiopathic epilepsy* is the diagnosis of many cases of generalized seizures without known cause, especially in cases of typical absence attacks associated with interictal and ictal 3 Hz spike-and-wave patterns, and in cases of generalized tonic-clonic seizures.

In practice, this diagnosis requires exclusion of organic disorders known to cause generalized seizures. Organic lesions must be suspected in patients who have (a) EEG findings of asynchronous and asymmetrical generalized epileptiform activity and of abnormal background activity; (b) a history of cerebral injuries or neurological disorders at any time from before birth to before the onset of seizures; (c) abnormal findings on neurological examination; (d) a general medical condition capable of causing generalized seizures. *Normal subjects* may rarely show specific patterns of generalized epileptiform activity (18.2.1; 18.4).

18.5.7 *Infectious diseases* produce generalized epileptiform activity only rarely and then mainly in the form of periodic complexes seen in subacute sclerosing panencephalitis, Jakob–Creutzfeldt diseases and herpes simplex encephalitis (19.3) or of infantile patterns (19.2).

18.5.8 *Psychiatric diseases* are not characterized by generalized epileptiform activity although widespread interictal discharges have been reported in small fractions of large groups of patients with various diseases. The possibility of causes other than non-organic psychiatric disorders must be evaluated in every case.

REFERENCES

Ajmone-Marsan, C. and Zivin, L.S. (1970) Factors related to the occurrence of typical paroxysmal abnormalities in the EEG records of epileptic patients. Epilepsia 11: 361–381.

Bancaud, J., Talairach, J., Morel, P., Besson, M., Bonis, A., Geier, S., Hemon, E. and Buser, P. (1974) 'Generalized' epileptic seizures elicited by electrical stimulation of the frontal lobe in man. Electroenceph. Clin. Neurophysiol. 37: 275–282.

Binnie, C.D. (1987) Electroencephalography and epilepsy. In: A. Hopkins (Ed.), Epilepsy. Demos, New York, pp. 169–200.

Blume, W.T. and Lemieux, J.F. (1988) Morphology of spikes in spike-and-wave complexes. Electroenceph. Clin. Neurophysiol. 69: 508–515.

Brenner, R.P. and Atkinson, R. (1982) Generalized paroxysmal fast activity: electroencephalographic and clinical features. Ann. Neurol. 11: 386–390.

Chabolla, D.R. and Cascino, G.D. (1996) Interpretation of extracranial EEG. In: E. Wyllie (Ed.), The Treatment of Epilepsy: Principles and Practice, 2nd Edition. Williams and Wilkins, Baltimore, pp. 264–279.

Daly, D.D. and Pedley, T.A. (1990) Current Practice of Clinical Neurophysiology: Electroencephalography. 2nd Edition. Raven Press, New York.

Dieter, J. (1989) Juvenile myoclonic epilepsy. Cleve. Clin. J. Med. 56 (Suppl. 1): S23–33.

Ellis, J.M. and Lee, S.I. (1978) Acute prolonged confusion in later life as an ictal state. Epilepsia 19: 119–128.

Fisch, B.J. (1996) Generalized tonic-clonic seizures. In: E. Wyllie (Ed.), The Treatment of Epilepsy: Principles and Practice, 2nd Edition. Williams and Wilkins, Baltimore, pp. 502–521.

Fisch, B.J. and Pedley, T.A. (1987) Generalized tonic-clonic epilepsies. In: H. Lüders and R.P. Lesser (Eds.), Epilepsy: Electroclinical Syndromes. Springer, New York, pp. 151–187.

Forster, F.M. (1977) Reflex Epilepsy, Behavioral Therapy and Conditional Reflexes. Thomas, Springfield, IL.

Fromm, G.H. (1987) The brain stem and seizures: summary and synthesis. In: G.H. Fromm, C.L. Faingold, R.A. Browning and W.M. Burning (Eds.), Epilepsy and the Reticular Formation. Liss, New York, pp. 203–218.

Gloor, P. (1979) Generalized epilepsy with spike-and-wave discharge: a reinterpretation of its electrographic and clinical manifestations. Epilepsia 20: 571–588.

Goldensohn, E.S., Legatt, A.D., Koszer, S. and Wolf, S.M. (1999) Goldensohn's EEG Interpretation: Problems of Overreading and Underreading. Second Edition. Futura Publishing Company, Armonk, NY.

Gomez, M.R. and Westmoreland, B.F. (1987) Absence seizures. In: H. Lüders and R. Lesser (Eds.), Epilepsy: Electroclinical Syndromes. Springer, New York, pp. 105–129.

Guberman, A., Cantu-Reyna, G., Stuss, D. and Broughton, R. (1986) Nonconvulsive generalized status epilepticus: clinical features, neuropsychological testing, and long-term follow-up. Neurology 36: 1284–1291.

Loiseau, P., Pestre, M., Dartigues, J.F., Commenges, D., Barberger-Gateau, C. and Cohadon, S. (1983) Long-term prognosis in two forms of childhood epilepsy: typical absence seizures and epilepsy with rolandic (centrotemporal) EEG foci. Ann. Neurol. 13: 642–648.

Lombroso, C.T. and Erba, G. (1970) Primary and secondary bilateral synchrony in epilepsy. Arch. Neurol. 22: 321–334.

Lüders, H., Lesser, R.P., Dinner, D.S. and Morris, H.H. (1984) Generalized epilepsies: a review. Cleve. Clin. Q., 51: 205–226.

Mancardi, G.L., Primavera, A., Leonardi, A., De Martini, I., Salvarani, S. and Bugiani, O. (1979) Tendency to periodic recurrence of EEG changes in Lafora's disease. Eur. Neurol. 18: 129–135.

Niedermeyer, E. (1993) Abnormal EEG patterns: epileptic and paroxysmal. In: E. Niedermeyer and F. Lopes da Silva (Eds.), Electroencephalography: Basic Principles, Clinical Applications and Related Fields. Urban and Schwarzenberg, Baltimore, pp. 217–240.

Niedermeyer, E., Fineyre, F., Riley, T. and Uematsu, S. (1979) Absence status (petit mal status) with focal characteristics. Arch. Neurol. 36: 417–421.

Niedermeyer, E., Rett, A., Renner, H., Murphy, M. and Naidu, S. (1986) Rett syndrome and the electroencephalogram. Am. J. Med. Genet. 24: 195–199.

Noriega-Sanchez, A., Martinez-Maldonado, M. and Haiffe, R.M. (1978) Clinical and electroencephalographic changes in progressive uremic encephalopathy. Neurology 28: 667–669.

Pedley, T.A. (1987) Epilepsy. In: A.M. Halliday, S.R. Butler and R. Paul (Eds.), A Textbook of Clinical Neurophysiology. Wiley, Chichester, pp. 231–267.

Penry, J.K., Porter, R.J. and Dreifuss, F.E. (1975) Simultaneous recording of absence seizures with video tape and electroencephalography. A study of 374 seizures in 48 patients. Brain 98: 427–440.

Rodin, E., Smid, N. and Mason, K. (1976) The grand mal pattern of Gibbs, Gibbs and Lennox. Electroenceph. Clin. Neurophysiol. 40: 401–406.

Salinsky, M., Kanter, R. and Dasheiff, R.M. (1987) Effectiveness of multiple EEGs in supporting the diagnosis of epilepsy: an operational curve. Epilepsia 28: 331–334.

Sperling, M.R. (1993) Intracranial electroencephalography. In: M.R. Sperling and R.R Clancy (Eds.), Atlas of Electroencephalography. Elsevier, Amsterdam.

Sperling, M.R. and Clancy, R.R. (1998) Ictal EEG. In: J. Engel, Jr. and T.A. Pedley (Eds.), Epilepsy. A Comprehensive Textbook. Vol. 2. Lippincott-Raven, Philadelphia, pp. 849–886.

Sperling, M.R. and Morrell, M.J. (1993) Pediatric and adult electroencephalography. In: M.R. Sperling and R.R. Clancy (Eds.), Atlas of Electroencephalography. Elsevier, Amsterdam.

Theodore, W.H., Sato, S. and Porter, R.J. (1984) Serial EEG in intractable epilepsy. Neurology 34: 863–867.

Tukel, K. and Jasper, H. (1952) The electroencephalogram in parasagittal lesions. Electroenceph. Clin. Neurophysiol. 4: 481–494.

Walczak, T.S. and Jayakar, P. (1998) Interictal EEG. In: J. Engel, Jr. and T.A. Pedley (Eds.), Epilepsy. A Comprehensive Textbook. Vol. 1. Lippincott-Raven, Philadelphia, pp. 831–848.

Westmoreland, B.F. (1985) The electroencephalogram in patients with epilepsy. In: M.J. Aminoff (Ed.), Electrodiagnosis, Neurologic Clinics. W.B. Saunders, Philadelphia, pp. 599–614.

Westmoreland, B.F., Reiher, J. and Klass, D.W. (1979) Recording small sharp spikes with depth electroencephalography. Epilepsia 20: 599–606.

Zivin, L. and Ajmone-Marsan, C. (1968) Incidence and prognostic significance of epileptiform activity in the EEG of non-epileptic subjects. Brain 91: 751–778.

19 Electrographic seizure patterns, pseudoperiodic patterns, and pseudo-epileptiform patterns

SUMMARY

This chapter joins several groups of interictal and ictal patterns that are clearly distinguished from the epileptiform patterns described in the preceding chapters.

(19.1) *Ictal patterns in neonates* are almost always focal or multifocal and often consist of rhythmical activity often without spike or sharp wave components. Ictal patterns in neonates frequently occur without obvious clinical manifestations.

(19.2) *Hypsarrhythmia, slow-spike-and-wave complexes and multifocal independent spikes* have features of both focal and generalized epilepti-form activity and appear at slightly different ages in infants and young children as the result of a great variety of organic brain disorders.

(19.3) *Pseudoperiodic patterns* are characterized by the fairly regular recurrence of paroxysmal activity of various forms.

(19.4) *Ictal patterns without spikes and sharp waves* occur in patients that also have focal and generalized interictal epileptiform patterns described in other sections.

(19.5) *Pseudoepileptogenic patterns* contain waveforms with epileptiform features that have no proven relation to epilepsy or seizures.

19.1   NEONATAL SEIZURES

19.1.1   In neonates spike or sharp wave abnormalities consist mainly of: (1) an increase in the number of multifocal sharp transients (MSTs) beyond that normally expected for a particular conceptual age; (2) persistent and frequent focal spikes involving a single head region in any state at any age; and (3) positive rolandic sharp waves. *Spikes and sharp waves are non-specific findings in neonates that occur in response to a wide variety of cerebral disturbances. They do not signify the presence of a potentially epileptogenic cerebral dysfunction.* In order to avoid 'overreading' epileptiform activity in neonatal EEGs it is important to recognize that similar shaped waveforms are normal at certain conceptual ages depending on their distribution, frequency of occurrence, and correlation with behavioral state (10.1). An abnormal increase in the abundance of MSTs represents a non-specific response to any encephalopathic process and does not specifically suggest the presence of a seizure disorder. If it is the only abnormal finding, then it should be considered a mild abnormality.

An invariant *suppression-burst pattern* in neonates or in early infancy is highly correlated with a poor prognosis for normal development or survival. When this pattern is associated with tonic spasms it is referred to as *Ohtahara's syn-*

TABLE 19.1

Special infantile and juvenile epileptiform patterns

Interictal epileptiform pattern	Ictal epileptiform pattern	Clinical seizure type	Underlying brain lesion
A. *Hypsarrhythmia:* Multiple spikes with shifting foci, on high amplitude, generalized asynchronous and bisynchronous slow waves	1. Sudden attenuation of amplitude, often preceded by a large slow wave or a sharp-and-slow-wave complex 2. A sharp-and-slow-wave complex or large slow wave only 3. Fast activity during amplitude attenuation	Infantile spasms Tonic seizures	*Prenatal* Prematurity Complicated pregnancy Meningocele Encephalocele Hydrocephalus Microcephaly Tuberous sclerosis Toxoplasmosis
B. *Slow spike-and-wave* ('Petit mal variant'): Spike-and-wave or sharp-and-slow-wave at 1.5–2.5 Hz; synchronous and symmetrical or not	1. Long slow-spike-and-wave discharge 2. Low voltage fast 3. Rhythmic 10 Hz discharge with increasing amplitude and decreasing frequency 4. Mixed fast and slow 5. Flattening 6. Slow waves 7. Pattern as in tonic-clonic seizures (Table 18.1)	Absences Bilateral massive epileptic myoclonus Tonic seizures Long atonic seizures Akinetic seizures Tonic-clonic seizures	Cerebromacular degeneration Phenylketonuria Sturge–Weber *Perinatal* Birth injury Anoxia Ischemia Hypoglycemia
C. *Independent multifocal spikes:* Spikes from more than two foci of constant location	Focal or generalized seizure discharges similar to those of adults (Tables 17.1, 18.1)	Partial simple seizures Partial complex seizures Generalized tonic, clonic, tonic-clonic seizures	*Postnatal* Infections Head injuries Cerebrovascular disease Metachromatic leukodystrophy Pyridoxine deficiency

drome of early infantile epileptic encephalopathy. Ohtahara's syndrome is often caused by cerebral dysgenesis or anoxic encephalopathy. *Early myoclonic encephalopathy* is characterized by the same EEG pattern but the clinical manifestations are not limited to tonic spasms, they include infantile spasms, myoclonus, and partial seizures. Early myoclonic encephalopathy is often caused by glycine encephalopathy or other inborn errors of metabolism.

Persistent focal spikes may occur with seizures or underlying structural abnormalities, particularly when accompanied by focal background slowing but their presence does not predict either electrographic or clinical seizures. Occasional spikes that occur in any location during wakefulness or active sleep after 42 weeks CA are abnormal, but are not specifically related to seizures.

Positive sharp waves (spikes with positive polarity) that: (1) occur over the rolandic and parasagittal head regions; (2) clearly stand out from both the ongoing background activity and other sharp transients; and (3) are accompanied by other EEG abnormalities, are thought to be associated with periventricular encephalomalacia (usually a consequence of intraventricular hemorrhage). However, this association has been questioned by some investigators. Currently, the presence of positive sharp waves should be noted and, particularly if they are associated with other EEG abnormalities, the question of an underlying structural abnormality such as periventricular encephalomalacia should be raised.

19.1.2 *Neonatal ictal patterns* are almost always focal or lateralized in onset. Generalized patterns are rarely seen possibly because intra- and interhemispheric cortical pathways are not sufficiently developed to allow for more widespread seizure propagation. The morphology of neonatal ictal patterns consists of either rhythmical, monomorphic waveforms or repetitive spikes or sharp waves (Fig. 19.1). Electrographic seizures are usually characterized by a buildup of activity that evolves in repetition rate and morphology. The duration of neonatal electrographic seizures may be less than 10 s or more than 30 min, but the majority last less than 1 min.

There is, in general, a poor correlation between specific ictal neonatal EEG patterns and clinical manifestations. Although it has been suggested that some patterns correlate with certain behaviors, such as rhythmic delta waves during tonic seizures and rhythmic alpha waves during apneic seizures, such correlations are not well established.

Neonatal electrographic seizures are frequently multifocal, often involve more than one hemisphere, and may overlap in time. A distinctive feature of neonatal electrographic seizures is the tendency for some to remain focal but gradually change location in the same hemisphere as the seizure progresses. In other cases the discharge may begin in one hemisphere and gradually move to the opposite hemisphere (Fig. 19.2).

Neonatal seizures are typically highly focal and may appear to involve only one electrode. However, prominent changes restricted to one electrode or abrupt rhythmic patterns involving one or more electrodes should always raise the question of

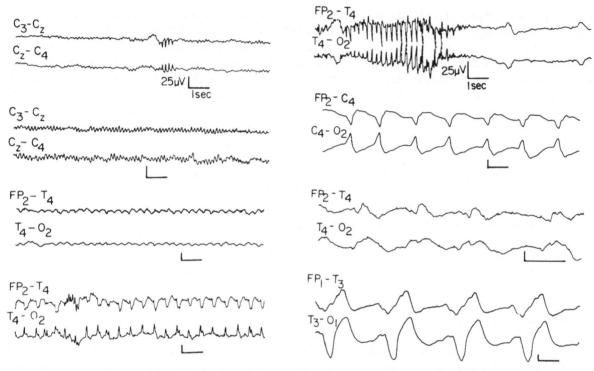

Fig. 19.1. Typical ictal patterns in premature and full-term infants. Except where otherwise indicated, calibration: 50 μV; 1 s. Courtesy B.R. Tharp, Electrodiagnosis in Clinical Neurology, 1986.

artifact. Certain rhythmical artifacts are characteristic findings in neonatal recordings and others occur commonly. Examples of common artifacts in neonatal recordings that could be confused with electrographic seizures are shown in Fig.

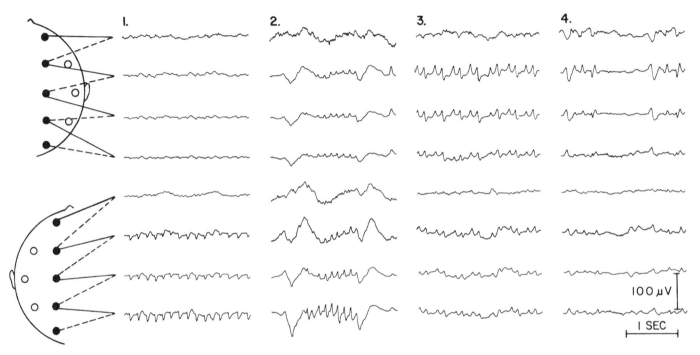

Fig. 19.2. Neonatal status epilepticus with seizure discharges on alternating sides in a 1-day-old full-term infant following an anoxic episode at birth. (1) Seizure discharge of rhythmical waves of 6–7 Hz, mainly on the left side. (2) One minute later, the left-sided seizure discharge consists of polyspikes, separated by high amplitude slow waves; similar discharges of lower amplitude appear on the right side. (3) Two minutes later, the seizure discharge on the left side abates and seizure discharges on the right side are at their height. (4) One minute later, the seizure discharge on the right side diminishes.

19.3.

Neonatal electrographic seizures may occur in the absence of clinical manifestations, so-called occult or subclinical seizures. Alternatively, the clinical change may be overlooked

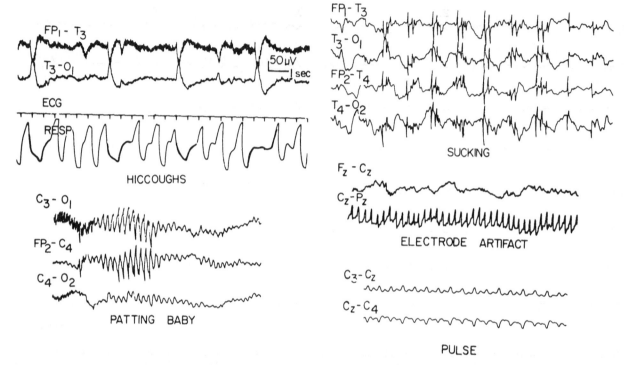

Fig. 19.3. Rhythmic artifacts which can be confused with ictal patterns. Calibration 50 μV, 1 s. Courtesy B.R. Tharp, Electrodiagnosis in Clinical Neurology, 1986.

because it does not represent an obvious departure from the neonate's baseline behavior. However, if the patient is carefully inspected during the electrographic seizure, then subtle clinical changes are usually detected. If clinical changes are not seen despite careful inspection, then the prognosis for normal development is currently thought to be poor.

312

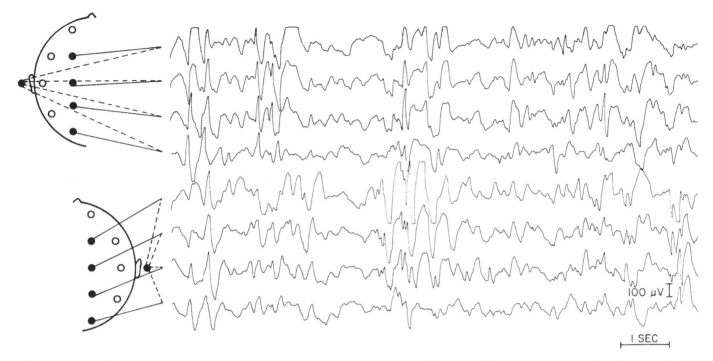

Fig. 19.4. Pattern of hypsarrhythmia. Interictal continuous spikes and slow waves of high amplitude in a shifting distribution. The patient is a 6-month-old infant with dysplasia of the left posterior fossa, hypotonia and infantile spasms.

Subclinical seizures have been shown to occur frequently in patients with or without any obvious impairment of consciousness. In general, if neonatal seizures are present, they occur frequently, with interictal periods usually lasting less than 10 min. Therefore, a typical neonatal recording (45–60 min in duration) is almost always sufficient to screen for the

313

presence of seizures. Also, since EEG recording is the most sensitive technique for detecting neonatal seizures, it should be liberally employed in all cases of suspected seizures. Once electrographic seizures are observed repeat recordings should be performed to monitor the efficacy of treatment.

19.2 THE INFANTILE AND JUVENILE PATTERNS OF HYPSARRHYTHMIA, SLOW-SPIKE-AND-WAVE DISCHARGES AND MULTIFOCAL INDEPENDENT SPIKES

These patterns (Table 19.1) are similar to each other in that (1) they usually have some focal or multifocal interictal features even though many of their ictal patterns are generalized from the start; (2) they are often associated with neurological abnormalities in the form of mental retardation and seizures; (3) they are the result of a great variety of prenatal, perinatal and postnatal pathological conditions most of which produce widespread or multifocal cerebral damage; (4) they depend more on the age of the patient and the severity of the underlying condition than on the particular type of the lesion. Hypsarrhythmia begins between the ages of 6 months to 2 years and may be replaced by one of the other patterns. The slow-spike-and-wave pattern begins at the age of 2–4 years and may continue through early childhood. The pattern of multifocal independent spikes may develop from either one of the other

patterns, or appear at the same ages as the other patterns in which case it usually represents less severe damage.

19.2.1 *Hypsarrhythmia.* Hypsarrhythmia is a term derived from the words 'hypselos', a Greek word which means 'high', and the word 'arrhythmia'. It thus describes a high voltage pattern (so high that it cannot be recorded at routine sensitivity settings) of a continuously irregular largely chaotic admixture of spikes, sharp waves, and slow waves (Fig. 19.4).

The classical pattern of hypsarrhythmia differs from other patterns of multifocal epileptiform discharges in that the locations of the focal spikes-and-sharp waves are not constant but shift from moment to moment. In addition, the spikes-and-sharp waves are often greatest in amplitude over the posterior head regions (a point which is sometimes helpful in distinguishing hypsarrhythmia from the early onset of the Lennox–Gastaut syndrome; 19.2.2).

Hypsarrhythmia is most pronounced during non-REM sleep and is often greatly attenuated or transiently abolished during REM sleep. Less often, wakefulness or arousal from non-REM sleep causes a reduction or transient disappearance of the pattern.

Modified hypsarrhythmia is a term used to describe commonly occurring variations of the classical hypsarrhythmia pattern. Modified hypsarrhythmic patterns include: (1) predominantly high voltage, generalized, asynchronous, slow wave activity; (2) unilateral or asymmetrical hypsarrhythmia; (3) a

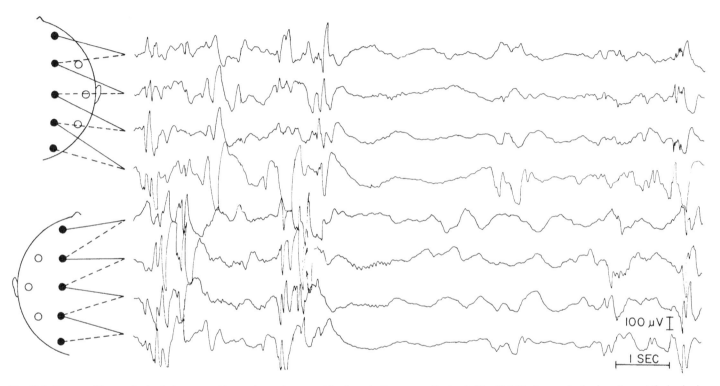

Fig. 19.5. Pattern of hypsarrhythmia interrupted by an electrodecremental seizure in the same patient as in Fig. 19.4. The hypsarrhythmic pattern at the beginning is abruptly replaced by very slow waves of much lower amplitude which were associated with mild spasmodic flexion of the arms.

discontinuous pattern with frequent epochs of widespread or localized attenuation similar in appearance to the suppression-burst pattern; and (4) hypsarrhythmia with increased interhemispheric synchrony. The suppression-burst variant in

315

particular carries a guarded prognosis with high mortality and little likelihood of normal development. The unilateral or asymmetric pattern is more likely to be non-idiopathic and to be associated with underlying localized structural or functional abnormalities.

The ictal patterns associated with hypsarrhythmia usually include: (1) the *electrodecremental pattern* (Fig. 19.5) characterized by a sudden attenuation of amplitude, often preceded by either a frontal dominant, high amplitude, paroxysmal slow wave or a generalized sharp and slow wave complex, (2) generalized sharp and slow wave complexes or generalized paroxysmal slow waves only, or (3) fast activity appearing during the period of amplitude attenuation. The most common ictal pattern is the electrodecremental pattern.

The clinical seizures consist mainly of infantile spasms (95% of cases) and tonic seizures. Infants and children with hypsarrhythmia and modified hypsarrhythmia often show an arrest of development of perceptual and motor skills. The combination of infantile spasms, mental retardation and hypsarrhythmia is referred to as *West syndrome*. Approximately 60% of children with infantile spasms demonstrate hypsarrhythmia. Although relative normalization of the EEG may occur in treated patients with hypsarrhythmia and infantile spasms, the infantile spasms may continue to occur. Thus, normalization of the EEG is a favorable sign, but it cannot be equated with effective therapy.

Clinical conditions causing hypsarrhythmia comprise a great variety of disorders of prenatal, perinatal or postnatal onset (Table 19.1, column 4). Most are due to diffuse or multifocal structural damage, but a few are due to metabolic disorders and are reversible, for instance hypoglycemia, pyridoxine deficiency and phenylketonuria. Rarely, local cerebral lesions such as the choroid plexus papilloma or the lesions seen in Sturge–Weber syndrome may be associated with hypsarrhythmia. In cases where there is a known and irreversible etiology for hypsarrhythmia with infantile spasms the long-term prognosis is poor. Only 5% of such patients develop normally or with only mild impairments. In contrast, the outcome is favorable in approximately 40% of idiopathic cases of hypsarrhythmia with infantile spasms.

19.2.2 *Slow-spike-and-wave pattern* (formerly called 'petit mal variant'). The slow-spike-and-wave pattern is an interictal pattern that consists of spike-and-wave complexes, polyspike-and-wave complexes or sharp-and-slow-wave complexes which occur intermittently or repeat at about 1.5–2.5 Hz for up to a few seconds (Fig. 19.6). The 'spike' component is usually more blunted than sharply contoured. The complexes may be symmetrical and bisynchronous, or asymmetrical and even asynchronous. They may have a focal onset. With sleep onset a wider variety of spikes, sharp waves and slow waves of varying distribution occur.

The ictal patterns that occur in patients with the slow-spike-and-wave pattern are generalized and consist of (1) repetition of the interictal discharges for more than a few seconds, often up to 1 min; (2) low amplitude fast activity of about 20 Hz with increasing amplitude; (3) rhythmical activity of about 10 Hz with increasing amplitude and decreasing frequency, occasionally interrupted by rhythmical slow waves and forming polyspike-and-wave or spike-and-wave complexes (Fig. 19.7); (4) a mixture of rhythmical slow waves and fast waves occasionally forming spike-and-wave patterns; (5) a simple reduction of amplitude leading to apparent flattening of the EEG; (6) generalized slow waves of delta or theta frequency; (7) a biphasic discharge of the type associated with generalized tonic-clonic seizures in adults. The slow-spike-and-wave pattern, even when occurring in a prolonged train (pattern 1), is often not associated with overt behavioral changes.

Clinical seizures are of various types. Absence attacks may occur with the ictal patterns (1), (2) or (3). These attacks are called 'atypical absences' in contrast to 'typical absences' (16.2) associated with bilaterally synchronous and symmetrical 3 Hz spike-and-wave discharges (18.1.2). Tonic, clonic and other generalized motor seizures occur with patterns (2)–(6). Pattern (7) is associated with tonic-clonic seizures similar to those of adults (16.2). Many patients have more than one type of seizure.

The combination of the EEG pattern of slow-spike-and-waves, intractable seizures and mental retardation is referred to as 'Lennox–Gastaut syndrome'.

Clinical conditions causing slow-spike-and-wave discharges are the same as those that in younger patients cause hypsarrhythmia. Subacute sclerosing panencephalitis may cause slow-spike-and-wave patterns in exceptional cases.

19.2.3 *Independent multifocal spikes. The interictal pattern* shows spikes arising independently from more than two foci (Fig. 19.8). In contrast to hypsarrhythmia, the foci of the spike discharges are constant, i.e. they do not shift in the same recording; the background shows less abnormal slow wave activity or is normal. Some spike foci may disappear and other, new, foci may appear from one recording to the next to give the appearance of migrating foci.

The ictal patterns vary widely and include both focal and generalized seizure discharges of all types seen in adults (Tables 17.1 and 18.1, column 2).

Clinical seizures also vary widely and include partial, secondary and primary generalized seizures of most types (Tables 17.1 and 18.1, column 3). Most patients have generalized motor seizures, and many have more than one type of seizure. As is true for patients with hypsarrhythmia and the slow-spike-and-wave pattern, the majority of patients with multifocal independent spikes suffer from a combination of seizures and mental retardation indicating severe and widespread cerebral damage.

Clinical conditions causing multiple independent focal spikes are the same as those causing hypsarrhythmia or slow-spike-and-wave patterns.

19.3 PSEUDOPERIODIC PATTERNS

The patterns described in this section (Table 19.2) are similar

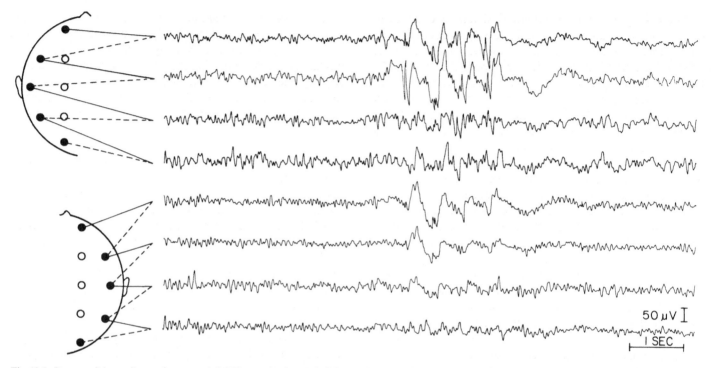

50 μV

1 SEC

Fig. 19.6. Pattern of slow spikes and waves at 1.5–2 Hz, maximal over the left anterior head. This 8-year-old girl has a history of generalized seizures of many types since birth; she is slightly retarded but without other neurological abnormalities.

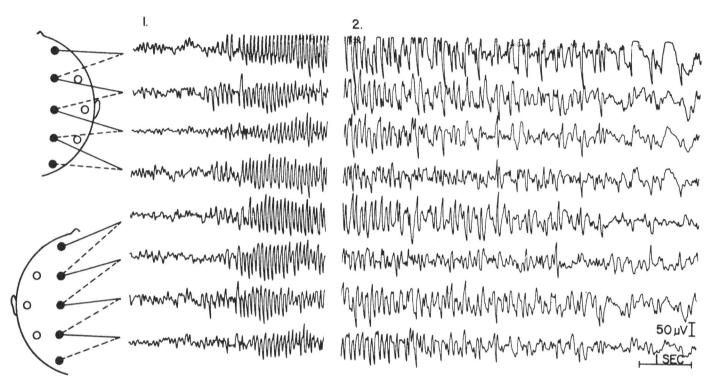

Fig. 19.7. Generalized seizure discharge in the same patient as in Fig. 19.6. (1) Generalized rhythm of high amplitude spikes at 12–14 Hz. (2) Fifteen seconds after the end of part 1, the frequency of the spikes has slowed and slow waves begin to interrupt the spikes. This episode was associated with a mild generalized tonic seizure.

to each other in that: (1) they consist of complexes which recur at fairly regular intervals on a background of slow waves of usually low amplitude; and (2) most of them are generalized or widespread in distribution and synchronous in timing over different parts of the head.

19.3.1 *Periodic lateralizing epileptiform discharges (PLEDs) and bilateral periodic lateralized epileptiform discharges (BI-PLEDs).* The EEG pattern shows complexes which consist of a di- or multiphasic spike or sharp wave and may include a slow wave (Fig. 19.9). Complexes usually last for only a fraction of a second. They commonly appear in a wide distribution on one side of the head. In some instances, they have a focal origin and in others they are bilateral but usually with a clear maximum on one side. They may have a different shape in different areas and they often vary in the same patient with time. The complexes recur every 1–2 s and are separated by low amplitude slow waves or by no detectable activity at regular gain. The background in regions not showing PLEDs is often abnormal. PLEDs may be interrupted by the appearance of a focal seizure discharge which may generalize. Electrographic seizure discharges evolve from the PLED pattern in one of two ways: either the PLEDs appear to evolve directly into an electrographic seizure pattern or an electrographic seizure pattern develops intermixed with the ongoing PLED pattern. In the latter situation the PLEDs usually persist for only a few seconds before disappearing as the seizure continues. The coexistence of PLEDs with a simultaneous and indepen-

dent appearing electrographic seizure pattern suggests that PLEDs may represent an interictal rather than ictal epileptiform pattern. PLEDs have been anatomically associated with localized increased metabolism seen on positron emission tomography in a patient who had had status epilepticus (Handforth et al., 1994) and presumably did not have ongoing seizure activity. For clinical purposes the PLED pattern is generally regarded as a highly epileptogenic interictal pattern.

PLEDs usually occur in the setting of an acute or subacute cerebral lesion. Among 170 reported cases etiologies included stroke (38%), neoplasm (20%), epilepsy (17%), and miscellaneous disorders including herpes encephalitis, sickle cell disease, hypoglycemia, electrolyte imbalance, subdural hematoma, tuberculoma, and unspecified infectious diseases (34%). Impaired consciousness was nearly always present, and seizures were evident in 77% of cases. The seizures were either partial or generalized and the partial seizures were always contralateral to the PLEDs. There are case reports of PLED patterns persisting for years.

Approximately 1% of all ischemic hemispheric non-lacunar infarctions are accompanied by PLEDs.

Therefore, any patient presenting with a hemispheric stroke and either fluctuating symptoms or spontaneous movements (e.g., finger or limb myoclonus, intermittent tonic posturing) should undergo EEG testing. More recently, PLEDs have been reported in mitochondrial encephalopathies (MERRF, MELAS) and in Jakob–Creutzfeldt disease (spongioform encephalopathies).

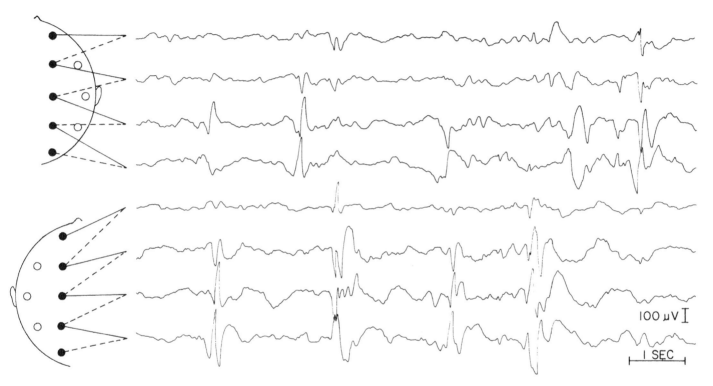

Fig. 19.8. Multifocal independent spikes. This EEG is of the same patient as in Figs. 19.1 and 19.2, now at an age of 13 months.

The individual epileptiform complexes of the PLED pattern are usually not associated with any convulsive activity, but in some cases they occur in synchrony with myoclonic jerks of the opposite side of the body. Focal or generalized electro-

TABLE 19.2

Periodic and pseudoperiodic complexes

Pattern name	Wave shape	Wave duration (s)	Interval activity	Interval duration (s)	Distribution	Clinical seizure manifestations	Common underlying disorders	Special features
1. Periodic lateralizing epileptiform discharges ('PLEDs')		0.06–0.5	Low amplitude delta, or no activity at regular gain	1–2	Unilateral or bilateral and asymmetric	Epilepsia partialis continua	Recent infarction, epilepsy, encephalitis, tumor, other cortical lesions	Rarely reactive to stimuli or changes in state; usually persist into sleep
2. Periodic generalized sharp waves, often associated with Jakob–Creutzfeldt disease	Mono-, di- or triphasic sharp waves	0.15–0.6	Low amplitude slow	0.5–2	Generalized, bisynchronous	Myoclonic jerks	Jakob–Creutzfeldt disease, postanoxic encephalopathy, fat embolism	Triggered by loud noise, flashes
3. Periodic generalized complexes, often associated with SSPE	One or more polyphasic sharp waves, with delta waves	0.5–3	Asynch. and bisynch. and delta; focal spikes and slow waves	3–20	Generalized, symmetrical, synchronous	Myoclonic jerks	SSPE, postanoxic myoclonus, Lennox–Gastaut syndrome, tuborous sclerosis, ketamine	Usually not triggered by stimuli; sleep may enhance or obscure the pattern
4. Suppression-burst	Irregular or regular slow waves, with or without sharp waves	1–3	Low amplitude delta, or no activity at regular gain	2 s–many min	Bilateral, unilateral, regional	None	Anesthesia, CNS depressant drugs, hypothermia, postanoxic encephalopathy, isolated cortex	Unreactive to stimuli
5. Triphasic waves	Major positive sharp wave, preceded and followed by minor negative waves	0.2–0.5	Asynchronous and bisynchronous slow waves	0.5–2	Generalized, maximal frontal or occipital	None	Hepatic, uremic and other metabolic encephalopathies, postanoxic encephalopathy	Incidence increases with age; rare under 20 years of age; may have longitudinal delay

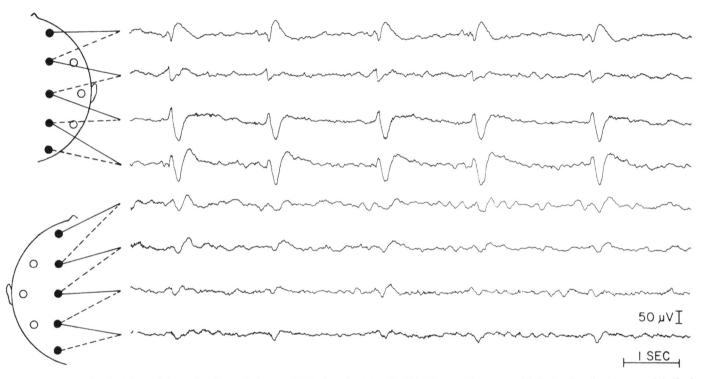

Fig. 19.9. Pattern of periodic lateralizing epileptiform discharges (PLEDs) on the right side. This 70-year-old woman suddenly developed weakness and rhythmical twitching of the left arm on the day of the recording; her condition was later diagnosed as a cerebral infarct.

50 μV

1 SEC

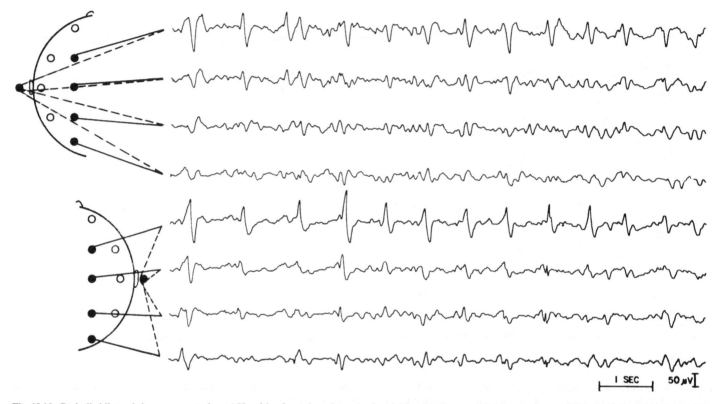

Fig. 19.10. Periodic bilateral sharp waves at about 1 Hz with a frontal maximum and variable posterior extension in a patient with Jakob–Creutzfeldt disease. This 83-year-old woman began to become confused 5 months earlier and then gradually developed dressing apraxia and illusions of a spatial distortion of objects in her left visual field. Startle myoclonus and spontaneous generalized myoclonus began soon after this EEG recording. She died 3 weeks later and her autopsy confirmed the clinical diagnosis of Jakob–Creutzfeldt disease.

graphic seizure patterns may appear to arise directly from PLEDs or they may occur simultaneously without interrupting the PLED pattern.

Although PLEDs are often considered to be continuous and invariant they may transiently attenuate or disappear during state changes, particularly during periods of arousal. The natural history of PLEDs consists of a gradual simplification of the morphology of complexes with increasingly longer repetition intervals and decreasing amplitude. This may occur over a period of days or weeks. Rarely, PLEDs may persist for years.

PLEDs may also occur independently over both hemispheres, a pattern referred to as bilateral independent periodic lateralized epileptiform discharges (BIPLEDs). BIPLEDs appear as approximately 0.5–1.5 Hz single or multiple wave complexes that vary in morphology from apiculate to blunted. Their amplitude in bipolar montages is usually between 40 and 150 μV. Thus, their appearance is similar to that of PLEDs except they appear over both hemispheres with a difference in timing that varies in a given recording between being approximately 0 ms to up to 500 ms. In patients exhibiting BIPLEDs, diffuse or bilateral multifocal cerebral diseases, rather than those with single focal lesions, are the rule. Thus, BIPLEDs are most often seen with infections (particularly herpes simplex encephalitis and other encephalitides), anoxic encephalopathy, epilepsy, and sickle cell anemia. As with PLEDs, myoclonus may sometimes accompany BIPLEDs either synchronously or independently. Although BI-

PLEDs are usually associated with a guarded prognosis, the author recently encountered a patient in coma with a BIPLED pattern with advanced AIDS (Fischer et al., 1997) who left the hospital several days later after treatment with anticonvulsants without apparent sequelae. The patient did not have a prior history of seizures and the etiology remained unknown.

19.3.2 *Periodic generalized sharp waves, often associated with Jakob–Creutzfeldt disease. The EEG pattern* is dominated by sharp waves which usually have one, two or three phases and last up to 0.6 s (Fig. 19.10). When fully developed, the sharp waves appear synchronously in a wide distribution over both hemispheres, sometimes with a frontal maximum; while they develop, they may be focal or unilateral. The background is usually highly abnormal and consists of generalized asynchronous slow waves of low amplitude. Sharp waves may be triggered by startling stimuli and by light flashes.

Clinical conditions causing these sharp waves include mainly Jakob–Creutzfeldt disease. The sharp waves appear usually within 12 weeks of the onset of clinical symptoms and are present during the fully developed disease in over 90% of all patients; they persist through the course of the disease and at the end become slower and disappear in a background of low amplitude. Similar sharp waves are occasionally seen in postanoxic encephalopathy and in cerebral fat embolism.

Seizure manifestations consist of widespread myoclonic jerks associated with the complexes. Startling and flash stimuli which produce sharp waves often also induce myoclonic jerks.

In the early stages of spongioform encephalopathy, even before mental symptoms predominate, the EEG may contain focal repetitive spikes or sharp waves, particularly over the parieto-occipital head regions. In such cases focal contralateral motor seizures are common. Indeed, in the early stages of the disease focal or lateralized epileptiform activity (including PLEDs) is more common than the generalized periodic pattern.

A recently described variant, so-called 'mad cow disease' in the United Kingdom, is not associated with prominent epileptiform or pseudoperiodic patterns.

19.3.3 *Periodic generalized complexes, often associated with subacute sclerosing panencephalitis (SSPE). The EEG pattern consists of high voltage (300–1500 µV) complexes containing one or more sharp waves and delta waves. Complexes last 0.5–3 s and recur every 3–20 s. The background consists of asynchronous and bisynchronous theta and delta waves; bisynchronous slow-spike-and-wave discharges, focal spikes and slow waves may also be present. Early in the course of the disease, the background may be fairly normal and the complexes may appear in a limited distribution. Later, however, the complexes usually become generalized, symmetrical and synchronous. Their shape may change with time and become disorganized before death. The complexes are usually not triggered by sensory stimuli. Sleep may enhance or obscure them.*

Seizure manifestations consist of myoclonic jerks occurring with the complexes. Tonic seizures may occur with electrodecremental ictal patterns (19.2).

Clinical conditions causing these complexes include mainly subacute sclerosing panencephalitis (SSPE). The complexes may appear at any stage of the disease. Similar complexes may be seen in postanoxic encephalopathy, after head injury, in drug intoxications, lipidoses, herpes simplex encephalitis, and tuberous sclerosis.

19.3.4 *Suppression-burst pattern* is seen only in comatose patients with reversible conditions (most commonly general anesthesia) or with irreversible conditions (most commonly cardiopulmonary arrest). The EEG pattern consists of bursts of irregular or rhythmic slow waves that may contain intermixed faster components. They are usually widespread and bisynchronous, but they may be limited to one hemisphere or part of it. Bursts last 1–3 s and are separated from each other by low amplitude delta waves or by periods of no activity recognizable at regular gain (Fig. 19.11). Successive bursts may vary in shape. The duration of the intervals between the bursts is often fairly regular in a given recording and ranges from 2 to 10 s depending on the severity of the cerebral dysfunction. The duration increases as the patient's condition worsens. Before death or with deepening anesthesia, bursts become shorter, simpler and of lower amplitude; periods of suppression become longer until complete electrocerebral silence supervenes. The complexes are not responsive to stimuli. When the

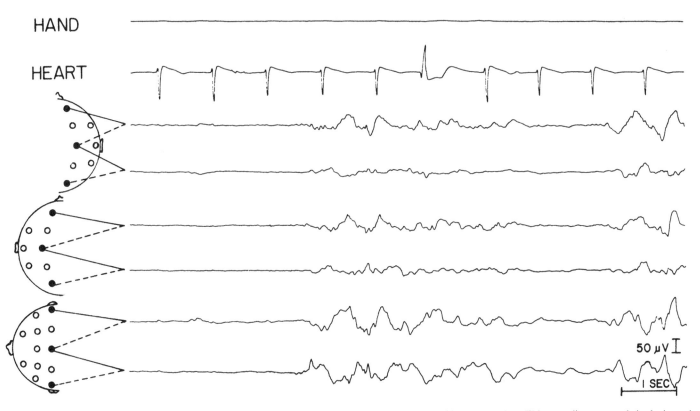

Fig. 19.11. Burst-suppression pattern recorded from a 60-year-old man in deep coma from a lethal barbiturate overdose. This recording was made in the intensive care unit with widely spaced electrodes and with monitoring of hand movement and heart beat.

bursts are longer in duration than the periods of suppression then the pattern is commonly referred to as a *burst-suppression* pattern rather than a suppression-burst pattern.

The underlying physiological changes that accompany the suppression-burst pattern during general anesthesia in animals consist of cortical neuronal inactivity during suppression, cortical depolarization during the burst, and cortical hyperpolarization just prior to the onset of suppression. Thalamic neurons (including those of the nucleus reticularis) during deep anesthesia are silent during suppression and depolarize during the burst. In light anesthesia with the suppression-burst pattern thalamic neuronal rhythmic firing at 1–4 Hz persists. These observations suggest that suppression-burst in general anesthesia involves thalamocortical interactions that have been modified by GABAergic inhibition. The pathophysiology of suppression-burst activity caused by other encephalopathic disorders (such as head trauma or anoxia) remains less clear. Surgical cortical isolation may produce a localized burst-suppression pattern, suggesting that the burst-suppression pattern is not necessarily dependent on thalamocortical interactions.

Seizure manifestations associated with this pattern are limited to myoclonus. However, a variety of behaviors have been associated with the bursts of activity, including chewing and tonic posturing.

Clinical conditions causing suppression-burst patterns include a variety of severe disorders of cerebral structure or function. Structural lesions include acute strokes, postanoxic encephalopathy, head injury, Wernicke's disease and encephalitis. Local burst-suppression patterns can be seen over abnormal cortical areas during surgical anesthesia. Commonly reversible disorders causing this pattern include deep anesthesia and coma due to barbiturates and other CNS depressant drugs, hypothermia and Reye's syndrome. The association of myoclonus, burst-suppression patterns and postanoxic coma suggests a very poor prognosis for survival.

19.3.5 *Triphasic wave pattern.* Triphasic waves are not associated with seizures but are included here because they frequently appear in an approximately periodic or pseudoperiodic pattern and are sometimes mistaken for epileptiform abnormalities. They consist of waveforms with 3 phases, each succeeding phase with longer duration than the one before, that clearly stand out from the background and other slow waves. The total duration of each triphasic wave complex varies between approximately 0.25 and 0.5 s. The second phase is positive in polarity and usually has the greatest amplitude of the 3 phases (Fig. 19.12). Occasionally a relatively low amplitude positive phase can be seen consistently proceeding the subsequent 3 phases. Triphasic waves may appear sporadically or periodically at 0.5–1 s intervals.

Although the amplitude distribution of triphasic waves varies in individual cases between either anterior or posterior dominance (with some individuals showing both simultaneously or at different times in the same record), in most cases triphasic waves are maximal over the anterior head regions.

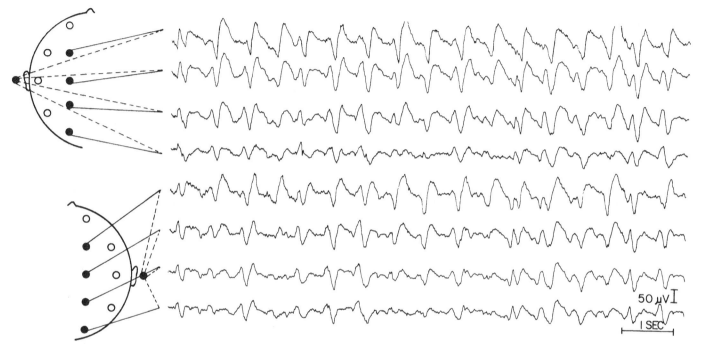

Fig. 19.12. Pattern of triphasic waves at 1–2 Hz with frontal maximum, recorded from a 68-year-old chronic alcoholic in hepatic coma.

In instances in which maximal amplitudes occur at Fp1 and Fp2, triphasic waves may closely resemble vertical eye movement artifact. In longitudinal bipolar recordings triphasic wave phase reversals may occur over the anterior or posterior head regions. In contrast, waves with 3 phases that have prominent phase reversals over the mid-temporal or central head regions suggest an electrographic disturbance other than the triphasic wave pattern.

In many cases there is an apparent phase lag (time delay) of the second phase when comparing the anterior and posterior derivations of longitudinal bipolar montages. This delay can occur in either the anterior to posterior or posterior to anterior direction and may last more than 100 ms. The majority of such phase lags are more apparent than real since they are far less common if reference montages (such as ipsilateral or linked ears) are used.

The pathophysiology of triphasic waves is poorly understood. As with other bisynchronous patterns, thalamic pacing probably plays an important role. Unilateral lesions that attenuate thalamically generated rhythms such as sleep spindles may also attenuate triphasic waves. It appears that triphasic wave generation is enhanced by biochemical and ultrastructural changes associated with aging: well developed triphasic wave patterns rarely occur in individuals less than 20 years of age, are infrequent before age 30, and increase in incidence thereafter.

Clinical conditions associated with the triphasic wave pattern are mainly metabolic/toxic disturbances with the most common being hepatic failure, renal failure and anoxia. Sporadic triphasic waves are also not uncommon in elderly individuals with clinically advanced dementing disorders. The triphasic wave pattern has also been associated with other disorders including: hypo- or hypernatremia, hypercalcemia, hypoglycemia, stroke, hypertensive encephalopathy, cerebral abscess, encephalitis, congestive heart failure, septic shock, lithium intoxication and postictal state. In the past a distinction was made between 'typical' and 'atypical' triphasic wave patterns because it was thought that 'typical' triphasic waves were highly characteristic of hepatic encephalopathy. This distinction is no longer considered valid. Indeed, the only feature that may be helpful in narrowing the list of diagnostic possibilities has been described by Fisch and Klass (1988) as severe background slowing characterized by mainly smoothly contoured background waveforms with little or no superimposed activity greater than 5 Hz. This combination of findings is almost always seen in the setting of either hepatic, renal or anoxic encephalopathy. Similarly, the prognosis for patients with triphasic waves is mainly dependent on the degree of background slowing, suppression or reduced reactivity, not the presence or absence of triphasic waves.

19.3.6 *The lateralized triphasic wave pattern*, described in a series of patients by Fisch and Klass (1988), is characterized by unilateral triphasic waves or triphasic waves with a consistent asymmetry greater than 50%. In anecdotal reports and in a series of 12 patients (Fisch et al., 1991) asymmetric triphasic waves have not been specifically associated with seizures and are therefore not considered an interictal epileptiform pattern. In contrast, focal triphasic waves (limited to 1–2 electrodes) are more likely to represent abnormal interictal epileptiform activity. Lateralized triphasic waves (as defined above) are almost always associated with an underlying structural abnormality. However, the involved hemisphere cannot be predicted from a relative increase or decrease in amplitude of the triphasic waves. Instead, underlying structural lesions are more accurately lateralized by background activity abnormalities and intermixed slower waveforms.

In contrast to the symmetric triphasic wave pattern, the lateralized triphasic wave pattern does not increase the likelihood of a coexistent metabolic/toxic disorder. As with symmetric triphasic waves, the prognostic implications depend more on background changes and impaired reactivity than on the presence or absence of triphasic waves. The lateralized triphasic wave pattern, like the symmetric pattern, is more likely to appear in older individuals.

19.4 ICTAL PATTERNS WITHOUT SPIKES AND SHARP WAVES

The patterns in this section (Table 19.3) are described in the chapters dealing with local and generalized epileptiform activity. They are joined here because they are related to each other in that they represent ictal activity which (1) has no spikes or sharp waves, (2) usually begins and ends abruptly, and (3) is often recognized only by its association with clinical seizure manifestations. Some of these patterns are local, others are generalized; some occur mainly with one type of interictal pattern or seizure, others occur with a variety of interictal patterns and seizure types.

19.4.1 *Generalized ictal slow waves. Rhythmical bisynchronous slow waves at 3 Hz* are occasionally seen instead of 3 Hz spike-and-wave discharges in absence attacks, especially in absence status. Similar slow waves may occur as interictal activity in patients with attacks of absences or of other primary generalized seizures.

Theta or delta waves, often irregular, asynchronous and arrhythmical, may be associated with tonic seizures which occur especially in patients with slow-spike-and-wave discharges.

Rhythmical 4–6 Hz waves or, occasionally, 2–10 Hz waves with a maximum in both temporal or frontotemporal regions are a common ictal pattern of complex partial seizures even though the seizures begin in one temporal lobe and the patient's interictal epileptiform spike activity may be restricted to one temporal lobe.

Various forms of periodic complexes may be associated with myoclonic jerks, for instance in subacute sclerosing panencephalitis. PLED patterns, particularly as they are beginning to disappear, often do not contain sharp waves or spikes but may still be associated with myoclonus.

19.4.2 *Local ictal slow waves. Rhythmical 4–6 Hz waves,* or 2–10 Hz waves, with a maximum in the temporal or frontotemporal regions of one hemisphere occur frequently in complex partial seizures.

Periodic or rhythmical slow waves are seen instead of PLEDs in some patients with epilepsia partialis continua.

TABLE 19.3
Ictal patterns without spikes and sharp waves

Ictal pattern	Distribution	Interictal patterns	Clinical seizure type
1. Three Hz rhythmical slow waves	Generalized	3 Hz spike-and-wave, 3 Hz slow waves, or normal	Absence, absence status, generalized seizures
2. Theta or delta waves	Generalized	Slow spike-and-wave	Tonic seizures
3. Rhythmical 4–6 (2–10) Hz waves	Bilateral or unilateral, temporal or frontotemporal	Spikes or sharp waves in the temporal area	Complex partial seizures
4. Delta or theta waves in periodic complexes	Generalized	Complexes of SSPE	Myoclonic jerks
5. Periodic or rhythmical slow waves	Localized	None	Epilepsia partialis continua
6. Loss of amplitude ('electro-decremental seizures')	Generalized	Hypsarrhythmia, slow-spike-and-wave	Infantile spasms, tonic seizures
7. Paroxysmal low voltage	Temporal, frontotemporal, bilateral or unilateral	Spikes or sharp waves in the temporal area	Complex partial seizures
8. No change of background	–	Spikes or sharp waves in the temporal area	Complex partial seizures
9. No change of background	–	None	Epilepsia partialis continua
10. Alpha waves	Focal, unilateral	Spikes, sharp waves, abnormal newborn patterns	Neonatal seizures
11. Beta waves	Focal, unilateral	Spikes, sharp waves, abnormal newborn patterns	Neonatal seizures
12. Beta waves	Central	Spikes, polyspikes or normal	Action myoclonus
13. Beta waves (14–20 Hz)	Bilateral or unilateral, maximum temporal or frontotemporal	Spikes or sharp waves in the temporal area	Complex partial seizures

19.4.3 *Generalized decrease of amplitude.* The *electrodecremental pattern* appears as a sudden reduction of high amplitude background activity in hypsarrhythmia and in recordings showing slow-spike-and-wave activity. Electrodecremental activity is usually heralded by the sudden appearance of widespread, high amplitude, spike or slow wave followed by flattening of the record or low amplitude fast activity lasting several seconds. The electrodecremental pattern is seen during infantile spasms or tonic seizures. Electrodecremental events also occur in some adults during tonic seizures.

The sudden appearance of low voltage activity is also seen in the early stages of some complex partial seizures.

Sudden loss of amplitude or low voltage fast activity also occurs in non-epileptic attacks of decerebration, often called 'cerebellar fits' seen in the terminal stages of metabolic or toxic coma.

19.4.4 *No change of background activity* is occasionally seen in simple partial seizures and in epilepsia partialis continua.

19.4.5 *Alpha waves,* usually unilateral or focal in distribution, can be seen in newborn and very young infants with partial, unilateral and generalized seizures or status epilepticus; unilateral or bilateral waves of alpha frequency are also the ictal pattern of some patients with complex partial seizures.

19.4.6 *Beta waves* may appear instead of lower frequency activity in some newborn infants. Fast waves of 14–20 Hz may appear with a maximum in the temporal or frontotemporal regions in complex partial seizures at any age after infancy. Central rhythmic beta activity, with or without spikes, may be associated with movement-activated myoclonus in adults, usually as a result of cerebral anoxia.

19.5 EPILEPTIFORM PATTERNS WITHOUT PROVEN RELATION TO SEIZURES ('PSEUDOEPILEPTIFORM PATTERNS')

These patterns (Table 19.4) are similar to each other in that they (1) consist of epileptiform activity of usually short duration, (2) have no corresponding ictal patterns, and (3) are not known to be associated with seizures or neurological diseases. Prior to the advent of controlled studies many of these benign patterns were considered indicative of neurological or psychiatric disorders. Their main importance now is that they can be easily misinterpreted with important consequences for the patient. Clinical electroencephalographers need to memorize each of these patterns and their variants and consider them when confronted by possible epileptiform abnormalities.

19.5.1 *Six-per-second spike-and-wave discharges* ('phantom spike-wave') consist of a 4–7 Hz repetitive spike-and-wave complex with a relatively low amplitude (less than 40 μV), fast spike (less than 30 ms) followed by a 5–7 Hz wave of equal or greater amplitude. Each burst usually appears in a bisynchronous fashion, lasts less than 1 s and occurs during drowsiness or during eye closure at rest. This pattern is most often seen in young adults.

Two different forms of the 6/s spike-and-wave discharge have been described. The classical form is relatively low in amplitude and is maximal over the posterior head regions (Fig. 19.13). Its incidence in normal individuals is increased

TABLE 19.4

Pseudoepileptiform patterns

Pattern name	Wave shape	Duration	Distribution	Age	Vigilance
1. Six Hz spike-and-slow-wave ('wave and spike phantom')	Miniature spike-and-wave at 4–7 Hz	Less than 1 s	Generalized, maximum often posterior	Adults, less often adolescents	Drowsy, awake
2. Fourteen and 6 Hz positive bursts	Repetitive positive spikes arch-shaped	Less than 1–2 s	Posterior temporal, parietal, bilaterally independent or synchronous	Adolescents, children; less often adults	Sleep, drowsiness
3. Rhythmical mid-temporal discharge ('RMTD') ('psychomotor variant')	6 (4–7) Hz negative sharp waves with notched or flat positive phases	Up to a few seconds	Midtemporal, unilateral, bilateral, independent or bisynchronous	Slightly more in middle-aged females	Sleep
4. Small sharp spikes ('SSS'),benign epileptiform transients of sleep ('BETS')	Short spikes, usually small	Less than 50 ms for single phase	Mid- and anterior temporal, often shifting in distribution; unilateral, bilaterally independent or bisynchronous	Adults, adolescents	Sleep
5. Wicket spikes	Often repetitive spikes forming arches	Repeating up to a few seconds	Anterior and middle temporal	Mainly adults	Awake, asleep
6. Occipital spikes and sharp waves of blind persons	Focal spikes and sharp waves	Up to 200 ms	Occipital, unilateral or bilateral	Often children	Awake, asleep
7. SREDA	Mono- or biphasic sharp wave(s) followed by rhythmic 4–7 Hz waves	Less than 10 s to more than 5 min; usually 40–80 s	Often symmetrical and posterior temporal and parietal maximal but may be unilateral or asymmetric	Adults	Awake, asleep
8. Paroxysmal hypnogogic hypersynchrony	3–5 Hz moderate to high amplitude rhythmic bursts with intermixed spikes	1–6 s	Generalized, maximum anterior or posterior	Children	Drowsy
9. Midline theta rhythms (of Cigánek)	4–7 Hz rhythmic trains with sinusoidal, spiky or arciform shape	Typically 4–20 s	Midline, usually central	Children and adults	Awake, drowsy

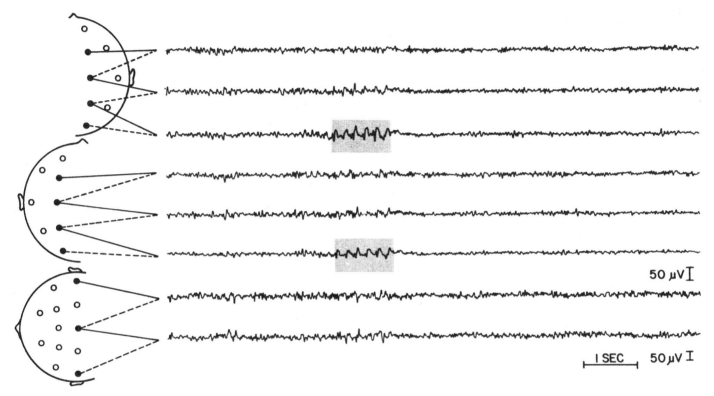

Fig. 19.13. Pattern of 6 Hz spike-and-slow-waves. A brief burst (shaded) appears in the posterior head regions during drowsiness. This 40-year-old woman has a history of headaches, no abnormal findings.

significantly by intravenous diphenhydramine and it is clearly not associated with seizures.

The second form is frontally dominant, often moderate or high in amplitude, but the spikes appear with lower amplitude than intervening waves. This form of 6/s spike-and-wave discharge overlaps with abnormal generalized atypical spike-and-wave patterns with rapid repetition rates. Four to 6 Hz anterior dominant rhythmic spike and slow wave patterns are often seen in patients with juvenile myoclonic epilepsy. The likelihood that frontally dominant rapid spike-and-wave discharges are associated with seizures increases if the repetition rate is less than 5 Hz or the spikes are clearly much greater in amplitude than the intervening slow waves. The interpretation of anterior dominant spike-and-wave patterns with rapid repetition rates therefore requires careful consideration.

19.5.2 *Fourteen and 6 Hz positive bursts* (also referred to as 'ctenoids' or 14 and 6 Hz positive spikes) consist of brief runs (usually less than 1 s) of positive spikes repeating at approximately 14 or 6 Hz. The amplitude is somewhat variable but rarely exceeds 75 μV using an ipsilateral ear reference montage. This pattern occurs either bisynchronously or unilaterally (usually involving both hemispheres at different times). It may be difficult to recognize in bipolar montages and is best seen in ear reference montages or those with long interelectrode distances. The 14 Hz component is more commonly seen than the 6 Hz component, but both may occur simultaneously (Fig. 19.14). The 14 Hz pattern often looks like a sleep spindle with a sharp positive phase, although its location is quite different; it is greatest in amplitude over the posterior temporal head regions. The sharp components often have a negative polarity in nasopharyngeal recordings.

Fourteen and 6/s positive spikes are most likely to occur during sleep in adolescents. Their peak incidence (which some investigators have found to be as high as 25% in normal subjects) occurs between ages 12 and 13. An unexplained finding is 14 and 6/s positive spikes in comatose patients with acute Reye's syndrome and in other disorders associated with hepatic failure. Less often it appears in comatose patients with other metabolic and postanoxic encephalopathies and occasionally in head trauma. In such cases the pattern may differ from that seen in normal individuals in that the frequency is often more variable, relatively low in amplitude and the bursts can be elicited by alerting stimuli.

19.5.3 *Rhythmical midtemporal discharges* (formerly also called 'psychomotor variant') are bursts of rhythmical sharp waves at about 6 Hz (range of 4–7 Hz) which often have a top which is flat or notched by a small 10–12 Hz component (Fig. 19.15). These bursts may last for up to a few seconds. They often begin and end with a gradual increase and decrease of amplitude but, unlike abnormal electrographic seizure activity, their overall frequency remains very stable throughout their appearance (they do not show much evidence of acceleration or deceleration). They occur in the midtemporal regions, either on one side or on both, either independently or simultaneously. Less often they spread to involve most head regions. They are mostly seen in young adults during light sleep. These bursts are distinguished from ictal discharges in patients with interictal temporal lobe spikes in that they do

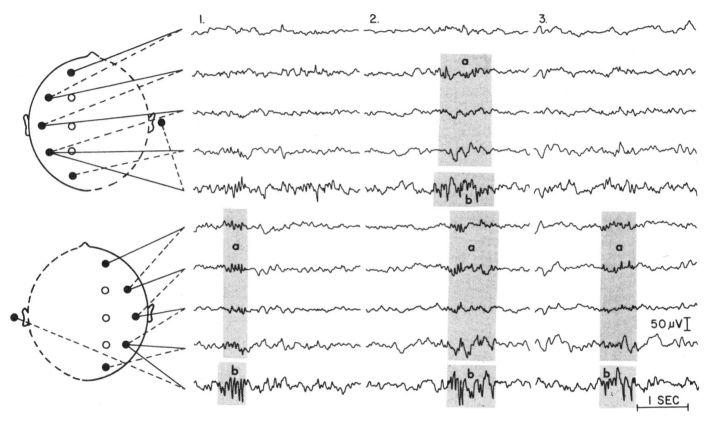

Fig. 19.14. Pattern of 14 and 6 Hz positive bursts. 1, 2 and 3 were recorded within a few minutes of each other during light sleep. Note that the bursts are barely distinguishable in conventional bipolar linkages between adjacent electrodes (a), but are greatly enhanced by the use of long interelectrode distances between posterior temporal electrodes and the opposite ear (b). This 12-year-old girl had a slight concussion 4 days earlier; the neurological examination is normal.

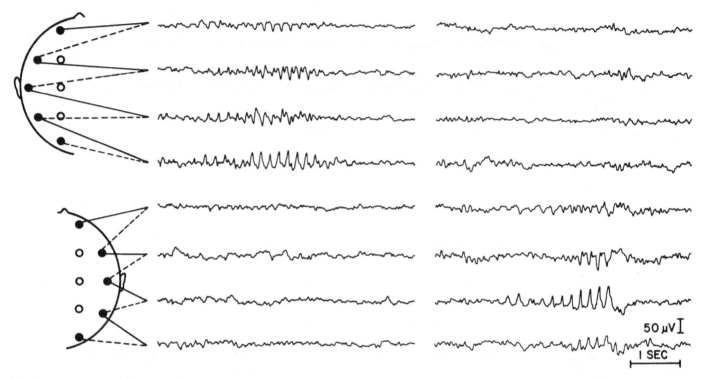

Fig. 19.15. Rhythmical midtemporal discharges (RMTD) at about 6 Hz, occurring independently on either side during light sleep. The patient is a 19-year-old girl with one seizure 5 years earlier, now normal.

not vary much in duration and wave shape and thus resemble neither interictal single spikes nor the ictal, sustained and changing discharges of temporal lobe foci.

19.5.4 *Small sharp spikes.* Small sharp spikes, also referred to as *benign epileptiform transients of sleep* ('BETS') or benign sporadic sleep spikes (BSSS), are sharply contoured mono- or

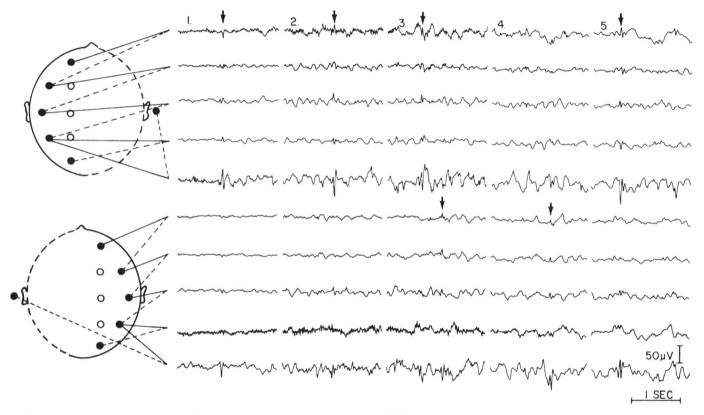

Fig. 19.16. Pattern of small sharp spikes (SSS) or benign epileptiform transients of sleep (BETS) occurring independently in the temporal regions during light sleep. 1–5 were recorded within 5 min. Note that the amplitude of the spikes (arrows) is greatly increased in interelectrode linkages from the posterior temporal electrodes to the opposite ears. This 15-year-old girl complains of dizziness which is probably due to hyperventilation.

biphasic (rarely tri- or quadriphasic) low amplitude, very brief duration (less than 65 ms) waveforms (Fig. 19.16) sometimes immediately followed by a waveform in the theta or alpha frequency range creating the appearance of a small spike and slow wave complex. Identifying features of small sharp spikes include their typically widespread horizontal dipole distribution that occurs in the absence of any apparent disruption of the ongoing background activity. Although they are often greatest in amplitude over the temporal head regions (as shown in depth electrode recordings), they are characteristically difficult to localize precisely and often appear in both hemispheres either independently or bisynchronously. They frequently demonstrate an opposite polarity in the anterior to posterior direction in a single hemisphere or, when they occur bisynchronously, transversely between hemispheres (i.e., a horizontal dipole configuration; true phase reversals). Another distinguishing feature of small sharp spikes is that they rarely repeat with the same distribution and morphology more than once per 0.5 s. Although the name 'small' suggests they are very low in amplitude, this may not be the case, particularly in montages with long interelectrode distances or in nasopharyngeal electrode recordings.

19.5.5 *Wicket spikes* occur in the anterior or middle temporal areas with a negative polarity and an amplitude of up to more than 200 μV. They differ from other, abnormal, spikes in that they appear not only intermittently but also repetitively in trains of arch-shaped rhythms resembling mu rhythm.

Wicket spikes result from an apparent sudden accentuation in amplitude of the ongoing background activity. When they occur and are immediately surrounded by similar frequency lower amplitude sharply contoured waveforms they are relatively easy to identify. Difficulty sometimes arises when they appear in isolation during drowsiness or sleep on an otherwise relatively low amplitude featureless background. In such cases they can be identified by comparison with other similarly shaped waveforms that make up part of the normal background.

Wicket spikes are most likely to occur in individuals whose background activity contains sharply contoured waveforms. Although wicket spikes were originally described as temporal in location and mainly occurring in older individuals, it is important to be aware that similar isolated sharply contoured waveforms may occur over *any* head region where there is sharply contoured background activity.

19.5.6 *Occipital spikes of blind persons* may occur after lesions of the visual path anterior to the occipital cortex early in life. Epileptiform spikes arising from the occipital lobes in such individuals are not likely to be associated with clinical seizures. Associated abnormalities that may be seen are disorganization of alpha rhythm, loss of photic responses and absence of lambda waves and POSTs. Occipital spikes that occur in older individuals with cerebral blindness due to bilateral occipital lesions that were acquired later in life (usually from stroke or trauma) are much more likely to be associated with seizures.

19.5.7 *Paroxysmal hypnogogic hypersynchrony* is a variant of hypnogogic hypersynchrony and therefore occurs in normal children during drowsiness or arousal from sleep. It consists of low amplitude spikes intermixed with rhythmical moderate to high amplitude 3–5 Hz bisynchronous bursts. The spike-like components most often take the form of a simple notch-

ing of the slow waves (Fig. 19.17). In other cases they are irregularly intermixed with the slow waves or may form brief runs with the appearance of multiple spike complexes (Fig. 19.18). A distinguishing feature of the irregularly intermixed spike components is their superimposed appearance; there is an in-

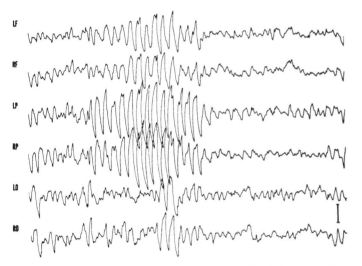

Fig. 19.17. Paroxysmal hypnogogic hypersynchrony. Notched pattern. Courtesy P. Kellaway, Current Practice of Clinical Electroencephalography, 1979.

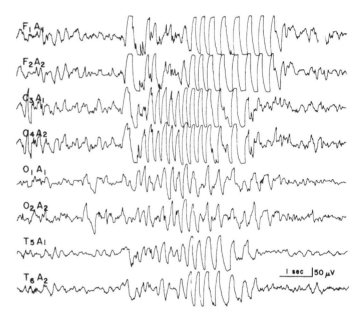

Fig. 19.18. Paroxysmal hypnogogic hypersynchrony. Irregular intermixed spike patterns. Courtesy P. Kellaway, Current Practice of Clinical Electroencephalography, 1979.

consistent time relationship between the spikes and the slow waves.

19.5.8 Subclinical rhythmic EEG discharge of adults (SREDA).

Like rhythmical midtemporal discharges (RMTD), SREDA is likely to be misinterpreted as an ictal epileptiform pattern. Unlike RMTD, SREDA occurs mainly in elderly individuals during wakefulness (in nearly all cases), during or shortly after hyperventilation (in some individuals only during hyperventilation), and occasionally during sleep. It also differs from RMTD in its topographic distribution and because it usually does not contain prominent harmonically related waveforms. Since SREDA invariably occurs while the patient is awake, response testing can be performed to demonstrate that, in contrast to most widespread epileptic events, consciousness and mentation are preserved. Other distinctive characteristics of this pattern are: (1) its tendency to occur several times in a single routine recording (over 15 times in some reported cases); (2) its tendency to be present in subsequent EEGs, even when more than 12 years have elapsed between recordings; (3) its relative lack of evolution in frequency, morphology or distribution compared to most abnormal seizure patterns; and (4) the absence of "postictal" EEG changes.

SREDA typically begins abruptly (Fig. 19.19) or is delayed 1 to several seconds after a single high amplitude mono- or biphasic sharp or slow wave component (Fig. 19.20). Once established, the pattern may consist of repetitive monophasic

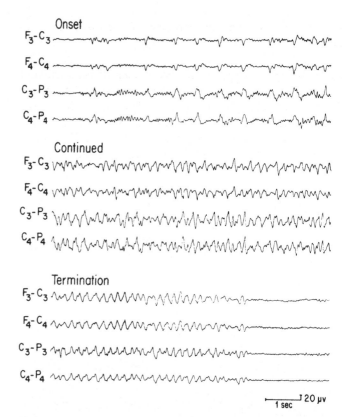

Fig. 19.19. Subclinical rhythmic EEG discharge of adults (SREDA) in a 60-year-old woman during wakefulness with abrupt onset and gradual evolution to 5 Hz rhythmic activity. Courtesy, B.F. Westmoreland, Electroenceph. Clin. Neurophysiol. 1981, 51: 186–191.

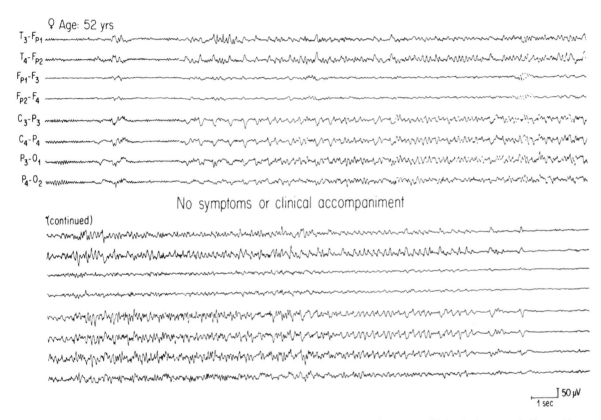

Fig. 19.20. Subclinical rhythmic EEG discharge of adults (SREDA) in a 52-year-old woman with headaches preceded by a widespread, moderate to high amplitude, biphasic waveform. Courtesy, B.F. Westmoreland, Electroenceph. Clin. Neurophysiol. 1981, 51: 186–191.

sharp waveforms (approximately 150–300 ms in duration) that repeat every 1–2 s and gradually evolve into a sustained sinusoidal 4–7 Hz pattern (usually 5–6 Hz). The pattern may either end abruptly or gradually diminish and merge with the background.

In approximately two-thirds of cases the discharges are bisynchronous and symmetrically distributed and are maximal over the parietal and posterior temporal regions. In other cases it is either asymmetric or unilateral. The average duration of the discharge is typically 40–80 s, but it may be less than 10 s or more than 5 min. In most cases it replaces the ongoing background activity. In other cases the background may persist. For example, during wakefulness reactivity of the alpha rhythm may be discernible and during sleep vertex waves and sleep spindles may be seen.

Although SREDA usually occurs in the elderly there are reports of the pattern occurring in individuals in the fourth decade of life. SREDA has not been specifically associated with any clinical diagnosis and patients followed up to 35 years have not developed seizure disorders. SPECT scanning performed in one patient with focal SREDA did not show any evidence of the blood flow changes typical for focal seizures.

REFERENCES

Aicardi, J. (1986) Epilepsy in Children. Raven Press, New York.
Aicardi, J. and Gomes, A.L. (1989) The myoclonic epilepsies of childhood.
Cleve. Clin. J. Med. 56 (Suppl. 1): S34–S39.
Aminoff, MA. (1998) Do nonconvulsive seizures damage the brain? – No. Controversies in neurology. Arch. Neurol. 55: 119–120.
Blume, W.T. (1978) Clinical and electroencephalographic correlates of the multiple independent spike foci pattern in children. Ann. Neurol. 4: 541–547.
Blume, W.T. (1987) Lennox–Gastaut syndrome. In: H. Lüders and R.P. Lesser (Eds.), Epilepsy: Electroclinical Syndromes. Springer, New York, pp. 73–92.
Blume, W.T. and Kaibara, M. (1995) Atlas of Adult Electroencephalography. Raven Press, New York.
Catani, P., Salzarulo, P. and Findji, F. (1978) Occipital spikes and eye movement activity during paradoxical sleep in visually defective children. Electroenceph. Clin. Neurophysiol. 44: 782–784.
Celesia, G.G. (1973) Pathophysiology of periodic EEG complexes in subacute sclerosing panencephalitis (SSPE). Electroenceph. Clin. Neurophysiol. 35: 293–300.
Chabolla, D.R. and Cascino, G.D. (1996) Interpretation of extracranial EEG. In: E. Wyllie (Ed.), The Treatment of Epilepsy: Principles and Practice, 2nd Edition. Williams and Wilkins, Baltimore, pp. 264–279.
Charlton, M.H. (1975) Myoclonic Seizures. Excerpta Medica, Amsterdam.
Chatrian, G.E., Shaw, C.M. and Leffman, H. (1964) The significance of periodic lateralized epileptiform discharges in EEG: an electrographic, clinical and pathological study. Electroenceph. Clin. Neurophysiol. 17: 177–193.
Ch'ien, L.T., Boehm, R.M., Robinson, H., Liu, C. and Frenkel, L.D. (1977) Characteristic early electroencephalographic changes in herpes simplex encephalitis. Clinical and virologic studies. Arch. Neurol. 34: 361–364.
Chiofalo, N., Fuentes, A. and Galves, C. (1980) Serial EEG findings in 27 cases of Creutzfeldt–Jakob disease. Arch. Neurol. 37: 143–145.
Clancy, R.R. and Legido, A. (1987) The exact ictal and interictal duration of electroencephalographic neonatal seizures. Epilepsia 28: 537–541.
Clancy, R.R., Legido, A. and Lewis, D. (1988) Occult neonatal seizures. Epilepsia 29: 256–261.

Cobb, W.A. (1979) Evidence on the periodic mechanism in herpes simplex encephalitis. Electroenceph. Clin. Neurophysiol. 46: 345–350.

Daly, D.D. and Pedley, T.A. (1990) Current Practice of Clinical Neurophysiology: Electroencephalography. 2nd Edition. Raven Press, New York.

De la Paz, D. and Brenner, R.P. (1981) Bilateral independent periodic lateralized epileptiform discharges. Arch. Neurol. 38: 713–715.

Drury, I. (1989) Epileptiform patterns of children. J. Clin. Neurophysiol. 6: 1–39.

Drury, I., Klass, D.W., Westmoreland, B.F. and Sharbrough, F.W. (1985) An acute syndrome with psychiatric symptoms and EEG abnormalities. Arch. Neurol. 35: 911–914.

Eeg-Olofsson, O. (1971) The development of the electroencephalogram in normal children from the age of 1 through 15 years. 14 and 6 Hz positive spike phenomenon. Neuropaediatrie 2: 405–427.

Fisch, B.J. (1996) Generalized tonic-clonic seizures. In: E. Wyllie (Ed.), The Treatment of Epilepsy: Principles and Practice, 2nd Edition. Williams and Wilkins, Baltimore, pp. 502–521.

Fisch, B.J. and Klass, D.W. (1988) The diagnostic specificity of triphasic wave patterns. Electroenceph. Clin. Neurophysiol. 70: 1–8.

Fisch, B.J. and Pedley, T.A. (1985) Evaluation of focal cerebral lesions. Role of electroencephalography in the era of computerized tomography. In: M.J. Aminoff (Ed.), Electrodiagnosis. Neurologic Clinics. Saunders, Philadelphia, pp. 649–662.

Fisch, B.J., Rosenstein, R., Ramirez-Lassepas and Hauser, W.A. (1986) The electroencephalogram as a predictor of epilepsy following occlusive cerebrovascular insult. Epilepsia 27: 615.

Fisch, B.J., Perez, J., Lemos, M.S., Garofalo, M. and Brust, J.C.M. (1991) The asymmetric triphasic wave pattern. Annual Meeting of the American EEG Society, Philadelphia, PA.

Fischer, M., Mader, Jr., E. and Fisch, B.J. (1997) HIV encephalopathy, seizure, and BIPLEDs. J. Clin. Neurophysiol. 15: 276.

Gabor, A.J. and Seyal, M. (1986) Effect of sleep on the electroencephalographic manifestations of epilepsy. J. Clin. Neurophysiol. 3: 23–38.

Gibbs, F.A. and Gibbs, E.L. (1952) Atlas of Electroencephalography. Vol. 2. Epilepsy. Addison-Wesley, Cambridge, MA.

Goldensohn, E.S., Legatt, A.D., Koszer, S. and Wolf, S.M. (1999) Goldensohn's EEG Interpretation: Problems of Overreading and Underreading. Second Edition. Futura Publishing Company, Armonk, NY.

Gurvitch, A.M., Zarzhetsky, Y.V., Trush, V.D. and Zonov, V.M. (1984) Experimental data on the nature of post-resusitation alpha frequency activity. Electroenceph. Clin. Neurophysiol. 58: 426–437.

Handforth, A., Cheng, J.T., Mandelkern, M.A. and Treiman, D.A. (1994) Markedly increased mesiotemporal lobe metabolism in a case with PLEDs: further evidence that PLEDs are a manifestation of partial status epilepticus. Epilepsia 35: 876–881.

Harrison, A., Lairy, G.C. and Leger, E.M. (1970) EEG et privation visuelle. Electroenceph. Clin. Neurophysiol. 29: 20–37.

Hrachovy, R.A. and Frost, Jr., J.D. (1989) Infantile spasms. Cleve. Clin. J. Med. 56 (Suppl. 1): S10–S16.

Hrachovy, R.A., Frost, Jr., F.D. and Kellaway, P. (1984) Hypsarrhythmia: variations on the theme. Epilepsia 25: 317–325.

Kaplan, P.W. (1996) Nonconvulsive status epilepticus in the emergency room. Epilepsia 37: 643–650.

Kellaway, P. and Mizrahi, E.M. (1987) Neonatal seizures. In: H. Lüders and R.P. Lesser (Eds.), Epilepsy: Electroclinical Syndromes. Springer, New York, pp. 151–187.

Kellaway, P., Hrachovy, R.A., Frost, Jr., J.D. and Zion, R. (1979) Precise characterization and quantification of infantile spasms. Ann. Neurol. 6: 214–218.

Klass, D.W. and Westmoreland, B.F. (1985) Nonepileptogenic epileptiform electroencephalographic activity. Ann. Neurol. 18: 627–635.

Krumholz, A., Sung, G.Y., Fisher, R.S., Barry, E., Berggey, G. and Grattan, L. (1995) Complex partial status epilepticus accompanied by serious morbidity and mortality. Neurology 45: 1494–1504.

Kuroiwa, Y. and Celesia, G.G. (1980) Clinical significance of periodic EEG patterns. Arch. Neurol. 37: 15–20.

Lai, C.W. and Gragasin, M.E. (1988) Electroencephalography in herpes simplex encephalitis. J. Clin. Neurophysiol. 5: 87–103.

Lee, S.I. (1983) Electroencephalography in infantile and childhood epilepsy. In: F.E. Dreifuss (Ed.), Pediatric Epileptology. John Wright, Boston, pp. 33–64.

Lee, S.I. and Kirby, D. (1988) Absence seizure with generalized rhythmic delta activity. Epilepsia 29: 262–267.

Lee, S.I. and Schauwecker, D.S. (1988) Regional cerebral perfusion in PLEDs: A case report. Epilepsia 29: 607–611.

Levy, S.R., Chiappa, K.H., Burke, C.J. and Young, R.R. (1986) Early evolution and incidence of electroencephalographic abnormalities in Creutzfeldt–Jakob disease. J. Clin. Neurophysiol. 3: 1–21.

Lipman, I.J. and Hughes, J.R. (1969) Rhythmic mid-temporal discharges. An electroclinical study. Electroenceph. Clin. Neurophysiol. 27: 43–47.

Lombroso, C.T. (1987) Neonatal electroencephalography. In: E. Niedermeyer and F. Lopes da Silva (Eds.), Electroencephalography: Basic Principles, Clinical Applications and Related Fields. Urban and Schwarzenberg, Baltimore, pp. 725–762.

Lombroso, C.T., Schwartz, I.H., Clark, D.M., Muench, H. and Barry, J. (1966) Ctenoids in healthy youths. Controlled study of 14- and 6-per-second positive spiking. Neurology 16: 1152–1158.

MacGillivray, B.B. (1976) Section III. The EEG in liver disease. In: A. Rémond (Ed.), Handbook of Electroenceph. Clin. Neurophysiol., Vol. 15C. Elsevier, Amsterdam, pp. 26–50.

Markand, O.N. and Panszi, J.G. (1975) The electroencephalogram in subacute sclerosing panencephalitis. Arch. Neurol. 32: 719–726.

Maulsby, R.L. (1979) EEG patterns of uncertain diagnostic significance. In: D.W. Klass and D.D. Daly (Eds.), Current Practice of Clinical Electroencephalography. Raven Press, New York, pp. 411–419.

McCutchen, C.B., Coen, R. and Iragui, V.J. (1984) Periodic lateralized epileptiform discharges in asphyxiated neonates. Electroenceph. Clin. Neurophysiol. 61: 210–217.

Miller, C.R., Westmoreland, B.F. and Klass, D.W. (1985) Subclinical rhythmic EEG discharge of adults (SREDA): further observations. Am. J. EEG Technol. 25: 217–224.

Mizrahi, E.M. and Kellaway, P. (1998) Diagnosis and Management of Neonatal Seizures. Lippincott-Raven, Philadelphia.

Mizrahi, E.M. and Tharp, B.A. (1982) A characteristic EEG pattern in neonatal herpes simplex encephalitis. Neurology 32: 1215–1220.

Mokran, V., Cigánek, L. and Kabatnik, Z. (1971) Electroencephalographic theta discharges in the midline. Eur. Neurol. 5: 288–293.

Niedermeyer, E. (1987) Epileptic seizure disorders. In: E. Niedermeyer and F. Lopes da Silva (Eds.), Electroencephalography: Basic Principles, Clinical Applications and Related Fields. Urban and Schwarzenberg, Baltimore, pp. 405–510.

Noriega-Sanchez, A. and Markand, O.N. (1976) Clinical and electroencephalographic correlation of independent multifocal spike discharges. Neurology 26: 667–672.

PeBenito, R. and Cracco, J. (1979) Periodic lateralized epileptiform discharges in infants and children. Ann. Neurol. 6: 47–50.

Pedley, T.A. (1981) EEG patterns that mimic epileptiform discharges but have no association with seizures. In: C. Henry (Ed.), Current Clinical Neurophysiology. Elsevier, Amsterdam, pp. 307–336.

Pettit, R.E. (1987) Pyridoxine dependency seizures: report of a case with unusual features. J. Child Neurol. 2: 38–40.

Pohlmann-Eden, B., Hoch, D.B., Cochius, J.I. and Chiappa, K.H. (1996) Periodic lateralized epileptiform discharges – a critical review. J. Clin. Neurophysiol. 13: 519–530.

Reeves, A.L., Westmoreland, B.F. and Klass, D.W. (1997) Clinical neurophysiology accompaniments of the burst-suppression pattern. J. Clin. Neurophysiol. 14: 150–153.

Reiher, J. and Lebel, M. (1977) Wicket spikes: clinical correlates of a previously undescribed EEG pattern. Can. J. Neurol. Sci. 4: 39–47.

Reiher, J., Rivest, J., Grand'Maison, F. and Leduc, C.P. (1991) Periodic lateralized epileptiform discharges with transitional rhythmic discharges: association with seizures. Electroenceph. Clin. Neurophysiol. 78: 12–17.

Risinger, M.W., Engel, Jr., J., Van Ness, P.C., Henry, T.R. and Crandall, P.H. (1989) Ictal localization of temporal lobe seizures with scalp sphenoidal recordings. Neurology 39: 1288–1293.

Rose, A.L. and Lombroso, C.T. (1970) Neonatal seizure states. A study of clinical, pathological, and electroencephalographic features in 137 full-term babies with long-term follow-up. Pediatrics 45: 404–425.

Schraeder, P.L. and Singh, N. (1980) Seizure disorders following periodic lateralized epileptiform discharges. Epilepsia 21: 647–653.

Schwartz, M.S., Prior, P.F. and Scott, D.F. (1973) The occurrence and evolution in the EEG of a lateralized periodic phenomenon. Brain 96: 613–622.

Shibasaki, H., Yamashita, Y. and Kuroiwa, Y. (1978) Electroencephalographic studies of myoclonus. Myoclonus-related cortical spikes and high amplitude somatosensory evoked potentials. Brain 101: 447–460.

Smith, J.B., Westmoreland, B.F., Reagan, T.J. and Sandok, B.A. (1975) A distinctive clinical EEG profile in herpes simplex encephalitis. Mayo Clin. Proc. 50: 469–474.

Snodgrass, S.M., Tsuburaya, K. and Ajmone-Marsan, C. (1989) Clinical significance of periodic lateralized epileptiform discharges: relationship with status epilepticus. J. Clin. Neurophysiol. 6: 159–172.

Sperling, M.R. and Clancy, R.R. (1998) Ictal EEG. In: J. Engel, Jr. and T.A. Pedley (Eds.), Epilepsy. A Comprehensive Textbook. Vol. 2. Lippincott-Raven, Philadelphia, pp. 849–886.

Steriade, M., Amzica, F. and Contreras, D. (1994) Cortical and thalamic cellular correlates of electroencephalographic burst-suppression. Electroenceph. Clin. Neurophysiol. 90: 1–16.

Swartz, B.E., Walsh, G.O., Delgado-Escueta, A.V. and Zolo, P. (1991) Surface ictal electroencephalographic patterns in frontal vs temporal lobe epilepsy. Can. J. Neurol. Sci. 18: 649–662.

Tharp, B.R. (1986) Neonatal and pediatric electroencephalography. In: M.J. Aminoff (Ed.), Electrodiagnosis in Clinical Neurology. Churchill/Livingstone, New York, pp. 77–124.

Thomas, J.E. and Klass, D.W. (1968) Six-per-second spike-and-wave pattern in the electroencephalogram: a reappraisal of its clinical significance. Neurology 18: 587–593.

Thomas, J.E., Reagan, T.J. and Klass, D.W. (1977) Epilepsia partialis continua. Arch. Neurol. 34: 266–275.

Towne, A., Pellock, J., Ko, D. and De Lorenzo, R. (1994) Determinants of mortality in status epilepticus. Epilepsia 35: 27–34.

Trieman, D. (1995) Electroclinical features of status epilepticus. J. Clin. Neurophysiol. 12: 343–362.

Trieman, D., Walton, N. and Kendrick, C. (1990) A progressive sequence of electroencephalographic and changes during generalized convulsive status epilepticus. Epilepsy Res. 5: 49–60.

Walczak, T.S. and Jayakar, P. (1998) Interictal EEG. In: J. Engel, Jr. and T.A. Pedley (Eds.), Epilepsy. A Comprehensive Textbook, Vol. 1. Lippincott-Raven, Philadelphia, pp. 831–848.

Walsh, J.M. and Brenner, R.P. (1987) Periodic lateralized epileptiform discharges: long term outcome in adults. Epilepsia 28: 533–536.

Werner, S.S., Stockard, J.E. and Bickford, R.G. (1977) Atlas of Neonatal EEG. Raven Press, New York.

Westmoreland, B.F. (1996) Epileptiform electroencephalographic patterns. Mayo Clin. Proc. 71: 501–511.

Westmoreland, B.F. and Gomez, M.R. (1987) Infantile spasms (West syndrome). In: H. Lüders and R.P. Lesser (Eds.), Epilepsy: Electroclinical Syndromes. Springer, New York, pp. 49–72.

Westmoreland, B.F. and Klass, D.W. (1981) A distinctive rhythmic EEG discharge of adults. Electroenceph. Clin. Neurophysiol. 51: 186–191.

Westmoreland, B.F. and Klass, D.W. (1986) Midline theta rhythm. Arch. Neurol. 43: 139–141.

Westmoreland, B.F. and Klass, D.W. (1997) Unusual variants of subclinical rhythmic electrographic discharge of adults (SREDA). Electroenceph. Clin. Neurophysiol. 102: 1–4.

Westmoreland, B.F., Groover, R.V. and Sharbrough, F.W. (1979a) Electrographic findings in three types of cerebromacular degeneration. Mayo Clin. Proc. 54: 12–21.

Westmoreland, B.F., Reiher, J. and Klass, D.W. (1979b) Recording small sharp spikes with depth electroencephalography. Epilepsia 20: 599–606.

Westmoreland, B.F., Sharbrough, F.W. and Donat, J.R. (1979c) Stimulus-induced EEG complexes and motor spasms in subacute sclerosing pancencephalitis. Neurology 29: 1154–1157.

Westmoreland, B.F., Klass, D.W. and Sharbrough, F.W. (1986) Chronic periodic lateralized epileptiform discharges. Arch. Neurol. 27: 729–733.

Westmoreland, B.F., Frere, R.C. and Klass, D.W. (1997) Periodic epileptiform discharges in the midline. J. Clin. Neurophysiol. 14: 495–498.

White, J.C., Langston, J.W. and Pedley, T.A. (1977) Benign epileptiform transients of sleep. Neurology 27: 1061–1068.

Yamada, T., Young, S. and Kimura, J. (1977) Significance of positive spike bursts in Reye syndrome. Arch. Neurol. 34: 376–380.

Young, G.B. and Jordan, K.G. (1998) Do nonconvulsive seizures damage the brain? – yes. Controversies in neurology. Arch. Neurol. 55: 117–119.

20 Localized slow waves

SUMMARY

(20.1) Localized (focal) slow waves have a frequency under 8 Hz and a limited distribution; they are usually restricted to one or a few neighboring electrodes, i.e., to a focus of slow waves; less often, they occupy an entire hemisphere.

(20.2) *The cause* of local slow waves is a circumscribed abnormality located superficially or deeply in a hemisphere. Commonly the abnormality is a structural lesion that has an acute onset or a progressive course. In the case of acute lesions, the slow waves develop at the time of the damage and persist for weeks or months. Slow waves may also occur as a result of transient local abnormalities such as seizures or ischemia and then outlast the transient event by several hours or a few days.

(20.3) *Other EEG abnormalities* are often associated with focal slow waves and may further clarify the location and type of the underlying lesion.

(20.4) *Mechanisms* generating focal slow waves include functional or partial structural interruption of corticocortical and corticosubcortical fiber connections.

(20.5) *Specific disorders* associated with focal slow waves include a variety of structural lesions such as tumors, infarcts, hemorrhages, abscesses and transient abnormalities such as transient ischemic attacks, migraine, partial seizures and hypertensive encephalopathy.

20.1 DESCRIPTION OF PATTERN

Localized (focal) slow waves consist of waves of less than 8 Hz which commonly appear at mainly one or a few electrodes, i.e. in a focal distribution (Figs. 20.1; 20.3; 20.4); less common are slow waves which are distributed over an entire hemisphere, i.e. unilateral slow waves (Fig. 20.2). Individual slow waves are often irregular in appearance and successive slow waves often are arrhythmical, i.e. composed of different frequencies. Focal irregular delta activity is commonly referred to as focal polymorphic delta activity.

The slow waves at the center of a focus of slow wave activity are usually more persistent and usually of lower frequency than slow waves at the periphery; foci of delta waves are often surrounded by theta waves. The amplitude of slow waves does not always have a maximum at the center; the surrounding slow waves may be larger. Focal slow waves often do not entirely replace the background activity (Figs. 20.1–20.4). Indeed, focal slow waves of low amplitude may at times be difficult to distinguish from normal background activity. Irregular focal delta waves usually show little attenuation with eye opening and alerting and may not be facilitated by hyperventilation, whereas surrounding slow waves of theta frequency often do respond to such maneuvers. Local slow waves are

349

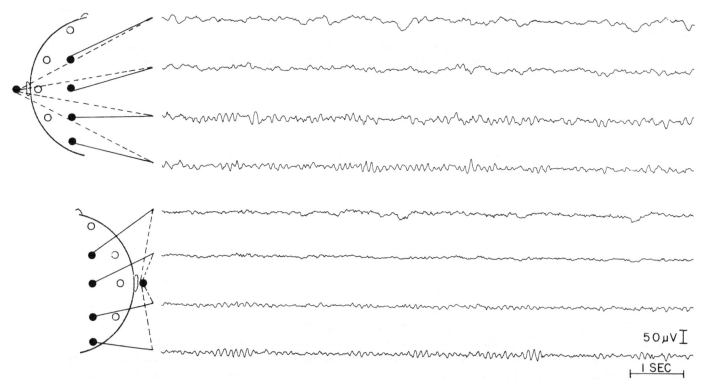

Fig. 20.1.   Left fronto-central slow wave focus; the right frontal slow waves are largely due to eye movements. The patient is a 53-year-old man with a 3 year history of partial complex seizures which begin with olfactory hallucinations. A left frontal oligodendroglioma was removed surgically a few days after this EEG recording.

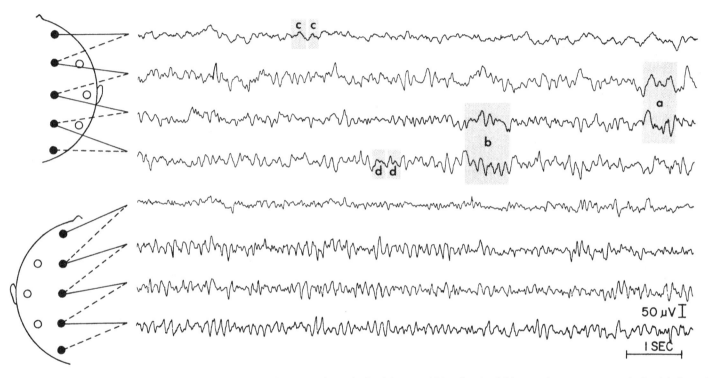

Fig. 20.2. Right centro-parietal slow wave focus. Delta waves have a maximum in the right central (a) and parietal (b) areas; theta waves appear in the right frontal (c) and occipital (d) areas. Occipital alpha rhythm on the right is slower than that on the left. This 76-year-old man had a large cerebral infarct in the distribution of the right middle cerebral artery 2 days before the EEG.

most conspicuous during transitions between wakefulness and light sleep and may persist into stage II non-REM sleep.

20.2 CLINICAL SIGNIFICANCE OF FOCAL SLOW WAVES

20.2.1 *Types of underlying lesions. Focal slow waves* indicate a circumscribed lesion which may be due to either lasting structural damage or a transient disturbance in an area of the subcortical white matter or in the thalamic nuclei; however, lesions of the meninges or the subdural space that invade or compress the underlying hemisphere can also cause focal slow waves. Beyond these general characteristics, focal slow waves do not indicate the specific nature of the local lesion and may thus be due to a variety of conditions.

The classic electrographic sign of a focal disturbance in cerebral function is focal delta activity. A structural lesion is most likely if the delta activity is continuously present, shows variability in waveform, amplitude, duration, and morphology (so-called *polymorphic delta activity),* and persists during changes in physiologic state. Delta waves that are suppressed with eye opening (or other alerting maneuvers), or fail to persist into sleep, are less likely to indicate structural (neuroimaging) pathology.

Transient cerebral disorders which can cause episodic focal slow waves are transient ischemic attacks, migraine attacks associated with focal neurological signs, hypertensive and metabolic encephalopathies, some partial seizures, postictal depression, and mild local head injuries. The slow waves should disappear within hours or a few days of the acute disorder; slow waves which persist longer suggest that lasting microstructural damage has occurred.

20.2.2 *The evolution of slow waves arising from structural damage is variable.* Focal slow waves appear immediately and maximally at the onset of sudden structural damage. Thus, if an acute lesion is going to give rise to local slow waves, it will do so at the onset. That is why in hemispheric non-lacunar stroke with cortical involvement the EEG is far more likely to be abnormal (i.e., show local slow waves over the area of involvement) than computerized tomography during the first 24 h. Indeed, EEG may show localizing slow waves in some patients who present with stroke who never develop clear signs of stroke on MRI. However, the somewhat predictable evolution of the appearance of an acute lesion on neuroimaging is not so clear with EEG. Focal slow waves may partially or completely resolve weeks or months after acute damage even though clinical signs and neuroimaging evidence persist; this discrepancy suggests that further clinical improvement is unlikely. Slow waves may also persist after neurological signs have cleared; this apparent dissociation indicates a higher likelihood of finding structural abnormalities using neuroimaging.

In many slowly progressive structural lesions, slow waves appear only at or after the onset of clinical signs; however, in some cases focal slow waves associated with tumors may be seen at a time when the patient has only vague symptoms.

20.2.3 *The spatial relationship between focal slow waves and the underlying cerebral lesion varies.* Slow waves in superficial lesions generally are fairly precise indicators of the site of the abnormality. However, in some cases, the slow wave focus may appear in a more lateral and anterior location than that of the cerebral lesion. Rarely do slow wave foci appear far away from the lesion. Lesions that are small and deep, for instance infarctions of the internal capsule, do not produce continuous irregular focal delta activity in the EEG even though the patient may show considerable neurological abnormalities.

The localizing value of focal delta is increased when it is topographically discrete or associated with a depression of intermixed faster background frequencies. Superficial lesions tend to produce more restricted EEG changes, whereas deep cerebral lesions may result in hemispheric, or even bilateral, delta. *Lesions involving the central and parietal areas are less likely to present with a circumscribed delta focus, and are also more apt to produce delta activity falsely localized to the temporal areas.*

Focal delta is usually, but by no means always, maximal over the lesion. If sufficient destruction of the cortex has occurred, the amplitude of delta activity may actually be reduced over the area of maximal cortical involvement and thus be higher in the areas bordering the lesion. If two or more delta foci are present, the one that is most persistent, least rhythmic, and contains less activity above 4 Hz indicates the site of the major lesion, regardless

of voltage. The observation that delta activity directly over a lesion is least likely to contain intermixed waveforms over 4 Hz gave rise to the term, *flat polymorphism*; the absence of intermixed faster waveforms gives the delta activity directly overlying a structural abnormality a 'flattened' (i.e., smooth) appearance.

Focal slow waves over an abnormality in one hemisphere may be associated with similar slow waves, usually of lower amplitude, in the opposite hemisphere, particularly in cases of frontal (Fig. 20.1) and occipital lesions. This phenomenon has several possible explanations: (a) an acute infarction or a tumor may produce compression, edema or ischemia in neighboring parts of the opposite hemisphere; (b) impulses from slow wave foci in one hemisphere may travel via commissural fibers to the corresponding area of the other hemisphere to produce slow waves there; (c) the electrical field of a slow wave focus may be conducted through the volume of the interposed tissue to the electrodes over the opposite hemisphere. In the first two instances, bilateral asynchronous frontal or occipital slow wave foci may make it difficult to distinguish between unilateral and bilateral cerebral lesions. In such cases, slight differences in the distribution and timing of slow waves may indicate the area of the primary abnormality. In the case of volume conduction, slow waves in the opposite hemisphere are perfectly synchronized, attenuated, copies of the slow waves of the major focus.

Lesions in the posterior fossa cause focal slow waves only very rarely. Infratentorial lesions may produce arrhythmical slow waves in the occipital regions; these waves are usually bilateral, sometimes asymmetrical and rarely focal. They may be due to pressure on, or ischemia of, the occipital lobes, caused by the infratentorial lesion.

20.3 OTHER EEG ABNORMALITIES ASSOCIATED WITH FOCAL SLOW WAVES

In many cases of focal slow waves, the EEG shows other abnormalities which may be helpful in making the clinical diagnosis. In a few instances such abnormalities precede the appearance of focal slow waves and thus become the earliest indication of a local lesion; this is particularly true in cases of cerebral tumors.

20.3.1 *Widespread asynchronous slow waves* are commonly seen in a hemisphere having a delta focus, or in both hemispheres (Fig. 20.2). They are more common in acute than in chronic lesions and suggest cerebral disturbances due to such possible mechanisms as local distortion of brain tissue, vascular, metabolic or other changes. Widespread slow waves can accompany the reduction of alertness that occurs in some deeply located hemispheric strokes and tumors. The generalized slow waves may become so prominent as to obscure the focal slow waves.

20.3.2 *Bilaterally synchronous slow waves* usually appear intermittently and in a wider distribution than the more persistent focal slow waves (Fig. 20.3). The bisynchronous slow waves may be larger or more persistent on the side of the focal slow waves

but often have a frontal maximum independent of the distribution of the focal slow waves. Bisynchronous slow waves often suggest that the lesion causing focal slow waves has involved deep midline structures in the anterior, middle or posterior fossa, especially the mesencephalon or diencephalon, by directly invading these structures, by compressing or distorting them or by rendering them ischemic. Indeed, *the combination of frontal or occipital dominant intermittent rhythmic delta activity (FIRDA or OIRDA) and continuous focal irregular delta activity is the classic electrographic sign of impending cerebral herniation* from a focal structural lesion. The referring physician should, therefore, be informed immediately if this combination of patterns is present. However, the same combination of patterns may also be seen in patients with focal structural lesions and co-existent toxic or metabolic encephalopathies.

20.3.3 *Focal spikes and sharp waves* may be caused by the same lesion that causes the focal slow waves (Fig. 20.4). On the other hand, slow waves associated with focal spikes or sharp waves may simply be a component of the ongoing epileptiform activity (20.6.6). Epileptiform activity, of course, does not arise within the substance of a structural lesion but at the periphery where cortical structures are affected but not destroyed.

20.3.4 *Asymmetry and reduced reactivity of the alpha rhythm* often accompany reduction of the frequency (Fig. 20.2) of the alpha rhythm in the hemisphere showing focal slow waves. This happens more often with lesions in the posterior parts of the

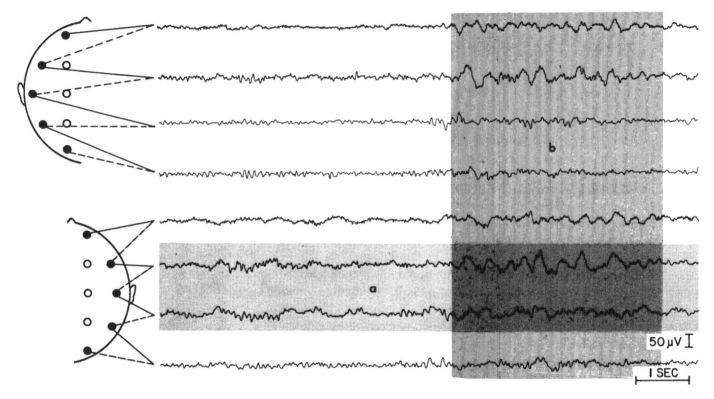

Fig. 20.3. Pattern of combined focal and bisynchronous slow waves. Focal slow waves of 0.5–2 Hz (a) occur continuously in the right temporal area; a burst of bisynchronous slow waves of 2–3 Hz (b) appears with a maximum in the anterior head regions, slightly greater on the right. The patient is a 62-year-old woman with a history of syncope and a decreased left nasolabial fold. Further workup was prompted by the EEG findings and revealed a right sphenoid wing meningioma.

hemisphere than with anterior lesions, possibly as a result of compression of the posterior structures involved in the production of the alpha rhythm. Occasionally, the alpha rhythm is reduced on the side opposite to a slow wave focus, perhaps due to compression, or interference with blood supply, of that hemisphere.

20.3.5 *Asymmetries of the beta rhythm, mu rhythm, vertex waves, K complexes, sleep spindles, FIRDA, OIRDA, and triphasic waves* may be due to a reduction of all EEG activity in the vicinity of a lesion producing a slow wave focus, especially a lesion near the central regions. An isolated depression of beta activity is a reliable localizing sign. In exceptional cases beta activity may be increased in the head region overlying a tumor. Beta activity increased ipsilateral to a lesion is almost always due to an underlying skull defect (causing a breach rhythm).

20.4 MECHANISMS CAUSING FOCAL SLOW WAVES

Clinical and experimental observations indicate that continuous, irregular, delta activity (i.e., polymorphic delta) results primarily from lesions affecting cerebral white matter. Involvement of superficial cortex is not essential and, indeed, rare lesions restricted to the cortical mantle do not generally produce significant focal delta activity. It is likely that partial functional or anatomic deafferentation of cortex, rather than a change in cortical metabolic rate, is critical. Total cortical deafferentation is not an effective means of producing focal polymorphic delta activity. Experimentally, localized or lateralized irregular delta activity can also be produced by ipsilateral lesions of the thalamus or midbrain reticular formation. In humans focal polymorphic delta rarely arises from lesions of the posterior fossa. Cerebral edema alone, even when extensive, does not appear to make a substantial contribution to the production of delta waves unless it causes a functionally significant compression of midline structures. Lesser degrees of focal slowing such as intermittent irregular theta activity probably have a similar pathogenesis, although the mechanism of cortical deafferentation is more likely to be due to transient disturbances or relatively small lesions.

20.5 SPECIFIC DISORDERS CAUSING FOCAL SLOW WAVES

20.5.1 *Degenerative, developmental and demyelinating diseases.* Degenerative diseases produce focal slow waves so rarely that prominent focal slowing raises the question of another disorder. Exceptions are the temporal slow wave foci which may appear in Alzheimer's dementia and local slow waves which occur at the beginning of Jakob-Creutzfeldt disease. Developmental diseases cause focal slow waves infrequently even if there is focal cerebral damage. This may be due to the fact that these lesions begin early in life, at a time

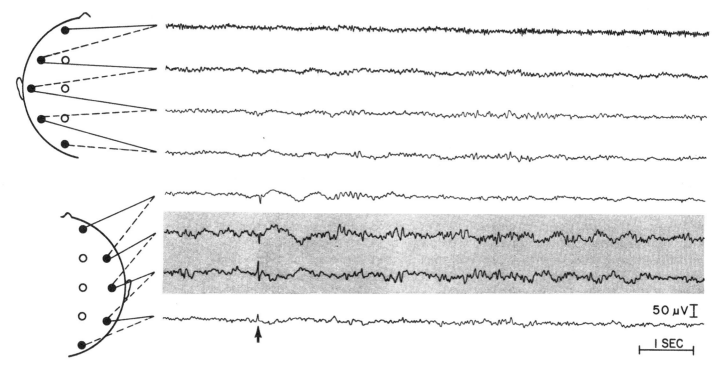

Fig. 20.4. Pattern of combined focal slow waves and focal spikes. Focal slow waves of 1–3 Hz (shaded) appear continuously in the right temporal region; a spike (arrow) appears in the same distribution. The recording was made during drowsiness. The patient is the same as in Fig. 20.3, 1 year after surgical removal of the meningioma; she had one generalized seizure 10 days before this EEG recording.

357

when local damage produces distortions of background and specific epileptiform patterns (19.1). Later in life, the residual cerebral damage is rarely reflected by discrete focal slow waves.

Senile and presenile dementia (Alzheimer's disease) may be associated with an exaggeration of the intermittent focal slow waves that appear in the temporal areas, particularly on the left side, with advancing age (13.4). However, these focal slow waves are a less reliable indicator of dementia than are generalized asynchronous slow waves.

Jakob-Creutzfeldt disease may show slow waves locally for a short period before they become generalized and before focal epileptiform or generalized periodic complexes appear (19.3).

Normal pressure hydrocephalus occasionally produces local or generalized asynchronous slow waves.

Hydrocephalus in children may be associated with focal slow waves in addition to other abnormalities; focal slow waves are more common at the site of shunt insertions.

Porencephaly, tuberous sclerosis, and perinatal cerebral damage may cause residual local slow waves in the EEG after causing generalized abnormalities in infancy.

Holoprosencephaly may cause focal slow waves and focal spikes, emanating from islands of preserved brain tissue.

Multiple sclerosis and Schilder's disease cause focal slow waves much less often than they cause widespread slow waves and other abnormalities.

Bilateral retrobulbar neuritis in children, causing significant visual loss, may lead to occipital slow waves in addition to spikes (17.5).

20.5.2 *Metabolic and toxic encephalopathies.* Focal slow waves are seen in these disorders much less often than are generalized slow waves. Focal slow waves may appear on a background of generalized slow waves during metabolic coma or emerge from generalized slow waves after metabolic coma as a result of local vascular complications, namely transient cerebral ischemia or infarction. Very few metabolic disorders cause focal slow waves without causing generalized slow waves and coma. Focal slow waves may occur in: hypoglycemia, hypoxia and CO poisoning, hyperosmolar coma, for instance in non-ketotic hyperglycemia, hyper-parathyroidism, porphyria, vitamin B12 deficiency and Wilson's disease. Focal slow waves may occur after myelography with metrizamide.

20.5.3 *Cerebrovascular diseases.* Strokes of the cerebral hemispheres caused by ischemia, embolism or hemorrhage are common causes of focal slow waves. Infarction in the distribution of the middle cerebral artery often causes local slow waves in the temporal, frontal, central and parietal areas (Fig. 20.2). Occlusion of the anterior cerebral artery, especially at the origin of the artery at the base of the brain, may cause frontal intermittent delta activity (22.2), even though this activity is more often due to frontal tumors than to infarctions. A cerebral infarct in the distribution of the posterior cerebral arteries is likely to cause focal slow waves in the occipital and posterior temporal areas. Infarction of the brainstem rarely produces focal slow waves over the posterior head. Brainstem infarctions may produce generalized bisynchronous and asynchronous slow waves if they involve the reticular formation in the core of the midbrain or alpha coma patterns if they involve the pontine reticular formation (25.3.2).

Multiple infarctions may be the cause of more than one slow wave focus. Slow wave foci are often acquired in sequence by patients who have successive strokes. Multiple small infarcts responsible for the lacunar state in hypertensive patients often cause no sharply defined slow wave foci but rather result in generalized slow waves. Cerebral air and fat emboli also usually cause generalized rather than focal slow waves.

Transient ischemic attacks of the cerebral hemispheres may cause local slow waves or reductions of amplitude (23.6.3). An EEG is rarely recorded during the attack, but slow waves may persist for many hours after the attack, or longer if an infarct has occurred.

Occlusion of the carotid artery is produced intentionally during surgical repair of a partially occluded artery (carotid endarterectomy). Sudden clamping of the artery may reduce the cerebral blood flow to a level below that needed to prevent infarction. Imminent infarction can be recognized by the appearance of severe attenuation or focal or unilateral slow waves within a few minutes after clamping; the slow waves are often followed by loss of amplitude. Monitoring of the EEG during carotid endarterectomy can thus help to determine the need for shunting and detect the occurrence of intraoperative stroke.

Migraine attacks can produce local slow waves, especially if the attacks are associated with unilateral neurological abnormalities other than visual symptoms. The slow waves are presumably due to local cerebral ischemia or spreading depression during the attack. If they persist for hours or a few days after the attack, the slow waves may be due to local cerebral ischemia; if they persist longer, they can be presumed to be due to infarction. Attacks of basilar artery migraine may be associated with focal slow waves in the posterior head regions on one or both sides, or with generalized slow waves. Slow wave foci in patients with headaches unexplained by a recent attack of migraine are sufficiently rare to warrant a workup for mass lesions or vascular malformations.

Chronic subdural hematoma commonly causes focal slow waves even though a regional reduction of amplitude is a more classic and suggestive finding. Bilateral subdural hematomas may be associated with any combination of unilateral and bilateral slow waves and asymmetries, including slow waves on one side and amplitude reductions on the other.

Subarachnoid hemorrhage produces focal slow waves only occasionally and by one of several possible mechanisms. The hemorrhage may damage the brain locally. Spasm of the bleeding vessel may cause local ischemia or infarction. Bleeding may come from an aneurysm or a vascular malformation which locally compresses the brain. Slow wave foci in the central head region suggest bleeding from an aneurysm of the middle cerebral artery; foci in the posterior temporal region have no localizing value. Subarachnoid hemorrhage may cause ipsilateral decrease of amplitude and decrease of alpha frequency; when associated with a lowered level of consciousness, generalized slow waves are practically always present. As first demonstrated by Labar et al. (1991), EEG monitoring following subarachnoid hemorrhage can be used to detect the onset of vasospasm, in some cases prior to the development of obvious clinical signs.

20.5.4 *Cerebral trauma. Head injuries* may lead to focal slow waves in addition to the more common initial decrease of amplitude and subsequent widespread slow waves. In many cases, focal slow waves after head injury are transient, variable in distribution and unassociated with focal neurological signs. They therefore probably do not represent local structural damage but may be explained by temporary local changes of cerebral circulation or compression from edema. In other instances, they last longer and are due to contusions, intracerebral hemorrhages, or acute traumatic subdural or epidural hematoma.

Progressive traumatic encephalopathy may produce one or more slow wave foci initially before leading to generalized slow waves.

Brain surgery involving the cerebral hemispheres is often followed by focal slow waves. They suggest local brain damage. However, this must be distinguished from the effects of a skull defect which can locally increase the amplitude of generalized slow waves (23.4).

Hemispherectomy may cause unilateral slow waves in addition to amplitude reductions.

20.5.5 *Brain tumors. Supratentorial brain tumors* are among the most important causes of focal slow waves, and focal slow waves are the most characteristic sign of a supratentorial tumor (Figs. 20.1 and 20.3). Focal slow waves of tumors may be associated with other EEG abnormalities such as focal epileptiform activity (Fig. 20.4) and generalized slow waves (Fig. 20.3) which have the implications described earlier (20.3).

Studies of the EEG in patients with brain tumors have revealed several important pieces of clinical information. Frontal tumors tend to produce a considerable amount of focal slow wave activity not only on the side of the tumor but also on the opposite side (Fig. 20.1). Tumors deep in the parietal lobe may cause focal parietal theta rhythm. Multiple metastases occasionally cause more than one slow wave focus. Tumors in older persons are more likely to produce bisynchronous slow waves than are tumors in persons of other ages. Infratentorial tumors, while often causing bisynchronous slow waves, produce local slow waves in the posterior head regions only rarely in adults and slightly more commonly in children. Slow wave foci in the temporal region may arise from temporal lobe tumors but may also arise as a falsely localizing sign from tumors located adjacent to the temporal lobe.

20.5.6 *Seizure disorders.* Postictal continuous irregular focal delta waves often appear after a single isolated seizure of focal onset, but rarely persist more than 20 min unless an underlying structural abnormality is present. In a patient who is known to have had a recent seizure but who shows no epileptiform activity in the EEG, focal slow waves can suggest a focal origin of the seizure and indicate the region of the brain where the seizure originated.

Interictal focal slow waves raise the suspicion of a local lesion such as a tumor, stroke, injury or malformation which can both damage subcortical tissue, giving rise to the slow waves, and irritate cortical tissue, producing epileptiform activity. However, focal slow waves, mixed with focal spikes or sharp waves, can be seen in stationary epileptogenic lesions as part of the ongoing epileptiform activity.

Ictal focal slow waves are rarely the only EEG manifestation of an ongoing seizure; this may be seen in seizures and status epilepticus of partial seizures and in epilepsia partialis continua (19.3.2). Ictal patterns, however, are always rhythmical whereas local slow waves arising from a non-epileptic functional or structural lesion are almost always irregular.

20.5.7 *Infectious diseases. Abscesses* of the cerebral hemispheres are more commonly associated with focal slow waves than with other EEG abnormalities such as focal spikes and sharp waves, periodic lateralizing epileptiform discharges, or local reductions of amplitude. Bisynchronous slow waves are more common with deeply located abscesses. Asynchronous generalized slow waves invariably appear when the level of alertness decreases.

Meningitis and encephalitis produce focal slow waves only rarely and when the infection involves one part of the hemispheres more than others. This is usually the case in the acute necrotizing encephalitis of herpes simplex which produces focal slow waves in one or both temporal areas early in the disease (19.3.1).

Progressive multifocal leukoencephalopathy may begin locally and be associated with focal slow waves before generalized asynchronous slow waves supervene.

20.5.8 *Psychiatric diseases. Focal slow waves* have been reported in a great variety of psychiatric disorders. However, this occurrence is so rare and without clear relation to specific diseases that focal slow waves cannot be accepted as a manifestation of psychiatric disease and a local cerebral lesion must be excluded by other examinations. This is especially true for patients whose symptoms include dementia where the finding of a slow wave focus in any part of the brain would be strong presumptive evidence for a structural cerebral lesion.

REFERENCES

Blume, W.T. and Kaibara, M. (1995) Atlas of Adult Electroencephalography. Raven Press, New York.

Daly, D.D. and Markand, O.N. (1990) Focal brain legions. In: D. Daly and T. Pedley (Eds.), Current Practice of Clinical Electroencephalography, Second Edition. Raven Press, New York, pp. 335–370.

Fisch, B.J. and Pedley, T.A. (1985) Evaluation of focal cerebral lesions. Role of electroencephalography in the era of computerized tomography. In: M.J. Aminoff (Ed.), Electrodiagnosis, Neurologic Clinics. Saunders, Philadelphia, pp. 649–662.

Fischer-Williams, M. (1987) Brain tumors and other space occupying lesions (with a section on oncological CNS complications). In: E. Niedermeyer and F. Lopes da Silva (Eds.), Electroencephalography: Basic Principles, Clinical Applications and Related Fields. Urban and Schwarzenberg, Baltimore, pp. 163–182.

Gambardella, A., Gotman, J., Cendes, F. and Andermann, F. (1995) Focal intermittent delta activity in patients with mesiotemporal atrophy: a reliable marker of the epileptogenic focus. Epilepsia 36: 122–129.

Gilmore, P.C. and Brenner, R.P. (1981) Correlation of EEG, computerized tomography, and clinical findings: study of 100 patients with focal delta activity. Arch. Neurol. 38: 371–372.

Gloor, P., Ball, G. and Schaul, N. (1977) Brain lesions that produce delta waves in the EEG. Neurology 27: 326–333.

Goldensohn, E.S. (1979) Use of the EEG for evaluation of focal intracranial lesions. In: D.W. Klass and D. Daly (Eds.), Current Practice of Clinical Electroencephalography. Raven Press, New York, pp. 307–342.

Goldensohn, E.S., Legatt, A.D., Koszer, S. and Wolf, S.M. (1999) Goldensohn's EEG Interpretation: Problems of Overreading and Underreading, Second Edition. Futura Publishing Company, Armonk, NY.

Klass, D.W. and Brenner, R.P. (1995) Electroencephalography of the elderly. J. Clin. Neurophysiol. 12: 116–131.

Klass, D.W. and Westmoreland, B.F. (1996) Electroencephalography: general principles and adult electroencephalograms. In: J. Daube (Ed.), Clinical Neurophysiology. F.A. Davis, Philadelphia, pp. 73–103.

Labar, D.R., Fisch, B.J., Pedley, T.A., Fink, M.E. and Solomon, R.A. (1991) Quantiative EEG monitoring for patients with subarachnoid hemorrhage. Electroenceph. Clin. Neurophysiol. 78: 325–332.

MacDonnell, R.A.L., Donnan, G.A., Bladin, P.F., Berkovic, S.F. and Wriedt, C.H.R. (1988) The electroencephalogram and acute ischemic stroke. Distinguishing cortical from lacunar infarction. Arch. Neurol. 45: 520–524.

Marshall, D., Brey, R.L. and Morse, M.W. (1988) Focal and/or lateralized polymorphic delta activity. Arch. Neurol. 45: 33–35.

Michel, B., Gastaut, J.L. and Bianchi, L. (1979) Electroencephalographic cranial computerized tomographic correlations in brain abscess. Electroenceph. Clin. Neurophysiol. 46: 256–273.

Newmark, M.E., Theodore, W.H., Sato, S., De la Paz, R., Patronas, N., Brooks, R., Jabbari, B. and Di Chiro, G. (1983) EEG, transmission computed tomography, and positron emission tomography with fluorodeoxyglucose ^{18}F: their use in adults with gliomas. Arch. Neurol. 40: 607–610.

Normand, M.M., Wszolek, Z.K. and Klass, D.W. (1995) Temporal intermittent rhythmic delta activity in electroencephalograms. J. Clin. Neurophysiol. 12: 280–284.

Petty, G.W., Labar, D.R., Fisch, B.J., Pedley, T.A., Mohr, J.P. and Khandji, A. (1995) Electroencephalography in lacunar infarction. J. Neurol. Sci. 134: 47–50.

Schaul, N., Gloor, P. and Gotman, J. (1981) The EEG in deep midline lesions. Neurology 31: 157–167.

Schaul, N., Green, L., Peyster, R. and Gotman, J. (1986) Structural determinants of electroencephalographic findings in acute hemispheric lesions. Arch. Neurol. 20: 703–711.

Sharbrough, F.W. (1993) Nonspecific abnormal EEG patterns. In: E. Niedermeyer and F. Lopes da Silva (Eds.), Electroencephalography: Basic Principles, Clinical Applications and Related Fields, Third Edition. Williams and Wilkins, Baltimore, pp. 197–215.

Sharbrough, F.W., Messick, J.M. and Sundt, T.M. (1973) Correlation of continuous electroencephalograms with cerebral blood flow measurements during carotid endarterectomy. Stroke 4: 674–683.

Steriade, M., Gloor, P., Llinás, R.R. and Lopes da Silva, F.H. (1990) Basic mechanisms of cerebral rhythmic activities. Electroenceph. Clin. Neurophysiol. 76: 481–508.

Van der Drift, J.H.A. and Kok, N.K.D. (1972) Section II. The EEG in cerebrovascular disorders in relation to pathology. In: A. Rémond (Ed.), Handbook of Electroenceph. Clin. Neurophysiol., Vol. 14A. Elsevier, Amsterdam, pp. 12–64.

Vignaendra, V., Ghee, L.T. and Chawla, J. (1975) EEG in brain abscess: its value in localization compared to other diagnostic tests. Electroenceph. Clin. Neurophysiol. 38: 611–622.

21 Generalized asynchronous slow waves

SUMMARY

(21.1) The *pattern* of generalized asynchronous slow waves consists of waves of less than 8 Hz which occur over both hemispheres in such a way that the waves on one side have no constant time relationship with the waves on the other side. Asynchronous slow waves usually vary in frequency and often have irregular shapes. They may be reduced by eye opening and alerting and increased by hyperventilation. They may have a local maximum, i.e. an area of higher amplitude and incidence, over some head regions; this pattern differs from a slow wave focus surrounded by generalized slow waves in that focal slow waves are usually lower in frequency and sometimes lower in amplitude than the surrounding slow waves and react less to eye opening, alerting and hyperventilation.

(21.2) *Causes* of generalized asynchronous slow waves include many normal and abnormal conditions. In general, these slow waves are present in all normal subjects during drowsiness and sleep. During wakefulness, slow waves are part of the normal background in subjects of all ages ex-

cept adults. In adults, a mild excess of generalized slow waves during wakefulness, although an electrographic abnormality, is found in 5–10% of otherwise normal subjects. A mild amount of asynchronous generalized slow waves in a wakeful adult can therefore only suggest that a person is somewhat more likely to have a cerebral abnormality. However, a marked amount of these slow waves always indicates a cerebral abnormality. The etiology remains unspecified: generalized asynchronous slow waves occur in such a great variety of widespread cerebral disorders that they are the most common and least specific EEG abnormality.

(21.3) *Other EEG abnormalities* associated with generalized asynchronous slow waves are usually of greater diagnostic significance.

(21.4) *Mechanisms* causing generalized asynchronous slow waves interfere with the structure or function of both hemispheres and often involve subcortical white matter.

21.1 DESCRIPTION OF PATTERN

Generalized asynchronous slow waves have a frequency under 8 Hz and occur over most or all parts of both hemispheres (Figs. 21.1; 21.2; 21.3). The slow waves in one area have no constant time relationship with slow waves in the corresponding area on the other side of the head. For example, slow waves may appear in some areas when there are no slow waves in other areas; slow waves appearing in different areas at the same time may have different frequency; waves of similar frequency appearing simultaneously in different areas may have varying phase relationship. Even though individual slow waves may often have a fairly regular shape, their rate of repetition usually varies by at least 2–3 Hz, i.e. they are often arrhythmical. The slow waves are reduced by eye opening and alerting, and increased by relaxation and hyperventila-

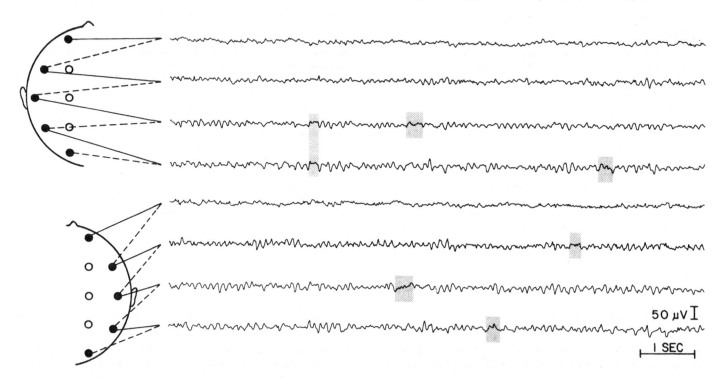

Fig. 21.1. Pattern of generalized asynchronous slow waves with a maximum in the posterior head regions. The slow waves are mainly in the theta range and of low or medium amplitude; a few slow waves are indicated by shading. The slow waves of much lower frequency in the prefrontal regions are eye movement artifacts. The patient is a 53-year-old woman with a schizoid personality disorder and several psychotic episodes, currently treated with 100 mg chlorpromazine every 4 h.

tion. In some comatose patients, alerting stimuli may paradoxically increase slow waves (Fig. 25.4). In general, the reactivity of generalized asynchronous slow waves is greater than that of focal slow waves and less pronounced than that of bisynchronous generalized slow waves. Generalized asynchronous slow waves are best recognized during wakefulness be-

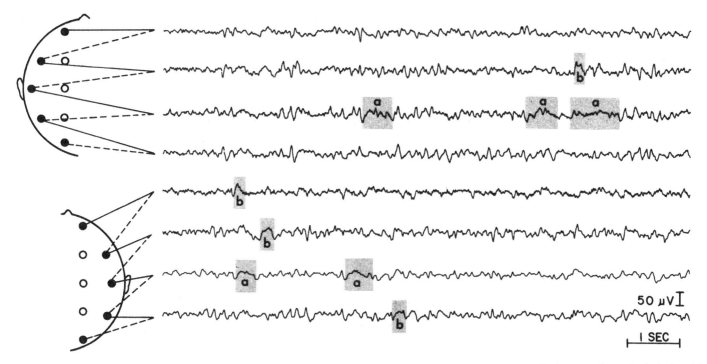

Fig. 21.2. Pattern of generalized asynchronous slow waves of delta (a) and theta (b) frequency and of moderate amplitude. Intermittent rhythmical occipital background activity has a frequency of 5–6 Hz. This 73-year-old man has fairly severe senile dementia.

cause during sleep they are usually obscured by the generalized slow waves of normal sleep patterns. Although distributed widely, generalized asynchronous slow waves may be more prominent in some areas than in others (Fig. 21.1). They may have a maximum of amplitude and incidence in corresponding parts of both hemispheres or in one area. This local prominence can usually be distinguished from focal slow waves which appear on a background of generalized slow waves since focal waves arising from a focal structural abnormality usually have a lower frequency, and sometimes lower amplitude, than the surrounding slow waves and they are less reactive to eye opening, alerting and hyperventilation than are generalized asynchronous slow waves.

21.2 GENERAL CLINICAL SIGNIFICANCE OF GENERALIZED ASYNCHRONOUS SLOW WAVES

21.2.1 *Normal generalized asynchronous slow waves* occur in drowsiness and sleep at all ages. During wakefulness, they are prominent in infants, gradually diminish in children and adolescents, and reach a minimum in adults; slightly greater amounts appear in older persons. The slow waves are therefore abnormal only if they exceed the normal range for the age of the patient.

21.2.2 *Abnormal amounts of generalized asynchronous slow*

waves in normal subjects occur in the waking record of 5–10% of adults and in perhaps even a greater percentage of subjects of other ages; a mild excess is far more common than a moderate one. Generalized asynchronous slow waves thus distinguish less sharply between normal and abnormal subjects than do other EEG patterns. Therefore, this finding can only suggest that a patient is more likely to have a cerebral abnormality than a patient with a normal EEG. A marked excess of generalized asynchronous slow waves in the waking EEG indicates a cerebral abnormality in every adult, teenager and child.

21.2.3 *Abnormal generalized asynchronous slow waves* are due to a wide variety of conditions and are the most common and least specific abnormal EEG pattern. However, an EEG showing only an excess of generalized asynchronous slow waves has a certain negative diagnostic value: the absence of other abnormalities reduces the likelihood of a recent focal brain lesion of the hemispheres considerably, and it reduces the probability of a convulsive disorder slightly.

21.3 OTHER EEG ABNORMALITIES ASSOCIATED WITH GENERALIZED ASYNCHRONOUS SLOW WAVES

21.3.1 *Attenuation, slowing and disorganization of alpha rhythm* often occur with mild and moderate generalized slow waves (Fig. 20.1). Marked generalized slow waves replace alpha rhythm completely (Fig. 20.3).

21.3.2 *Bisynchronous slow waves* often appear intermittently in bursts which usually have higher amplitude and restricted distribution and therefore stand out against a background of asynchronous generalized slow waves. Many cerebral abnormalities that eventually lead to bisynchronous slow waves initially cause disorganization of alpha rhythm and mild or moderate asynchronous slow waves, and later produce mixtures of bisynchronous and asynchronous slow waves. The bisynchronous slow waves usually are of greater diagnostic importance than the asynchronous slow waves.

21.3.3 *Focal slow waves, generalized epileptiform activity, periodic complexes and other abnormal patterns* of greater diagnostic significance than asynchronous generalized slow waves often appear on a background of these slow waves.

21.4 MECHANISMS CAUSING GENERALIZED ASYNCHRONOUS SLOW WAVES

Generalized asynchronous slow waves may be produced by various mechanisms. Most of them interfere with structure or function of both hemispheres and involve subcortical white matter or thalamocortical and corticothalamic pathways in a wide distribution; rarely are the generalized slow waves an extension of focal slow waves. Widespread interruption or disorganization of cortical input from the brainstem reticular formation may be an important factor in many cases; brainstem lesions cause widespread asynchronous slow waves in some cases although they are equally likely to produce bisynchronous slow waves. Children are more likely to produce asynchronous slow waves in response to mild cerebral or metabolic disorders (such as high fever) than are adults.

21.5 SPECIFIC DISORDERS CAUSING GENERALIZED ASYNCHRONOUS SLOW WAVES

21.5.1 *Degenerative, developmental and demyelinating diseases.* Most of the degenerative diseases that produce generalized asynchronous slow waves are those that involve the cerebral hemispheres and cause dementia. Degenerative diseases involving the cerebellum, sub-thalamic brainstem and spinal cord do not produce EEG abnormalities.

(1) *Alzheimer's disease* is often associated with an exaggeration of age-related EEG changes (13) and thus leads to: (a) excessive generalized asynchronous slow waves; (b) marked slowing, reduction of amplitude and disorganization of alpha rhythm (Fig. 21.2); (c) fairly frequent bursts of focal slow waves, often with sharp contours, appearing in the temporal regions, most often on the left side; and (d) the appearance of bilaterally synchronous slow waves. While excessive generalized asynchronous slow waves correlate better with dementia than do the other EEG abnormalities, Alzheimer's dementia usually becomes quite obvious before the EEG becomes definitely abnormal. Indeed, *prominent EEG abnormalities occurring early in the course (e.g., within the first 6 months) of a dementia, particularly one that is rapid in onset, argue strongly against the diagnosis of Alzheimer's disease.* Once the dementing illness is well established EEG abnormalities are expected and help to differentiate Alzheimer's disease from other disorders such as the pseudodementia of depression.

(2) *Pick's disease* which can usually not be distinguished from Alzheimer's disease on clinical grounds often produces few EEG abnormalities even in the presence of rather severe dementia.

(3) *Parkinson's disease* is associated with a mild or moderate amount of generalized asynchronous slow wave activity in less than half of all patients. This is not of great clinical importance because the diagnosis is not based on the EEG; however, it is worth noting that the finding of generalized asynchronous slow waves in a patient with Parkinson's disease should cause no alarm. Cerebral slow waves (focal, multifocal or generalized) in the EEG of a patient with Parkinson's disease must be distinguished from artifacts consisting of intermittent or continuous rhythmical 4–6 Hz waves produced by tremor of the head or neck. Rarely, these slow waves may fall in phase with motor unit action potentials from nearby scalp muscles and generate patterns resembling spike-and-wave discharges.

(4) *Progressive supranuclear palsy* may lead to generalized slow waves in advanced cases, but the initial abnormalities of sleep patterns and asynchronous slow waves in the waking record are diagnostically more important.

(5) *Huntington's chorea* may be associated with generalized asynchronous slow waves, but the generalized reduction of amplitude is a more important diagnostic feature.

(6) *Jakob–Creutzfeldt disease* or *spongioform encephalopathy* is characterized by progressive and widespread slowing of the EEG and by disintegration of alpha rhythm. Moderate or marked slow waves replace all normal background activity in advanced cases. In the end stage of the disease, the amplitude of all activity may decrease and the EEG may become nearly flat and featureless. Periodic sharp waves, appearing in the early or middle stages of the disease, are the most characteristic abnormal pattern in this disease (19.3).

(7) *Normal pressure hydrocephalus* often produces no EEG abnormality but may be associated with mild or moderate generalized slow waves or with focal slow waves. The generalized slow waves are asynchronous in most cases, in contrast to

bisynchronous slow waves that may appear in obstructive hydrocephalus.

(8) *Hydrocephalus in children,* regardless of its cause, may be associated with asynchronous generalized slow waves and other abnormalities including bisynchronous slow waves, focal slow waves, and spike foci.

(9) *Tuberous sclerosis* in adults can cause asynchronous generalized slow waves in addition to bisynchronous slow waves and focal spikes; infants and young children show different abnormalities.

(10) *Other degenerative and developmental diseases* may produce generalized asynchronous slow waves as the only abnormality or as one of several abnormalities in some patients; other patients with the same diseases may have normal EEGs. These diseases include: Leber's hereditary optic atrophy, Riley-Day syndrome, Seitelberger's disease, Leigh's disease, microcephaly with or without microgyria, macrogyria or agyria, holoprosencephaly, cerebral palsy, infantile hemiplegia, myotonic dystrophy, trisomy 21, MERRF, and MELAS.

(11) *Multiple sclerosis* produces generalized asynchronous slow waves, reduction of amplitude and other abnormalities in approximately one-half of all cases. The incidence of abnormalities varies widely in different groups of patients, probably depending on acuteness, duration and rate of progression of the disease. Longer duration of the disease may account for higher incidences of abnormalities in some studies of multiple sclerosis.

21.5.2 *Metabolic and toxic encephalopathies.* Generalized asynchronous slow waves may occur in any of these conditions when they cause significant encephalopathy and therefore do not distinguish these conditions from each other or from other conditions. Mild or moderate slow waves, often associated with a disorganization of the background, are usually the first abnormality in the EEG and marked slow waves may be the only abnormality found in the severest stages. Asynchronous slow waves in these encephalopathies may combine with bisynchronous slow waves and other abnormalities in adults and children, and with special patterns in infants (19.1.2). *Moderate to severe toxic or metabolic encephalopathies are often associated with the diagnostically suggestive pattern of nearly absent beta activity and relatively smoothly contoured asynchronous theta and delta waveforms.*

(1) *Congenital encephalopathies such as phenylketonuria, amaurotic familial idiocy, metachromatic and other leukodystrophies (Krabbe's and Pelizaeus–Merzbacher's diseases)* often cause hypsarrhythmia, slow spikes and waves or multifocal independent spikes (19.2) in infancy and early childhood, but only excessive slow waves at later ages. Thus, the three infantile epileptiform patterns are often found in the infantile (Tay–Sachs) and late infantile (Bielschowski–Jansky) storage diseases in the juvenile (Spielmeyer–Vogt) and adult (Kufs) forms of ceroid lipofuscinosis that show only asynchronous generalized slow waves and occasional bisynchronous slow waves.

(2) *Wilson's disease* produces generalized asynchronous or focal slow waves in about one-half of all patients, especially those with significant liver disease.

(3) *Acquired metabolic encephalopathies* such as those due to hepatic failure (e.g., hepatitis, alcoholic liver disease, or Reye's syndrome), renal failure, hypoglycemia, hypoxia and electrolyte imbalances often have an initial phase of generalized asynchronous slow waves and disorganized background followed by combinations of these slow waves with prominent bilaterally synchronous slow waves and other abnormalities. Asynchronous slow waves in these encephalopathies are usually present when the patient begins to become confused and somnolent. As the encephalopathy progresses to the point where the prognosis is poor the EEG loses virtually all activity over 5–6 Hz and periods of widespread flattening appear creating a discontinuous pattern somewhat like burst suppression. In patients who recover, residual slow waves may persist suggesting widespread residual cerebral damage. Metabolic encephalopathies and their corresponding EEG abnormalities are listed in Table 22.1. Hypothyroidism leads to a decrease of the frequency of alpha rhythm and a generalized reduction of overall amplitude whereas hyperthyroidism causes an increase of alpha rhythm frequency (25.6) and an excess of fast activity.

(4) *Toxic encephalopathies* commonly produce generalized asynchronous slow waves in acute intoxications, especially those associated with reduced levels of alertness. Common examples are intoxications by alcohol, barbiturates, and other drugs depressing the central nervous system. However, slow waves induced by drugs are not always accompanied by clinical manifestations of encephalopathy: intravenous administration of atropine, chronic intake of sedatives and psychotropic drugs, or myelography with metrizamide can induce generalized slow waves without producing overt mental changes.

Alcohol. Acute alcohol intoxication may cause generalized asynchronous slow waves, decrease of alpha frequency and increase of central beta activity.

Chronic alcoholism itself produces no EEG abnormalities, but asynchronous generalized slow waves may be found when chronic alcoholism is associated with cerebral atrophy in patients over 60 years of age.

Acute withdrawal syndrome, delirium tremens, and Korsakoff's psychosis usually induce no more than mild or moderate generalized slow waves; only a few cases of Korsakoff's psychosis show more prominent generalized slow waves similar to those of Wernicke's disease. The more common pattern seen in alcohol withdrawal consists of relatively low amplitude background activity in the beta frequency range that is usually composed of cerebral beta activity and intermixed muscle artifact (also referred to as the low voltage fast pattern).

Wernicke's encephalopathy usually produces prominent generalized asynchronous slow waves and often also causes bisynchronous slow waves and a decrease of the alpha rhythm.

Hepatic encephalopathy and subdural hematoma can be indirect results of alcoholism that usually are associated with asynchronous slow waves but often with more characteristic abnormalities such as triphasic waves in hepatic encephalopathy (19.3) or focal slow waves and asymmetries of amplitude in subdural hematoma.

Barbiturates acutely produce prominent central or generalized beta activity and a decrease of alpha rhythm at low or medium blood levels. At higher levels, beta waves and frontal 10–12 Hz waves may persist as generalized asynchronous theta and delta waves emerge and become more prominent until non-reactive delta waves predominate. Then periods of low amplitude activity or of complete electrical silence of a few seconds in duration begin to interrupt the delta waves at short intervals, creating burst-suppression patterns (19.3). With deepening coma, the quiet periods increase in duration and the delta waves in the bursts decrease in amplitude and eventually disappear completely. Electrocerebral silence may persist and ultimately indicate cerebral death although the patient and the EEG may sometimes recover after more than 24 h without recordable EEG.

EEG and clinical recovery from barbiturate intoxication may be protracted, lasting several days or longer, depending on the severity of intoxication. This is also true for short acting barbiturates, such as pentobarbital, whose half-life and toxic effects can increase dramatically with prolonged use.

Chronic intake of barbiturates may either cause excessive beta activity or produce no effect on the EEG.

Barbiturate withdrawal can produce asynchronous slow waves along with bursts of high amplitude bisynchronous theta waves. Photoparoxysmal responses and spontaneous generalized epileptiform activity may also occur.

Phenothiazines, haloperidol and *rauwolfia derivatives* may produce generalized asynchronous slow waves and slowing of alpha rhythm at moderate doses. Toxic overdoses can induce bisynchronous slow waves, prominent beta activity, and bilateral spike-and-wave or multiple spike-and-wave patterns.

Tricyclic antidepressants may produce generalized asynchronous or bisynchronous slow waves, and bilateral spikes or spike-and-wave discharges.

Carbon monoxide and other poisons causing widespread structural brain damage may produce generalized asynchronous slow waves.

Lithium commonly causes varying degrees of generalized asynchronous slowing and less often alpha rhythm slowing, intermittent rhythmic delta activity (FIRDA, OIRDA), or triphasic waves. The likelihood of these abnormalities occurring correlates poorly with lithium serum levels.

Other toxic agents of many different types can produce generalized asynchronous slow waves. These include: carbon disulfide, methyl chloride and bromide, organic solvents, manganese, mercury, tin, strontium, lead, arsenic, bismuth, lithium, monoamine oxidase inhibitors, opiates, chloralose. Some of these are associated with a slowing of alpha frequency and bisynchronous slow waves, others with epileptiform activity. Most vitamin deficiencies causing asynchronous slow waves also cause bisynchronous slow waves.

21.5.3 *Cerebrovascular diseases*

(1) *Syncope of various causes including Stokes–Adams attacks, transient ischemic attacks of the brainstem,* and other conditions causing transitory reductions of blood flow to the entire brain or to the brainstem produce generalized slow waves as consciousness becomes impaired; bisynchronous slow waves may be added. If interruption of blood flow continues then the EEG quickly evolves to electrocerebral inactivity. The slow waves disappear within minutes or hours after recovery from these conditions; persistence of slow waves suggests that structural damage has occurred.

(2) *Postanoxic encephalopathy* is often the direct result of cardiac and respiratory arrest, or the indirect result of metabolic encephalopathy, intracerebral or subarachnoid hemorrhage, or of severe cerebral injury which causes widespread structural cerebral damage and generalized asynchronous slow waves. Depending on the severity of the underlying damage, asynchronous slow waves show higher amplitude and lower frequency (Fig. 21.3) and may be associated with, or replaced by: (a) bursts of bisynchronous slow waves; (b) rhythmical, widespread and unreactive alpha or theta activity;

(c) reduced amplitude; (d) spikes or sharp waves; (e) burst-suppression patterns; or (f) electrocerebral silence (24.6.3).

The prognostic value of the EEG during the first 6 h after the anoxic insult is uncertain. Later, the persistence of electrocerebral silence indicates cerebral death whereas the return of a normal EEG has a good prognosis. Between these extremes, the EEG does not clearly predict the outcome. A non-reactive unchanging pattern of diffuse slowing or a burst suppression pattern suggests a very poor outcome. The presence of elements of normal sleep activity and of any EEG response to alerting stimuli suggests less severe damage and a better prognosis.

(3) *Midbrain* strokes due to thrombosis, embolism or hemorrhage which damage the reticular formation in the central parts of the midbrain reduce the patient's alertness and produce generalized asynchronous slow waves with or without superimposed bisynchronous slow waves. Infarcts in the central parts of the pons may produce coma associated with alpha or theta activity, while infarcts involving the lateral parts of the midbrain or pons usually do not produce EEG abnormalities or alterations of consciousness.

(4) *Multiple cerebral infarcts, lacunar state, fat and air embolism* commonly produce generalized asynchronous slow waves.

(5) *Chronic subdural hematoma* commonly produces generalized asynchronous slow waves, but focal slow waves and asymmetries (23.2) often overshadow this abnormality and always are of greater diagnostic significance.

(6) *Migraine and other headaches* are associated with an abnormally high incidence of generalized asynchronous slow waves and other abnormalities between attacks. Additional abnormalities may appear during migrainous attacks.

21.5.4   *Cerebral trauma*

(1) *Mild head injuries* that cause only a brief loss of consciousness or no unconsciousness at all may produce diffuse asynchronous theta and delta waves and a decrease of alpha amplitude and frequency; the abnormalities usually disappear within hours or days but may persist for weeks even in patients who recover without complications. The abnormalities are generally more severe in children than in adults.

(2) *Severe head injuries* that cause longer periods of unconsciousness are associated with marked generalized asynchronous slow waves and may also be associated with (a) generalized decrease of amplitude, (b) focal decrease of amplitude, (c) focal slow waves, (d) bisynchronous generalized slow waves, (e) early or late focal epileptiform activity, and (f) absence of sleep patterns.

(3) *Progressive traumatic encephalopathy* of boxers and other persons exposed to repeated head injuries is often associated with generalized asynchronous and bisynchronous slow waves; these abnormalities are usually preceded by slowing of alpha rhythm and the appearance of focal slow waves.

21.5.5   *Brain tumors*

(1) *Solitary brain tumors* produce asynchronous generalized slow waves only indirectly, namely when they invade or compress midbrain and diencephalic structures so that alertness is reduced. Focal slow waves or bisynchronous slow waves may precede this development.

(2) *Multiple metastases* cause asynchronous generalized slow waves as the result of initially discrete slow wave foci or as the result of diencephalic or mesencephalic lesions that reduce consciousness.

21.5.6   *Seizure disorders*

(1) *Postictal generalized asynchronous slow waves* may persist for up to several days after a cluster of two or more generalized seizures; they may remain for a few weeks after electro-convulsive treatment or following status epilepticus. Asynchronous slow waves usually resolve completely within hours or remain mild following a single generalized tonic-clonic seizure.

(2) *Interictal generalized asynchronous slow waves* are found in a higher percentage of subjects with epilepsy with generalized tonic-clonic seizures than in the asymptomatic population; the incidence of interictal slow waves is especially high in patients whose seizures are associated with widespread cerebral damage.

(3) *Ictal generalized asynchronous slow waves* are very rare.

21.5.7 *Infectious diseases*

(1) *High fever* can lead to generalized asynchronous slow waves and slowing of alpha rhythm, particularly in children, in keeping with a reduction of alertness. However, slow waves in patients with only moderate fever may be the expression of a cerebral infection.

(2) *Meningitis* is more likely to produce EEG abnormalities if it extends into the brain; generalized slow waves are more common in children than in adults.

(3) *Encephalitis* produces generalized asynchronous slow waves as a signal of widespread involvement of cerebral structure or function. Bisynchronous slow waves may be added as the result of toxic or metabolic complications or of predominant involvement of cortical and subcortical gray matter. Focal slow waves can appear when there is more localized damage, especially that produced by herpes simplex encephalitis and abscesses.

Subacute sclerosing panencephalitis, a late complication of measles infection, initially often produces generalized asynchronous slow waves as a background on which the characteristic periodic complexes later develop.

(4) *Progressive multifocal leukoencephalopathy* produces generalized asynchronous slow waves that may be preceded in onset by focal slow waves.

(5) *Sydenham's chorea,* associated with streptococcal infections, in many cases produces asynchronous generalized slow waves in excess of those of normal children at the same age and in some cases produces bisynchronous slow waves or spikes and sharp waves.

(6) *General paresis due to syphilis* produces asynchronous and, occasionally, bisynchronous rhythmic slow waves in slightly over one-half of all cases whereas patients with other forms of neurosyphilis usually have a normal EEG.

(7) *AIDS dementia complex* or *encephalopathy* is characterized in the early stages by mild degrees of background slowing with widespread bisynchronous and asynchronous waveforms predominantly in the theta frequency range. This may occur at a time when neuroanatomical imaging studies and evoked potential studies are normal. As the disease progresses slowing becomes more prominent. A characteristic EEG pattern has not been identified, however, the author has noted anterior displacement of the normal posterior dominant background resulting in a diffuse or anterior dominant amplitude gradient as a common finding in a number of cases. Milder degrees of background disorganization and slowing may be detectable with serial studies in patients at risk. Asymptomatic HIV infection does not cause EEG abnormalities.

21.5.8 *Psychiatric diseases.* The incidence of generalized asynchronous slow waves is slightly higher in patients with various psychiatric diseases than in the general population (Fig. 21.1). This is most evident in schizophrenia where slow waves are seen most often in the catatonic form and least in the paranoid form. Depression may also be associated, infrequently, with mild degrees of background slowing. In general, the slowing seen in uncomplicated psychiatric disorders occurs infrequently, is usually mild, and can often be attributed to medications, particularly butyrophenones and phenothiazines. Such findings or lack of findings are diagnostically helpful to the extent that: (a) the absence of other abnormalities in the EEG may help to exclude gross organic disease, and (b) the presence of moderate to severe generalized asynchronous slow waves is more likely to occur with organic disorders.

REFERENCES

Bauer, G. (1993) Drug effects and central nervous system poisoning. In: E. Niedermeyer and F. Lopes da Silva (Eds.), Electroencephalography: Basic Principles, Clinical Applications and Related Fields. Third Edition. Williams and Wilkins, Baltimore, pp. 631–642.

Blume, W.T. and Kaibara, M. (1995) Atlas of Adult Electroencephalography. Raven Press, New York.

Brenner, R.P. (1985) The electroencephalogram in altered states of consciousness. In: M.J. Aminoff (Ed.), Electrodiagnosis, Neurologic Clinics. Saunders, Philadelphia, pp. 615–629.

Brenner, R.P. (1993) EEG and dementia. In: E. Niedermeyer and F. Lopes da Silva (Eds.), Electroencephalography: Basic Principles, Clinical Applications and Related Fields. Third Edition. Williams and Wilkins, Baltimore, pp. 339–349.

Courjon, J. (1972) Traumatic disorders. In: A. Rémond (Ed.), Handbook of Electroenceph. Clin. Neurophysiol., Vol. 14B. Elsevier, Amsterdam.

Farrell, D.F. (1969) The EEG in progressive multifocal leukoencephalopathy. Electroenceph. Clin. Neurophysiol. 26: 200–205.

Forstl, H., Sattel, H., Besthorn et al. (1996) Longitudinal cognitive, electroencephalographic, and morphological brain changes in aging and Alzheimer's disease. Br. J. Psychiatr. 168: 280–286.

Giel, R., De Vlieger, M. and Van Vliet, A.G.M. (1966) Headache and the EEG. Electroenceph. Clin. Neurophysiol. 21: 492–495.

Gloor, P., Kalabay, O. and Giard, N. (1968) The electroencephalogram in diffuse encephalopathies: electroencephalograpic correlates of gray and white matter lesions. Brain 91: 779–802.

Hansotia, P., Harris, R. and Kennedy, J. (1969) EEG changes in Wilson's disease. Electroenceph. Clin. Neurophysiol. 27: 523–528.

Johannesson, G., Brun, A., Gustafson, L. and Ingvar, D.H. (1977) EEG in presenile dementia related to cerebral blood flow and autopsy findings. Acta Neurol. Scand. 56: 89–103.

Johannesson, G., Hagberg, B., Gustafson, L. and Ingvar, D.H. (1979) EEG and cognitive impairment in presenile dementia. Acta Neurol. Scand. 59: 225–240.

Kaszniak, A.W., Garron, D.C., Fox, J.H., Bergen, D. and Huckman, M. (1979) Cerebral atrophy, EEG slowing, age, education, and cognitive functioning in suspected dementia. Neurology 29: 1273–1279.

Klass, D. and Westmoreland, B. (1996) Electroencephalography: general principles and adult electroencephalograms. In: J. Daube (Ed.), Clinical Neurophysiology. F.A. Davis, Philadelphia, pp. 73–103.

Kurtz, D. (1976) Section VII. The EEG in acute and chronic drug intoxications. In: A. Rémond (Ed.), Handbook of Electroenceph. Clin. Neurophysiol., Vol. 15C. Elsevier, Amsterdam, pp. 88–104.

Levic, Z.M. (1978) Electroencephalographic studies in multiple sclerosis. Specific changes in benign multiple sclerosis. Electroenceph. Clin. Neurophysiol. 44: 471–478.

Markand, O.N. (1990) Organic brain syndromes and dementias. In: D.D. Daly and T.A. Pedley (Eds.), Current Practice of Clinical Neurophysiology: Electroencephalography. 2nd Edition. Raven Press, New York, pp. 371–400.

Mellerio, F. and Kubicki, S. (1977) Section VII. B. Encephalopathy due to poisoning. In: A. Rémond (Ed.), Handbook of Electroenceph. Clin. Neurophysiol., Vol. 15A. Elsevier, Amsterdam, pp. 108–135.

Nuwer, M.R., Miller, E.N., Visscher, B.R. et al. (1992) Asymptomatic HIV infection does not cause EEG abnormalities: results from the Multicenter AIDS Cohort Study (MACS). Neurology 42: 1214–1219.

Olejniczak, P. and Fisch, B.J. (1999) Metabolic encephalopathies and brain death. In: R. Evans (Ed.), Diagnostic Testing in Neurology. Neurologic Clinics. W.B. Saunders, Philadelphia, Chapter 9.

Radermecker, F.J. (1977a) Infections and inflammatory reactions, allergy and allergic reactions; degeneralive diseases. In: A. Rémond (Ed.), Handbook of Electroenceph. Clin. Neurophysiol., Vol. 15A. Elsevier, Amsterdam, pp. 1–108.

Radermecker, F.J. (1977b) Degenerative diseases of the nervous system. In: A. Rémond (Ed.), Handbook of Electroenceph. Clin. Neurophysiol., Vol. 15A. Elsevier, Amsterdam, pp. 162–191.

Robinson, D.J., Merskey, H., Blume, W.T. et al. (1994) Electroencephalography as an aid in the exclusion of Alzheimer's disease. Arch. Neurol. 51: 280–284.

Rumpl, E., Lorenzi, E., Hackl, J.M., Gerstenbrand, F. and Hengl, W. (1979) The EEG at different stages of acute secondary traumatic midbrain and bulbar brain syndromes. Electroenceph. Clin. Neurophysiol. 46: 487–497.

Sharbrough, F.W. (1993) Nonspecific abnormal EEG patterns. In: E. Niedermeyer and F. Lopes da Silva (Eds.), Electroencephalography: Basic Principles, Clinical Applications and Related Fields. Third Edition. Williams and Wilkins, Baltimore, pp. 197–216.

Silverman, D. (1975) Section VII. The electroencephalogram in anoxic coma. In: A. Rémond (Ed.), Handbook of Electroenceph. Clin. Neurophysiol., Vol. 12. Elsevier, Amsterdam, pp. 81–94.

Soininen, H., Partanen, J., Laulumaa, V. et al. (1991) Serial EEG in Alzheimer's disease: 3 year follow-up and clinical outcome. Electroenceph. Clin. Neurophysiol. 79: 342–348.

Stevens, J.R., Sachdev, K. and Milstein, V. (1968) Behavior disorders of childhood and the electroencephalogram. Arch. Neurol. 18: 160–177.

Stigsby, B., Johannesson, G. and Ingvar, D.H. (1981) Regional EEG analysis and regional cerebral blood flow in Alzheimer's and Pick's diseases. Electroenceph. Clin. Neurophysiol. 51: 537–547.

Tarrier, N., Cooke, E.C. and Lader, M.H. (1978) The EEGs of chronic schizophrenic patients in hospital and in the community. Electroenceph. Clin. Neurophysiol. 44: 669–673.

Vas, G.A. and Cracco, J.B. (1990) Diffuse encephalopathies. In: D.D. Daly and T.A. Pedley (Eds.), Current Practice of Clinical Neurophysiology: Electroencephalography. 2nd Edition. Raven Press, New York, pp. 371–400.

Volavka, J., Feldstein, S., Abrams, R., Dornbush, R. and Fink, M. (1972) EEG and clinical change after bilateral and unilateral electroconvulsive therapy. Electroenceph. Clin. Neurophysiol. 32: 631–639.

Westmoreland, B.F. (1993) The EEG in cerebral inflammatory processes. In: E. Niedermeyer and F. Lopes da Silva (Eds.), Electroencephalography: Basic Principles, Clinical Applications and Related Fields. Third Edition. Williams and Wilkins, Baltimore, pp. 291–304.

Westmoreland, B.F. and Saunders, M.G. (1979) The EEG in the evaluation of disorders affecting the brain diffusely. In: D.W. Klass and D. Daly (Eds.), Current Practice of Clinical Electroencephalography. Raven Press, New York, pp. 307–342.

22 Bilaterally synchronous slow waves

SUMMARY

(22.1) *Bisynchronous slow wave patterns* contain waveforms that have a frequency of less than 8 Hz that appear at the same time in corresponding areas of the left and right hemispheres. These waves may be distributed over the entire head or be limited to one or a few bilateral electrodes; in many cases, their distribution shifts from one moment to the next. They usually appear as intermittent trains of waves on a background of lower amplitude. Bisynchronous slow waves commonly are monomorphic, but may be irregular and arrhythmical. These waves are reduced or blocked by eye opening or alerting; they are increased by hyperventilation and drowsiness. Bisynchronous slow waves frequently appear as the characteristic pattern known as frontal intermittent rhythmical delta activity (FIRDA), also called 'monorhythmic frontal delta' (MFD). FIRDA consists of bursts of high amplitude sinusoidal 2–3 Hz waves over the bifrontal head regions.

(22.2) *Bisynchronous slow waves occur in several normal and abnormal conditions*. Normal bisynchronous slow waves are seen in infants and children during wakefulness and sleep, and in adults during drowsiness and sleep and during and after hyperventilation. Bisynchronous slow waves are abnormal in alert resting adults. Bisynchronous slow waves often result from the projection of an abnormality from distant, subcortical structures, especially from the brainstem reticular system and its rostral connections deep at the midline of the posterior, middle and anterior fossa, to the site of EEG production in the cerebral cortex. These abnormalities include (1) diffuse encephalopathies that involve subcortical and cortical cerebral gray matter more than cerebral white matter; (2) structural lesions that directly or indirectly involve the mesencephalon, diencephalon, orbital and mesial surfaces of the frontal lobe; and (3) metabolic, toxic and endocrine encephalopathies.

(22.3) *Other EEG abnormalities* include a background of generalized asynchronous slow waves from which bisynchronous slow waves are often difficult to distinguish; however, the special diagnostic implications of bisynchronous slow waves justify the attempt to discriminate between these two varieties of generalized slow waves.

(22.4) *Mechanisms* underlying bisynchronous slow waves involve thalamocortical and interhemispheric interactions.

(22.5) *Specific disorders* include many diseases impairing structure and function of deep midline structures and those which produce a widespread involvement of cortical and subcortical structures.

22.1 DESCRIPTION OF PATTERN

Bisynchronous slow waves have a frequency of less than 8 Hz and appear simultaneously in corresponding parts of the two hemispheres. Individual waves are commonly sinusoidal or at least regular (Fig. 22.1). They are usually rhythmical, i.e., they repeat at the same rate and vary by no more than a few hertz over the course of time. They are usually intermittent, lasting for a few seconds and forming trains that begin and end at about the same time on the two sides of the head. The wave

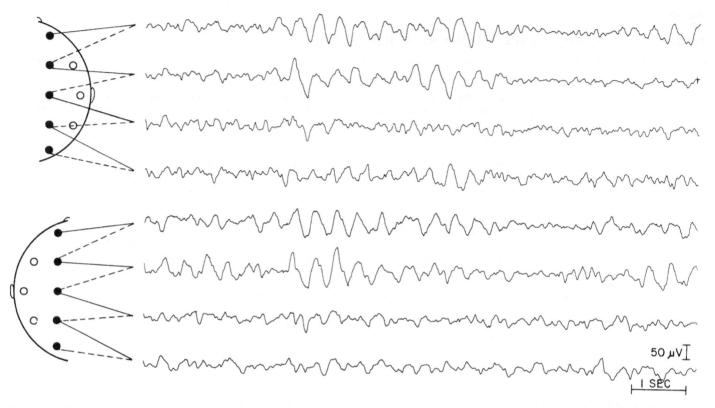

50 µV

1 SEC

Fig. 22.1.   Pattern of frontal intermittent rhythmical delta activity (FIRDA). Trains of bisynchronous slow waves of 2–3 Hz and of high amplitude appear with a maximum in the frontal regions on a background of diffuse slow waves of low to medium amplitude. The patient is an 18-year-old girl who sustained a severe head injury 2 weeks earlier. She had been in coma initially, then was confused and irritated until 2 days before the recording. At the time of the recording, her neurological examination was normal; there were no gross mental symptoms. Follow-up EEGs 7 weeks and several months later were entirely normal; the patient recovered without deficit. The final diagnosis was brainstem contusion.

peaks in one area do not always coincide with the peaks in another area of the same hemisphere, but waves of the same frequency in different areas are usually synchronous on the two sides. In contrast to most other slow waves, bisynchronous slow waves may occur sporadically, separated from each other by periods of entirely normal activity.

Bisynchronous slow waves may be generalized or restricted; they may have a maximum in the same portions of both hemispheres or may be more prominent on one side from moment to moment. They are abolished or reduced on both sides by eye opening or alerting; they are increased during eye closure, hyperventilation and drowsiness. Abnormal bisynchronous slow waves disappear in the background of normal bisynchronous slow waves that occur during sleep stages I–IV, but may reappear in REM sleep.

There are 2 main categories of bisynchronous slow waves: (1) delta frequency, medium to high amplitude and regular and rhythmical (Fig. 22.1); and (2) delta or theta frequency, low to medium amplitude, irregular and arrhythmical (Figs. 22.2 and 22.3). Discrete trains of rhythmical delta waves, i.e. intermittent rhythmical delta activity ('IRDA') (Fig. 22.1), may occur maximally in the frontal areas (frontal intermittent rhythmical delta activity, 'FIRDA') or in the occipital areas (occipital intermittent rhythmical delta activity, 'OIRDA'). Because these waves usually are of only a single frequency, they have also been called 'monorhythmic frontal or occipital delta' (MFD, MOD) activity. Other names, implicating their origin, are 'rythmes à distance' or 'projected slow waves'.

FIRDA and OIRDA often occur at a frequency of 2.5 Hz and may have a slight notch on the descending phase of the waveform. In some cases FIRDA and OIRDA patterns merge or co-exist with generalized triphasic waves.

22.2 CLINICAL SIGNIFICANCE OF BISYNCHRONOUS SLOW WAVES

22.2.1 *Normal bisynchronous slow waves* are seen (1) during drowsiness and sleep at any age; (2) during wakefulness in subjects under the age of 20 years; (3) in response to hyperventilation at any age, especially childhood; (4) in adults having the rare patterns of slow alpha variant and of posterior slow waves (11.7).

22.2.2 *Abnormal bisynchronous slow waves* are those occurring under conditions other than the ones listed above and usually reflect abnormalities located deeply in the brain or at some distance from the recording site. These abnormalities may be diffuse or circumscribed structural lesions, or disorders of cerebral function.

Diffuse structural damage may produce bisynchronous slow waves if it involves gray matter of subcortical structures alone or in combination with cortical gray matter, especially when the gray matter is damaged more than the hemispheric white matter. This is the presumed cause of bisynchronous slow waves in some degenerative encephalopathies.

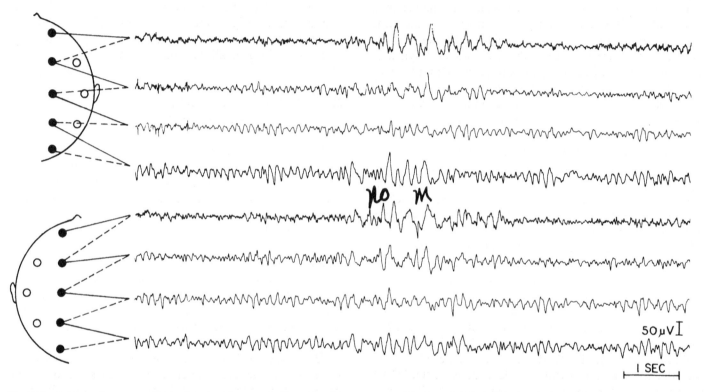

Fig. 22.2. Pattern of paroxysmal bisynchronous slow waves of irregular shape on a normal background. Technician's comment (NO M) means that the patient did not move during this paroxysm. This 58-year-old woman had a parathyroidectomy 18 years earlier. For several weeks before the recording she felt increasingly tired and experienced an episode of nearly fainting. Chvostek and Trousseau signs were positive, serum calcium was decreased at 5.6 mg% and phosphorus was increased at 6.3 mg%.

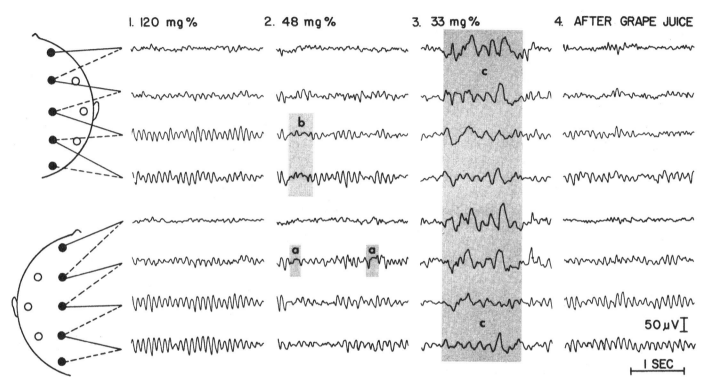

Fig. 22.3. Bisynchronous slow waves induced by hypoglycemia which developed during a glucose tolerance test. (1) Before the beginning of the test, the EEG was normal. (2) At a blood sugar level of 48 mg%, the EEG showed low to medium amplitude diffuse theta (a) and delta (b) waves of low to medium amplitude. (3) At a blood sugar level of 33 mg%, bursts of high amplitude bisynchronous delta and theta waves appeared with a maximum in the frontal regions (c). (4) After the patient drank some grapefruit juice, the EEG returned almost completely to normal. This recording is of an 18-year-old boy with two episodes of nearly fainting several hours after the last meal.

Circumscribed structural lesions may cause bisynchronous slow waves either directly or indirectly. Lesions which are located near the midline at the base of the brain may directly involve the brainstem, diencephalon or the orbital and mesial surfaces of the frontal lobes (Fig. 22.1); lesions located near these structures may secondarily invade, compress, or distort them or render them ischemic or edematous (Fig. 20.3). While increased intracranial pressure by itself does not alter the EEG until it reaches the range of the arterial blood pressure, expanding temporal lobe lesions can produce herniation of the uncus of the temporal lobe which distorts the brainstem and thereby induces bisynchronous slow waves.

Disorders of cerebral function include mainly encephalopathies of toxic and metabolic etiology (Figs. 22.2; 22.3; 22.4; 22.5). The bisynchronous slow waves in these encephalopathies usually disappear when the underlying abnormality is reversed. Transient bisynchronous slow waves may also be seen during and after generalized seizures, in attacks of vertebral-basilar migraine, vertebral-basilar ischemia, in syncope and in some cases of transient global amnesia.

22.3   OTHER EEG ABNORMALITIES ASSOCIATED WITH BISYNCHRONOUS SLOW WAVES

22.3.1   *Reduction, slowing and disorganization of alpha rhythm* may occur with mild or moderate bisynchronous slow waves (Fig. 22.3).

22.3.2   *Generalized asynchronous slow waves* may be so prominent as to obscure bisynchronous slow waves. They usually are not seen in cases of uncomplicated deep circumscribed lesions.

22.3.3   *Focal slow waves, local reduction of amplitude or focal epileptiform activity* suggest either a local lesion which primarily produces focal EEG abnormalities and secondarily involves subcortical structures producing bisynchronous slow waves (Fig. 20.3), or a metabolic or toxic encephalopathy which primarily produces bisynchronous slow waves and is associated with local cerebral damage producing focal EEG abnormalities.

22.4   MECHANISMS CAUSING BISYNCHRONOUS SLOW WAVES

The bilaterally synchronous appearance of slow waves, like that of bilaterally synchronous epileptiform activity, is commonly thought to be due to an abnormal interaction between the cortex and the rostral brainstem and thalamic structures that project diffusely to the cortex (1.2). The involvement of this diffusely projecting system allows the slow waves to be generated with a high degree of interhemispheric synchrony. This may explain why three very different types of basic cerebral pathology, namely diffuse damage to subcortical and cortical gray matter, local lesions near deep midline structures,

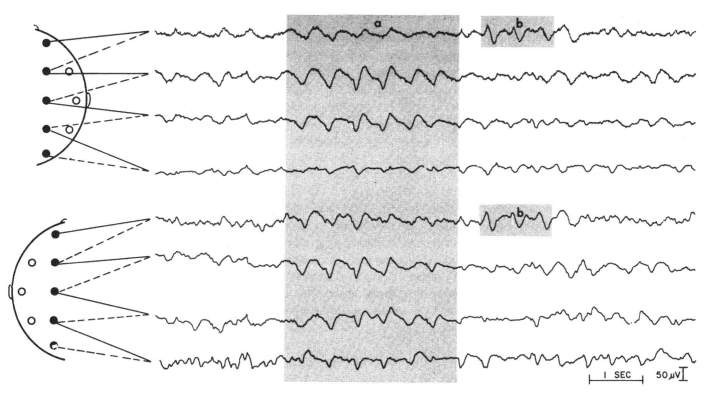

Fig. 22.4.   Pattern of bisynchronous slow waves of the triphasic wave pattern demonstrating an apparent longitudinal time delay of the second phase (downgoing phase) over the more posterior head regions compared to the anterior head regions. The recording is from a 54-year-old in hepatic coma who died several days later.

383

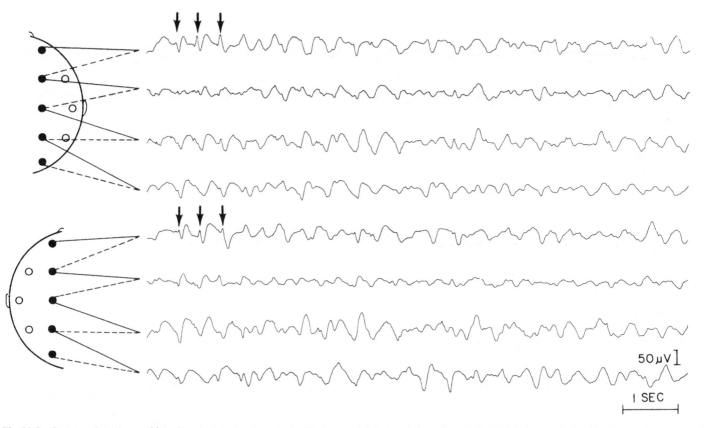

Fig. 22.5. Pattern of continuous bisynchronous slow waves mixed with sharp waves (arrows), sometimes referred to as an atypical triphasic wave pattern. This 26-year-old woman was in delirium due to water intoxication with metabolic acidosis and hyponatremia. Her EEG 5 days later was normal; she had completely recovered.

and metabolic and toxic encephalopathies, all cause bisynchronous slow waves. Diffuse damage to subcortical and cortical gray matter may cause bisynchronous slow waves by damaging both the subcortical and cortical components. Local damage to deep midline structures may directly or indirectly interfere with rostral projections to the cerebral cortex. Metabolic and toxic encephalopathies are known to preferentially affect the function of mesencephalic and diencephalic centers, especially those responsible for alertness.

22.5 SPECIFIC DISORDERS CAUSING BILATERALLY SYNCHRONOUS SLOW WAVES

22.5.1 *Degenerative, developmental and demyelinating diseases*

(1) *Alzheimer's disease* is in some cases associated with bifrontal synchronous slow waves. Asynchronous slow waves and slowing of the alpha rhythm are more common findings. Infrequently, sporadic bilateral triphasic waves occur, usually over the occipital head regions.

(2) *Parkinson's disease* is rarely associated with bisynchronous slow waves; asynchronous slow waves are more common.

(3) *Progressive supranuclear palsy* may produce bisynchronous slow waves, usually after the sleep EEG has become abnormal.

(4) *Other diseases* may induce bisynchronous slow waves in some cases: Leber's hereditary optic atrophy, Ramsey–Hunt's cerebellar myoclonic dyssynergia, myotonic dystrophy, tuberous sclerosis, hydrocephalus, and others.

(5) *Multiple sclerosis* causes bisynchronous slow waves in some patients, often in combination with asynchronous slow waves.

22.5.2 *Metabolic and toxic encephalopathies. Bisynchronous slow waves* occur in the mild or moderate stages of many of these disorders (Table 22.1 and Figs. 22.2; 22.3, part 3) and are commonly associated with other abnormalities, namely slowing of the alpha rhythm and generalized asynchronous slow waves, and less often with focal slow waves and generalized or focal spikes and sharp waves.

In acute encephalopathies, EEG abnormalities appear in a sequence that roughly parallels the severity of the disorder. At the mildest stage, bisynchronous slow waves do not appear spontaneously but may be induced by hyperventilation. The alpha rhythm first decreases in frequency and later in prominence (Fig. 22.3, part 2). Spontaneous bisynchronous slow waves appear first in short bursts (Fig. 22.3, part 3; Fig. 22.2), later in long trains or continuously (Fig. 22.1). Asynchronous

TABLE 22.1

	Decreased alpha frequency	Generalized asynchronous slow waves	Focal slow waves	Triphasic waves	Spikes
ACTH, cortisone Rx	+	+			(+)
Acute anoxia, pulmonary insufficiency	+	+		+ +	
Addison's disease	+	+			(+)
Cerebromacular degenerations		+ +			
CO poisoning		+		(+)	
Dialysis encephalopathy	+	+	(+)	+	+
Hepatic encephalopathy (Fig. 22.2)	+	+		+ +	
Hydration (hyponatremia, Fig. 22.3)		+		+	+
Hyperglycemia without ketoacidosis					+
Hyperparathyroidism (hypercalcemia)	+	+	(+)	+	
Hypoglycemia	+	+	+	+	+
Hypokalemia (alkalosis)	+	+			
Hypoparathyroidism pseudohypo-parathyroidism (hypocalcemia, Fig. 22.4)	+	+			+
Hypopituitarism		+			
Porphyria	+	+	+		+
Renal encephalopathy		+	+	+ +	+
Thyrotoxicosis		+		+	+
Vitamin B12 deficiency	+	+	+		
Wernicke's encephalopathy	+	+			
Wilson's disease		+	+	(+)	

generalized slow waves may appear as soon as the alpha rhythm becomes disorganized; these slow waves become prominent and replace the alpha rhythm when alertness becomes impaired. Other abnormalities that may appear at this stage are focal slow waves and focal, unilateral or generalized spikes or sharp waves. With increasing severity, generalized asynchronous slow waves obscure all other abnormalities; the patient then is usually in deep coma. Death is often preceded by activity of low amplitude which may be interrupted by bursts of slow waves to form suppression burst patterns. If the underlying metabolic or toxic abnormality is reversed at any point, the EEG abnormalities may regress in reverse sequence. Generalized slow waves may persist to indicate that widespread cerebral damage has resulted, or focal slow waves may appear to indicate that local structural damage has occurred.

Most chronic metabolic encephalopathies produce bisynchronous slow waves, slowing of alpha rhythm and generalized asynchronous slow waves.

22.5.3 *Cerebrovascular diseases*

(1) *Transient ischemia* of the brain in general and of the brainstem in particular (e.g., syncope, transient brainstem ischemia, or basilar artery migraine) can lead to bisynchronous slow waves which appear when consciousness begins to decline and abate when consciousness is regained. If they do not completely disappear in a few days, lasting damage is likely to have occurred.

(2) *Strokes* due to thrombosis, embolism or hemorrhage involving the central parts of the upper midbrain and diencephalon can lead to bisynchronous slow waves, often associated with asynchronous slow waves. Large hemispheric strokes, especially hypertensive hemorrhages, may lead to edema and to compression of the brainstem and thereby produce bisynchronous slow waves mixed with focal and asynchronous generalized slow waves. Even strokes in the distribution of the anterior cerebral artery, causing damage to deep parts of the frontal lobe, are capable of producing bisynchronous intermittent frontal delta activity.

(3) *Postanoxic encephalopathy* may be associated with bisynchronous slow waves as one of many abnormalities and indicate involvement of deep structures of the brain.

(4) *Chronic subdural hematoma* may produce intermittent bisynchronous slow waves, especially in cases with fluctuating levels of consciousness; focal slow waves and asymmetric amplitude changes are more common and more characteristic of subdural hematoma.

(5) *Subarachnoid hemorrhage* may be associated with bisynchronous slow waves in addition to asynchronous slow waves in patients with impaired consciousness; focal slow waves may be present and reflect local damage.

(6) *Moyamoya disease in children* may be associated with bisynchronous posterior slow waves.

22.5.4 Cerebral trauma

(1) *Head injury* may produce bisynchronous slow waves either at the onset of unconsciousness when the EEG shows reduction of amplitude, or as patients emerge from deep coma when the EEG shows asynchronous slow waves and other abnormalities due to local or widespread cerebral damage. Bisynchronous slow waves indicate a relatively light stage of post-traumatic coma. Intermittent bisynchronous slow waves may persist for days or weeks after either severe (Fig. 22.1) or seemingly mild head injuries.

(2) *Epidural and acute subdural hematoma* may initially produce bisynchronous slow waves. Focal delta waves and reduction of amplitude may develop more slowly.

(3) *Functional neurosurgery,* for instance coagulation of the anterior parts of the internal capsule or of the thalamus and internal globus pallidus may produce bisynchronous frontal intermittent delta activity, presumably by interrupting subcortical connections to the frontal cortex.

(4) *Progressive traumatic encephalopathy* may produce bisynchronous slow waves, in addition to asynchronous slow waves.

22.5.5 Brain tumors

(1) *Infratentorial tumors* (such as ependymomas or pineal tumors) may cause bisynchronous slow waves if they invade or compress the midbrain or distort the diencephalon. In contrast, tumors located at some distance from these structures, for instance cerebellar tumors and meningiomas of the posterior fossa, may grow to considerable size without compressing the brainstem and producing bisynchronous slow waves. Tumors of the lower brainstem, such as pontine gliomas, do not usually cause EEG abnormalities.

(2) *Supratentorial tumors* are likely to cause bisynchronous slow waves if they are located in or near the diencephalon or the mesial and orbital parts of the frontal lobe. Tumors in other locations may cause bisynchronous slow waves by secondarily involving the deep midline structures. Other associated EEG abnormalities are described above (22.3). Combinations of bisynchronous slow waves with focal slow waves (Fig. 20.3) and focal epileptiform activity are particularly suggestive of deeply located supratentorial tumors. Bisynchronous slow waves as a manifestation of supratentorial tumor are more likely to be found in old persons than in young adults.

(3) *Pseudotumor cerebri* or benign intracranial hypertension shares with cerebral tumors only the name but not the pathology or EEG abnormalities. In contrast to obstructive hydrocephalus, it produces no EEG abnormality in most patients, but bisynchronous slow waves may occasionally be seen.

22.5.6 Seizure disorders

(1) *Interictal* bisynchronous slow waves appear in some patients with primary generalized seizures. In particular, patients with absence attacks often show interictal bisynchronous rhythmical waves of 3 Hz. Interictal slow waves may be only indirectly related to seizures: they may be the manifestation of diseases causing seizures, for instance metabolic encephalopathies or myoclonus epilepsy, or they may be the result of disorders caused by seizures, for instance subdural hematomas or brainstem contusions.

(2) *Ictal* bisynchronous slow waves are rarely the only manifestation of a seizure.

(3) *Postictal* bisynchronous slow waves, including triphasic waves, may occur in addition to asynchronous postictal slow waves.

22.5.7 Infectious diseases

(1) *Fever, reduced alertness, metabolic abnormalities* and electrolyte imbalances associated with infections may cause bisynchronous slow waves, particularly in children and adolescents or the elderly, even if the brain is not infected.

(2) *Meningitis and encephalitis* may cause bisynchronous slow waves in conditions in which they cause asynchronous slow waves.

(3) *Sydenham's chorea* causes bisynchronous slow waves in many cases; asynchronous slow waves may also appear.

22.5.8 Psychiatric diseases

(1) *Personality disorders, behavior disturbances and schizophrenia* are occasionally associated with bisynchronous slow waves. However, this abnormality, like other abnormal EEG patterns, is not common in psychiatric diseases. Therefore, organic causes for this abnormality have to be excluded, particularly treatable conditions such as metabolic and toxic encephalopathies, frontal, hypothalamic and pituitary tumors which all may cause psychiatric symptoms.

(2) *Kleine–Levin syndrome* during attacks may be associated with bursts of bisynchronous slow waves on a background of asynchronous slow waves; these abnormalities are not entirely explained by drowsiness and sleep.

REFERENCES

Allen, E.M., Singer, F.R. and Melamed, D. (1970) Electroencephalographic abnormalities in hypercalcemia. Neurology 20: 15–22.

Bingley, T. and Persson, A. (1978) EEG studies on patients with chronic obsessive-compulsive neurosis before and after psychosurgery (stereotaxic bilateral anterior capsulotomy). Electroenceph. Clin. Neurophysiol. 44: 691–696.

Blume, W.T. and Kaibara, M. (1995) Atlas of Adult Electroencephalography. Raven Press, New York.

Cordeau, J.P. (1959) Monorhythmic frontal delta activity in the human electroencephalogram: a study of 100 cases. Electroenceph. Clin. Neurophysiol. 11: 733–746.

Daly, D., Whelen, J.L., Bickford, R.G. et al. (1953) The electroencephalogram in cases of tumors of the posterior fossa and third ventricle. Electroenceph. Clin. Neurophysiol. 5: 203–216.

Dow, R.S. (1961) The electroencephalographic findings in acute intermittent porphyria. Electroenceph. Clin. Neurophysiol. 13: 425–437.

Gastaut, H. and Fischer-Williams, M. (1957) Electroencephalographic study of syncope. Its differentiation from epilepsy. Lancet ii: 1018–1025.

Glaser, G.H. (1976) Metabolic, endocrine and toxic diseases. In: A. Rémond (Ed.), Handbook of Electroenceph. Clin. Neurophysiol., Vol. 15C. Elsevier, Amsterdam.

Gloor, P. (1976) Section IV. Generalized and widespread bilateral paroxysmal activities. In: A. Rémond (Ed.), Handbook of Electroenceph. Clin. Neurophysiol., Vol. IIB. Elsevier, Amsterdam, pp. 52–87.

Gloor, P., Kalaby, O. and Giard, N. (1968) The electroencephalogram in diffuse encephalopathies: electroencephalographic correlates of grey and white matter lesions. Brain 91: 779–802.

Goldensohn, E.S., Legatt, A.D., Koszer, S. and Wolf, S.M. (1999) Goldensohn's EEG Interpretation: Problems of Overreading and Underreading. Second Edition. Futura Publishing Company, Armonk, NY.

Harner, R.N. and Katz, R.I. (1975) Section IV. Electroencephalography in metabolic coma. In: A. Rémond (Ed.), Handbook of Electroenceph. Clin. Neurophysiol., Vol. 12. Elsevier, Amsterdam, pp. 47–62.

Hasegawa, K. and Aird, R.B. (1963) An EEG study of deep-seated cerebral and subtentorial lesions in comparison with cortical lesions. Electroenceph. Clin. Neurophysiol. 15: 934–946.

Heller, G.L. and Kooi, K.A. (1962) The electroencephalogram in hepato-lenticular degeneration (Wilson's disease). Electroenceph. Clin. Neurophysiol. 14: 520–526.

Johannesson, G., Brun, A., Gustafson, L. and Ingvar, D.H. (1977) EEG in presenile dementia related to cerebral blood flow and autopsy findings. Acta Neurol. Scand. 56: 89–103.

Klass, D.W. and Westmoreland, B.F. (1996) Electroencephalography: general principles and adult electroencephalograms. In: J. Daube (Ed.), Clinical Neurophysiology. F.A. Davis, Philadelphia, pp. 73–103.

Markand, O.N. (1984) Electroencephalography in diffuse encephalopathies. J. Clin. Neurophysiol. 1: 357–407.

Martinius, J., Matthes, A. and Lombroso, C.T. (1968) Electroencephalographic features in posterior fossa tumors in children. Electroenceph. Clin. Neurophysiol. 25: 128–139.

Schaul, N., Gloor, P. and Gotman, J. (1981a) The EEG in deep midline lesions. Neurology 31: 157–167.

Schaul, N., Lueders, H. and Sachdev, K. (1981b) Generalized bilaterally synchronous bursts of slow waves in the EEG. Arch. Neurol. 38: 690–692.

Sharbrough, F.W. (1993) Nonspecific abnormal EEG patterns. In: E. Niedermeyer and F. Lopes da Silva (Eds.), Electroencephalography: Basic Principles, Clinical Applications and Related Fields. Third Edition. Williams and Wilkins, Baltimore, pp. 197–215.

Sidell, A.D. and Daly, D.D. (1961) The electroencephalogram in cases of benign intracranial hypertension. Neurology 11: 413–417.

Su, P.C. and Goldensohn, E.S. (1973) Progressive supranuclear palsy. Arch. Neurol. 29: 183–186.

Van der Drift, J.H.A. and Magnus, O. (1962) The EEG with space occupying intracranial lesions in old patients. Electroenceph. Clin. Neurophysiol. 14: 664–673.

Wallace, P.W. and Westmoreland, B.F. (1976) The electroencephalogram in pernicious anemia. Mayo Clin. Proc. 51: 281–285.

Westmoreland, B.F. and Saunders, M.G. (1979) The EEG in the evaluation of disorders affecting the brain diffusely. In: D.W. Klass and D. Daly (Eds.), Current Practice of Clinical Electroencephalography. Raven Press, New York, pp. 307–342.

Wilkus, R.J. and Chiles, J.A. (1975) Electrophysiological changes during episodes of the Kleine–Levin syndrome. J. Neurol. Neurosurg. Psychiat. 38: 1225–1231.

23 Localized and lateralized changes of amplitude: asymmetries

SUMMARY

(23.1) Asymmetry is characterized by differences in amplitude of the EEG recorded from the two sides of the head. Differences in amplitude may involve the entire background or only certain background patterns. Local reduction of the amplitude of a rhythmical background pattern in some cases is associated with a 0.5–2 Hz reduction in frequency. A consistent asymmetry of beta activity of greater than 35% is considered abnormal and an asymmetry of greater than 50% is considered abnormal for the alpha rhythm.

(23.2) *Causes* of asymmetry are either unilateral lesions (most of which are superficial) or changes in the conducting medium (such as subdural hematomas, skull defects, or local scalp edema) between the cortex and recording electrodes. The amplitude of activity in the alpha and beta frequency range is usually reduced on the side of the lesion. Cerebrovascular disease may sometimes result in a seemingly paradoxical ipsilateral increase in background amplitude. Amplitude may be reduced by local cortical damage (e.g., superficial infarctions, tumors and head injuries) or by transient disturbances of cerebral function (e.g., transient ischemic attacks and migraine). Extracerebral lesions can also change EEG amplitude. Subdural hematomas may reduce it and skull defects may increase it. The alpha rhythm may be reduced by lesions of thalamocortical connections. In some instances, the alpha rhythm is reduced by anterior lesions.

(23.3) *Other EEG abnormalities,* if limited to one side, may further help to indicate the site of the underlying cerebral abnormality.

(23.4) *Mechanisms* of asymmetries involve either changes of cortical EEG production, as in the case of structural or functional cortical lesions, or alterations of the media between cortex and recording electrodes, such as fluid collections or skull defects.

(23.5) *Specific disorders* causing asymmetries include many clinically important diseases.

(23.6) *Asymmetries of alpha, beta, mu and other rhythms* are seen in a variety of clinical conditions.

23.1 DESCRIPTION OF PATTERN

Asymmetry consists of a difference in the amplitude of activity recorded from corresponding areas on the two sides of the head (Figs. 23.1; 23.2; 23.3). Asymmetries usually affect all types of background activity during wakefulness and sleep, but sometimes affect mainly one frequency band or waveform pattern (Fig. 23.1). Thus, an asymmetry may involve only the alpha rhythm, beta rhythm, mu rhythm, responses to photic stimulation and hyperventilation, or certain sleep patterns, such as sleep spindles. A local decrease in the amplitude of alpha rhythm is often associated with a decrease of alpha frequency.

Lesions which cause an asymmetry of normal background activity may also cause an asymmetry of abnormal activity. This can produce difficulties in identifying the side of the ab-

393

normality. For instance, a superficial lesion reducing the amplitude of the EEG on the same side may also cause bilateral abnormalities such as slow waves or epileptiform activity. This combination makes the abnormal activity appear with a higher amplitude on the uninvolved side and falsely suggests that the uninvolved side is the abnormal one (Fig. 23.2). To correctly identify the involved side in these cases, the EEG reader must carefully search for the following signs:

(1) normal patterns which should be reduced in amplitude on the abnormal side (Fig. 23.1);

(2) subtle (1–2 Hz) differences in the peak frequency of the background rhythm (with the slower frequency indicating the more abnormal side);

(3) reduced reactivity on the abnormal side; and

(4) additional abnormalities that may be limited to the abnormal side.

Asymmetries of activity involving large parts of the hemispheres can be recognized with referential recordings. However, asymmetries between small areas are better detected with bipolar linkages between closely spaced electrodes. Asymmetry of amplitude can be accepted as having an intra-

TABLE 23.1

Asymmetries

Abnormal patterns	Causes	Mechanisms	Examples of diseases
Decreased amplitude of all types of activity	Local cortical damage	Decreased cortical EEG production	Cortical infarct, Sturge–Weber syndrome
	Local disorder of cortical function	As above	Local cortical ischemia
	Unilateral increase of media between cortex and recording electrodes	Decreased electrical impedance within the conducting media	Subdural hematoma
		Increased electrical impedance between cortex and recording electrodes	Skull hyperostosis
Of alpha, beta, mu rhythm, sleep patterns	Defect may be distant, at presumed site of pacemaker	Decreased rhythmical input to cortex	Cerebral infarcts, tumors, injuries, without reliable relation to location of rhythm
Increased amplitude	Skull defects	Decreased electrical impedance between cortex and electrodes	Postoperative skull defect

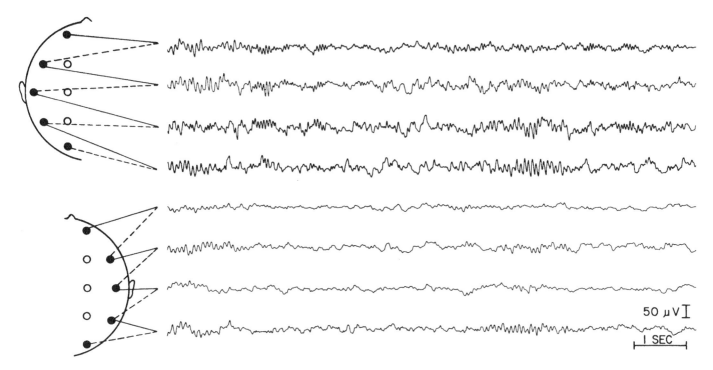

Fig. 23.1.   Pattern of asymmetry of normal background activity. Sleep spindles and slow waves of sleep are attenuated over the right side. This 7-year-old boy has signs characteristic of Sturge–Weber syndrome: a right facial nevus, cerebral calcifications extending into the parietal and temporal areas, and left-sided and generalized motor seizures.

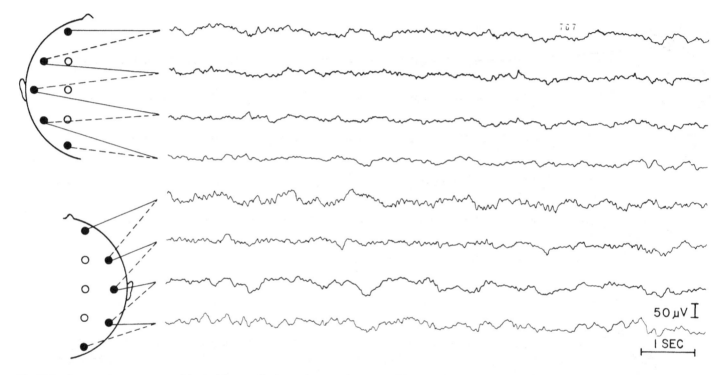

Fig. 23.2. Pattern of asymmetry combined with generalized asynchronous slow waves. The reduction of amplitude on the left side attenuates the generalized slow waves on that side and thereby makes them appear with higher amplitude on the right side, falsely suggesting a right-sided cerebral abnormality. The correct localization of an abnormality on the left side is suggested by the circumstance that the faster frontal rhythms are also reduced on the left side. The patient is a 37-year-old chronic alcoholic in coma. A large chronic subdural hematoma on the left side was evacuated a few hours after this EEG recording.

cranial cause only if errors in electrode placement, electrode impedance imbalances, differences in gain and filter settings, skull defects, and scalp edema have been excluded.

23.2 CLINICAL SIGNIFICANCE OF ASYMMETRIES

23.2.1 *Normal asymmetries* are those described earlier for the alpha rhythm and for photic driving. The mu rhythm typically occurs bilaterally with similar amplitude over the two hemispheres. But asymmetry of photic driving, POSTs or the mu rhythm alone, in the absence of other abnormalities, is of little clinical significance. A consistent asymmetry of beta activity of greater than 35% is considered abnormal and an asymmetry of greater than 50% is considered abnormal for the alpha rhythm.

23.2.2 *Abnormal asymmetries* are usually due to a decrease of amplitude on the side of the cerebral abnormality. Only rarely is the amplitude of activity above 8 Hz increased on the involved side causing activity of lower amplitude to appear on the normal side. However, in the absence of associated localizing abnormalities, or in the presence of bilateral abnormal EEG activity, it may be difficult to decide which side is abnormal (see above).

Asymmetries of all background activity. A decrease of amplitude of all types of activity in one area is due either to a reduction of cortical EEG production or to an increase of the media (e.g., subdural hematoma) separating the cortex from the recording electrodes. Reductions of cortical electrogenesis may be long-lasting and due to structural lesions such as cortical strokes, tumors and injuries. Transient amplitude reductions may follow focal seizures or be due to reversible conditions such as transient local ischemia or migraine.

An increase of amplitude of all types of activity in one area is much rarer than a decrease of amplitude. It is usually due to a local skull defect.

Asymmetry of alpha rhythm has lateralizing but little localizing value. A local decrease of the amplitude in the posterior head regions may be due (a) to a lesion of the underlying cortex; (b) to a lesion of the thalamus or its connections to the underlying cortex; or (c) to a lesion in the frontal and central regions.

Asymmetry of beta rhythm with reduction of amplitude is the earliest and most sensitive indicator of cortical dysfunction or a local cortical lesion. An increase may rarely be seen as the first sign of a superficial brain tumor, a decrease may be the last evidence of a long-standing atrophic scar.

Asymmetry of hyperventilation responses and sleep patterns may occur in an isolated fashion or in association with asymmetries of other patterns. When present they suggest a lesion of the hemisphere with lower amplitude.

23.3 OTHER ABNORMALITIES ASSOCIATED WITH ASYMMETRIES

23.3.1 *Focal slow waves* may appear in an area of reduced amplitude suggesting that white matter under the cortex is involved as well as the cortex itself. The center of the lesion may show waves of the slowest frequencies and of the lowest amplitude.

23.3.2 *Focal epileptiform activity* may appear in or near the area of depressed amplitude suggesting local irritation of the cortex. The combination of focal epileptiform activity and reduced amplitude may be the manifestation of a cortical epileptogenic lesion or the result of a very recent focal seizure.

23.3.3 *Generalized asynchronous and bisynchronous slow waves and generalized epileptiform activity* may be attenuated on the side of a lesion causing a reduction of amplitude and thus falsely suggest a lesion on the opposite side (see above).

23.4 MECHANISMS CAUSING LOCAL CHANGES OF AMPLITUDE

23.4.1 *Decreases of amplitude* are due to mechanisms that vary with the type of underlying lesion:

(1) *Reduction of cortical EEG production* may be due to structural damage reducing the total area of functioning cortical nerve cells, particularly of the large pyramidal neurons which are the major generators of the EEG (1.1). A temporary reduction of electrocortical potential changes may be due to a transient decrease of regional cerebral blood flow resulting in local hypoxia and hypoglycemia. These conditions may completely depolarize cortical neuronal membranes leaving them incapable of responding to excitatory and inhibitory input.

(2) *Interposition of material* between the cortical generators and the recording electrodes can attenuate the EEG by one of two mechanisms; the effect depends on the electrical properties of the interposed material. Substances of high impedance such as thickened skull or greasy scalp act as insulators and partly isolate the electrocortical potentials from the recording electrodes. Substances of low impedance such as subdural blood or spinal fluid act as conductors within the volume under the electrodes and shunt the potential differences before they reach the electrodes.

(3) *Selective decreases of the alpha rhythm* may be due to derangements of thalamocortical networks that produce the impulses that help to synchronize the cortical neurons in the posterior head regions (1.2). The mechanisms whereby frontal and central lesions reduce posterior alpha rhythm are unknown.

23.4.2 *Increases of amplitude* are commonly seen after craniotomy and are partly due to reduced impedance between the EEG generator and the recording electrodes; in addition, local cortical excitability may produce local increases in amplitude.

Seemingly paradoxical asymmetric increases in background activity amplitude may occur over the hemisphere affected by a pathological process. In the author's experience this occurs most commonly in cerebrovascular disease, particularly in middle cerebral artery territory ischemia and infarction. In such cases several other EEG features (23.1) often appear that help to identify the abnormal hemisphere:

(1) there may be a slight (0.5–1 Hz) slowing of the higher amplitude background activity, particularly during eye closure at rest,

(2) during drowsiness intermixed theta or delta waveforms may appear on the abnormal side, and

(3) background reactivity may be partially reduced on the abnormal side (23.1).

23.5 SPECIFIC DISORDERS CAUSING ASYMMETRIES OF AMPLITUDE

23.5.1 *Developmental, degenerative and demyelinating diseases*

(1) *Porencephaly, holoprosencephaly and other defects* due to developmental malformation, perinatal injury or disease may show reduced EEG amplitude in addition to focal slow waves and focal epileptiform activity over areas of atrophic brain defects.

(2) *Sturge–Weber syndrome* is commonly associated with a decrease of amplitude on the side of the nevus (Fig. 23.1). This decrease may be found in infancy before cortical calcium deposits develop. The EEG may also show focal slow waves and focal epileptiform activity in the same area; bilateral synchronous slow waves and widespread epileptiform activity may be present.

(3) *Paget's disease* may cause a local increase in the thickness of the skull and thereby decrease the amplitude of the EEG over the involved area.

(4) *Multiple sclerosis* may produce a local decrease of EEG amplitude with or without other abnormalities.

23.5.2 *Metabolic and toxic encephalopathies*

A local or unilateral decrease of amplitude is not a direct result of these diseases but may occur as the result of complications, especially of cortical infarcts in renal, hypertensive, hypoglycemic and anoxic encephalopathy, and of subdural hematoma in hepatic and Wernicke's encephalopathy.

23.5.3 *Cerebrovascular diseases*

(1) *Attacks of transient ischemia* involving the cortex of parts of the cerebral hemispheres may cause a local decrease of amplitude. The effects of acute local ischemia can be observed when EEG monitoring is used during carotid endarterectomies: a local reduction of amplitude, usually preceded by slow waves, may occur after clamping of the internal carotid artery.

(2) *Strokes* involving the cortex may cause a prolonged reduction of amplitude over the infarcted area. Focal slow waves may be present in the same area or in the surrounding parts during the acute stage but a reduction of amplitude may outlast other EEG abnormalities in the chronic stage.

Less often middle cerebral artery territory infarctions may produce a widespread increase in background activity. As noted above, this may be accompanied by other findings that include: (1) irregularities in amplitude and frequency; (2) a 0.5–2 Hz reduction in the peak background rhythm compared to homotopic head regions; (3) less well sustained rhythmic alpha and beta activity; and (4) reduced reactivity.

Lacunar infarction rarely causes moderate EEG changes but in 20–40% of cases may cause mild abnormalities such as a slight amplitude asymmetry or mild intermittent slowing (Petty et al., 1995). The main value of the EEG in lacunar infarction is that it demonstrates a great disparity between the mild or absent EEG changes and the severe degree of sensory impairment or hemiparesis. Strokes causing such symptoms by carotid occlusion or occlusion of a major branch of the anterior cerebral or middle cerebral artery always produce moderate to severe ipsilateral EEG abnormalities.

(3) *Chronic subdural hematoma* causes a unilateral or focal decrease of background amplitude in about one-half of all cases; alpha rhythm may be depressed more than other background activity. Focal slow waves are even more common than a decrease of amplitude in chronic subdural hematoma, but the decrease of amplitude is an important signal of a superficial lesion and should always raise the suspicion of a subdural hematoma.

(4) *Subarachnoid hemorrhage* may produce amplitude asymmetry especially if there is local cortical damage or significant vasospasm.

(5) *Migraine* may cause unilateral reduction of amplitude during attacks. Between attacks, patients with migraine may show persistent reductions of background amplitude, especially of alpha rhythm, possibly representing residues of vascular damage incurred during an attack.

23.5.4 *Cerebral trauma*

(1) *Head injuries* that are mild may lead to an immediate and transient decrease of amplitude that does not indicate definite cerebral damage. Severe head injuries can cause various EEG abnormalities initially and may later be followed by a long-lasting decrease of amplitude indicating residual structural damage due to contusions, intracerebral hemorrhage, epidural and acute subdural hematomas. Traumatic hemorrhages of newborn infants may be characterized by large areas of depressed amplitude.

(2) *Subgaleal hematoma,* a collection of blood between skull and scalp occurring mainly in infants with linear skull fractures, acts like a subdural or epidural hematoma in that it attenuates the amplitude of the EEG locally.

(3) *Scalp edema,* often caused by infiltration of intravenous fluids given through scalp veins to newborn infants, is a possible source of local attenuation of EEG amplitude.

(4) *Cranial defects* such as burrholes or larger defects remaining after neurosurgical operations are characterized by a local increase of background amplitude. These asymmetries appear not only in recordings from electrodes placed over the defect but also in recordings from electrodes on bone near the edges of the defect. Alpha rhythm of higher amplitude may be recorded on the side of bony defects near the posterior head regions. Beta activity may be found near bone defects in any part of the head; contralateral beta activity may be either absent or of lower amplitude. Bone defects near the central regions are often associated with a mu-like rhythm, local slow waves and sharply contoured waves, all of which block like mu rhythm (11.3); mu rhythm of lower amplitude is not always present on the other side (Fig. 23.3). The appearance of these unilateral rhythms near a bone defect raises the question whether they are due only to the bone defect. Bone defects cause a fairly selective reduction of electrical impedance for fast EEG rhythms. A cerebral abnormality is more likely if (a) the activity on the two sides differs not only in amplitude but also in waveform and frequency, (b) recording from electrodes at some distance from the edge of the bone defect also shows abnormally slow activity, and (c) differences of amplitude develop gradually after removal of the bone. While the reduction of an asymmetry after replacement of the bone (Fig. 23.3) suggests that the asymmetry was due to the bone defect, its persistence does not necessarily indicate that it is due to a cerebral abnormality because persisting gaps between skull and replacement may cause persistent asymmetries of impedance. Moreover, even if asymmetries are due to a cerebral abnormality, the abnormality may consist of no more than local meningo-cortical adhesions and cortical gliosis; only in the case of clear-cut focal slow waves and spikes would one suspect the recurrence of an underlying cerebral lesion such as a tumor or a subdural hematoma, or the development of an epileptogenic focus.

(5) *Hemispherectomy,* i.e., the partial or complete removal of a hemisphere, reduces the amplitude of the EEG on the operated side in most cases but causes little change in some.

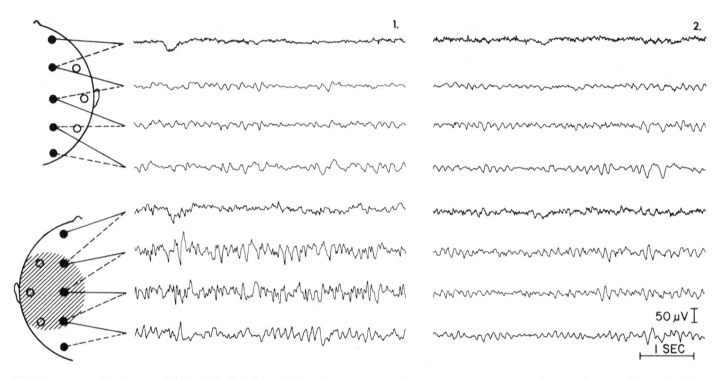

Fig. 23.3. Pattern of local amplitude changes due to a skull defect. (1) Theta waves resembling mu rhythm appear at the left central electrode which is located over a skull defect indicated by the hatched area in the diagram on the left. Frontal beta rhythm and occipital alpha rhythm are also larger on the left than on the right side. (2) After repair of the skull defect, both sides show symmetrical activity. This 48-year-old woman had an acute traumatic subdural hematoma evacuated 2 months before the recording in part 1; part 2 was recorded 3 months after repair of the skull defect. She had no neurological abnormalities at the time of either recording.

The EEG on the operated side is generated by the opposite hemisphere and by deep remnants of the operated hemisphere that are volume conducted to the recording electrodes on the operated side. The volume conducted EEG is attenuated by the electrical shunting effect of cerebrospinal fluid which usually accumulates in the operated space.

23.5.5 *Brain tumors. Primary and metastatic brain tumors* rarely first manifest by an asymmetry of amplitude in alpha, beta or mu rhythms.

23.5.6 *Seizure disorders*

(1) *Postictal* local reduction of amplitude, including delta activity, commonly appears immediately and only for a few seconds after a focal seizure discharge. Localized attenuation of alpha and beta frequency activity may persist for several minutes.

(2) *Interictal asymmetry* is usually due to the lesion causing the seizures, for instance an old cerebral infarction, residual damage after a head injury, Sturge–Weber syndrome or porencephaly.

(3) *Ictal* decreases of amplitude (19.4) are usually bilateral, even in partial complex seizures. However, a local reduction of amplitude often briefly precedes focal seizure discharges.

23.5.7 *Infectious diseases*

(1) *Encephalitis* of any etiology can produce a local reduction of amplitude in the area of maximum involvement. A lasting reduction indicates residual local damage.

(2) *Abscesses* can decrease the amplitude of all background activity or of alpha, beta or mu rhythms only.

(3) *Progressive multifocal leukoencephalitis* in its early stages may reduce the amplitude of background activity locally before causing generalized asynchronous slow waves.

(4) *Thrombophlebitis* of the cerebral venous sinuses may reduce the amplitude of all activity locally or unilaterally, especially in the acute phase when unilateral seizure discharges or status epilepticus are also likely to occur.

23.5.8 *Psychiatric diseases* without gross organic abnormalities are not associated with localized or lateralized reductions of EEG amplitude. Therefore, the finding of an asymmetry in a patient with psychiatric disease should prompt an investigation for an organic cerebral lesion.

23.6 ASYMMETRIES OF ALPHA, BETA, MU AND OTHER RHYTHMS

A decrease of the amplitude of one of these rhythms is usually part of an amplitude reduction involving all types of activity in one area. However, in a few conditions, the amplitude of one of these rhythms is reduced on one side or in one area while the amplitude of other activity remains symmetrical or is not reduced to the same extent. To be abnormal, an asymmetry of these rhythms must exceed their normal range of asymmetry (23.2.1). A selective asymmetry of alpha or theta rhythms alone does not indicate which is the abnormal side. However, clinically important asymmetries are often associated with a decrease of the frequency of that rhythm, or with other unilateral or focal EEG abnormalities that help to lateralize the underlying lesion correctly. In most instances, an asymmetry of the alpha rhythm is due to a posterior lesion and asymmetries of central beta and of mu rhythms are due to anterior lesions.

23.6.1 *Asymmetries of the alpha rhythm*

(1) *Chronic subdural hematoma* may show a preferential depression of alpha rhythm. This is seen more commonly with posterior than with anterior hematomas.

(2) *Hemispheric infarctions* may reduce the amplitude of alpha rhythm more than that of other activity; a decrease of alpha activity may be the last residual abnormality of old infarcts.

(3) *Migraine* may reduce alpha rhythm unilaterally acutely during the attack; alpha rhythm may be found to be asymmetrical in the interval between attacks without other evidence for infarction.

(4) *Head injuries* can lead to a unilateral decrease of the amplitude of alpha rhythm acutely. Asymmetry of alpha rhythm may be present while other EEG abnormalities due to the injury are also present; the alpha asymmetry may persist and be the last residual of severe head injuries or the only effect of mild head injuries.

(5) *Brain tumors and abscesses* involving the hemispheres, the thalamus or the floor of the third ventricle may selectively decrease alpha amplitude.

23.6.2 *Asymmetries of the beta and mu rhythms*

(1) *Developmental lesions* reduce beta activity if they lead to cortical defects such as those seen in porencephaly or local atrophy.

(2) *Degenerative diseases* may produce an asymmetrical reduction of beta and mu before producing generalized reductions of amplitude.

(3) *Vascular diseases* may cause atrophic lesions producing selective reductions of the beta and mu rhythms; *central fast activity activated by movement* may be seen in postanoxic action myoclonus.

(4) *Cerebral trauma and brain operations* leading to skull defects are followed by a local increase of fast activity or mu rhythm, often associated with other abnormalities.

(5) *Brain tumors and abscesses* may cause a reduction (or rarely an increase) in beta activity and the mu rhythm as the earliest EEG abnormality.

(6) *Ictal and interictal* beta activity may be produced by epileptogenic foci (19.4).

23.6.3 *Asymmetry and asynchrony* of sleep activity may persist in infants and children with perinatal cerebral abnormalities, particularly those with hydrocephalus. An asymmetry of sleep spindles can occur at any age as the result of hemispheric tumors, infarcts, Sturge–Weber's syndrome, leukotomy or other conditions, which involve either: (1) the reticular nucleus and other non-specific thalamic nuclei involved in the generation of sleep spindles, (2) the thalamocortical projections of the non-specific nuclei, or (3) the cortex which receives those projections. Sleep spindle asymmetry may accompany a similar asymmetry of abnormal patterns, such as

triphasic waves, OIRDA, and FIRDA, that are also dependent on thalamocortical projections.

REFERENCES

Binnie, C.D. (1987) Recording techniques: montages, electrodes, amplifiers and filters. In: A.M. Halliday, S.R. Butler and R. Paul (Eds.), A Textbook of Clinical Neurophysiology. Wiley, Chichester, pp. 3–22.

Chatrian, G.E., Somasundaram, M. and Foltz, E.L. (1969) EEG changes in subgaleal hematomas. Electroenceph. Clin. Neurophysiol. 26: 524–527.

Cobb, W. and Sears, T.A. (1960) A study of the transmission of potentials after hemispherectomy. Electroenceph. Clin. Neurophysiol. 12: 371–383.

Cobb, W.A., Guiloff, R.J. and Cast, J. (1979) Breach rhythm: the EEG related to skull defects. Electroenceph. Clin. Neurophysiol. 47: 251–271.

Coull, B.M. and Pedley, T.A. (1978) Intermittent photic stimulation: clinical usefulness of nonconvulsive responses. Electroenceph. Clin. Neurophysiol. 44: 353–363.

Fisch, B.J. and Pedley, T.A. (1985) Evaluation of focal cerebral lesions. Role of electroencephalography in the era of computerized tomography. In: M.J. Aminoff (Ed.), Electrodiagnosis, Neurologic Clinics. Saunders, Philadelphia, pp. 649–662.

Fisch, B.J., Pedley, T.A. and Keller, D.A. (1988) A topographic background symmetry display for comparison with routine EEG. Electroenceph. Clin. Neurophysiol. 69: 491–494.

Fukuyama, Y. and Tsuchiya, S. (1979) A study on Sturge–Weber syndrome. Report of a case associated with infantile spasms and electroencephalographic evolution in five cases. Eur. Neurol. 18: 194–204.

Goldensohn, E.S., O'Brien, J.L. and Ransohoff, J. (1961) Electrical activity of the brain. In patients treated with hemispherectomy or extensive decortication. Arch. Neurol. 5: 210–220.

Green, R.L. and Wilson, W.P. (1961) Asymmetries of beta activity in epilepsy, brain tumor, and cerebrovascular disease. Electroenceph. Clin. Neurophysiol. 13: 75–78.

Homan, R.W., Herman, J. and Purdy, P. (1987) Cerebral localization of international 10–20 system electrode placement. Electroenceph. Clin. Neurophysiol. 66: 376–382.

Jaffe, R. and Jacobs, L. (1972) The beta focus: its nature and significance. Acta Neurol. Scand. 48: 191–203.

Kellaway, P. (1979) An orderly approach to visual analysis: parameters of the normal EEG in adults and children. In: D.W. Klass and D.D. Daly (Eds.), Current Practice of Clinical Electroencephalography. Raven Press, New York, pp. 69–147.

Kelly, J.J., Sharbrough, F.W. and Westmoreland, B.F. (1978) Movement-activated central fast rhythms: an EEG finding in action myoclonus. Neurology 28: 1037–1040.

Labar, D.R., Fisch, B.J., Pedley, T.A., Fink, M.A. and Solomon, R.A. (1991) Quantitative EEG monitoring for patients with subarachnoid hemorrhage. Electroenceph. Clin. Neurophysiol. 78: 325–332.

Leissner, P., Lindholm, L.E. and Petersén, I. (1970) Alpha amplitude dependence on skull thickness as measured by ultrasound technique. Electroenceph. Clin. Neurophysiol. 29: 392–399.

Marshall, C. and Walker, A.E. (1950) The electroencephalographic changes after hemispherectomy in man. Electroenceph. Clin. Neurophysiol. 2: 147–156.

Nealis, J.G.T. and Duffy, F.H. (1978) Paroxysmal beta activity in the pediatric electroencephalogram. Ann. Neurol. 4: 112–116.

Petty, G.W., Labar, D.R., Fisch, B.J., Pedley, T.A., Mohr, J.P. and Khandji, A. (1995) Electroencephalography in lacunar infarction. J. Neurol. Sci. 134: 47–50.

24 Generalized changes of amplitude: symmetrically high and low amplitude

SUMMARY

(24.1) *The patterns* of generalized changes of amplitude consist of a bilateral symmetrical decrease or increase of amplitude of all types of normal activity or of specific patterns only. Such changes of amplitude are best recognized by comparison with previous recordings from the same subject because the amplitude of normal patterns differs widely in the general population. While abnormally low amplitude can be defined by voltage criteria, there is practically no upper limit for the amplitude of normal patterns. Instead the amplitude of activity in a given frequency range is judged as normal or abnormal according to its distribution and its amplitude in comparison to the activity in the other frequency bands.

(24.2) *Causes* of bilateral abnormally low amplitude are similar to those producing unilateral reductions of amplitude, namely bilateral superficial lesions which reduce cortical function transiently or in a lasting manner or which change the media between cortex and recording electrodes. Bilateral reductions of amplitude may also be due to widespread cerebral disorders such as Huntington's chorea, postanoxic encephalopathy, cerebral death or severe changes in cortical function caused by toxic and metabolic diseases.

(24.3) *Other EEG abnormalities* include generalized asynchronous slow waves and periodic complexes.

(24.4) *Mechanisms* causing bilateral amplitude reductions consist of either decreased cortical activity or an alteration of the electrical impedance of the media between cortex and recording electrodes. Selective changes of the amplitude of specific rhythms are more likely to be due to selective involvement of distant structures controlling the production of these rhythms by the cortex.

(24.5) *Specific disorders* reducing overall amplitude include those associated with a wide variety of structural and functional abnormalities.

(24.6) *A bilateral decrease of the alpha rhythm* may result from toxic and metabolic conditions or simply from anxiety.

(24.7) *Generalized increased beta activity* is seen mainly as a result of tranquilizers and sedatives.

(24.8) *Sleep patterns* may be changed in amplitude by drugs and metabolic disorders.

24.1 DESCRIPTION OF PATTERNS

24.1.1 *Abnormally low amplitude* consists of cerebral activity not exceeding 20 μV in any channel in any montage during relaxed wakefulness while the eyes are closed (Figs. 24.1; 24.2). The low amplitude must be sustained. Transient reductions of amplitude due to transient anxiety, mental effort, eye opening or an intermittent increase or decrease of alertness are not abnormal. Because amplitude increases with interelectrode distances up to about 10 cm, the diagnosis of abnormally low amplitude requires the use of similar interelectrode distances. Correct gain settings, calibration signals and elec-

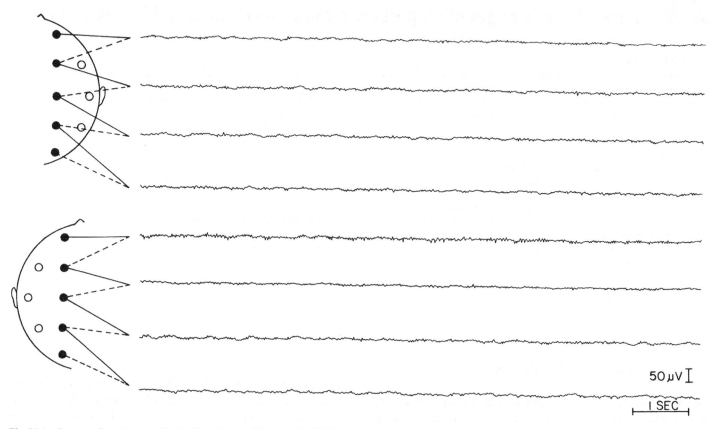

Fig. 24.1. Pattern of very low amplitude. There is no activity over 10 μV. The patient is a 66-year-old woman with a family history of Huntington's disease who has had progressive chorea and dementia for over 12 years.

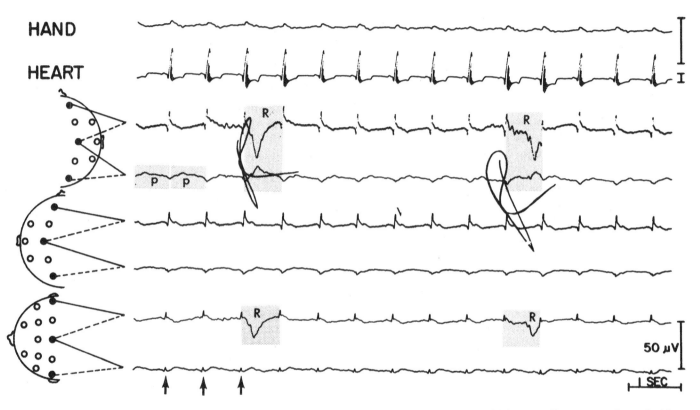

Fig. 24.2.   Pattern of electrocerebral silence. The recording is made with widely spaced electrodes and high sensitivity. The artifacts commonly seen in this type of recording are due to heart beat (arrows), pulse waves (p) and movement by artificial respiration (R). This recording is from a 65-year-old woman who had a cardiac arrest 3 days earlier and was in postanoxic coma without spontaneous respiration and brainstem mediated reflexes since then. EEG and clinical condition did not change over the next 24 h and she was pronounced cerebrally dead.

trode impedances are essential to make the diagnosis of low amplitude. Special recording methods are needed to establish the absence of all electrocerebral activity (5.3).

24.1.2 *Abnormally low amplitude of specific patterns* can be diagnosed only by comparison with previous recordings from the same subject because of the great variability of the amplitude of normal patterns between subjects. A complete absence of the alpha rhythm in children and teenagers or an absence of sleep spindles in a prolonged recording between the ages of 6 and 8 months is abnormal.

24.1.3 *Abnormally high amplitude* of all types of activity cannot be well defined. Even though activity of 100 μV is uncommon in wakeful adults, it is only considered abnormal on the basis of frequency, morphology, or distribution rather than amplitude alone.

24.1.4 *Abnormally high amplitude of specific patterns* can usually be determined only by comparison with previous records from the same individual. The common exception is prominent, sustained, rhythmic, generalized beta activity.

24.2 CLINICAL SIGNIFICANCE OF HIGH AND LOW AMPLITUDE

24.2.1 *Normal* high amplitude occurs in the waking record of children and in deep stages of sleep at any age. Normal low amplitude of under 20 μV occurs transiently as a result of eye opening, mental effort, anxiety, alerting or drowsiness.

24.2.2 *Abnormally low amplitude of all activity. Low amplitude in normal subjects* can be seen in about 5–10% of adults but is not acceptable as normal in younger persons. The reduction of amplitude is usually mild in degree, i.e. the waking record contains some activity of 10–20 μV. Such low voltage patterns (11.8) in adults are similar to slight excesses of generalized asynchronous slow waves in that they do not sharply distinguish between normal and abnormal subjects. This does not affect the significance of a moderate and marked reduction of overall amplitude (>10 μV) which is abnormal at any age.

Abnormally low amplitude in abnormal conditions may be either transient and due to acute anoxic, toxic and metabolic factors, head injury, postictal state, or permanent and due to lasting damage resulting from these conditions or from other diseases significantly involving the cortex, such as Huntington's chorea. As the severity of a diffuse acute or subacute encephalopathy progresses the EEG may demonstrate brief, 1 to several second intervals of diffuse attenuation that give the record a somewhat discontinuous appearance. This is a regular occurrence in severe hepatic and renal encephalopathy. An increase in material between cortex and recording electrodes such as that caused by bilateral subdural hematoma may produce a bilateral reduction of amplitude.

24.2.3 *Abnormal reduction of specific patterns* is presumably due to abnormalities involving specific afferent input to the cortex. For instance, interruption of either projections from nucleus reticularis of the thalamus or thalamocortical pathways may attenuate or abolish the alpha rhythm or sleep spindles.

24.2.4 *Abnormal increases of specific patterns* of clinical importance are the increases of beta rhythms produced by toxic and metabolic conditions, especially by barbiturates, benzodiazepines, high dose chloral hydrate and other sedatives, tranquilizers and by hyperthyroidism.

24.3 OTHER EEG ABNORMALITIES ASSOCIATED WITH HIGH AND LOW AMPLITUDE

24.3.1 *Generalized asynchronous slow waves* are often produced by the same conditions that reduce amplitude.

24.3.2 *Bursts of periodic sharp waves and slow waves* may alternate with activity of low amplitude in burst-suppression and other special patterns (19.3).

24.4 MECHANISMS CAUSING GENERALIZED CHANGES OF AMPLITUDE

24.4.1 *Reduction of cortical potentials* may be caused by structural abnormalities (e.g., infarction, trauma, tumor), or by metabolic abnormalities (e.g., ischemia, hypoglycemia, renal or hepatic failure, postictal depression, general anesthesia).

24.4.2 Reduced amplitude bilaterally can arise from the same mechanisms that cause local decreases of amplitude (23.4.1).

24.4.3 *Selective decreases of amplitude of patterns* over both sides of the head may be due to interference with distant structures that control the production of these patterns in the cortex. Thus, bilateral reduction of alpha rhythm may be due to bilateral interruption of the input from thalamic nuclei that modulates the alpha rhythm in the cortex or to an increase in the activity of diencephalic and mesencephalic structures which normally abolishes alpha rhythm under conditions of increased and decreased alertness. As stated above, reduction of sleep spindles may also be due to an abnormality of thalamic or thalamocortical pathway function. The term 'desynchronization' is sometimes used to describe replacement of widespread activity of medium or high amplitude, for instance the alpha rhythm or slow waves, by low amplitude irregular activity. It is thought that the disappearance of these patterns, which often occurs in response to alerting stimuli, may be due, in part, to a failure in the synchronization of the underlying neuronal potentials (1.2).

24.4.4 *High amplitude of all types of activity* may, in some cases, be due to relatively short distances between cortex and recording electrodes or to a thin or absent skull. Other causes for high amplitude of normal activity in adults are unknown. Although abnormally low cerebral metabolism causes low amplitude and normal metabolism is required for maintenance of normal amplitude, an increase of metabolism does not increase the amplitude of activity under 13 Hz.

24.4.5 *High amplitude beta activity* seen in some toxic and metabolic conditions is poorly understood.

24.5 SPECIFIC DISORDERS CAUSING A GENERALIZED DECREASE OF AMPLITUDE OF ALL TYPES OF ACTIVITY

24.5.1 *Degenerative, developmental and demyelinating diseases*

(1) *Huntington's chorea* is characterized by activity of very low amplitude that correlates with the severity of cortical atrophy observed in this disease (Fig. 24.1). In the early stages of the disease when background features are still distinguishable, alpha rhythm becomes disorganized, asynchronous generalized slow waves appear, and sleep spindles and K complexes disappear. The EEG of family members at risk does not predict later development of the disease.

(2) *Jakob–Creutzfeldt disease* leads to a decrease of overall amplitude in the advanced stages, i.e. after generalized asynchronous slow waves have vanished. Activity of very low amplitude is also present during the intervals between periodic generalized sharp waves.

(3) *Alzheimer's disease* is associated with a decrease of background amplitude in some cases; alpha and beta activity are usually affected most. Generalized slow waves are a more reliable indicator of dementia.

(4) *Microcephaly* may cause low amplitude of the EEG in addition to other abnormalities.

(5) *Multiple sclerosis* in malignant, progressive cases may be associated with a generalized reduction of amplitude although generalized asynchronous slow waves are a more common abnormality in this disease.

24.5.2 *Metabolic and toxic encephalopathies.* Many of these encephalopathies reduce the amplitude of the EEG by reducing cerebral blood flow, oxygen supply and metabolism. Hypo- or hyperthermia can also decrease EEG amplitude.

(1) *Acute cerebral anoxia* immediately results in asynchronous and bilaterally synchronous slow waves which may be followed by a generalized decrease of amplitude and electrocerebral silence within less than 1 min if anoxia persists.

(2) *Hypothermia* leads to a decrease of EEG amplitude and frequency beginning at about 25°C. Electrocerebral activity disappears completely between 10 and 20°C. Because reduction of amplitude even after long periods of hypothermia is reversible, hypothermia must be excluded as a cause or contributing factor in cases of electrocerebral silence in the determination of cerebral death. *It is generally accepted that EEGs for this purpose be recorded only if the body temperature is above 90°F (32.2°C).*

(3) *Hyperthermia* of over 42°C reduces the amplitude of the EEG. Moderate hyperthermia can increase the overall amplitude of the EEG; slow waves appear when consciousness becomes clouded.

(4) *Hypothyroidism* usually reduces the frequency and organization of alpha rhythm and characteristically leads to an overall reduction of amplitude. Generalized asynchronous slow waves may also be present and sleep spindles are often reduced or absent.

(5) *Hypoparathyroidism and pseudohypoparathyroidism* may lead to a reduction of amplitude in general and of the alpha rhythm in particular as one of several abnormalities.

(6) *Renal and hepatic encephalopathy* may reduce the amplitude of all activity or of the alpha rhythm in the intermediate stages; in advanced hepatic encephalopathy, an acute decrease of amplitude is often associated with sudden clinical deterioration. Bisynchronous slow waves and other abnormalities are most common in the intermediate stages (Table 24.1).

(7) *Intoxication with barbiturates and other drugs* depressing the central nervous system leads to loss of amplitude preterminally. However, electrocerebral silence may develop long before cerebral death: partial or complete recovery of EEG and cerebral function is possible even after more than 24 h of electrocerebral silence. However, iatrogenic electrocerebral silence (as in barbiturate coma for status epilepticus) for more than 1 h should be avoided because of the often fatal consequences. Intoxication with barbiturates and other central nervous system depressant drugs must be excluded in the evaluation of electrocerebral silence as an indicator of cerebral death.

24.5.3 *Cerebrovascular diseases*

(1) *Syncope, Stokes–Adams attacks and other conditions* producing a generalized reduction of cerebral blood flow, like acute anoxia from other causes, produce first generalized slow waves and then a generalized decrease of amplitude.

(2) *Postanoxic encephalopathy* causes generalized asynchro-

TABLE 24.1

Generalized changes of amplitude

Abnormal patterns	Causes	Mechanisms	Examples of diseases
Decreased amplitude of all types of activity	Bilateral cortical damage	Decreased cortical EEG production	Bilateral cortical infarcts, postanoxic encephalopathy
	Widespread cerebral damage, involving cortex and sub-cortex	Decreased cortical EEG pro-duction, decreased rhythmical input to cortex	Huntington's chorea, Jakob–Creutzfeldt disease, postanoxic encephalopathy
	Widespread disturbance of cortical function	Same as above	Anoxia, hypothermia, hypothyroidism, preterminal toxic-metabolic encephalop-athies, head injury, postictal coma, anxiety
	Bilateral increase of media between cortex and recording electrodes	Decreased electrical impedance within the conducting media	Bilateral subdural hematomas
		Increased electrical impedance between cortex and recording electrodes	Dry scalp, Paget's disease
of alpha rhythm	Mild metabolic disturbances	Decreased cortical EEG production	Early hepatic, hypothyroid, hypo-parathyroid encephalopathy
	Functional subcortical dis-turbance	Decreased rhythmical input to cortex	Anxiety
of sleep patterns	Structural brainstem damage	As above	Progressive supranuclear palsy, pontine lesions
	Functional brainstem dis-turbance	As above	Phenylketonuria, hypothyroidism, uremia
Increased amplitude of all types of activity	No known pathological cause		
of beta rhythm	Functional disturbance	Unknown	Sedatives and tranquilizers, hyper-thyroidism, anxiety
of sleep patterns	As above	Increased input to cortex	Tricyclic antidepressants, flurazepam

nous slow waves and other EEG abnormalities. Low amplitude may occur either early, i.e. during the first few hours or days, or late, i.e. as a residual after other EEG abnormalities have abated. If low amplitude of early onset persists, the prognosis is poor.

(3) *Cerebral death* is often the immediate result of cerebral anoxia which is most often caused by cardiac or respiratory arrest; toxic, metabolic and traumatic disorders can cause cerebral death directly or through cardiopulmonary arrest.

(4) *Bilateral subdural hematomas* may reduce the amplitude of the EEG over wide parts of both hemispheres and are often associated with focal slow waves.

(5) *Vertebrobasilar insufficiency* seems to be associated with an increase in the incidence of low voltage EEG patterns between attacks.

(6) *Air embolism* may suddenly reduce the amplitude of the EEG or induce generalized slow waves, occasionally more on the right side than the left, possibly because of the more direct arterial pathway.

24.5.4 *Cerebral trauma. Head injury,* if mild, may produce a brief decrease of amplitude with or without loss of consciousness. Severe head injuries that lead to coma may be associated with prolonged or progressive reduction of amplitude which carries a poor prognosis. A decrease of amplitude may occur during recovery in comatose patients who initially demonstrated high amplitude generalized slow waves.

24.5.5 *Brain tumors.* Tumors do not reduce overall amplitude directly; pituitary tumors may cause low amplitude by producing hypothyroid encephalopathy.

24.5.6 *Seizure disorders*

(1) *Ictal decreases of amplitude* over all head regions may occur at the beginning of a generalized seizure. A sudden localized decrease in amplitude is frequently seen in direct cortical recordings from the area of ictal onset. Less often this same localized 'flattening' of the EEG may be seen in routine scalp electrodes. A reduction of amplitude may be the only ictal manifestation in some forms of seizures (for example, electro-decremental electrographic seizures). Flattening of the EEG, or low amplitude fast activity, also occurs during 'cerebellar fits' which, despite their name and paroxysmal character, are not seizures but attacks of decerebration; the underlying mechanisms are not yet fully understood but probably involve a sudden increase in intracranial pressure, generalized cortical ischemia, or an abrupt change of the function of the brainstem reticular formation.

(2) *Postictal depression* of amplitude appears immediately after most generalized seizures and lasts a few minutes until

slow waves supervene. Localized amplitude depression over the area of seizure onset may also be seen immediately (within the first 5 s) after complex partial (focal onset) seizures.

24.5.7 *Infectious diseases*

(1) *Encephalitis and meningitis* can reduce overall EEG amplitude during the acute phase of the disease. Persistence of reduced amplitude indicates residual widespread cerebral damage.

(2) *Progressive multifocal leukoencephalopathy* may reduce amplitude widely or induce generalized asynchronous slow waves.

24.5.8 *Psychiatric diseases.* Anxiety reduces overall amplitude mainly by reducing alpha rhythm.

24.6 GENERALIZED DECREASE OR ABSENCE OF ALPHA RHYTHM

24.6.1 *Normal attenuation of alpha rhythm* occurs with eye opening, alerting, mental effort, anxiety, and decreased alertness to the level of drowsiness. A slight degree of anxiety is a normal reaction of many subjects to their first EEG recording and usually disappears during the course of the recording, particularly after hyperventilation. The transient nature of these normal patterns of alpha attenuation distinguishes them from the low voltage patterns and from the effects of pathological anxiety.

24.6.2 *Acute and chronic anxiety reactions* of psychiatric relevance produce commonly a persistent reduction of alpha rhythm leaving mainly cerebral beta activity or a low voltage fast pattern.

24.7 GENERALIZED INCREASE OF BETA RHYTHM

24.7.1 *Normal* prominence of beta activity varies widely; beta activity is very prominent in some normal subjects and absent in others. However, the persistence of increased beta activity throughout the recording is abnormal.

24.7.2 *Hyperthyroidism* produces prominent fast activity either in the central regions or in a wide distribution. This activity mixes with, or replaces, alpha rhythm. The frequency of alpha rhythm is often increased. The beta activity stands out in part because of the relative absence of activity in the other frequency ranges.

24.7.3 *Barbiturates, benzodiazepines, other sedatives and tranquilizers* acutely induce widespread fast activity with a maximum in the central and frontal regions. This persists during wakefulness and becomes more conspicuous during drowsiness when the alpha rhythm disappears. Barbiturates in doses producing coma may cause non-reactive frontal or widespread 10–12 Hz rhythms (25.3.2). Many patients chronically taking barbiturates lose this fast activity. Beta activity induced by barbiturates does not directly depend on the involvement of subthalamic brainstem centers. Beta activity is produced acutely (within 3 min) and unilaterally following a single intracarotid injection of barbiturate medication in the absence of sleep induction (as frequently observed during WADA testing). This unilateral beta may then be easily seen to persist for 25–50 min.

24.7.4 *Acute and chronic anxiety* are usually associated with an increase of fast activity in addition to the reduction of alpha activity. In many cases, however, this activity may be largely due to muscle artifact.

24.8 CHANGES OF AMPLITUDE OF SLEEP PATTERNS

In general, any disorder that causes a diffuse decrease in amplitude during wakefulness causes a similar depression of sleep patterns. Some disorders, however, have earlier or more selective effects on certain sleep patterns.

24.8.1 *Phenylketonuria* may be associated with absent, jagged or sharp spindles and K complexes during sleep while the waking record may show hypsarrhythmia, multifocal independent spikes or slow spikes and waves.

24.8.2 *Progressive supranuclear palsy* may cause reduction of sleep spindles, V waves and K complexes and disturbances of sleep cycles (25.4.5) even before the waking record shows abnormalities.

24.8.3 *Hypothyroidism, hypoparathyroidism, uremia and chlorpromazine intake* are among other conditions which reduce sleep spindles more than overall amplitude.

24.8.4 *Tricyclic antidepressants, benzodiazepines, barbiturates and other hypnotics,* notably flurazepam, increase sleep spindles.

24.8.5 *Alzheimer's disease,* which involves the degeneration of cholinergic pathways, early in its course reduces the number of rapid eye movements that normally occur in REM sleep. This is consistent with the observation that REM sleep is neurochemically a cholinergic state.

REFERENCES

Alvarez, L.A., Moshe, S.L., Belman, A.L., Maytal, J., Resnick, T.J. and Keilson, M. (1988) EEG and brain death determination in children. Neurology 38: 227–230.

Arfel, G., Casanova, C., Naquet, R., Passelecq, J. and Dubost, C. (1967) Etude électro-clinique de l'embolie gazeuse cérébrate en chirurgie cardiaque. Electroenceph. Clin. Neurophysiol. 23: 101–122.

Bauer, G. (1987) Coma and brain death. In: E. Niedermeyer and F. Lopes da Silva (Eds.), Electroencephalography: Basic Principles, Clinical Applications and Related Fields. Urban and Schwarzenberg, Baltimore, pp. 391–404.

Beecher, H.K. (1968) A definition of irreversible coma. JAMA 205: 337–340.

Brenner, R.P., Schwartzman, R. and Richey, E. (1975) Prognostic significance of episodic low amplitude or relatively isoelectric EEG patterns. Dis. Nerv. Syst. 36: 582.

Cabral, R., Prior, P.F., Scott, D.F. and Brierley, J.B. (1977) Reversible profound depression of cerebral electrical activity in hyperthermia. Electroenceph. Clin. Neurophysiol. 42: 697–701.

Celesia, G.G. and Andermann, F. (1964) Some observations on the electrographic correlates of the decerebrate attack. Electroenceph. Clin. Neurophysiol. 16: 295–300.

Chatrian, G.E. (1986) Electrophysiologic evaluation of brain death: a critical appraisal. In: M.J. Aminoff (Ed.), Electrodiagnosis in Clinical Neurology. Churchill/Livingstone, New York, pp. 669–736.

Jørgensen, E.O. (1974) EEG without detectable cortical activity and cranial nerve areflexia as parameters of brain death. Electroenceph. Clin. Neurophysiol. 36: 70–75.

Klass, D.W. and Westmoreland, B.F. (1996) Electroencephalography: general principles and adult electroencephalograms. In: J. Daube (Ed.), Clinical Neurophysiology. F.A. Davis, Philadelphia, pp. 73–103.

Leestma, J.E., Hughes, J.R. and Diamond, E.R. (1984) Temporal correlates in brain death. Arch. Neurol. 41: 147–152.

Niedermeyer, E. (1963) The electroencephalogram and vertebrobasilar artery insufficiency. Neurology 13: 412–422.

Rae-Grant, A.D., Strapple, C. and Barbour, P.J. (1991) Episodic low-amplitude events: an underrecognized phenomenon in clinical electroencephalography. J. Clin. Neurophysiol. 8: 203–211.

Schultz, M.A., Schulte, F.J., Akiyama, Y. and Parmelee, A.H. (1968) Development of electroencephalograph sleep phenomena in hypothyroid infants. Electroenceph. Clin. Neurophysiol. 25: 351–358.

Scott, D.F., Heathfield, K.W.G., Toone, B. and Margerison, J.H. (1972) The EEG in Huntington's chorea: a clinical and neuropathological study. J. Neurol. Neurosurg. Psychiat. 35: 97–102.

Sharbrough, F.W. (1993) Nonspecific abnormal EEG patterns. In: E. Niedermeyer and F. Lopes da Silva (Eds.), Electroencephalography: Basic Principles, Clinical Applications and Related Fields. Third Edition. Williams and Wilkins, Baltimore, pp. 197–215.

Sharbrough, F.W., Messick, J.M. and Sundt, T.M. (1973) Correlation of continuous electroencephalograms with cerebral blood flow measurements during carotid endarterectomy. Stroke 4: 674–683.

Sishta, S.K., Troupe, A., Marszalek, K.S. and Kremer, L.M. (1974) Huntington's chorea: an electroencephalograph and psychometric study. Electroenceph. Clin. Neurophysiol. 36: 387–393.

Trewby, P.N., Casemore, C. and Willians, R. (1978) Continuous bipolar recording of the EEG in patients with fulminant hepatic failure. Electroenceph. Clin. Neurophysiol. 45: 107–110.

25 Deviations from normal patterns

SUMMARY

Several patterns are abnormal due to features other than those described in the preceding chapters. These patterns include: (1) abnormal slowing of the alpha rhythm; (2) abnormal reactivity of the alpha rhythm; (3) activity of theta, alpha and beta frequency in coma and seizures; (4) abnormal reactivity in coma; and (5) abnormal timing and incidence of sleep patterns.

25.1 ABNORMAL FREQUENCY OF THE ALPHA RHYTHM

25.1.1 *Description of patterns.* A unilateral decrease in the frequency of the alpha rhythm is abnormal if it results in a consistent left–right difference of over 0.5 Hz. Left–right differences in alpha frequency of less than 1 Hz are difficult to appreciate by routine visual inspection but can be detected using signal analysis methods such as spectral analysis. The underlying abnormality is always located on the side with the lower alpha frequency.

A bilateral increase or decrease in the frequency of the alpha rhythm can be diagnosed with certainty only by comparing records from the same patient. To qualify as abnormal, the alpha frequency should be consistently lowered by more than 2 Hz between recordings performed with the patient in a similar level of alertness. The chances of reliably detecting such changes in older children and adults are considerably increased by the routine practice of asking specific alerting questions during the recording (e.g., time, date, mental calculation, etc.). It is obvious, however, that without a previous record for comparison many patients with an abnormal reduction of the alpha frequency will escape detection because significant decreases in frequency may occur without falling below the lower normal value of 8 Hz. Even so, it is important to be aware that an alpha rhythm of 8–8.5 Hz is likely to represent an abnormal decline in frequency, even in elderly individuals. A bilateral increase of the frequency of alpha rhythm ⩾ 16 Hz usually represents a normal fast alpha variant, i.e. a beta rhythm that has a similar distribution and reactivity as the alpha rhythm.

25.1.2 *Clinical significance of frequency changes of alpha rhythm. Bilateral decrease of alpha frequency* is often due to conditions which slow the metabolism of the brain. Many of these conditions are associated with a decrease of alertness,

419

memory, awareness and orientation. Some of these conditions are transient, for instance toxic or metabolic encephalopathies; others are associated with long-standing damage, for instance cerebral atrophy or bilateral subdural hematomas. Generalized slowing of alpha rhythm may be an early signal of various types of abnormalities that later produce other, more specific, abnormalities. Reduced cardiac output, as in severe congestive heart failure, is regularly associated with a 1–2 Hz slowing of the alpha rhythm and of background activity in general. Once the low cardiac output condition is treat-

TABLE 25.1

Deviations from normal patterns

Abnormal patterns	Causes	Examples of diseases
1. Bilateral decrease of alpha frequency	Generalized disturbance of cerebral function:	
	Metabolic disorders	Hypothyroidism, hepatic and renal encephalopathy
	Change of rhythmical input to cortex	Reduced alertness
	Bilateral structural damage to occipital cortex or its thalamic input	Alzheimer's disease, multiple infarcts, subdural hematoma
2. Unilateral decrease of alpha frequency	Unilateral disturbance of function of occipital cortex or its thalamic input	Transient ischemic attack, condition after mild head injury
	Unilateral structural damage to occipital cortex or its thalamic input	Unilateral chronic subdural hematoma, condition after severe head injury, cerebral infarct
3. Bilateral increase of alpha frequency	Metabolic disorders	Hyperthyroidism, fever
4. Unilateral failure of alpha blocking	Parietal or temporal lobe lesions	Tumors, infarcts
5. Bilateral failure of alpha blocking on monocular input	Disorders of one eye or optic nerve	Monocular blindness
6. Absence of alpha rhythm, presence of occipital spikes (Table 19.4)	Long-standing diseases of both eyes or central visual path	Congenital or early acquired binocular blindness
7. Alpha frequency coma	Central pontine lesions	Infarcts, head injuries
	Widespread cerebral damage	Postanoxic encephalopathy
8. Ictal activity of alpha or beta frequency (Table 19.3)	Local or widespread cerebral damage in newborns	Infantile partial or generalized seizures or status epilepticus
	Irritative temporal lobe lesions	Partial complex seizure activity

ed, the alpha rhythm and background activity increase in frequency.

Unilateral decrease of alpha frequency usually occurs in conditions that also cause a unilateral decrease of the amplitude of alpha rhythm. Such decreases may be the only residual EEG abnormality in mild or old vascular or traumatic lesions of the posterior head regions, but they occasionally appear early in expanding tumors and in lesions of the central and frontal areas.

Bilateral increase of alpha frequency occurs in some conditions of increased cerebral metabolism.

25.1.3 *Other EEG abnormalities associated with abnormal frequency of alpha rhythm.* An abnormal reduction in alpha rhythm frequency may be the only abnormal finding (e.g., high therapeutic or toxic levels of phenytoin), or it may occur in association with asynchronous or synchronous slow waves, or epileptiform abnormalities.

25.1.4 *Mechanisms causing an abnormal frequency of the alpha rhythm* are not well established but probably involve changes in metabolism of non-specific thalamic nuclei, thalamocortical projections, or cortical neurons that produce or modulate the alpha rhythm.

25.1.5 *Specific disorders causing unilateral or bilateral decrease of alpha frequency*

(1) *Degenerative, developmental and demyelinating diseases. Alzheimer's disease* (senile and presenile dementia) causes abnormal slowing of the alpha rhythm which is of less diagnostic importance than are asynchronous generalized slow waves.

Myotonic dystrophy may cause slowing of the alpha rhythm; this may be due to the endocrine disturbances characteristic of this disease.

(2) *Metabolic and toxic encephalopathies.* Many of these encephalopathies produce early slowing of alpha frequency before causing other abnormalities and disappearance of alpha rhythm. The most important encephalopathies in this group are due to acute anoxia, hyponatremia, vitamin B12 deficiency, hypoglycemia, hepatic and renal failure, porphyria, Addison's disease, hyper- and hypoparathyroidism, Wernicke's disease, acute intoxication with barbiturates, phenytoin, alcohol, antipsychotics, amphetamines, lithium and other psychotropic drugs. Hypothyroidism may cause slowing of alpha rhythm often followed by reduction of amplitude without other abnormalities. Prior to the advent of serum level testing for phenytoin (Dilantin), neurologists determined the presence of high therapeutic or toxic levels according to the degree of alpha rhythm slowing.

(3) *Cerebrovascular diseases.* Local or generalized slowing of alpha rhythm occurs temporarily in transient local or generalized cerebral ischemia. Persistent slowing of alpha rhythm may be seen in bilateral or multiple cerebral infarcts, lacunar state of hypertensives, unilateral and bilateral subdural hematomas, thalamic infarcts, mesencephalic infarcts, postanoxic encephalopathy, subarachnoid hemorrhage with obtundation and in conditions associated with reduced cardiac output (e.g. coronary artery disease and congestive heart failure).

(4) *Cerebral trauma. Head injuries* of mild intensity may produce no more EEG abnormalities than a slowing of alpha rhythm, with or without a reduction of its amplitude. Patients recovering from more severe head injuries may show a decrease of alpha frequency, amplitude, or both as the last residual EEG abnormality. Repeated head injuries, for instance those of boxers, may produce lasting and progressive reduction of the frequency of alpha rhythm in addition to generalized slow waves.

(5) *Brain tumors. Infratentorial tumors* may reduce alpha frequency and amplitude bilaterally in addition to producing bisynchronous slow waves and asynchronous slowing. *Supratentorial tumors,* especially those in the parietal or occipital lobes or thalamus, may decrease alpha frequency and amplitude ipsilaterally in addition to producing focal or lateralized slow waves.

(6) *Seizure disorders. Ictal discharges* sometimes consist of rhythmical waves of alpha or slower frequency which are easily distinguished from alpha rhythm.

Postictal slowing in the alpha frequency range may persist longer than other postictal changes.

(7) *Infectious diseases. Non-specific slowing of the alpha rhythm* may occur in many infectious diseases including those not directly involving the brain; this slowing is commonly associated with fever and mental status changes.

Cerebral infections causing widespread cerebral damage (encephalitis or meningoencephalitis) may produce slowing of the alpha rhythm, in addition to other abnormalities.

25.1.6 *Specific disorders causing a bilateral increase of the alpha frequency*

(1) *Hyperthyroidism,* including that induced by treatment, is commonly associated with an increase in alpha frequency; the absolute amount of the alpha rhythm may also be reduced. Other abnormalities are often present. Many patients show increased beta activity, some have diffuse spikes and sharp waves, and a few have prominent generalized asynchronous slow waves. Treatment of the hyperthyroidism gradually reverses all abnormalities except for the asynchronous slow waves.

(2) *Fever* may transiently increase the alpha rhythm frequency.

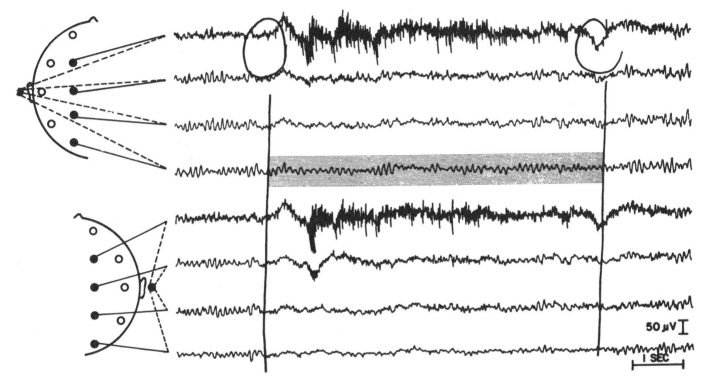

Fig. 25.1.   Unilateral failure of blocking of alpha rhythm. Before eye opening (O) and after eye closing (C), alpha rhythm is present and symmetrical on the two sides. While the eyes are open, alpha rhythm is blocked normally on the right side but persists on the left (shaded). This 32-year-old woman sustained a head injury without loss of consciousness 9 days before the EEG recording and had some receptive aphasia which cleared gradually.

423

25.2 ABNORMAL REACTIVITY OF THE ALPHA RHYTHM

25.2.1 *Unilateral failure of alpha blocking* on eye opening, often referred to as *Bancaud's phenomenon,* occurs with lesions of the parietal and temporal lobe on the side which fails to block (Fig. 25.1). This sign may be present in the absence of any other EEG abnormality and therefore may be the earliest indicator of lesions in those areas. More recently, Westmoreland and Klass (1998) described a series of 120 patients who demonstrated an abnormal asymmetry of the alpha rhythm during the performance of mental arithmetic problems in the eyes closed condition. As with the Bancaud phenomenon, attenuation was reduced ipsilateral to the abnormal hemisphere. The majority of patients did not have the classical Bancaud's phenomenon but the clinical implications of abnormal reactivity were similar. Therefore, it is recommended that mental alerting with calculation tasks be performed with the subjects' eyes closed during routine recording. Other mild background abnormalities may be present on careful inspection of the record, such as a slight reduction in the peak frequency of alpha activity on the abnormal side.

25.2.2 *Bilateral failure of alpha blocking*

(1) *Normal subjects* show great variability of alpha blocking (Fig. 13.2) and may have only very brief reductions of alpha amplitude in response to eye opening and alerting.

(2) *Unilateral cerebral lesions* located in the frontal or temporal lobes that abolish the blocking of alpha activity are usually associated with an impairment of consciousness, prominent neurological deficits, or both. In contrast, lesions located in the parietal or occipital lobes that abolish blocking of the alpha rhythm are often not associated with impaired consciousness or severe deficits.

(3) *Binocular blindness,* when acquired after the development of alpha, leads to a loss of the reactivity of alpha rhythm to eye opening. The alpha rhythm in this condition may have a central or unusually wide distribution. Like congenitally blind persons, persons with acquired blindness may have no alpha rhythm and may develop occipital spikes even in the absence of occipital lesions.

(4) *Monocular blindness* or loss of discriminative vision can cause failure of alpha blocking in both hemispheres when the blind eye is opened; opening of the seeing eye produces normal bilateral alpha blocking.

25.3 RHYTHMICAL ACTIVITY OF THETA, ALPHA AND BETA FREQUENCY IN COMA AND REACTIVITY IN COMA

25.3.1 The terms *theta coma, alpha coma, alpha-theta coma and beta coma pattern* are often used to denote patterns of

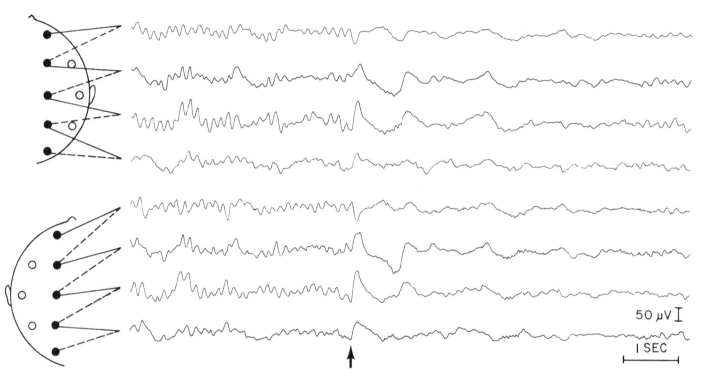

Fig. 25.2.   Pattern of alpha frequency coma in a patient with a presumed pontine lesion. Sinusoidal 7 Hz waves, superimposed on delta waves, are seen in a wide distribution in the left part of the figure. Pinching of the left arm (arrow) blocks the sinusoidal waves promptly for several seconds. This 25-year-old woman sustained a severe head injury in a motorcycle accident 3 days before this recording and was in coma since then with papillary and other signs suggestive of a pontine contusion.

rhythmical waves which have theta, alpha or beta frequency but differ from normal rhythms in that they occur in isolation without other accompanying waveforms in comatose patients. In addition, they usually do not demonstrate spontaneous variability or reactivity to sensory stimulation. Their topography (distribution over the head) is usually abnormal in that neither the alpha or theta activities have a posterior dominant amplitude gradient and beta patterns are widespread. These waves show little variation in frequency and are either the only activity present or are clearly the dominant activity. Variants of these coma patterns occur with less stable dominant frequency and with intermixed generalized slow waves. *The beta coma pattern usually indicates a high likelihood of recovery from coma whereas the other coma patterns are more often associated with poor outcome.*

Regardless the dominant frequency of the pattern seen, in the absence of general anesthesia, hypotension, or hypothermia, *non-reactivity and lack of spontaneous variability are the most important predictors of poor outcome.* Reactivity in coma takes two main forms: (1) attenuation of the ongoing pattern, or (2) a sudden accentuation of amplitude, usually consisting of an admixture of slower waveforms. Currently, there is no known prognostic difference between these two reactive patterns or between patterns that show mild vs. dramatic reactivity.

25.3.2   Two kinds of *alpha coma pattern* have been distinguished which loosely correspond with different anatomical distributions of pathological involvement.

(1)   *The posterior dominant alpha coma pattern* shows either no reaction or, rarely, a variable attenuation or increase in amplitude following alerting maneuvers. This pattern is usually encountered in patients with brainstem lesions, particularly pontine infarction (Fig. 25.2). It is important to attempt to differentiate patients with similarly located lesions who are in the so-called 'locked-in state' from those who are comatose. A posterior dominant alpha background activity that attenuates with alerting in patients with little other evidence of response to stimulation (or in some cases only vertical eye movements) is indicative of the 'locked-in state'. Such patients may have nearly complete awareness, but are immobilized by an interruption of corticospinal motor pathways.

(2)   *Generalized or predominantly frontal alpha activity* without reaction to alerting stimuli can be seen in patients with widespread cerebral damage, especially that following cardiac or respiratory arrest, prolonged hypoglycemia or bilateral destruction of midline thalamic nuclei (Fig. 25.3). Variants present with intermixed focal or generalized slow waves or amplitude abnormalities. This alpha pattern is usually seen for up to 5 days after the insult and is then replaced by other abnormalities. The prognosis for complete recovery or survival is generally considered to be poor, particularly in cases of anoxic encephalopathy. However, complete recovery has been

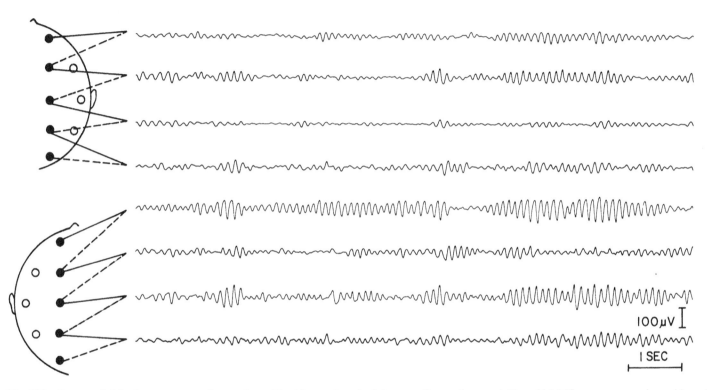

Fig. 25.3. Pattern of alpha frequency coma in a patient with widespread cerebral damage after cardiac arrest. Sinusoidal 8 Hz waves appear in a wide and asymmetrical distribution. They did not react to loud noises or noxious stimuli. This 27-year-old man was in postanoxic coma for 2 days after a cardiac arrest. A follow-up EEG 9 days later showed generalized slow waves of very low amplitude. The patient then was unresponsive and in a decerebrate posture and had roving vertical eye movements. He died 3 weeks later without regaining consciousness.

427

reported to occur frequently in cases of electrical injury and sedative intoxication uncomplicated by anoxia. Alpha coma patterns in patients who have overdosed with sedative medications usually contain asynchronous and bisynchronous delta activity. As noted above, an alpha coma pattern without spontaneous variability or reactivity suggests a much worse prognosis than a reactive alpha pattern or a record with spontaneously changing patterns.

25.3.3   The *theta coma pattern* is characterized by generalized monorhythmic activity in the theta frequency range that shows little or no evidence of either spontaneous variability or reactivity to noxious stimulation. The clinical correlates of the theta coma pattern are similar to those of the generalized or frontal dominant alpha coma pattern. Interestingly, it is not unusual for the alpha coma pattern to be replaced by the theta coma pattern. Such transitions indicate a poor prognosis for normal recovery or survival. As with the alpha coma pattern, the theta coma or mixed alpha-theta coma patterns are not as reliable for predicting a poor outcome as the absence of reactivity and spontaneous variability.

25.3.4   The *beta coma pattern* consists of a generalized, sometimes frontal dominant, pattern of mainly rhythmic beta waveforms. It usually occurs in coma caused by or complicated by barbiturate or benzodiazepine intoxication. Unlike the alpha and theta coma patterns, the beta coma pattern is usually associated with a favorable outcome, because in most cases it is a demonstration of the ability of cortical structures to generate a 'normal' response to pharmacological stimulation.

25.3.5   The *spindle coma pattern* is so named because it consists of recognizable sleep spindles occurring in patients who are either in a vegetative state or in coma. It is often accompanied by other sleep patterns such as vertex waves or K complexes and appears to represent a sleep stage with impaired arousal. It is usually associated with a favorable outcome, but is not as good an electrographic prognostic sign as a reactive beta coma pattern. It is often seen following head trauma but has also been observed in patients recovering from anoxic encephalopathy or encephalitis.

25.4   ABNORMAL TIMING AND INCIDENCE OF SLEEP PATTERNS

25.4.1   *Sleep activity in comatose patients* is occasionally superimposed on the slow waves or the abnormal alpha activity caused by the underlying disorder or it may simply contain abundant sleep spindles (i.e., the spindle coma pattern). Sleep activity seems inappropriate in these patients insofar as they do not exhibit cycles of wakefulness and sleep. However, the appearance of sleep activity in such patients indicates a better prognosis than does its absence.

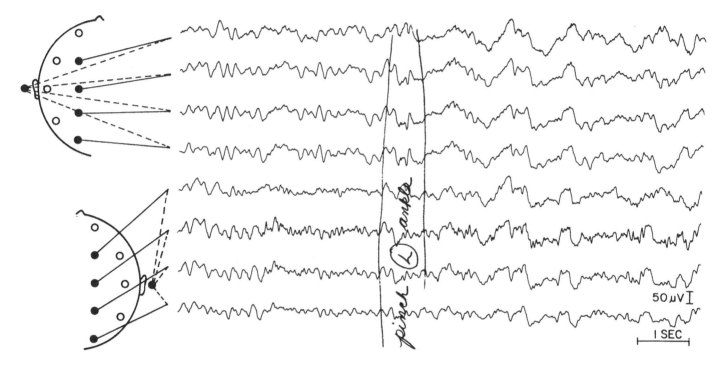

Fig. 25.4. Paradoxical slow wave response to alerting stimuli in an obtunded patient. Rhythmical 4–5 Hz waves at rest are replaced by generalized delta waves after pinching of the left ankle. This 70-year-old woman had repeated subarachnoid hemorrhages from an aneurysm on the left posterior communicating artery 2–3 weeks before this recording and began to recover from coma at the time of the recording.

25.4.2 *Paradoxical slow wave response to alerting stimuli* consists of a transient increase or appearance of generalized slow waves on a background of slow waves of lower amplitude or of alpha activity in patients with reduced alertness (Fig. 25.4). It is analogous to the paradoxical alpha rhythm.

25.4.3 *Sleep onset REM periods (SOREMPs) and short latency to sleep onset* of less than 5 min on the multiple sleep latency test occur in patients with narcolepsy, and Kleine–Levin syndrome and in REM deprived patients (e.g., obstructive sleep apnea).

25.4.4 *Reduction of REM sleep* can occur as the result of diseases causing structural damage, for instance mongolism, and Pelizaeus–Merzbacher disease, and as an effect of various drugs, for instance alcohol, barbiturates, tricyclic antidepressants and various other neuroleptic drugs.

25.4.5 *Disordered sleep cycles* occur in narcolepsy, sleep apnea, progressive supranuclear palsy and children or adults with episodic sleep disturbances or abnormal behaviors during sleep (i.e., parasomnias).

25.4.6 *Loss of muscle atonia during REM sleep* is a diagnostic finding in *REM behavior disorder*. EMG monitoring, using skin surface electrodes during polysomnography, reveals excessive muscle activity during REM sleep. Affected individuals, unprotected by normal paralysis during REM sleep, physically act out their dreams, often with violent consequences.

25.5 IMMATURE PATTERNS

Immature patterns are those found at an age when these patterns normally have disappeared. In neonates a retrogression of EEG patterns occurs as a non-specific response to transient or long-lasting cerebral disorders. In older individuals the persistence of immature patterns (e.g. posterior slow waves of youth seen in adults) is of uncertain clinical significance.

REFERENCES

Austin, E.J., Wilkus, R. and Longstreath, W.T. (1988) Etiology and prognosis of alpha coma. Neurology 38: 773–777.

Bancaud, J., Hacaen, H. and Lairy, G.C. (1955) Modifications de la réactivité EEG, troubles des functions symboliques et troubles confusionnels dans les lésions hémisphériques localisées. Electroenceph. Clin. Neurophysiol. 7: 179–192.

Bauer, G. (1987) Coma and brain death. In: E. Niedermeyer and F. Lopes da Silva (Eds.), Electroencephalography: Basic Principles, Clinical Applications and Related Fields. Urban and Schwarzenberg, Baltimore, pp. 391–404.

Benoit, O., Goldenberg-Leygonie, F., Lacombe, J. and Marc, M.E. (1978) Sommeil de l'enfant présentant des manifestations épisodiques du sommeil: comparaison avec l'enfant normal. Electroenceph. Clin. Neurophysiol. 44: 502–512.

Brenner, R.P. (1985) The electroencephalogram in altered states of consciousness. In: M.J. Aminoff (Ed.), Electrodiagnosis, Neurologic Clinics. Saunders, Philadelphia, pp. 615–629.

Britt, Jr., C.W., Raso, E. and Gerson, P. (1980) Spindle coma, secondary to primary traumatic midbrain hemorrhage. Electroenceph. Clin. Neurophysiol. 49: 406–408.

Cadilhac, J. (1976) Section V. EEG in thyroid dysfunction. In: A. Rémond (Ed.), Handbook of Electroenceph. Clin. Neurophysiol., Vol. 15C. Elsevier, Amsterdam, pp. 70–76.

Carroll, W.M. and Mastaglia, F.L. (1979) Alpha and beta coma in drug intoxication uncomplicated by cerebral hypoxia. Electroenceph. Clin. Neurophysiol. 46: 95–105.

Chatrian, G.E. (1975) Section V. Electrographic and behavioral signs of sleep in comatose states. In: A. Rémond (Ed.), Handbook of Electroenceph. Clin. Neurophysiol., Vol. 12. Elsevier, Amsterdam, pp. 63–77.

Chatrian, G.E. (1990) Coma, other states of altered responsiveness and brain death. In: D. Daly and T. Pedley (Eds.), Current Practice of Clinical Electroencephalography, Second Edition. Raven Press, New York, pp. 425–488.

Chokroverty, S. (1975) 'Alpha-like' rhythms in electroencephalograms in coma after cardiac arrest. Neurology 25: 655–663.

Fukuyama, Y. and Hayashi, M. (1979) Sleep electroencephalograms and sleep stages in hypoparathyroidism. Eur. Neurol. 18: 38–48.

Glass, J.D. (1977) Alpha blocking: absence in visuobehavioral deprivation. Science 198: 58–60.

Grindal, A., Suter, C. and Martinez, A. (1977) Alpha-pattern coma: 24 cases with 9 survivors. Ann. Neurol. 1: 371–377.

Gross, R.A., Spehlmann, R. and Daniels, J.C. (1978) Sleep disturbances in progressive supranuclear palsy. Electroenceph. Clin. Neurophysiol. 45: 16–25.

Gurvitch, A.M., Zarzhetsky, Y.V., Trush, V.D. and Zonov, V.M. (1984) Experimental data on the nature of post-resuscitation alpha frequency activity. Electroenceph. Clin. Neurophysiol. 58: 426–437.

Hansotia, P., Gottschalk, P., Green, P. and Zais, D. (1981) Spindle coma: incidence clinicopathologic correlates, and prognostic value. Neurology 31: 83–87.

Harner, R.N. (1975) EEG evaluation of the patient with dementia. In: D.F. Benson and D. Blumer (Eds.), Psychiatric Aspects of Neurological Disease. Grune and Stratton, New York, pp. 63–82.

Homan, R.W. and Jones, M.G. (1981) Alpha coma pattern in a 2-month-old child. Ann. Neurol. 9: 611–613.

Hulihan, Jr., J.F. and Syna, D.R. (1994) Electroencephalographic sleep patterns in postanoxic stupor and coma. Neurology 44: 758–760.

Jeavons, P.M. and Harding, G.F.A. (1975) Photosensitive epilepsy: a review of the literature and a study of 460 patients. Clin. Dev. Med. 56: 1–121.

Klass, D.W. and Westmoreland, B.F. (1996) Electroencephalography: general principles and adult electroencephalograms. In: J. Daube (Ed.), Clinical Neurophysiology. F.A. Davis, Philadelphia, pp. 73–103.

Knauss, T.A. and Carlson, C.B. (1978) Neonatal paroxysmal monorhythmic alpha activity. Arch. Neurol. 35: 104–107.

Laffont, F., Autret, A., Minz, M., Beillevaire, T., Gilbert, A., Cathala, H.P. and Castaigne, P. (1979) Etude polygraphique du sommeil dans 9 cas de maladie de Steele–Richardson. Rev. Neurol. 135: 127–142.

Newmark, M.E. and Penry, J.K. (1979) Photosensitivity and Epilepsy: A Review. Raven Press, New York.

Pfurtscheller, G., Maresch, H. and Schuy, S. (1977) Inter- and intrahemispheric differences in the peak frequency of rhythmic activity within the alpha band. Electroenceph. Clin. Neurophysiol. 42: 77–83.

Rae-Grant, A.D., Strapple, C. and Barbour, P.J. (1991) Episodic low-amplitude events: an underrecognized phenomenon in clinical electroencephalography. J. Clin. Neurophysiol. 8: 203–211.

Schwartz, M.S. and Scott, D.F. (1978) Pathological stimulus-related slow wave arousal responses in the EEG. Acta Neurol. Scand. 57: 300–304.

Sorenson, K., Thomassen, A. and Wernberg, M. (1978) Prognostic significance of alpha frequency EEG rhythm in coma after cardiac arrest. J. Neurol. Neurosurg. Psychiat. 41: 840–842.

Stockard, J.J., Werner, S.S., Aalbers, J.A. and Chiappa, K.H. (1976) Electro-encephalographic findings in phencyclidine intoxication. Arch. Neurol. 33: 200–203.

Van Hufflen, A.C., Poortvliet, D.C.J. and Van der Wulp, C.J.M. (1984) Quantitative electroencephalography in cerebral ischemia. Detection of abnormalities in 'normal' EEGs. In: G. Pfurtscheller, E.J. Jonkman and F.H. Lopes da Silva (Eds.), Brain Ischemia: Quantitative EEG and Imaging Techniques. Elsevier, Amsterdam, pp. 3–28.

Westmoreland, B.F. and Klass, D.W. (1998) Defective alpha reactivity with mental concentration. J. Clin. Neurophysiol. 15: 424–428.

Westmoreland, B.F., Klass, D.W., Sharbrough, F.W. and Reagan, T.J. (1975) Alpha-coma. Electroencephalographic, clinical, pathologic, and etiologic correlations. Arch. Neurol. 32: 713–718.

Young, G.B., Blume, W.T., Campbell, V.M., Demelo, J.D., Leung, L.S., McKeown, M.J., McLachlan, R.S., Ramsay, D.A. and Schieven, J.R. (1994) Alpha, theta, and alpha-theta coma: a clinical outcome study utilizing serial recordings. Electroenceph. Clin. Neurophysiol. 91: 93–99.

Zander Olsen, P., Stoier, M., Siersbaek-Nielsen, K., Molholm Hansen, J., Schioler, M. and Kristensen, M. (1972) Electroencephalographic findings in hyperthyroidism. Electroenceph. Clin. Neurophysiol. 32: 171–177.

Zaret, B.S. (1985) Prognostic and neurophysiological implications of concurrent burst suppression and alpha patterns in the EEG of post-anoxic coma. Electroenceph. Clin. Neurophysiol. 61: 199–209.

26 The EEG report

SUMMARY

The EEG report should include:

(26.1) *A simple brief description* of the essential features of normal and abnormal activity observed under various conditions of recording, namely resting wakefulness, hyperventilation, photic stimulation and sleep.

(26.2) *An EEG summary* or *impression* listing the major significant abnormal findings and events.

(26.3) *An interpretation* that explains the EEG impression and clinical correlation in the light of the patient's problems and referring physician's reason for requesting the study.

26.1 DESCRIPTION OF THE RECORD

The report should describe the essential normal and abnormal patterns appearing under the various recording conditions so that a person with some knowledge of EEG can envisage the findings on which diagnosis and interpretation are based. Sufficient detail should be given to enable the reader of a later EEG to estimate whether the major features of the two recordings are similar or different. The report should not be exhaustive in describing normal detail but should include those rare or unusual features in the record which may have clinical significance. As far as possible, the report should use the terms defined in the glossary of the International Federation of Societies for EEG and Clinical Neurophysiology (9). Judgments like 'good' and 'poor' should be used only sparingly and only to characterize the overall composition of a record, but not to rate individual rhythms: persons not familiar with the EEG cannot know that 'poor' driving has no different clinical significance than has 'good' or even 'excellent' driving. Similary, the EEG should not be anthropomorphisized. There is no such thing as an *irritable EEG*, whereas there may be waveforms that suggest cortical irritability. Patterns should be described by indicating the frequency, amplitude and distribution of the component waves. Wave shape, rhythmicity, symmetry, synchrony, persistence, reactivity and periodicity may be important for the description of abnormal patterns. Because the frequency of a rhythm often varies, it is usually indicated in terms of a frequency range or band of a few hertz in width rather than in terms of a single frequency. In most instances, it is not sufficient to use only the wide bands of delta, theta, alpha and beta frequency to describe the frequencies of waves in a record; the frequency of alpha and beta rhythms and of theta and delta waves observed in a recording should be specified in narrower bands. Amplitude may be reported in absolute or relative measurements, preferably with the montage specified. Absolute units must be used in the diagnosis of electrocerebral silence in which no cerebral activity of over 2 μV should be present. Even if activity of very low amplitude over 2 μV is found in these cases, the amplitude should be specified to indicate the severity of the abnormality and to provide a basis for comparison with subsequent recordings. In most other instances, it is sufficient to characterize amplitude as low, medium or high.

To avoid omitting important features in the report, one should adhere to a standard sequence of reporting.

26.1.1 Although many electroencephalographers do not include a summary of the clinical history, it is advisable to briefly state the referring complaint and any other information that is immediately relevant to the interpretation of the recording under a separate heading such as *"History"*. This provides the referring physician with feedback as to the electroencephalographers' understanding of the referring complaint, facilitates future review of the EEG report, and helps in the interpretation of subsequent EEGs. It is also an important exercise for those who are training to become electroencephalographers.

The general level of consciousness of the patient, other behavioral abnormalities (such as lack of cooperation, or persistent movement causing excessive artifact), the equipment used (e.g., digital or analog), the recording environment (e.g., outpatient, bedside, ICU, patient ventilator dependent), and whether or not sedation was given (e.g., chloral hydrate) should either be stated under a separate heading, such as *"Conditions of the Recording"*, or in the opening of the general body of the descriptive report.

26.1.2 *The resting record*

(1) *Description of normal background. Alpha, beta, mu and other rhythms and patterns,* if present, are described in terms of their frequency range, relative amplitude and distribution. Wave shape, rhythmicity, symmetry, distribution, persistence and reactivity should be mentioned if they are abnormal. Excessive beta activity and unilateral blocking of the alpha rhythm must be reported.

(2) *Description of abnormal patterns. Epileptiform activity* is characterized by its shape, amplitude, repetition rate, persistence, distribution, synchrony, symmetry, relationship between focal and generalized discharges and any other feature of possible clinical significance including the association with behavioral seizure manifestations.

Slow waves are described in terms of frequency, amplitude, shape, rhythmicity, regularity, persistence, distribution, symmetry, synchrony and any other parameter of clinical importance. If more than one type of slow wave is present, the specifications for each type must be given. Abnormal generalized asynchronous slow waves must be distinguished by amplitude, frequency, distribution and persistence from the range of asynchronous slow waves normally seen at the age of the patient.

Asymmetries and generalized changes of amplitude are usually noted when describing the normal background.

Deviations from normal must be described by indicating the specific features which make a pattern abnormal, for instance the appearance of alpha activity which has a frontal maximum, lacks reactivity and is associated with coma.

26.1.3 *Hyperventilation. Normal responses* can be described in one short sentence, for instance 'Hyperventilation produced no change' or 'Hyperventilation produced bilaterally synchronous slow waves' or 'Hyperventilation did not elicit any abnormalities.' The performance of the patient may be mentioned. Symptoms induced by hyperventilation should be reported, particularly if the symptoms resemble episodic symptoms for which the patient is examined. Changes in the patient's behavior, such as jerking movements or loss of responsiveness, must be reported.

Abnormal responses such as an asymmetrical buildup, enhancement of abnormalities of the resting record and induction of new abnormalities must be described in detail.

26.1.4 *Photic stimulation.* Normal responses can be described briefly by stating 'Photic stimulation did not elicit a driving response' or 'Photic stimulation elicited a symmetric driving response.'

Abnormal responses such as significant asymmetries and photoparoxysmal responses must be described.

26.1.5 *Sleep.* It is helpful to either briefly describe the major EEG findings during sleep or simply list the deepest stage of sleep that occurred. If the patient was referred for the evaluation of a possible seizure disorder and epileptiform activity did not occur, then the depth and duration of sleep will be of particular importance. The report should also indicate whether sleep was induced with a sedative or occurred spontaneously.

Abnormalities during sleep should be described in detail. Most important is the appearance of epileptiform activity. Other abnormalities of clinical significance include persistence of abnormal patterns seen in the waking record, abnormal sleep patterns and sleep onset REM periods. Patterns of doubtful clinical significance such as 6 Hz spike-and-slow-wave, 14 and 6 Hz positive bursts, small sharp spikes and rhythmical midtemporal discharges may be mentioned, but their uncertain significance must be stressed in the description and summary to avoid confusion with clinically significant EEG abnormalities.

26.2   EEG SUMMARY IMPRESSION

It is helpful to summarize the diagnostically important features of the EEG under a separate heading. Although this can be done using descriptive prose, in the author's experience it is preferable to provide a terse enumeration of clinically or electrographically important findings. This can be done using either a grading system, such as that developed at the Mayo Clinic, or by providing a numerical list of the pertinent findings using a telegraphic writing style. A succinct approach to summarization serves several purposes. First, it creates a distillation of relevant findings that tends to eliminate confusion. Second, it allows individuals with some understanding of electroencephalography to quickly review the relevant findings. Third, it allows the electroencephalographer to quickly review the salient features of prior EEG reports. Finally, it forces the reader to focus clearly on the major findings and summarize them succinctly. Summary writing is therefore an extremely useful teaching exercise for residents and fellows who are learning to read EEGs. The summary of electrographic findings can be used in combination with the interpretation to form a preliminary report that can be read over the phone or quickly sent out in electronic media. Laboratories that use grading systems require an environment where all the referring neurologists are familiar with that grading system.

If a grading system is not used, then EEG summaries should be stated with the least number of terms needed to describe the major findings. It is helpful to organize the wording of findings in the following order: *major finding; amplitude; persistence, reactivity, activation; location;* and *behavioral state.* For example, an EEG that contains focal left anterior temporal continuous irregular delta activity that does not disappear with alerting and persists during wakefulness and sleep and also has epileptiform spikes that appear with the highest amplitude over the left anterior temporal head region during sleep, could be summarized as follows:

Summary of findings:

(1) Epileptiform spikes; left anterior temporal; during sleep only.
(2) Irregular delta activity; moderate amplitude; continuous, non-reactive; left anterior temporal maximal.

In the interpretation the reader may choose to refer to the summary and then state the clinical correlation. For example, in the EEG described above the interpretation might read as follows:

Interpretation: The EEG is moderately abnormal due to the above summarized findings. These findings indicate the presence of a potentially epileptogenic focal cerebral dysfunction involving the left anterior temporal area and strongly suggest the presence of an underlying structural abnormality. These findings are consistent with the clinical impression of a partial seizure disorder.

26.3 CLINICAL CORRELATION

26.3.1 *Normal records* generally do not need an interpretation. Exceptions should be made in cases of apparent discrepancies between the EEG and the clinical condition of the patient. This is especially true if the patient has clinical abnormalities during the recording as in the example of a report given below. Other interpretations of normal reports may be of interest to some, but not all, recipients of EEG reports; the EEG reader should try to tailor his reports to the needs of the referring physician. Thus, in the case of a patient with dementia, the interpretation may include the statement that 'a normal EEG may be seen in mild or less often in moderately advanced cases of Alzheimer's dementia'. The proper use of the terms *cerebral dysfunction, indicative, suggestive,* and *compatible* are discussed in the Guidelines for Writing EEG Reports in Appendix II.

26.3.2 *Abnormal findings* must be interpreted. Without interpretation, the report of an abnormal EEG finding is similar to a radiology report that lists opacities and translucencies of the bone but does not say whether they indicate a fracture. To interpret an abnormal EEG, the reader should take into consideration each abnormal pattern and mentally scan its general pathological and specific clinical correlates as outlined in the preceding chapters and tables. To arrive at a meaningful interpretation, he must compare the many possible clinical correlates of the EEG patterns with the clinical presentation of the case and must select the diagnoses most likely to satisfy both (15.3). Clearly, the interpretation will improve with the amount of clinical information given to the EEG reader and with the reader's ability to match the abnormal patterns with the clinical presentation.

26.3.3 *Recommendations for further diagnostic testing* may be appropriate in some cases. Repeat EEG recordings may help to answer questions whether focal slow waves are postictal, i.e. whether they disappear after several days without seizures. The failure to obtain a sleep recording in a patient suspected of having partial complex seizures may lead to the suggestion to have the patient return sedated. A patient with a suspected seizure disorder who shows no epileptiform activity in his first EEG including a sleep recording may show epileptiform discharges in a second or third EEG recording. Repeat recordings may better evaluate the condition of patients with acute and transient changes resulting from head injuries, cardiorespiratory arrest or drug effects. The presence of muscle artifact preventing the interpretation of an EEG of a patient with suspected cerebral death may lead to the proposal to use neuromuscular blocking agents during the recording. The multiple sleep latency test may be indicated for patients with a possible diagnosis of narcolepsy or simultaneous respiratory monitoring during prolonged sleep may be indicated for those suspected of having severe sleep apnea. Unexplained focal slowing may prompt the recommendation of further diagnostic studies.

26.3.4 *The following sample EEG report* is based on the recording of a 15-year-old girl referred with a history of four attacks of dizziness during the preceding 3 months. The referring physician requested the EEG to investigate the possibility of a convulsive disorder.

Description: The EEG during wakefulness contains an approximately symmetric, medium amplitude, 10–11 Hz, posterior dominant activity that attenuates with eye opening. During eye closure at rest a medium amplitude intermittent 9.5–10.5 Hz mu rhythm is present. Occasional 5–7 Hz theta waves are present over most head regions.

Hyperventilation did not elicit any abnormalities. During hyperventilation the patient complained of feeling dizzy and faint in a manner similar to that experienced during her recent attacks.

Photic stimulation elicited a symmetric driving response.

Sleep occurred following sedation with chloral hydrate and was characterized by the appearance of generalized slowing, vertex waves, POSTs, and sleep spindles.

Summary of findings: Hyperventilation induced a sensation of dizziness characteristic of the patient's attacks and was not associated with any EEG abnormalities.

Interpretation: The EEG is normal with the patient recorded in the awake and sleep states. Hyperventilation produced a sensation of dizziness which the patient describes as similar to that which she experienced during her previous attacks. The absence of epileptiform activity suggests that her attacks of dizziness are probably not a seizure manifestation. If a chronic seizure disorder is strongly suspected, then a repeat recording in the awake and sleep states may provide additional information.

26.3.5 The Guidelines for Writing EEG Reports recommended by the American EEG Society complement the information provided in this chapter and the reader is encouraged to review them. They are reproduced in Appendix II.

REFERENCES

American EEG Society Guidelines in Electroencephalography, Evoked Potentials and Polysomnography (1994) Guideline Eight: Guidelines for writing EEG reports. J. Clin. Neurophysiol. 11: 37–39.
Schneider, J. (1977) Section IV. The EEG report. In: A. Rémond (Ed.), Handbook of Electroenceph. Clin. Neurophysiol., Vol. IIA. Elsevier, Amsterdam, pp. 97–109.

Appendix I

A GLOSSARY OF TERMS MOST COMMONLY USED BY CLINICAL ELECTROENCEPHALOGRAPHERS[1,2,3,4]

G.E. CHATRIAN (Chairman), L. BERGAMINI, M. DONDEY[†], D.W. KLASS, M. LENNOX-BUCHTHAL and I. PETERSÉN

Absence. Use of term discouraged when describing EEG patterns. Terms suggested, whenever appropriate: 3 Hz spike-and-slow-waves; atypical repetitive spike-and-slow-waves.

Abundance. Use of term discouraged. Term suggested: quantity (not a synonym).

Activation. (1) Any procedure designed to enhance or elicit normal or abnormal EEG activity, especially paroxysmal activity. Examples: hyperventilation; photic stimulation; sleep; injection of convulsant drugs. (2) EEG pattern consisting of a low voltage record which becomes apparent upon blocking of EEG rhythms by physiological or other stimuli such as electrical stimulation of the brain (use discouraged).

Active electrode. Use of term discouraged. *Cf.*, exploring electrode (not a synonym).

Activity, EEG. Any EEG wave or sequence of waves.

After-discharge. (1) EEG seizure pattern following repetitive electrical stimulation of a discrete area of the brain via cortical or intracerebral electrodes.

[1]The following annotations are used throughout the glossary:

*American.

**British.

***Cf. Report of the Committee on Methods of Clinical Examination in Electroencephalography. *Electroenceph. Clin. Neurophysiol.*, **1958**, *10*: 370–375.

****Cf. Report of the Committee on EEG Instrumentation Standards. *Electroenceph. Clin. Neurophysiol.*, **1974**, *37*: 549–553.

[2]The Report of the Committee on Terminology, page 529, to which this glossary is an appendix, should be consulted.

[3]Enquiries regarding reprints should be addressed to the President of the Federation, Dr. R.J. Ellingson, Nebraska Psychiatric Institute, 602 South 44th Avenue, Omaha, NE 68105, U.S.A.

[4]This Appendix is an official document of the International Federation of Societies for Electroencephalography and Clinical Neurophysiology. As such it has not been subject to editorial review, nor are the editors of the EEG Journal responsible for its contents.

(2) Burst of rhythmic activity following a transient such as an evoked potential or a spike.

Alpha band. Frequency band of 8–13 Hz. Greek letter: α.

Alpha rhythm. Rhythm at 8–13 Hz occurring during wakefulness over the posterior regions of the head, generally with higher voltage over the occipital areas. Amplitude is variable but is mostly below 50 μV in the adult. Best seen with the eyes closed and under conditions of physical relaxation and relative mental inactivity. Blocked or attenuated by attention, especially visual, and mental effort. Comment: use of term alpha rhythm must be restricted to those rhythms which fulfil all these criteria. Acitivities in the alpha band which differ from the alpha rhythm as regards their topography and/or reactivity either have specific appellations (for instance, the mu rhythm) or should be referred to as *rhythms of alpha frequency*. *Cf.*, rhythm of alpha frequency.

Alpha variant rhythms. Term applies to certain characteristic EEG rhythms which are recorded most prominently over the posterior regions of the head and differ in frequency but resemble in reactivity the alpha rhythm. *Cf.*, fast alpha variant rhythm; slow alpha variant rhythms.

Alpha wave. Wave with duration of 1/8–1/13 s.

Alphoid rhythm. Use of term discouraged.

Amplitude. Voltage of EEG waves. Generally expressed in microvolts (μV). Measured peak-to-peak. Comment: amplitude of EEG waves recorded from the surface of the head is influenced to a major degree by extracerebral factors including the impedances of the meninges, cerebrospinal fluid, skull, scalp and electrodes.

Antiphase signal**. *Cf.*, out-of-phase signal*.

Aperiodic. Applies to: (1) EEG waves or complexes occurring in a sequence at an irregular rate. (2) EEG waves or complexes occurring intermittently at irregular intervals.

Apotentiality, Record of cerebral. Use of term discouraged. Term suggested: record of electrocerebral inactivity. *Cf.*, inactivity, record of electrocerebral.

Application, Electrode. The process of establishing connection between an electrode and the subject's scalp or brain.

Arceau rhythm. Use of term discouraged. Term suggested: mu rhythm. Arousal. Use of term discouraged when describing EEG pattern.

Array. A regular arrangement of electrodes over the scalp or brain or within the brain substance.

Arrhythmic activity. A sequence of waves of inconstant period. *Cf.*, rhythm.

Artifact (artefact). (1) Any potential difference due to an extracerebral source, recorded in EEG tracings. (2) Any modification of the EEG caused by extracerebral factors such as alterations of the media surrounding the brain, instrumental distortion or malfunction, and operational errors.

Asymmetry. (1) Unequal amplitude and/or form and frequency of EEG activities over homologous areas on opposite sides of the head. (2) Unequal development of EEG waves about the baseline.

Asynchrony. The non-simultaneous occurrence of EEG activity regions on the same or opposite sides of the head.

Attenuation. (1) Reduction in amplitude of EEG activity. May occur transiently in response to physiological or other stimuli, such as electrical stimulation of the brain, or result from pathological conditions. *Cf.*, blocking. (2) Reduction of sensitivity of an EEG channel, i.e., decrease in output pen deflection by operation or sensitivity or filter controls. Customarily expressed as relative reduction of sensitivity at certain stated frequencies. *Cf.*, sensitivity; high frequency filter; low frequency filter****.

Atypical repetitive spike-and-slow-waves. Term refers to paroxysms consisting of a sequence of spike-and-slow-wave complexes which occur bilaterally synchronously but do not meet one or more of the criteria of 3 Hz spike-and-slow-waves. *Cf.*, 3 Hz spike-and-slow-waves.

Augmentation. Increase in amplitude of electrical activity.

Average potential reference. Average of the potentials of all or many EEG electrodes, used as a reference. Synonym: Goldmann–Offner reference (use discouraged).

Background activity. Any EEG activity representing the setting in which a given normal or abnormal pattern appears and from which such pattern is distinguished. Comment: not a synonym of any individual rhythm such as the alpha rhythm.

Balanced amplifier. An amplifier which consists essentially of two identical single-ended amplifiers operated as a pair and in opposite phases.

Band. Portion of EEG frequency spectrum. *Cf.*, delta, theta, alpha, beta bands.

Bandwidth, EEG channel. Range of frequencies between which the response of an EEG channel is within stated limits. Determined by the frequency response of the amplifier-writer combination and the frequency filters used. Comment: the manner in which the EEG channel bandwidth is specified by different manufacturers is not standardized at present. For instance, in a given instrument, a bandwidth of 0.5–50 Hz may indicate that frequencies of 0.5 and 50 Hz are attenuated 30% (3 dB), or another stated per cent, with intermediate frequencies being attenuated less****.

Basal electrode. Any electrode located in proximity to the base of the skull. *Cf.*, nasopharyngeal electrode; sphenoidal electrode.

Baseline. (1) Strictly: line obtained when an identical voltage is applied to the two input terminals of an EEG amplifier or when the instrument is in the calibrate position but no calibration signal is applied. (2) Loosely: imaginary line corresponding to the approximate mean values of the EEG activity assessed visually in an EEG derivation over a period of time.

Beta band. Frequency band over 13 Hz. Greek letter: β. Comment: practically, most electroencephalographs using pen writers appreciably attenuate frequencies higher than 75 Hz. The customary use of relatively slow paper speeds further limits the electroencephalographer's ability to resolve visually waves of frequencies higher than 35 Hz. However, this does not justify limiting unduly the high frequency response of the EEG channels for EEG waves include transients such as spikes and sharp waves with components at frequencies above 50 Hz.

Beta rhythm. In general: any EEG rhythm over 13 Hz. Most characteristically: a rhythm from 13 to 35 Hz recorded over the fronto-central regions of the head during wakefulness. Amplitude of fronto-central beta rhythm is variable but is mostly below 30 μV. Blocking or attenuation by contralateral movement or tactile stimulation is especially obvious in electrocorticograms. Other beta rhythms are most prominent in other locations or are diffuse.

Bilateral. Involving both sides of the head.

Biparietal hump. Use of term discouraged. Term suggested: vertex sharp transient.

Biphasic wave. Use of term discouraged. Term suggested: diphasic wave.

Bipolar depth electrode. Use of term discouraged. Term suggested: dual-electrode (or multi-electrode) lead.

Bipolar derivation. Recording from a pair of exploring electrodes ***. *Cf.*, exploring electrode; bipolar montage.

Bipolar montage. Multiple bipolar derivations, with no electrode being common to all derivations. In most instances, bipolar derivations are linked, i.e., adjacent derivations from electrodes along the same array have one electrode in common, connected to the input terminal 2 of one amplifier and to the input terminal 1 of the following amplifier***. *Cf.*, referential montage.

Bisynchronous. Abbreviation for: bilaterally synchronous (use discouraged).

Black lead*.** Use of term discouraged. Term suggested: input terminal 1.

Blocking. (1) Apparent, temporary obliteration of EEG rhythms in response to physiological or other stimuli such as electrical stimulation of the brain.

Cf., attenuation. (2) A condition of temporary unresponsiveness of the EEG amplifier, caused by major overload. Manifested initially by extreme, flat-topped pen excursion(s) lasting up to a few seconds. *Cf.*, overload; clipping.

Brain wave. Use of term discouraged. Term suggested: EEG wave.

Buffer amplifier. An amplifier, generally with a voltage gain of 1, a high input impedance and a low output impedance, used to isolate the input signal from the loading effects of an immediately following circuit. In some electroencephalographs, each input is connected to a buffer amplifier located in the jack box to reduce cable artifact and interference.

Build-up. Colloquialism. Employed to describe progressive increase in voltage of the EEG or appearance of waves of increasing amplitude, frequently associated with decrease in frequency. Sometimes applied to hyperventilation or seizure discharges (use discouraged).

Burst. A group of waves appear and disappear abruptly and are distinguished from background activity by differences in frequency, form and/or amplitude. Comments: (1) Term does not imply abnormality. (2) Not a synonym of paroxysm. *Cf.*, paroxysm.

Burst-suppression. Pattern characterized by burst of theta and/or delta waves, at times intermixed with faster waves, and intervening periods of relative quiescence. Comment: term should be used to describe the EEG effects of some anesthetic drugs at certain levels of anesthesia.

Calibration. (1) Procedure of testing and recording the responses of EEG channels to voltage differences applied to the input terminals of their respective amplifiers. Comment: DC (usually) or AC voltages of magnitude comparable to the amplitudes of EEG waves are used in this procedure***·****. (2) The procedure of testing the accuracy of paper speed by means of a time marker. Comment: some electroencephalographs provide time marks throughout recording. *Cf.*, common EEG input test.

Cap, Head. A cap which is fitted over the head to hold pad electrodes in position.

Channel. Complete system for the detection, amplification and display of potential differences between a pair of electrodes. Comment: electroencephalographs generally consist of several EEG channels***·****.

Chopper. A device consisting of a mechanical or electronic switch used in some EEG amplifiers for interrupting (chopping) DC, and low frequency AC, signals and converting them into square waves of relatively high frequency. The same device may provide synchronous rectification of these square waves after amplification to reconvert them to the form of the original signal at the output.

Chopper amplifier. A direct current amplifier in which a chopper interrupts DC, and low frequency AC, signals and converts them into square waves of relatively high frequency. These are magnified by an AC amplifier and then reconverted by synchronous rectification to the form of the original signal at the output.

Circumferential bipolar montage. A montage consisting of derivations from pairs of electrodes along circumferential arrays.

Clipping. Distortion of EEG waves which makes them appear flat-topped in the write-out. Caused by overload.

Comb rhythm. Use of term discouraged. Term suggested: mu rhythm.

Common EEG input test. Procedure in which the same pair of EEG electrodes is connected to the two terminals of all channels of the electroencephalograph***. Comment: used as adjunct to calibration procedure. *Cf.*, calibration.

Common mode rejection. A characteristic of differential amplifiers whereby they provide markedly reduced amplification of common mode signals, compared to differential signals. Expressed as common mode rejection ratio, i.e., ratio of amplifications of differential and common mode signals. Example:

$$\frac{\text{amplification, differential}}{\text{amplification, common mode}} = \frac{20,000}{1} = 20,000{:}1.$$

Common mode signal. Common component of the two signals applied to the two respective input terminals of a differential EEG amplifier. Comment: in EEG recording, external interference frequently occurs as common mode signal.

Common reference electrode. A reference electrode connected to the input terminal 2 of several or all EEG amplifiers.

Common reference montage. Several referential derivations sharing a single reference electrode***. *Cf.*, referential derivation; reference electrode.

Complex. A sequence of two or more waves having a characteristic form or recurring with a fairly consistent form, distinguished from background acitivity.

Coronal bipolar montage. A montage consisting of derivations from pairs of electrodes along coronal (transverse) arrays. Synonym: transverse bipolar montage***.

Cortical electrode. Electrode applied directly upon or inserted in the cerebral cortex.

Cortical electroencephalogram. *Cf.*, electrocorticogram.

Cortical electroencephalography. *Cf.*, *electrocorticography.*

Corticogram. Abbreviation for: electrocorticogram (use discouraged).

Corticography. Abbreviation for: electrocorticography (use discouraged).

Cycle. The complete sequence of potential changes undergone by individual components of a sequence of regularly repeated EEG waves or complexes.

Cycles per second. Unit of frequency. Abbreviation: c/s. Synonym: hertz (Hz) preferred.

c/s. Abbreviation for cycles per second. Equivalent: Hz preferred.

DEEG. Abbreviation for: depth electroencephalogram and depth electroencephalography .

Delta band. Frequency band under 4 Hz. Greek letter δ. Comment: DC potential differences are not monitored in conventional EEGs.

Delta rhythm. Rhythm under 4 Hz.

Delta wave. Wave with duration over 0.25 s.

Depression. Use of term discouraged when describing EEG patterns.

Depth electrode. Electrode implanted within the brain substance.

Depth electroencephalogram. Record of electrical activity of the brain by means of electrodes implanted within the brain substance itself. Abbreviation: DEEG. *Cf.*, stereotactic (stereotaxic) depth electroencephalogram.

Depth electroencephalography. Technique of recording depth electroencephalograms. Abbreviation: DEEG.

Derivation. (1) The process of recording from a pair of electrodes in an EEG channel. (2) The EEG record obtained by this process.

Desynchronization. Use of term discouraged when describing EEG change. Terms suggested: blocking; attenuation.

Desynchronized. Use of term discouraged when describing EEG pattern. *Cf.*, low voltage EEG.

Diffuse. Occurring over large areas of one or both sides of the head. *Cf.*, generalized.

Differential amplifier. An amplifier whose output is proportional to the voltage difference between its two input terminals. Comment: electroencephalographs make use of differential amplifiers in their input stages.

Differential signal. Difference between two unlike signals applied to the respective two input terminals of a differential EEG amplifier.

Diphasic wave. Wave consisting of two components developed on alternate sides of the baseline.

Direct-coupled amplifier. An amplifier in which successive stages are connected (coupled) by devices which are not frequency-dependent.

Direct current amplifier. An amplifier which is capable of magnifying DC (zero frequency) voltages and slowly varying voltages. Comment: the di-

443

rect-coupled amplifier and the chopper amplifier are direct current amplifiers. *Cf.*, direct-coupled amplifier; chopper amplifier.

Disk electrode. Metal disk attached to the scalp with an adhesive such as collodion, a paste or wax***.

Discharge. Interpretive term commonly used to designate such paroxysmal patters as epileptiform patterns and seizure patterns. *Cf.*, epileptiform pattern; seizure pattern, EEG.

Disorganization. Gross alteration in frequency, form, topography and/or quantity of physiologic EEG rhythms in an individual record, relative to previous records in the same subject or the rhythms of homologous regions on the opposite side of the head.

Distortion. An instrument alteration in waveform. *Cf.*, artifact.

Duration. (1) The interval from beginning to end of and individual wave or complex. Comment: the duration of the cycle of individual components of a sequence of regularly repeating waves or complexes is referred to as the period of the wave or complex. (2) The time that a sequence of waves or complexes or any other distinguishable feature lasts in an EEG record.

Dysrhythmia. Use of term discouraged.

Earth connection**. *Cf.*, synonym: ground connection*.

ECoG. Abbreviation for: electrocorticogram and electrocorticography.

EEG. Abbreviation for: electroencephalogram and electroencephalography.

Electrocorticogram. Record of EEG activity obtained by means of electrodes applied directly over or inserted in the cerebral cortex. Abbreviation: ECoG.

Electrocorticography. Technique of recording electrical activity of the brain by means of electrodes applied over or implanted in the cerebral cortex. Abbreviation: ECoG.

Electrode, EEG***. Strictly: a conducting device applied over or inserted into a region of the scalp or brain. Loosely: synonym of lead.

Electrode impedance. Opposition to the flow of an AC current through the interface between an electrode and the scalp or brain. Measured between pairs of electrodes or, in some electroencephalographs, between each individual electrode and all other electrodes connected in parallel. Expressed in ohms (generally kilohms, kΩ). Comments: (1) Over the EEG frequency range, because the capacitance factor is small, electrode impedance is usually numerically equal to electrode resistance. (2) Not a synonym of input impedance of EEG amplifier. *Cf.*, electrode resistance; input impedance.

Electrode resistance. Opposition to the flow of a DC current through the interface between an EEG electrode and the scalp or brain. Measured between pairs of electrodes or, in some electroencephalographs, between each individual electrode and all the other electrodes connected in parallel. Expressed in ohms (generally kilohms, kΩ). Comment: measurement of electrode resistance with DC currents results in varying degrees of electrode polarization. *Cf.*, electrode impedance.

Electroencephalogram. Record of electrical activity of the brain taken by means of electrodes placed on the surface of the head, unless otherwise specified.

Electroencephalograph. Instrument employed to record electroencephalograms.

Electroencephalography. (1) The science relating to the electrical activity of the brain. (2) The technique of recording electroencephalograms. Abbreviation: EEG.

Electrogram. Use of term discouraged.

Electrography. Use of term discouraged.

Epidural electrode. Electrode located over the dural covering of the cerebrum.

Epileptic pattern. Use of term discouraged. *Cf.*, epileptiform pattern.

Epileptiform pattern. Interpretive term. Applies to distinctive waves or complexes, distinguished from background activity, and resembling those recorded in a proportion of human subjects suffering from epileptic disorders and in animals rendered epileptic experimentally. Epileptiform patterns include spikes and sharp waves, alone or accompanied by slow waves, occurring singly or in bursts lasting at most a few seconds. Comment: (1) Term refers to inter-ictal paroxysmal activity and not to seizure patterns. *Cf.*, seizure pattern. (2) Probability of association with clinical epileptic disorders is variable.

Epoch. A period of time in an EEG record. Duration of epochs is determined arbitrarily. Example: a 10 s epoch.

Equipotential. Applies to regions of the head or electrodes which are at the same potential at a given instant in time.

Equipotential line. Imaginary line joining a series of points which are at the same potential at a given instant in time.

Evoked potential. Wave or complex elicited by and time-locked to a physiological or other stimulus, for instance an electrical stimulus, delivered to a sensory receptor or nerve, or applied directly to a discrete area of the brain. Comment: computer summation techniques are especially suited for the detection of these and other event-related potentials from the surface of the head.

Evoked response. Tautology. Use of term discouraged. Term suggested: evoked potential.

Exploring electrode. Any electrode over the scalp or brain or within the brain substance, intended to detect EEG activity. Such an electrode is customarily connected to either the input terminal 1 or the input terminal 2 of an EEG amplifier in bipolar derivations and to the input terminal 1 of an EEG amplifier in referential derivations. *Cf.*, bipolar derivation; referential derivation.

Extracerebral potential. Any potential which does not originate in the brain, referred to as an artifact in EEG. May arise from: electrical interference external to the subject and recording system; the subject; the electrodes and their connections to the subject and the electroencephalograph; and electroencephalograph itself. *Cf.*, artifact.

Fast activity. Activity of frequency higher than alpha, *i.e.*, beta activity.

Fast alpha variant rhythm. Characteristic rhythm at 14–20 Hz, detected most prominently over the posterior regions of the head. May alternate or be intermixed with alpha rhythm. Blocked or attenuated by attention, especially visual, and mental effort.

Fast wave. Wave with duration shorter than alpha waves, i.e., under 1/13 s.

Flat EEG. Use of term discouraged. *Cf.*, low voltage EEG; inactivity, record of electrocerebral.

Focus. A limited region of the scalp, cerebral cortex or depth of the brain displaying a given EEG activity, whether normal or abnormal.

Form. Shape of a wave. Synonym: waveform; morphology.

Fourteen and 6 Hz positive burst. Burst of arch-shaped waves at 13–17 Hz and/or 5–7 Hz but most commonly at 14 and/or 6 Hz, seen generally over the posterior temporal and adjacent areas of one or both sides of the head during sleep. The sharp peaks of its component waves are positive with respect to other regions. Amplitude varies but is generally below 75 μV. Comments: (1) Best demonstrated by referential recording using contralateral earlobe, or other remote, reference electrodes. (2) The clinical significance of this pattern, if any, is controversial.

Fourteen and 6 Hz positive spikes. Use of term discouraged. Term suggested: 14 and 6 Hz positive burst.

Frequency. Number of complete cycles of repetitive waves or complexes in 1 s. Measured in hertz (Hz), a unit preferred to its equivalent, cycles per second (c/s).

Frequency response. *Cf.*, bandwidth; low frequency response; high frequency response****.

Frequency response curve. A graph depicting the relationships between output pen deflection or amplifier output and input frequency in an EEG channel, for a particular setting of low and high frequency filters****.

Frequency spectrum. Range of frequencies composing the EEG. Divided into 4 bands termed delta, theta, alpha and beta. *Cf.*, delta; theta; alpha; beta bands.

Frontal intermittent rhythmic delta activity. Fairly regular or approximately sinusoidal waves, mostly occurring in bursts at 1.5–3 Hz over the frontal areas of one or both sides of the head. Comment: caution should be exercised to differentiate this acitivity from potential changes generated by vertical eye movements.

G1*. Abbreviation for grid 1 (use of term discouraged).

G2*. Abbreviation for grid 2 (use of term discouraged).

Gain. Ratio of output signal voltage to input signal voltage of an EEG channel. Example:

$$\text{gain} = \frac{\text{output voltage}}{\text{input voltage}} = \frac{10 \text{ V}}{10 \text{ } \mu\text{V}} = 1,000,000$$

often expressed in decibels (dB), a logarithmic unit. Example: a voltage gain of 10 = 20 dB, of 1000 = 60 dB, of 1,000,000 = 120 dB. *Cf.*, sensitivity.

Gamma rhythm. Use of term discouraged. *Cf.*, beta rhythm (not a synonym).

Generalization. Propagation of EEG activity from limited areas to all regions of the head.

Generalized. Occurring over all regions of the head.

Goldman–Offner reference. Use of term discouraged. Term suggested: average potential reference.

Grand mal. Use of term discouraged when describing EEG pattern.

Grid 1*. Use of term discouraged. Term suggested: input terminal 1****.

Grid 2*. Use of term discouraged. Term suggested: input terminal 2****.

Ground connection*. Conducting path between the subject and the electroencephalograph, and the electroencephalograph and earth****. Synonym: earth connection**.

Harness, Head. A combination of straps which are fitted over the head to hold pad electrodes in position.

Hertz. Unit of frequency. Abbreviation: Hz. Preferred to synonym: cycles per second.

High frequency filter. A circuit which reduces the sensitivity of the EEG channel to relatively high frequencies. For each position of the high frequency filter control, this attenuation is expressed as per cent reduction in output pen deflection at a given frequency, relative to frequencies unaffected by the filter, i.e., in the mid-frequency band of the channel. Comment: at present, high frequency filter designations and their significance are not standardized for instruments of different manufacture. For instance, for a given instrument, a position of the high frequency filter control designated as 35 Hz may indicate a 30% (3 dB), or other stated per cent, reduction in sensitivity at 35 Hz, compared to the sensitivity, for example at 10 Hz***·****.

High frequency response. Sensitivity of an EEG channel to relatively high frequencies. Determined by the high frequency response of the amplifier-writer combination and the high frequency filter used. Expressed as per cent reduction in output pen deflection at certain specific high frequencies, relative to other frequencies in the mid-frequency band of the channel****.

High pass filter. *Cf.*, synonym: low frequency filter.

Hyperexcitability, Neuronal. Use of term discouraged when describing EEG patterns.

Hypersynchrony. Use of term discouraged when describing EEG patterns.

Hyperventilation. Deep and regular respiration performed for a period of several minutes***. Used as activation procedure. Synonym: overbreathing. *Cf.*, activation.

Hypsarrhythmia. Pattern consisting of high voltage arrhythmic slow waves interspersed with spike discharges, without consistent synchrony between the two sides of the head or different areas on the same side.

Hz. Abbreviation for hertz. Preferred to equivalent: c/s.

Impedance meter. An instrument used to measure impedance. *Cf.*, electrode impedance.

Inactive electrode. Use of term discouraged. *Cf.*, reference electrode (not a synonym).

Inactivity, Record of electrocerebral. Absence over all regions of the head of indentifiable electrical activity of cerebral origin, whether spontaneous or induced by physiological stimuli and pharmacological agents. Comment: determination of electrocerebral inactivity requires advanced instrumentation and stringent technical precautions. Tracings of electrocerebral inactivity should be held in clear contradistinction to low voltage EEGs and records displaying delta activity of low amplitude. *Cf.*, low voltage EEG.

Independent (temporally). *Cf.*, Synonym: asynchronous.

Index. Per cent time an EEG activity is present in an EEG sample. Example: alpha index.

Indifferent electrode. Use of term discouraged. Term suggested: reference electrode (not a synonym).

In-phase discrimination. Use of term discouraged. Term suggested: common mode rejection (not a synonym).

In-phase signals. Waves with no phase difference between them. *Cf.*, common mode signal (not a synonym).

Input. The signal fed into an EEG amplifier. *Cf.*, input terminal 1; input terminal 2****.

Input terminal 1. The input terminal of the differential EEG amplifier at which negativity, relative to the other input terminal, produces an upward pen deflection****. Synonyms: "grid 1" (G1)*, black lead*** (use discouraged). *Cf.*, polarity convention. Comment: in diagrams, the connection of

an electrode to the input terminal 1 of the EEG amplifier is represented as a solid line.

Input terminal 2. The input terminal of the differential EEG amplifier at which negativity, relative to the other input terminal, produces a downward pen deflection****. Synonyms: "grid 2" (G2)*, white lead*** (use discouraged). *Cf.*, polarity convention. Comment: in diagrams, the connection of an electrode to the input terminal 2 of the EEG amplifier is represented as a dotted or dashed line.

Input circuit. System consisting of the EEG electrodes and intervening tissues, the electrode leads, jack box, input cable and electrode selectors.

Input impedance. Impedance that exists between the two inputs of an EEG amplifier. Measured in ohms (generally megohms, $M\Omega$) with or without the additional specification of input shunt capacitance (measured in picofarads, pF)****. Comment: not a synonym of electrode impedance.

Input voltage. Potential difference between the two input terminals of a differential EEG amplifier.

Instrumental phase reversal. Simultaneous pen deflections in opposite directions caused by a wave in two bipolar derivations. This inversion is purely instrumental in nature, i.e., due to the same signal being simultaneously applied to the input terminal 2 of one differential amplifier and to the input terminal 1 of the other amplifier. Comment: when observed in two linked bipolar derivations, phase reversal indicates that the potential field is maximal or, less frequently, minimal at or near the electrode common to such derivations. Hence, this phenomenon is used to localize EEG activities, whether normal or abnormal. *Cf.*, true phase reversal; bipolar montage; differential amplifier.

Inter-electrode distance. Spacing between pairs of electrodes. Comment: distances between adjacent electrodes placed according to the standard 10–20 system or more closely spaced electrodes are frequently referred to as *short* or *small* inter-electrode distances. Larger distances such as the double or triple distance between standard electrode placements are often termed *long* or *large* inter-electrode distances***.

Inter-hemispheric derivation. Recording between a pair of electrodes located on opposite sides of the head.

Intracerebral electrode. *Cf.*, synonym: depth electrode.

Intracerebral electroencephalogram. *Cf.*, depth electroencephalogram.

Irregular. Applies to EEG waves and complexes of inconstant period and/or uneven countour.

Isoelectric. (1) The record obtained from a pair of equipotential electrodes. *Cf.*, equipotential. (2) Use of term discouraged when describing record of electrocerebral inactivity. *Cf.*, inactivity, record of electrocerebral.

Isolated. Occurring singly.

K complex. A burst of somewhat variable appearance, consisting most commonly of a high voltage diphasic slow wave frequently associated with a sleep spindle. Amplitude is generally maximal in proximity of the vertex. K complexes occur during sleep, apparently spontaneously or in response to sudden sensory stimuli, and are not specific for any individual sensory modality. *Cf.*, vertex sharp transient.

Kappa rhythm. Rhythm consisting of bursts of alpha or theta frequency occurring over the temporal areas of the scalp of subjects engaged in mental activity. Comments: (1) Best recorded between electrodes located lateral to the outer canthus of each eye. (2) The cerebral origin of this rhythm is regarded as unproven.

Lambda wave. Sharp transient occurring over the occipital regions of the head of waking subjects during visual exploration. Mainly positive relative to other areas. Time-locked to saccadic eye movement. Amplitude varies but is generally below 50 μV. Greek letter λ.

Lambdoid wave. Use of term discouraged. Term suggested: positive occipital sharp transient of sleep.

Larval spike-and-slow-waves. Use of term discouraged. Term suggested: 6 Hz spike-and-slow-waves.

Lateralized. Involving mainly the right or left side of the head. *Cf.*, unilateral.

Lead. Strictly: wire connecting an electrode to the electroencephalograph. Loosely: synonym of electrode.

Linkage. The connection of a pair of electrodes to the two respective input terminals of a differential EEG amplifier. *Cf.*, derivation.

Longitudinal bipolar montage. A montage consisting of derivations from pairs of electrodes along longitudinal, usually antero-posterior, arrays***.

Low frequency filter. A circuit which reduces the sensitivity of the EEG channel to relatively low frequencies***. For each position of the low frequency filter control, this attenuation is expressed as per cent reduction of output pen deflection at a given stated frequency, relative to frequencies unaffected by the filter, i.e., in the mid-frequency band of the channel. Comment: at present, low frequency filter designations and their significance are not standardized for instruments of different manufacture. For instance, in a given instrument, a position of the low frequency filter control designated 0.5 Hz may indicate at 30% (3 dB) or other stated per cent, reduction in sensitivity at 0.5 Hz, compared to the sensitivity, for example, at 10 Hz. The same position of the low frequency filter control also may be designated by the time constant. Synonym: high pass filter. *Cf.*, time constant****.

Low frequency response. Sensitivity of an EEG channel to relatively low frequencies. Determined by the low frequency response of the amplifier and by the low frequency filter (time constant) used. Expressed as per cent reduction in output pen deflection at certain stated low frequencies, relative to other frequencies in the mid-frequency band of the channel. *Cf.*, low frequency filter; time constant****.

Low pass filter. *Cf.*, synonym: high frequency filter.

Low voltage EEG. A waking record characterized by activity of amplitude not greater than 20 μV over all head regions. With appropriate instrumental sensitivities this activity can be shown to be composed primarily of beta, theta and, to a lesser degree, delta waves, with or without alpha activity over the posterior areas. Comments: (1) Low voltage EEGs are susceptible to change under the influence of certain physiological stimuli, sleep, pharmacological agents and pathological processes. (2) They should be held in clear contradistinction to the tracings of electrocerebral inactivity, records which consist primarily of delta waves of relatively low voltage, and tracings which display low voltages over limited regions of the head.

Low voltage fast EEG. Use of term discouraged. Term suggested: low voltage EEG.

Machine, EEG. Use of term discouraged. Term suggested: electroencephalograph .

Monomorphic. Use of term discouraged when describing EEG patterns.

Monophasic wave. Wave developed on one side of the baseline.

Monopolar. Use of term discouraged. Term suggested: referential. *Cf.*, also unipolar.

Monorhythmic. Use of term discouraged when describing EEG patterns.

Monorhythmic sinusoidal delta activity. Use of term discouraged. *Cf.*, delta rhythm: frontal (occipital) intermittent rhythmic delta activity.

Montage. The particular arrangement by which a number of derivations are displayed simultaneously in an EEG record***.

Morphology. (1) The study of the form of EEG waves. (2) The form of EEG waves.

Mu rhythm. Rhythm at 7–11 Hz, composed of arch-shaped waves occurring over the central or centro-parietal regions of the scalp during wakefulness. Amplitude varies but is mostly below 50 μV. Blocked or attenuated most clearly by contralateral movement, thought of movement, readiness to move or tactile stimulation. Greek letter: μ. Synonyms: *arceau,* wicket, comb rhythms (use discouraged).

Multiple foci. Two or more spatially separated foci.

Multiple spike-and-slow-wave complex. A sequence of two or more spikes associated with one or more slow waves. Preferred to synonym: polyspike-and-slow-wave complex.

Multiple spike complex. A sequence of two or more spikes. Preferred to synonym: polyspike complex.

Nasopharyngeal electrode. Rod electrode introduced through the nose and placed against the nasopharyngeal wall with its tip lying near the body of the sphenoid bone.

Needle electrode. Small needle inserted into the subdermal layer of the scalp.

Neutral electrode. Use of term discouraged. Term suggested: reference electrode (not a synonym).

Noise, EEG channel. Small fluctuating output of an EEG channel recorded, when high sensitivities are used, even if there is no input signal. Measured in microvolts (μV), referenced to the input***·****.

Notch filter. A filter which selectively attenuates a very narrow frequency band thus producing a sharp notch in the frequency response curve of an EEG channel. A 60 (50) Hz notch filter is used in some electroencephalographs to provide attenuation of 60 (50) Hz interference under extremely unfavorable technical conditions.

Occipital intermittent rhythmic delta activity. Fairly regular or approximately sinusoidal waves, mostly occurring in bursts at 2–3 Hz over the occipital areas of one or both sides of the head. Frequently blocked or attenuated by opening the eyes.

Ohmmeter. An instrument used to measure resistance. *Cf.*, electrode resistance.

Organization. The degree to which physiologic EEG rhythms conform to certain ideal characteristics displayed by a proportion of subjects in the same age group, free from personal and family history of neurologic and psychiatric diseases, and other illnesses that might be associated with dysfunction of the brain. Comments: (1) The organization of physiologic EEG rhythms progresses from birth to adulthood. (2) Poor organization of EEG rhythms such as the alpha rhythm does not necessarily imply abnormality.

Out-of-phase signals*. Two waves of opposite phases. *Cf.*, differential signal (not a synonym).

Output voltage. The voltage across the writer of an EEG channel.

Overbreathing. *Cf.*, synonym: hyperventilation.

Overload. Condition resulting from the application to the input terminals of an EEG amplifier of voltage differences larger than the channel is designed or set to handle. Causes clipping of EEG waves and/or blocking of the amplifier, depending on its magnitude. *Cf.*, clipping; blocking.

Pad electrode. Metal electrode covered with a cotton or felt and gauze pad, held in position by a head cap or harness.

Paper speed. Velocity of movement of EEG paper. Expressed in centimeters per second (cm/s)***.

Paroxysm. Phenomenon with abrupt onset, rapid attainment of a maximum and sudden termination, distinguished from background activity. Comment: commonly used to refer to epileptiform patterns and seizure patterns. *Cf.*, epileptiform pattern; seizure pattern, EEG.

Pattern. Any characteristic EEG activity.

Peak. Point of maximum amplitude of a wave.

Pen galvanometer. *Cf.*, synonym: pen writer.

Pen motor. *Cf.*, synonym: pen writer.

Pen writer. A writer using ink delivered by a pen. Synonym: pen galvanometer; pen motor.

Period. Duration of complete cycle of individual component of a sequence of regularly repeated EEG waves or complexes. Comment: the period of the individual components of an EEG rhythm is the reciprocal of the frequency of the rhythm.

Periodic. Applies to: (1) waves or complexes occurring in a sequence at an approximately regular rate. (2) EEG waves or complexes occurring intermittently at approximately regular intervals, generally of 1 to several seconds.

Petit mal. Use of term discouraged when describing EEG patterns. Terms suggested, whenever appropriate: 3 Hz spike-and-slow-waves; Atypical repetitive spike-and-slow-waves; repetitive sharp-and-slow-waves.

Petit mal variant. Use of term discouraged when describing EEG patterns. Terms suggested whenever appropriate: atypical repetitive spike-and-slow-waves; repetitive sharp-and-slow-waves.

Phantom spike-and-waves. Use of term discouraged. Terms suggested: 6 Hz spike-and-slow-waves.

Phantom spike-and-slow-waves. Use of term discouraged. Term suggested: 6 Hz spike-and-slow-waves.

Phase. (1) Time or polarity relationships between a point on a wave displayed in a derivation and the identical point on the same wave recorded simultaneously in another derivation. (2) Time or angular relationships between a point on a wave and the onset of the cycle of the same wave. Usually expressed in degrees or radians****.

Phase reversal. *Cf.*, instrumental phase reversal; true phase reversal.

Photic driving. Physiologic response consisting of rhythmic activity elicited over the posterior regions of the head by repetitive photic stimulation at frequencies of about 5–30 Hz. Comments: (1) Term should be limited to activity time-locked to the stimulus and of frequency identical or harmonically related to the stimulus frequency. (2) Photic driving should be held in contradistinction to the visual evoked potentials elicited by isolation flashes of light or flashes repeated at very low frequencies.

Photic stimulation. Delivery of intermittent flashes of light to the eyes of a subject. Used as EEG activation procedure***.

Photic stimulator. Device for delivering intermittent flashes of light. Synonym: stroboscope (discouraged).

Photo-convulsive response. *Cf.*, synonym: photo-paroxysmal response (preferred).

Photo-myoclonic response. *Cf.*, synonym: photo-myogenic response (preferred).

Photo-myogenic response. A response to intermittent photic stimulation characterized by the appearance in the record of brief, repetitive muscular spikes over the anterior regions of the head. These often in crease gradually in amplitude as stimuli are continued and cease promptly when the stimulus is withdrawn. Comment: this response is associated frequently with flutter of the eyelids and vertical oscillations of the eyeballs and sometimes with discrete jerking mostly involving the musculature of the face and head. Preferred to synonym: photomyoclonic response.

Photo-paroxysmal response. A response to intermittent photic stimulation characterized by the appearance in the record of spike-and-slow-wave and multiple spike-and-slow-wave complexes. These are bilaterally synchronous, symmetrical and generalized and may outlast the stimulus by a few seconds. Comment: this response may be associated with impairment of consciousness and brisk jerks involving the musculature of the whole body, most prominently that of the upper extremities and head. Preferred to synonym: photo-convulsive response.

Polarity convention. International agreement whereby differential EEG amplifiers are constructed so that negativity at the input terminal 1 relative to the input terminal 2 of the same amplifier produces an upward pen deflec-tion***·****. Comment: this convention is contrary to that prevailing in some other biological and non-biological fields.

Polarity, EEG wave. Sign of potential difference existing at a given instant in time between an electrode affected by a given potential change and another electrode not appreciably, or less, affected by the same change. *Cf.*, polarity convention.

Polygraphic recording. Simultaneous monitoring of multiple physiological measures such as the EEG, respiration, electrocardiogram, electromyogram, eye movement, galvanic skin resistance, blood pressure, etc.

Polymorphic activity. Use of term discouraged when describing EEG pattern.

Polyphasic wave. Wave consisting of two or more components developed on alternating sides of the baseline. *Cf.*, diphasic wave; triphasic wave.

Polyrhythmic activity. Use of term discouraged when describing EEG pattern.

Polyspike-and-slow-wave complex. *Cf.*, synonym: multiple spike-and-slow-wave complex (preferred).

Polyspike complex. *Cf.*, synonym: multiple spike complex (preferred).

Positive occipital sharp transient of sleep. Sharp transient maximal over the occipital regions, positive relative to other areas, occurring apparently spontaneously during sleep. May be single or repetitive. Amplitude varies but is generally below 50 μV.

Positive occipital spike-like wave of sleep. Use of term discouraged. Term suggested: positive occipital sharp transient of sleep.

Potential. (1) Strictly: voltage. (2) Loosely: synonym of wave.

Potential field. Amplitude distribution of an EEG wave at the surface of the head or cerebral cortex or in the depth of the brain, measured at a given instant in time. Represented in diagrams by equipotential lines.

Projected patterns. Abnormal EEG activities believed to result from a disturbance at a site remote from the recording electrodes. Description of specific EEG patterns preferred.

Provocation procedure. Use of term discouraged. Term suggested: activation.

Pseudo-periodic. Use of term discouraged. Term suggested: quasi-periodic.

Psychomotor variant. Use of term discouraged when describing EEG pattern. Term suggested: rhythmic temporal theta burst of drowsiness.

Quantity. Amount of EEG activity with respect to both number and amplitude of waves.

Quasi-periodic. Applies to EEG waves or complexes occurring at intervals only approaching regularity.

R-C coupled amplifier. Abbreviation for: resistance-capacitance coupled amplifier.

Reactivity. Susceptibility of individual rhythms or the EEG as a whole to change following sensory stimulation or other physiologic actions.

Record. The end product of the EEG recording process.

Recording. (1) The process of obtaining an EEG record. Synonym: tracing. (2) The end product of the EEG recording process, most commonly traced paper. Synonyms: record; tracing.

Reference electrode. (1) In general: any electrode against which the potential variations of another electrode are measured. (2) Specifically: a suitable reference electrode is any electrode customarily connected to the input terminal 2 of an EEG amplifier and so placed as to minimize the likelihood of pickup of the same EEG activity recorded by an exploring electrode, usually connected to the input terminal 1 of the same amplifier, or of other activities. Comments: (1) Whatever the location of the reference electrode, the possibility that it might be affected by appreciable EEG potentials should always be considered. (2) A reference electrode connected to the input terminal 2 of all or several EEG amplifiers is referred to as a *common reference electrode.*

Referential derivation. Recording from a pair of electrodes consisting of an exploring electrode generally connected to the input terminal 1 and a refer-

ence electrode usually connected to the input terminal 2 of an EEG amplifier***. *Cf.,* exploring electrode; reference electrode; referential montage; common reference montage.

Referential montage. A montage consisting of referential derivations. Comment: a referential montage in which the reference electrode is common to multiple derivations is referred to as a common reference montage***. *Cf.,* referential derivation.

Regular. Applies to waves or complexes of approximately constant period and relatively uniform appearance.

Resistance-capacitance coupled amplifier. An amplifier in which successive stages are connected (coupled) by networks consisting of capacitors and resistors. Abbreviation: R-C coupled amplifier.

Rhythm. EEG activity consisting of waves of approximately constant period.

Rhythm of alpha frequency. (1) In general, any rhythm in the alpha band. (2) Specifically: term should be used to designate those activities in the alpha band which differ from the *alpha rhythm* as regards their topography and/or reactivity and do not have specific appellations (such as mu rhythm). *Cf.,* alpha rhythm.

Rhythmic temporal theta burst of drowsiness. Characteristic burst of 4–7 Hz waves frequently notched by faster waves, occurring over the temporal regions of the head during drowsiness. Synonym: psychomotor variant pattern (use discouraged). Comment: the clinical significance of this pattern, if any, is controversial.

Run. Colloquialism. Use of term discouraged. Term suggested: montage.

Scalp electrode. Electrode held against, attached to or inserted into the scalp.

Scalp electroencephalogram. Record of electrical activity of the brain by means of electrodes placed on the surface of the head. Abbreviation: SEEG. Comment: term and abbreviations should be used only to distinguish between scalp and other electroencephalograms such as depth electroencephalograms. In all other instances, a scalp electroencephalogram should be referred to simply as an electroencephalogram (EEG).

Scalp electroencephalography. Technique of recording scalp electroencephalograms. Abbreviation: SEEG. Comment: term and abbreviation should be used only to distinguish between this and other recording techniques such as depth electroencephalography. In all other instances scalp electroencephalography should be referred to simply as electroencephalography (EEG).

SDEEG. Abbreviation for stereotactic (stereotaxic) depth electroencephalography.

SEEG. Abbreviation for scalp electroencephalogram and scalp electroencephalography.

Seizure pattern, EEG. Phenomenon consisting of repetitive EEG discharges with relatively abrupt onset and termination and characteristic pattern of evolution, lasting at least several seconds. The component waves or complexes vary in form, frequency and topography. They are generally rhythmic and frequently display increasing amplitude and decreasing frequency during the same episode. When focal in onset, they tend to spread subsequently to other areas. Comment: EEG seizure patterns unaccompanied by clinical epileptic manifestations detected by the recordist and/or reported by the patient should be referred to as "subclinical". *Cf.*, epileptiform pattern..

Sensitivity. Ratio of input voltage to output pen deflection in an EEG channel****. Sensitivity is measured in microvolts per millimeter (μV/mm)***. Example:

$$\text{sensitivity} = \frac{\text{input voltage}}{\text{output pen deflection}} = \frac{50\ \mu\text{V}}{10\ \text{mm}} = 5\ \mu\text{V/mm}.$$

Sharp wave. A transient, clearly distinguished from background activity, with pointed peak at conventional paper speeds and duration of 70–200 ms, i.e., over 1/14–1/5 s, approximately. Main component is generally negative relative to other areas. Amplitude is variable. Comments: (1) Term does not apply to (a) distinctive physiologic events such as vertex sharp transients, lambda waves and positive occipital sharp transients of sleep, (b) sharp transients poorly distinguished from background activity and sharp-appearing individual waves of EEG rhythms. (2) Sharp waves should be differentiated from spikes, i.e., transients having similar characteristics but shorter duration. However, it is well to keep in mind that this distinction is largely arbitrary and serves primarily descriptive purposes. Practically, in ink-written EEG records taken at 3 cm/s, sharp waves occupy more than 2 mm of paper width and spikes 2 mm or less. *Cf.*, spike.

Sharp-and-slow-wave complex. A sequence of a sharp wave and a slow wave. Comment: hyphenation facilitates use of term in plural form: sharp-and-slow-wave complexes or sharp-and-slow-waves.

Sigma rhythm. Use of term discouraged. Term suggested: sleep spindles.

Silence, Record of electrocerebral. Use of term discouraged. Term suggested: record of electrocerebral inactivity. *Cf.*, inactivity record of electrocerebral.

Simultaneous. Occurring at the same time. Synonym: synchronous.

Sine wave. Wave having the form of a sine curve.

Single-ended amplifier. An amplifier that operates on signals which are asymmetric with respect to ground.

Sinusoidal. Term applies to EEG waves resembling sine waves.

Six Hz spike-and-slow-waves. Spike-and-slow-wave complexes at 4–7 Hz, but mostly at 6 Hz, occurring generally in brief bursts bilaterally synchronously, symmetrically or asymmetrically, and either confined to or of larger amplitude over the posterior or anterior regions of the head. Amplitude is variable but generally smaller than that of spike-and-slow-wave complexes repeating at slower rates. Comment: the clinical significance of this pattern, if any, is controversial.

Sleep spindle. Burst at 11–15 Hz, but mostly at 12–14 Hz, generally diffuse but of higher voltage over the central regions of the head, occurring during sleep. Amplitude is variable but is mostly below 50 μV in the adult. Synonym: sigma rhythm (use discouraged).

Sleep stages. Distinctive phases of sleep, best demonstrated by polygraphic recordings of the EEG and other variables, including at least eye movements and activity of certain voluntary muscles.

Slow alpha variant rhythms. Characteristic rhythms at 3.5–6 Hz but mostly at 4–5 Hz, recorded most prominently over the posterior regions of the head. Generally alternate, or are intermixed, with alpha rhythm to which they often are harmonically related. Amplitude is variable but is frequently close to 50 μV. Blocked or attenuated by attention, especially visual, and mental effort. Comment: slow alpha variant rhythms should be held in contradistinction to posterior slow waves characteristic of children and adolescents and occasionally seen in young adults.

Slow activity. Activity of frequency lower than alpha, i.e., theta and delta activities.

Slow spike. Use of term discouraged. Term suggested: sharp wave.

Slow spike-and-wave complex. Use of term discouraged. Term suggested: sharp-and-slow-wave complex.

Slow wave. Wave with duration longer than alpha waves, i.e., over 1/8 s.

Special electrode. Any electrode other than standard scalp electrode.

Sphenoidal electrode. Needle or wire electrode inserted through the soft tissues of the face below the zygomatic arch with its tip lying near the base of the skull in the region of the foramen ovale.

Spike. A transient, clearly distinguished from background activity, with pointed peak at conventional paper speeds and a duration from 20 to under 70 ms, i.e., 1/50–1/40 s, approximately. Main component is generally negative relative to other areas. Amplitude is variable. Comments: (1) EEG spikes should be differentiated from sharp waves, i.e., transients having similar characteristics but longer durations. However it is well to keep in mind that this distinction is largely arbitrary and serves primarily descriptive purposes. Practically, in ink-written EEG records taken at 3 cm/s, spikes occupy 2 mm or less of paper width and sharp waves more than 2 mm. (2) EEG spikes should be held in clear contradistinction to the brief unit spikes recorded from single cells with microelectrode techniques. *Cf.*, sharp wave.

Spike-and-dome complex. Use of term discouraged. Term suggested: spike-and-slow-wave complex.

Spike-and-slow-wave complex. A pattern consisting of a spike followed by a slow wave. Comment: hyphenation facilitates use of term in plural form: spike-and-slow-wave complexes or spike-and-slow-waves.

Spike-and-slow-wave rhythm. Use of term discouraged. Term suggested, whenever appropriate: 3 Hz spike-and-slow-waves; atypical repetitive spike-and-slow-waves.

Spindle. Group of rhythmic waves characterized by a progressively increasing, then gradually decreasing, amplitude. *Cf.*, sleep spindle.

Spread. Propagation of EEG waves from one region of the scalp and/or brain to another. *Cf.*, generalization.

Standard electrode. Conventional scalp electrode. *Cf.*, disk electrode; needle electrode; pad electrode; special electrode.

Standard electrode placement. Scalp electrode location(s) determined by the ten–twenty system. *Cf.*, Ten–twenty system.

Status epilepticus, EEG. The occurrence of virtually continuous seizure activity in an EEG.

Stephenson–Gibbs reference. Use of term discouraged. Term suggested: sterno-spinal reference electrode.

Stereotactic (stereotaxic) depth electroencephalogram. Recording of electrical activity of the brain by means of electrodes implanted within the brain substance according to stereotactic (stereotaxic) measurements. Abbreviation: SDEEG.

Stereotactic (stereotaxic) depth electroencephalography. Technique of recording stereotactic (stereotaxic) depth electroencephalograms. Abbreviation: SDEEG.

Sterno-spinal reference. A non-cephalic reference achieved by interconnecting two electrodes placed over the right sterno-clavicular junction and the apophysis spinosa of the seventh cervical vertebra, respectively, and balancing the voltage between them by means of a potentiometer to reduce ECG artifact.

Stick-on electrode**. Colloquialism. Use of term discouraged. Term suggested: disk electrode.

Stigmatic electrode. Use of term discouraged. Term suggested: exploring electrode.

Subdural electrode. Electrode inserted under the dural covering of the cerebrum.

Suppression. Use of term discouraged when describing EEG patterns other than burst suppression pattern.

Symmetry. (1) Approximately equal amplitude, frequency and form of EEG activities over homologous areas on opposite sides of the head. (2) Approximately equal distribution of potentials of unlike polarity on either side of a zero isopotential axis. *Cf.*, true phase reversal. (3) Approximately equal distribution of EEG waves about the baseline.

Synchrony. The simultaneous occurrence of EEG waves over regions on the same or opposite sides of the head. Comment: term *simultaneous* only implies lack of delay measurable with ink writers at customary paper speeds.

Ten–twenty system. System of standardized scalp electrode placement recommended by the International Federation of Societies for Electroencephalography and Clinical Neurophysiology***. According to this system, electrode placements are determined by measuring the head from external landmarks and taking 10% or 20% of such measurements. Comment: the use of additional scalp electrodes, such as true anterior temporal electrodes, is indicated in various circumstances.

Theta band. Frequency band from 4 to under 8 Hz. Greek letter: θ.

Theta rhythm. Rhythm with a frequency of 4 to under 8 Hz.

Theta wave. Wave with duration of 1/4 to over 1/8 s.

Three Hz spike-and-slow-waves. Characteristic paroxysm consisting of a regular sequence of spike-and-slow-wave complexes which: (1) repeat at 3–3.5 Hz (measured during the first few seconds of the paroxysm), (2) are bilateral in their onset and termination, generalized and usually of maximal amplitude over the frontal areas, (3) are approximately synchronous and symmetrical on the two sides of the head throughout the paroxysm. Amplitude is variable but can reach values of 1000 μV (1 mV). *Cf.*, atypical repetitive spike-and-slow-waves.

Time constant, EEG channel. The product of the values of the resistance (in megohms, MΩ) and the capacitance (in microfarads, μF) which make up the time constant control of an EEG channel. This product represents the time required for the pen to fall to 37% of the deflection initially produced when a DC voltage difference is applied to the input terminals of the amplifier. Expressed in seconds (s). Abbreviation: TC. Comment: for a simple R-C coupling network, the TC is related to the per cent reduction in sensitivity of the channel at a given stated low frequency by the equation TC $= 1/2\pi f$, where f is the frequency at which a 30% (3 dB) attenuation occurs. For instance, for a TC of 0.3 s, an attenuation of 30% (3 dB) occurs at 0.5 Hz. Thus, either the time constant or the per cent attenuation at a given stated low frequency can be used to designate the same position of the low frequency filter of the EEG channel. *Cf.*, low frequency filter****.

Topography. Amplitude distribution of EEG activities at the surface of the head, cerebral cortex or in the depths of the brain.

Tracé alternant. EEG pattern of sleeping newborns, characterized by bursts of slow waves, at times intermixed with sharp waves, and intervening periods of relative quiescence.

Tracing. *Cf.*, synonyms: record; recording.

Transient, EEG. Any isolated wave or complex, distinguished from background activity.

Transverse bipolar montage. *Cf.*, synonym: coronal bipolar montage.

Triangular bipolar montage. A montage consisting of derivations from pairs of electrodes in a group of 3 electrodes arranged in a triangular pattern.

Triphasic wave. Wave consisting of 3 components alternating about the baseline.

True phase reversal. Simultaneous pen deflections in opposite directions occurring in two referential derivations using a suitable common reference electrode and displaying the same wave. Comments: (1) This phenomenon is rarely observed in scalp EEGs. (2) When demonstrated beyond doubt in appropriate recording conditions, it indicates a 180° change in phase of an EEG wave between adjacent areas of the brain, on either side of a zero isopotential axis. *Cf.*, instrumental phase reversal.

Unilateral. Confined to one side of the head. Comments: (1) Unilateral EEG activities may be focal or diffuse. (2) They are said to be lateralized to the right or left side of the head.

Unipolar. Use of term discouraged. Term suggested: referential.

Unipolar derivation. Use of term discouraged. *Cf.*, referential derivation.

Unipolar depth electrode. Use of term discouraged. Term suggested: single-electrode lead.

Unipolar montage. Use of term discouraged. Term suggested: referential montage.

Vertex sharp transient. Sharp potential, maximal at the vertex, negative relative to other areas, occurring apparently spontaneously during sleep or in response to a sensory stimulus during sleep or wakefulness. May be single or repetitive. Amplitude varies but rarely exceeds 250 μV. Abbreviations: V wave. *Cf.*, K complex.

Vertex sharp wave. Use of term discouraged when describing physiologic vertex sharp transient.

Voltage. *Cf.*, amplitude.

V wave. Abbreviation for: vertex sharp transient.

Wave. Any change of the potential difference between pairs of electrodes in EEG recording. May arise in the brain (EEG wave) or outside it (extra-cerebral potential).

Waveform. The shape of an EEG wave.

White lead***. Use of term discouraged. Term suggested: input terminal 2.

Wicket rhythm. Use of term discouraged. Term suggested: mu rhythm.

Writer. System for direct write-out of the output of an EEG channel. Most writers use ink delivered by a pen. In certain instruments, the ink is sprayed as a jet stream. In other recorders the pen writer uses carbon paper instead of ink****.

Zero potential reference electrode. Use of term discouraged. Term suggested: reference electrode (not a synonym).

Appendix II

American Clinical Neurophysiology Society recording guidelines

GUIDELINE ONE: MINIMUM TECHNICAL REQUIREMENTS FOR PERFORMING CLINICAL ELECTROENCEPHALOGRAPHY

INTRODUCTION

Although no single best method exists for recording EEGs under all circumstances, the following standards are considered the minimum for the usual clinical recording of EEGs in all age groups except the very young (see Guideline Two: Minimum Technical Standards for Pediatric Electroencephalography).

Recording at minimum standards should not give pride to the EEG department working at this level and cannot ensure a satisfactory test. Minimum standards provide barely adequate fulfillment of responsibilities to the patient and the referring physician.

To the minimum standards have been added recommenda-

This material originally appeared in *J Clin Neurophysiol* 1986; 3 (Suppl 1):1–6. © 1994 American Electroencephalographic Society, Vol. 11 (1): 2–5.

tions to improve standardization of procedures and also facilitate interchange of recordings and assessment among laboratories in North America.

1. Equipment

1.1 To find the distribution of EEG activity, it is necessary to record simultaneously from as many regions of the scalp as possible. When too few channels are used simultaneously, the chances of interpretive errors increase, and, conversely, when more channels are utilized, the likelihood of such errors decreases. This is particularly true for transient activity.

Eight channels of simultaneous recording are the minimum number required to show the areas producing most normal and abnormal EEG patterns, and 16 channels are now found to be necessary by most laboratories. Additional channels are often needed for monitoring other physiologic activities.

1.2 Alternating current (AC) wiring should meet the Underwriters Laboratories standards required for hospital service. Adequate grounding of the instrument must be provided by all AC receptacles. All equipment in each patient in area in the EEG laboratory must be grounded to a common point.

1.3 In the usual clinical setting, electrical shielding of the patient and equipment is not necessary, and such shielding need not be installed unless proven necessary.

1.4 Ancillary equipment should include a device for delivering rhythmic, high-intensity flash stimuli to the patient.

2. Electrodes

2.1 Recording electrodes should be free of inherent noise and drift. They should not significantly attenuate signals between 0.5 and 70 Hz. Experimental evidence suggests that silver–silver chloride or gold disk electrodes held on by collodion are the best, but other electrode materials and electrode pastes have been effectively used especially with contemporary amplifiers having high input impedances. High-quality electrodes are available from several manufacturers and are generally preferable to home-made electrodes.

To decrease noise, electrodes must be kept clean, with appropriate precautions taken after recording from patients with contagious diseases (viral hepatitis, Creutzfeldt-Jakob disease, acquired immunodeficiency syndrome) (AEEGS, 1984).

2.2 Needle electrodes are not recommended. If circumstances necessitate their use, they must be completely steril-

ized, and the technologist who employs them should have been taught the exact techniques, as well as the disadvantages and hazards, of their use. Parallel anteroposterior alignment of the needles is important; misalignment may cause artifactual amplitude asymmetries or distortions.

It is rarely appreciated that proper use of needle electrodes requires more care and expertise than for any other type of electrode. However, needle electrodes can be effectively utilized in comatose patients, in whom pain responses are usually minimal or absent, and who are in medical settings requiring efficient recording with a minimum of delay.

2.3 All 21 electrodes and placements recommended by the International Federation of Societies for EEG and Clinical Neurophysiology (Jasper, 1958, 1983) should be used. The 10–20 system is the only one officially recommended by the International Federation of Societies for EEG and Clinical Neurophysiology. It is the most commonly used existing system, and it should be used universally. The use of the term 'modified 10–20 system' is undesirable when it means that head measurements have not been made and placements have been estimated. In this case, the term 'estimated 10–20 placement' is more appropriate. (For neonates, refer to Guideline Two.)

An adequate number of electrodes is essential to ensure that EEG activity having a small area of representation on the scalp is recorded and to analyze accurately the distribution of more diffuse activity. Occasionally, additional electrodes, placed between or below those representing the standard placements, are needed in order to record very localized activity.

A grounding electrode always should be used, except in situations (e.g., intensive care units, operating rooms) in which other electrical equipment is attached to the patient. In such cases, double grounding must be avoided.

2.4 Interelectrode impedances should be checked as a routine prerecording procedure. Ordinarily, electrode impedance should not exceed 5 kΩ.

Electrode impedances should be rechecked during the recording when any pattern that might be artifactual appears.

3. Recordings

3.1 Montages should be designed in conformity with Guideline Seven: A Proposal for Standard Montages to Be Used in Clinical Electroencephalography. It is desirable that at least some montages in all laboratories be uniform to facilitate communication and comparison.

3.2 The record should have written on it as a minimum the name and age of the patient, the date of the recording, an identification number, and the name or initials of the technologist.

Identifications should be made at the time of recording. Failure to do so may result in errors that have adverse medical and legal consequences. A Basic Data Sheet, attached to every record, should include the time of the recording, the time and date of the last seizure (if any), the behavioral state of the patient, a list of all medications that the patient has been taking, including premedication given to induce sleep during EEG, and any relevant additional medical history.

3.3 Appropriate square-wave calibrations should be made at the beginning and end of every EEG recording. A recording with all channels connected to the same pair of electrodes should follow at the beginning (biologic calibration). At the outset, all channels should be adjusted, if necessary, so that they respond equally and correctly to the calibration signal. When doubt as to correct functioning of any amplifier exists, a repeat calibration run should be made.

The calibration is an integral part of every EEG recording. It gives a scaling factor for the interpreter and tests the EEG machine for sensitivity, high- and low-frequency response, noise level, and pen alignment and damping. It also gives information about the competence and care of the technologist. Calibration voltages must be appropriate for the sensitivities used.

In addition to the standard square-wave calibration, a biologic calibration ('bio-cal') may at times be of additional help in detecting errors in the montage selection process or in the pen-writing mechanism. For this purpose, an anteroposterior (fronto-occipital) derivation should be used, since it can include fast and alpha range patterns as well as eye movement activity in the delta range.

3.4 The sensitivity of the EEG equipment for routine recording should be set in the range of 5–10 μV/mm of pen deflection.

Sensitivity is defined as the ratio of input voltage to pen

deflection. It is expressed in microvolts per millimeter (μV/mm). A commonly used sensitivity is 7 μV/mm which, for a calibration signal of 50 μV, results in a deflection of 7.1 mm.

If the sensitivity is decreased (for example, from 7 to 10 μV/mm), the amplitude of the writeout of a given EEG on the paper also decreases. Conversely, if the sensitivity is increased (for example, from 7 to 5 μV/mm), the amplitude of the writeout of a given EEG increases.

When the sensitivity is less than 10 μV/mm (for example, 20 μV/mm), significant low-amplitude activity may become indiscernible. If the sensitivity is greater than 5 μV/mm (for example, 3 μV/mm), normal EEG activity may overload the system, causing a squaring off of the peaks of the writeout onto the paper.

Note that a sensitivity of 5 μV/mm means that, to obtain a pen deflection of 1 mm, a 5-μV input voltage is required (and correspondingly, to obtain a 10-mm deflection, an input of 50 μV is required). If the sensitivity is decreased to 10 μV/mm, the same 1-mm pen deflection now requires a larger input, i.e., 10 μV rather than 5 μV (and correspondingly, a 10-mm pen deflection now requires an input of 100 μV rather than 50 μV). Thus, as the sensitivity is increased, its numerical value becomes smaller. Conversely, as the sensitivity is decreased, its numerical value becomes larger. This perhaps seemingly paradoxical relationship is actually a logical consequence of the definition of sensitivity as input voltage per unit of pen deflection.

During calibration for routine recordings, the recorded signals should not be distorted but should be large enough to permit measurement to better than ±5% between any of the signals on the different channels.

No matter which sensitivity (within the above limits) is chosen prior to the recording, appropriate adjustments should be made whenever EEG activity encountered is of too high or low amplitude to be recorded properly.

3.5 For standard recordings, the low-frequency filter should be no higher than 1 Hz (-3 dB) corresponding to a time constant of at least 0.16 s. The high-frequency filter should be no lower than 70 Hz (-3 dB).

A low-frequency filter setting higher than 1 Hz should not be used routinely to attenuate slow-wave artifacts in the record. Vital information may be lost when pathologic activity in the delta range is present. Similarly, a setting lower than 70 Hz for the high-frequency filters can distort or attenuate spikes and other pathologic discharges into unrecognizable forms and can cause muscle artifact to resemble spikes. Production of a record with lost or inaccurate information is poor medical practice.

It must be emphasized, however, that judicious use of the low- or high-frequency filters – with appropriate annotation on the record – can emphasize or clarify certain types of patterns in the record. These filter controls, therefore, should be used selectively and carefully.

3.6 The 60-Hz (notch) filter can distort or attenuate spikes; it therefore should be used only when other measures against 60 Hz interference fail.

3.7 A paper speed of 3 cm/s should be utilized for routine recordings. A paper speed of 1.5 cm/s is sometimes used for EEG recordings in newborns, during polysomnograms, or in other special situations.

3.8 When instrument settings (sensitivities, filters, paper speed, montage) are changed during the recording, the settings should be clearly identified on the record at the time of the change. The final calibration(s) should include each sensitivity and filter settings used in the recording, and should include calibration voltages appropriate to the sensitivities actually used. It is especially important to record calibration signals at very high sensitivities when these settings have been used.

3.9 The baseline record should contain at least 20 min of technically satisfactory recording. Longer recordings are often more informative.

The EEG is a short sample in time from the patient's life. Within reasonable limits, the longer the recording, the better the chance of recording an abnormality or abnormalities demonstrating the variability of these. Experience in many centers shows that a very minimum of 20 min of artifact-free recording is necessary to assess baseline waking EEG activity. The addition of photic stimulation, hyperventilation, and especially sleep – which should be recorded whenever possible – often requires an increase of recording time.

3.10 The recordings should include periods when the eyes are open and when they are closed.

Proper EEG recordings requires examining the effect of stimuli upon the EEG. A comparison between the eyes-open and eyes-closed condition constitutes one important means for assessment. Some rhythms can be masked by the alpha activity and are visible only when the alpha rhythm has been attenuated by eye-opening. Certain forms of eye movement may appear to be frontal delta or theta activity but eye-opening and closing helps in differentiation. Finally, paroxysmal activity may appear only when the eyes are opened or only when the eyes are closed or at the times these conditions change. Thus, failure to record with eye-opening and closing as a routine procedure can reduce chances of obtaining potentially important information. This procedure is so simple that it is unjustifiable not to request eye-opening and closure whenever patient cooperation permits, or to manually open and close the eyes when it does not.

3.11 Hyperventilation should be used routinely unless medical other justifiable reasons (e.g., a recent intracranial hemorrhage, significant cardiopulmonary disease, sickle cell disease or trait, or patient inability or unwillingness to cooperate) contraindicate it. It should be performed for a minimum of 3 min with continued recording for at least 1 min after cessation of overbreathing. At times, hyperventilation must be performed for a longer period in order to obtain adequate activation of the EEG. To evaluate the effects of this activation technique, at least 1 min of recording with the same montage should be obtained before overbreathing begins. The record should contain an assessment of the quality of patient effort during hyperventilation. It is often helpful to record electro-

461

radiographic (ECG) activity directly on one EEG channel during this and other parts of the recording, particularly if spikes and sharp waves, or pulse or ECG artifact, are in question. With an additional (e.g., 17th) channel, the ECG can be monitored continuously.

3.12 Sleep recordings should be taken whenever possible but not to the exclusion of the waking record.

It is increasingly evident that considerable additional information can be obtained by recording during drowsiness and sleep. Some laboratories use sleep recording routinely. Sleep recording is usually essential for patients with suspected or known convulsive disorders.

3.13 The patient's level of consciousness (awake, drowsy, sleeping, or comatose), and any change thereof, should be noted by the technologist on the EEG recording. Any commands or signals to the patient, and any movement or clinical seizure activity or absence thereof, should also be noted on the recording. Careful observation of the patient with frequent notations is often essential, particularly when unusual waveforms are observed in the tracing. Abbreviations used should be standardized, with their definitions readily available to the reader.

In stuporous or comatose patients and those showing invariant EEG patterns of any kind, visual, auditory, and somatosensory stimuli should be applied systematically during recording. The stimuli and the patient's responses or failure to respond should be noted on the recording paper as near as possible to their point of the occurrence.

It is the responsibility of the electroencephalographer to recognize the patterns usually associated with different states of consciousness. However, observations by the technologist about the patient's clinical status can be of considerable interpretative value, particularly when discrepancies or unusual correlations occur.

To facilitate assessing awake background activity, it is important for the technologist to ascertain that the patient is maximally alert for at least a portion of the record.

3.14 Special procedures that are of some risk to the patient should be carried out only in the presence of a qualified physician, only in an environment with adequate resuscitating equipment, and with the informed consent of the patient or responsible relative or legal guardian.

3.15 EEGs for the evaluation of cessation of cerebral function ('cerebral death') require special procedures and extraordinary precautions (see Guideline Three: Minimum Technical Standards for EEG Recording in Suspected Cerebral Death).

REFERENCES

American Electroencephalographic Society. Infectious Diseases Committee Report. *J Clin Neurophysiol* 1984;1:437–41.

Jasper HH. The ten–twenty electrode system of the International Federation. *Electroencephalogr Clin Neurophysiol* 1958;10:371–3.

Jasper HH. The ten–twenty electrode system of the International Federation. In: *International Federation of Societies for Electroencephalography and Clinical Neurophysiology: Recommendations for the practice of clinical electroencephalography.* Amsterdam: Elsevier, 1983:3–10.

GUIDELINE TWO: MINIMUM TECHNICAL STANDARDS FOR PEDIATRIC ELECTROENCEPHALOGRAPHY

INTRODUCTION

These guidelines for clinical pediatric EEG should be considered in conjunction with the more general Guideline One: Minimum Technical Requirements for Performing Clinical Electroencephalography (MTR).

The basic principles of clinical EEG outlined in the MTR also apply to the very young and are reaffirmed. However, special considerations are pertinent to pediatric recordings and are discussed below. The numbers in parentheses in this Guideline refer specifically to sections of the MTR that must be modified in these special situations. Where a subject is not covered here, the recommendations of Guideline One remain appropriate and should be consulted.

Emphasis here will be on EEG in neonates, infants, and young children, since recording the EEGs of older children and adolescents differs little from recording the EEGs of adults. Because EEG recording in the newborn presents a number of special problems, this Guideline is divided into

This material originally appeared in *J Clin Neurophysiol* 1986;3(Suppl 1):7–11.
© 1994 American Electroencephalographic Society, Vol. 11 (1): 6–9.

two parts setting forth recommendations for children and for neonates separately.

1. Children

1.1 (MTR 2.1) Because children, especially young children, have a tendency to move a good deal during recording, electrode application should be performed with great care. Electrodes may be applied with paste or collodion, according to the preference of the laboratory, but their positions and impedances should be monitored carefully throughout the study. The inverted saucer-shaped silver–silver chloride electrode with a small hole for the injection of electrolyte solution is best. Needle electrodes are not needed and should not be used.

1.2 (MTR 2.3) All 21 electrodes of the international 10–20 system (Jasper, 1958) should be used for most purposes. The standard montages used for adults should be used for children.

1.3 (MTR 3.2) Before recording the EEGs of young inpatients, especially those in so precarious a condition that the recordings must be done at bedside, the technician should consult with the nursing staff concerning the patient's condition and any limitations on recording procedures.

1.4 (MTR 3.4) The voltage of EEG activity in many young children is higher than that of older children and adults, and appropriate reduction of sensitivity (to 10 μV/mm or even 15 μV/mm) should be used. However, at least a portion of the record should be run at a sensitivity (such as 7 μV/mm) adequate to display low-voltage fast activity. Otherwise, for patients beyond infancy, the same instrument control settings can be used as for adults in the same laboratory.

1.5 (MTR 3.9) Photic stimulation over the frequency range of at least 1–20 flashes/s should be used during wakefulness in appropriate patients.

1.6 (MTR 3.10) Whenever possible, recordings should include periods when the eyes are open and when they are closed. In infants over 3 months of age, passive eye closure (by placing the technician's hand over the patient's eyes) is often successful in producing the dominant posterior rhythm, as is the playing of a game such as peek-a-boo.

1.7 (MTR 3.12) Sleep recordings should be obtained whenever possible, but not to the exclusion of the awake record. The recording of the patient during drowsiness, initiation of sleep, and arousal is important. Natural sleep is preferred, but if the use of sedation is necessary, all efforts should still be made to record arousal at the end of the recording.

1.8 (MTR 3.13) The patient's condition should be clearly indicated at the beginning of the recording from every montage. Continuous observation by the technician, with frequent notations on the recording, is particularly important when recording young patients.

2. Neonates and young infants (up to 4–8 weeks post term)

2.1 (MTR 1.1) Sixteen-channel instruments should be used. Two, and often more, channels must be devoted to recording non-EEG 'polygraphic' variables, such as EKG and respiration. Consequently, the number of channels left for EEG recording on an 8-channel machine is unacceptable. Sixteen or more channels allow the necessary flexibility.

Because EEG patterns seen in the neonate are not as clearly related to stages of the wake–sleep cycle as are those of adults and older children, it is usually necessary to record polygraphic (non-EEG) variables along with the EEG in order to assess accurately the baby's state during the recording. Polygraphic recording is also helpful in identifying physiologic artifacts; for example, apparent monomorphic delta activity often turns out to be respiration artifact, since babies may have respiratory rates of up to 100/min. Moreover, variables other than the EEG may be directly pertinent to the patient's problems. For example, in those experiencing apneic episodes, breathing and heart rate changes are most relevant.

The parameters most frequently monitored along with EEG in infants are respirations, eye movements, and heartbeats. A recording of muscle movements, by submental electromyography (EMG) or movement transducer, also can be quite helpful.

Respirogram can be recorded by any of the following means: (1) abdominal and/or thoracic strain gauges, (2) changes in impedance between thoracic electrodes (impedance pneumogram), or (3) airway thermistors/thermocouples. In infants with respiratory problems, it is necessary to devote three or four channels to respiration in order to monitor both abdominal and thoracic movements, plus airflow in the upper airway. In infants without respiratory problems, one channel of abdominal or thoracic respirogram may be sufficient.

For recording eye movements, one electrode should be placed 0.5 cm above and slightly lateral to the outer canthus of one eye and another 0.5 cm below and slightly lateral to the outer canthus of the other eye. These can be designated E1 and E2. Both lateral and vertical eye movements can be detected by linking (referring) E1 to A1 and E2 to A1 (or E1-A2, E2-A2).

EKG should be recorded routinely if there is an available channel and is particularly needed when there are cardiac or respiratory problems or when rhythmic artifacts occur.

2.2 (MTR 2.1) Electrodes may be applied with either collodion or paste. The inverted saucer-shaped silver–silver chloride electrode with a small hole for the injection of electrolyte solution is best. For neonates, the fumes of acetone and ether may not be acceptable, and disk electrodes with electrolyte paste are preferable. Needle electrodes should never be used.

2.3 (MTR 2.3) It is a matter of individual preference whether or not a reduced array is routinely acceptable for neonates. Some electroencephalographers prefer the full 10–20 array; others prefer a reduced array. It is generally agreed that a reduced array is acceptable in premature infants with small heads or where, as in neonatal intensive care units, time or other circumstances may not allow application of the full array.

The following electrodes are suggested as a minimum reduced array: Fp1, Fp2, C3, Cz, C4, T3, T4, O1, O2, A1, and A2. If a baby's earlobes are too small, mastoid leads may be substituted and can be designated M1 and M2. Acceptable alternative frontal placements in the reduced array are Fp3 and Fp4 instead of Fp1 and Fp2. Fp3 and Fp4 are halfway between the Fp1 and F3, and the Fp2 and F4 positions, respectively. (Note that the use of Fp3 and Fp4 makes for unequal interelectrode distances in scalp–scalp montages.)

Determining electrode sites by measurement is just as important in infants and children as in adults. Deviation from this principle is permissible only in circumstances in which it is impossible or clinically undesirable to manipulate the child's head to make the measurements. If an electrode placement must be modified due to intravenous lines, pressure bolts, scalp hematomas, and the like, the homologous contralateral electrode placement should be similarly modified. If no measurements are made, the technologist should note this on the recording.

2.4 (MTR 2.4) Electrode impedances of less than 5 kΩ can be obtained regularly, although higher impedances may be allowed in order to avoid excessive manipulation or excessive abrasion of tender skin. It is most important that marked differences in impedances among electrodes be avoided.

2.5 (MTR 3.1) In neonates in whom two or more channels

must be devoted to polygraphic variables, the following montages are recommended:

Channel	A	B	C
1	Fp1-F3	Fp1-A1	FP1-C3
2	F3-C3	Fp2-A2	C3-O1
3	C3-P3	F3-A1	Fp1-T3
4	Fp2-F4	F4-A2	T3-O1
5	F4-C4	C3-A1	Fp2-C4
6	C4-P4	C4-A2	C4-O2
7	F7-T3	P3-A1	Fp2-T4
8	T3-T5	P4-A2	T4-O2
9	T5-O1	O1-A1	T3-C3
10	F8-T4	O2-A2	C3-Cz
11	T4-T6	T3-A1	Cz-C4
12	T6-O2	T4-A2	C4-T4

They are based on the assumption that a 16-channel instrument is used with 4 channels devoted to polygraphic variables, leaving 12 channels for EEG. Montages A and B are for full 10–20 system electrode arrays; Montage C for the reduced array. In Montages B and C, Fp3 and Fp4 may be substituted for Fp1 and Fp2, and M1 and M2 may be substituted for A1 and A2.

It is not implied that the above montages are the only ones that can be used. Rather, they should be considered standard montages, and at least one of them should be used for at least a portion of a neonate's EEG recording in all laboratories, to provide some standardization among laboratories. Since Montage C includes the midline, it can be particularly helpful when recording premature infants. In any case, Cz should always be included because positive 'rolandic' sharp waves (a common pathologic finding) may occur only at Cz in this population. Various other montages can be devised for special purposes. Even a montage combining referential and scalp–scalp derivations is acceptable for neonatal EEGs.

The use of a single montage throughout a recording of a neonate may be, and often is, sufficient and is preferred in many laboratories. It is not implied, however, that a single montage is always adequate. Even in laboratories preferring single montages, additional montages should be used when the need arises, for example, to better delineate unifocal abnormalities.

For recording polygraphic variables, the following derivations are recommended: (1) For eye movements (EOG): use E1-A1 and E2-A1 or E2-A1 and E1-A2. (2) For submental EMG: two electrodes under the chin, each 1–2 cm on either side of the midline. (3) For EKG, lead 1 (right arm–left arm) is preferred. If submental EMG is being recorded and if only heart rate is of interest, the EKG channel can often be omitted because the R wave is usually visible in the EMG channel.

2.6 (MTR 3.2) Before recording the EEGs of inpatients, especially those in so precarious a condition that the recording must be done at bedside, the technician should consult with the nursing staff concerning the patient's condition and any limitations on recording procedures.

The baby's gestational age at birth and conceptional age (gestational age at birth plus time since birth) on the day of recording, stated in weeks, are absolutely essential to interpretation and must be included, together with chronological age since birth, in the information available to the electroencephalographer. All other available relevant clinical information (including concentration of blood gases, serum electrolyte values, and current medications) should be noted for the electroencephalographer's use.

2.7 (MTR 3.4) In young infants' EEGs, the most appropriate sensitivity is usually 7 μV/mm, but adjustments up or down are more often needed than in the case of older patients. At least a portion of the recording should be run at a sensitivity adequate to display low-voltage fast activity. The low-frequency filter setting should be between 0.3 and 0.6 Hz (-3 dB) (time constants of 0.27–0.53 s), not the commonly used 1 Hz (0.16 s).

For EOG, a sensitivity of 7 μV/mm and the same time constant as for the concomitantly recorded EEG derivations are recommended. For respirogram, amplification should be adjusted to yield a clearly visible vertical deflection, and a low-frequency filter setting of 0.3–0.6 Hz, but not direct current (DC), should be used. For the submental EMG recording, a sensitivity of 3 μV/mm, a low-frequency filter setting of about 5 Hz (time constant of about 0.03 s), and a high-frequency filter setting of 70 Hz should be employed.

2.8 (MTR 3.0, 3.12) If possible, it is advantageous to schedule the EEG at feeding time and arrange to feed the child after the electrodes have been applied, but before beginning the recording, as babies tend to sleep after feedings.

Allow for extra recording time for the EEGs of neonates. Time is commonly lost due to a greater number of movement and other physiologic artifacts during wakefulness, and extra time is usually needed in order to obtain sufficient recording to permit evaluation of stages of the wake–sleep cycle and other states.

Except when the EEG is grossly abnormal, 20- or 30-min recordings are usually insufficient. In those neonates in whom patterns appear to be invariant, it may be necessary to obtain at least 60 min of recording to demonstrate that the tracings are not likely to change. In the rest, adequate sampling of both major sleep states is important. The initial sleep state in the neonate is usually active sleep, which may last a very short time or continue for many minutes. An adequate sleep tracing must include a full episode of quiet sleep.

It is never necessary or desirable to use sedation to obtain a sleep recording in a neonate.

Repetitive photic stimulation is rarely, if ever, clinically useful in neonates and is not recommended.

2.9 (MTR 3.13) The child's condition, including head and eyelid position, should be clearly indicated at the beginning of every montage. Continuous observations by the technologist, with frequent notations on the recording, are particularly important when recording from neonates.

In stuporous or comatose patients and in those showing invariant EEG patterns of any kind, visual, auditory, and somatosensory stimuli should be applied systematically during recording, but only toward the end of the recording period, lest normal sleep cycles be disrupted or unexpected arousal-produced artifact render the tracings unreadable thereafter. The stimuli and the patient's clinical responses or failure to respond should be noted on the recording paper as near as possible to their point of occurrence.

REFERENCE

Jasper HH. The ten–twenty electrode system of the International Federation. *Electroencephalogr Clin Neurophysiol* 1958;10:371–3.

GUIDELINE THREE: MINIMUM TECHNICAL STANDARDS FOR EEG RECORDING IN SUSPECTED CEREBRAL DEATH

INTRODUCTION

EEG studies for the determination of cerebral death are no longer confined to major laboratories. Many small hospitals have intensive care units and EEG facilities. The need for minimal standard guidelines has thus increased.

The first (1970) edition of Minimum Technical Standards for EEG Recording in Suspected Cerebral Death reflected the state of the art and the technique of the late 1960s. Substantially improved EEG instrumentation is now available, and many laboratories have had years of experience in this area. Equally important, there is now a much larger number of competent EEG technologists. Finally, the EEG results of a collaborative study of cerebral death that was being planned in 1970 have been published (Bennett et al., 1976).

The survey in the later 1960s by the American EEG Society's Ad Hoc Committee on EEG Criteria for the Determination of Cerebral Death revealed that, of 2650 cases of coma with presumably 'isoelectric' EEGs, only three whose records satisfied the committee's criteria showed any recovery of cere-

bral function. These three had suffered from massive overdoses of nervous system depressants, two from barbiturates, and one from meprobamate. Many of the reported 'isoelectric' records were, on review, either low-voltage records or obtained with techniques inadequate to bring out low-voltage activity. That is, inadequate technique alone gave the graphs the appearance of being 'flat'. It should be pointed out, however, that this study did not include children. Hence, the comparable data on which to base recommendations for this young age group do not exist at present. The 1970 committee recommended dropping nonphysiologic terms such as 'isoelectric' or 'linear' (the word 'flat' should likewise not be used) and renaming the state 'electrocerebral silence'. Subsequently, 'electrocerebral inactivity' was the term recommended in the Glossary of the International Federation of Societies for EEG and Clinical Neurophysiology (Chatrian et al., 1974).

The current Guideline includes an updating of the criteria for electrocerebral inactivity, reflecting what has been learned since the first appearance of these standards (Chatrian et al., 1974; Bennett et al., 1976; Chatrian, 1980; NINCDS, 1980; Medical Consultants, 1981; Walker, 1981).

At the present time, telephone transmission of EEG cannot be used for determination of electrocerebral silence in the di-

This material originally appeared in *J Clin Neurophysiol* 1986;3(Suppl 1):12–7.
© 1994 American Electroencephalographic Society, Vol. 11 (1): 10–13.

agnosis of brain death because of the inherent and unpredictable electrical noise present in telephone networks relative to the very low signal in the electrocerebral silence recording (see also Guideline Six: Recommendations for Telephone Transmission of EEGs).

Definition

Electrocerebral inactivity (ECI) or electrocerebral silence (ECS) is defined as no EEG activity over 2 μV when recording from scalp electrode pairs 10 or more cm apart with interelectrode impedances under 10,000 Ω, but over 100 Ω.

Ten guidelines for EEG recordings in cases of suspected cerebral death, with the rationale for each, are set forth with explanatory comments.

1. A minimum of eight scalp electrodes should be utilized

The major brain area must be covered to be certain that absence of activity is not a focal phenomenon. The use of a single-channel instrument such as is sometimes used for EEG monitoring of anesthetic levels is therefore unacceptable for the purpose of determining ECS. The frontal, central, occipital, and temporal areas are recommended as the minimal required coverage. A grounding electrode should be added. However, for recordings in intensive care units, a ground electrode should *not* be used if grounding from other electrical equipment is already attached to the patient.

Since, prior to the recording, one does not know whether an ECS record will be obtained, it is desirable to use a full set of scalp electrodes on the initial examination, as defined in Guideline One: Minimum Technical Requirements for Performing Clinical Electroencephalography, Section 2.3. In any event, the initial study should not use less than the routine coverage standard for the particular clinical laboratory. A full set of electrodes includes midline placements (Fz, Cz, Pz); these are useful for the detection of residual low-voltage physiologic activity and are relatively free from artifact. Since the EEGs of patients with suspected ECS actually may have EEG abnormalities other than ECS, the use of more complete, rather than less complete, electrode coverage is often essential.

2. Interelectrode impedances should be under 10,000 Ω but over 100 Ω

2.1 Unmatched electrode impedances may distort the EEG. When one electrode has a relatively high impedance compared to the second electrode of the pair, the amplifier becomes unbalanced and is prone to amplify extraneous signals unduly. This may result in the occurrence of 60-Hz interference or other artifacts. Situations characterized by low-voltage electrocerebral activity and high instrument sensitivity demand especially scrupulous electrode application.

2.2 There is a marked dropoff of potentials with impedances below 100 Ω and, of course, no potential at 0 Ω. Such an occurrence could be one possible reason for a false ECI record. A test of interelectrode impedances to assure that they are of adequate magnitude thus should be performed during the recording. When fixed arrays of electrodes ('electrode cap' or similar devices) are utilized, it is essential that excess jelly does not spread from one electrode to another, creating a shunt or short circuit, which would attenuate the signal.

Stable, low-impedance electrodes are absolutely essential for all bedside (i.e., away from the laboratory) studies.

2.3 Although not recommended for general use, needle electrodes have been used effectively in suspected ECI recordings. The greater impedance they may have is offset by a greater probability of similar values among different electrodes, so that the likelihood that artifact will occur in the record is not increased. (See also Guideline One: Minimum Technical Requirements for Performing Clinical Electroencephalography, Section 2.2.)

3. The integrity of the entire recording system should be tested

Ordinary instrumental calibration tests the operation of the amplifiers and writer units, but it does not exclude the possibility of shunting or an open circuit at the electrodes, electrode board, cable, or input of the machine. If, after recording on one montage at increased amplification, an EEG suggesting ECS is found, the integrity of the system may be tested by touching each electrode of the montage gently with a pencil point or cotton swab to create an artifact potential on the record. This test verifies that the electrode board is connected to the machine; records made with the electrode board inadvertently not connected can sometimes resemble low-amplitude EEG activity. The test further proves that the selector switch settings match the electrode placements.

4. Interelectrode distances should be at least 10 cm

In the international 10–20 system, the average adult interelectrode distances are between 6 and 6.5 cm. A record taken with average interelectrode distances at ordinary sensitivity may suggest ECS; however, if it were recorded using longer interelectrode distances, cerebral potentials might be seen in the tracing. Hence, with longitudinal or transverse bipolar montages, some double distance electrode linkages are recommended (e.g., Fp1-C3, F3-P3, C3-O1, etc.).

Ear reference recording is almost invariably too contaminated by EKG to be useful but a Cz reference may be satisfactory. In one study (Bennett et al., 1976), the best montage was: Fp2-C4, C4-O2, Fp1-C3, C3-O1, T4-Cz, Dz-T3, with one-channel EKG and one-channel noncephalic (hand). Occipital leads, however, are more difficult to attach in immobilized patients and are particularly susceptible to movement artifact induced by artificial respirators. A montage that includes F7-T5, F8-T6, F3-P3, F4-P4, and Fz-Pz may therefore yield a better record.

None of the foregoing should imply that the usual prese-lected laboratory montages could not also be used.

5. Sensitivity must be increased from 7 μV/mm to at least 2 μV/mm *for at least 30 min* **of the recording, with inclusion of appropriate calibrations**

5.1 This is undoubtedly the most important and the most often overlooked parameter. One has only to realize that at a sensitivity of 7 μV/mm a signal of 2 μV cannot be seen be-cause the average ink line is 0.25 mm in width, i.e., about the size of the signal one desires to see. Obviously, the criterion voltage of 2 μV will deflect the pen only 1 mm at a sensitivity of 2 μV/mm. Such a signal should be visible at 2 μV/mm, and more certainly so at a sensitivity of 1.5 or 1 μV/mm. However, very slow activity with gradual wave slopes still may be diffi-cult to see. Contemporary equipment permits extended re-cording at a sensitivity of 1.5 or 1 μV/mm. This 50–100% in-crease in sensitivity will allow a more confident assessment of the presence, or the absence, of a 2-μV signal.

5.2 Adequate and appropriate calibration procedures are essential. It is good practice to calibrate with a signal near the size or value of the EEG signal that has been recorded; thus, for electrocerebral silence, a calibration of 2 or 5 μV is appropriate. A 50-μV calibration signal at a sensitivity of 2 or 1 μV/mm is useless, since the pens block. The inherent noise level of the recording system also should be noted.

5.3 Self-limited periods of ECI of up to 20 min may occur in low-voltage records (Jørgensen, 1974), and, therefore, a sin-gle recording should be at least 30 min long to be certain that intermittent low-voltage cerebral activity is not missed.

6. Filter settings should be appropriate for the assessment of ECS

In order to avoid attenuation of low-voltage fast or slow activity, whenever possible, high-frequency filters should not be set below a high-frequency setting of 30 Hz, and low-fre-quency filters should not be set above a low-frequency setting of 1 Hz.

It is well known that short time constants attenuate slow potentials. In the situation approaching ECS, there may be potentials in the theta and delta ranges, so every effort should be made to avoid attenuation of these low frequencies. How-ever, it has been demonstrated that a low-frequency setting of 1 Hz is adequate for the determination of ECI (Jørgensen, 1974; Bennett et al., 1976). There need be no hesitation in the use of the 60-Hz notch filter.

7. Additional monitoring techniques should be employed when necessary

The EEG record is a composite of true brain waves, other physiologic signals, and artifacts (either internal or external to the machine, and of mechanical, electromagnetic, and/or electrostatic origin). When the sensitivity is increased, such artifacts are accentuated and therefore must be identified in order to accurately assess whether EEG is present. It should be emphasized that the best insurance against many artifacts is a stable, low-impedance electrode system.

The *Atlas of Electroencephalography in Coma and Cerebral Death* should be consulted for information about a wide range of artifacts (Bennett et al., 1976).

7.1 Since one rarely sees an ECI record without varying amounts of EKG artifact, an EKG monitor is essential.

7.2 If respiration artifact cannot be eliminated, the artifact must be documented by specific technician notation on the record or be monitored by transducer. Briefly disconnecting the respirator will allow definitive identification of the artifact.

7.3 Frequently, an additional monitor is needed for other artifact emanating from the patient or for artifact induced from the surroundings. The most convenient for this purpose is a pair of electrodes on the dorsum of the hand separated by about 6–7 cm.

7.4 It is now clear that some EMG contamination can persist in patients with ECI recordings. If EMG potentials are of such amplitude as to obscure the tracing, it may be necessary to reduce or eliminate them by use of a neuromuscular blocking agent such as pancuronium bromide (Pavulon) or succinylcholine (Anectine). This procedure should be performed under the direction of an anesthesiologist or other physician familiar with the use of the drug.

7.5 Machine noise and external interference may be conveniently checked by a 'dummy patient,' i.e., a 10,000-Ω resistor between input terminal 1 (G1) and input terminal 2 (G2) of one channel.

7.6 Even with good technique, however, an EEG recorded at the increased sensitivities required above can at times leave the electroencephalographer who interprets the recordings in considerable difficulty. An attempt must be made to determine what portion of the record results from noncerebral physiologic signals, or nonphysiologic artifacts, including the ongoing noise level of the complete system in the particular ICU as indicated, for example, by a recording from the hand. An estimate must then be made of whether or not the remaining activity exceeds 2 μV in amplitude. When this cannot be done with confidence, the EEG report must indicate the uncertainty, and the record cannot be classified as demonstrating ECI (see Section 10).

8. There should be no EEG reactivity to intense somatosensory, auditory, or visual stimuli

In the collaborative study, there was no instance of stimulus-related activity in routine recordings of patients with ECS (Bennett et al., 1986; NINCDS, 1980; Walker, 1981). Any apparent EEG activity resulting from the above stimuli or any others (airway suctioning and other nursing procedures can be potent stimuli) must be carefully distinguished from noncerebral physiologic signals and from nonphysiologic artifacts. For example, an electroretinogram can still persist in response to photic stimulation when there is ECS. Stimulation may be of help also in documenting the degree of reactivity of records found not to be characterized by ECS.

9.   Recordings should be made only by a qualified technologist

Great skill is essential in recording cases of suspected ECS. The recordings are frequently made under difficult circumstances and include many possible sources for artifact. Elimination of most artifacts and identification of all others can be accomplished by a qualified technologist.

Qualifications for a competent EEG technologist for ECS recordings include the requirement of supervised instruction in the techniques of recording in ICU settings. The technologist should work under the direction of a qualified electro-encephalographer (see Guidelines Four and Five).

10. A repeat EEG should be performed if there is doubt about ECS

In the Collaborative Study of Cerebral Death (Bennett et al., 1976; NINCDS, 1980; Walker, 1981), there were no patients who survived for more than a short period after an EEG showed ECS, provided that overdose of depressant drugs was excluded. This finding confirmed the results of the earlier survey, which were summarized in the Introduction. It is evident, therefore, that a single EEG showing ECS is a highly reliable procedure for the determination of cortical death. (For other guidelines to assist physicians in the determination of brain death, see the References.)

In the event that technical or other difficulties lead to uncertainty in the evaluation of the question of ECS, the entire procedure should be repeated after an interval, for example, after 6 h (see Section 7).

REFERENCES

Bennett DR, Hughes JR, Korein J, Merlis JK, Suter C. *An atlas of electroencephalography in coma and cerebral death.* New York: Raven Press, 1976.
Chatrian GE, Bergamini L, Dondey M, Klass DW, Lennox-Buchthal M, Petersén I. A glossary of terms most commonly used by clinical electroencephalographers. *Electroencephalogr Clin Neurophysiol* 1974;37:538–48.
Chatrian GE. Electrophysiologic evaluation of brain death: a critical appraisal. In: Aminoff MJ, ed. *Electrodiagnosis in clinical neurology.* New York: Churchill Livingstone, 1980.
Jørgensen EO. Requirements for recording the EEG at high sensitivity in suspected brain death. *Electroencephalogr Clin Neurophysiol* 1974;36:65–9.
The Medical Consultants on the Diagnosis of Death to the President's Commission for the Study of Ethical Problems in Medicine and Biomedical and Behavioral Research. Guidelines for the determination of death. *JAMA* 1981;246:2184–6.
The NINCDS Collaborative Study of Brain Death. NINCDS Monograph No. 24, NIH Publication No. 81–2286, December 1980.
Walker AE. *Cerebral death.* Baltimore: Urban & Schwarzenberg. 1981.

GUIDELINE FOUR: STANDARDS OF PRACTICE IN CLINICAL ELECTROENCEPHALOGRAPHY

1. Minimal qualifications for a clinical electroencephalographer

These standards are proposed for individuals entering the EEG field after 1978. Many highly competent electroencephalographers who entered the field before 1978 and currently interpret EEGs do not meet the requirements listed below.

1.1 The clinical electroencephalographer should be a physician with board eligibility or certification in neurology, pediatric neurology, neurosurgery, or psychiatry.

1.2 Training should meet the minimal requirements for examination by the American Board of Clinical Neurophysiology. Currently, these include board eligibility or certification in neurology, neurosurgery, or psychiatry and a minimum of 12 months supervised experience in EEG during or following the residency, of which at least 3 months must include full-time training in EEG and clinical neurophysiology.

Some of this material originally appeared in *J Clin Neurophysiol* 1986;3(Suppl 1): 18–9. © 1994 American Electroencephalographic Society, Vol. 11 (1): 14–15.

2. Qualifications of EEG technologists and technicians

2.1 The qualifications of EEG technologists shall be those set forth in Guideline Five: Recommendations for Writing Job Descriptions for Technologists and Samples.

2.2 In no case should a technician with less than 6 months of supervised clinical experience, following formal training, operate independently or in an unsupervised capacity.

3. Laboratory organization

3.1 Hospital laboratories should meet accreditation requirements of the American EEG Society's Clinical Neurophysiology, Laboratory Association Board (see Guidelines).

3.2 The chief electroencephalographer shall have the primary responsibility for the overall operations and policies of the laboratory. The policies of the laboratory should be documented in a policy and procedures manual. Under the supervision of the EEG laboratory director, the chief EEG technologist shall be responsible for the daily operation of the laboratory. The chief technologist, together with the laboratory director, shall maintain the highest standards of EEG technical practice.

3.3 All EEGs should be analyzed by, and official reports, including clinical interpretations, provided by a qualified electroencephalographer. Under no circumstances should a technologist, however well-qualified and experienced, have primary responsibility for clinical interpretation of EEGs.

Qualified technologists, however, should be able to give a descriptive technical report of the record.

3.4 Records should be maintained in an orderly manner and should be available for review by the patient's referring physician and other qualified persons.

4. Equipment

Technical standards recommended by the AEEGS Instrumentation Committee and the International Federation of Societies for EEG and Clinical Neurophysiology should form the basis for selection of clinical EEG equipment.

4.1 Basic recording equipment should conform to the recommendations of Guideline One: Minimum Technical Requirements for Performing Clinical Electroencephalography.

5. Statement on the administration of medications by EEG or EP technologists

The AEEGS endorses the use of qualified EEG or EP technologists to administer oral sedative medication as ordered by a referring physician or by the Medical Director of the EEG laboratory. The administering technologist should be under the direct supervision of a licensed physician. The technologist should be part of a continuing education program that documents the effects and risks of medication that they administer. The documentation of the continuing education is the responsibility of the Medical Director of the laboratory. The ordering physician and the Medical Director of the laboratory bear the ultimate responsibility for the safe administration of these medications by the technical staff. Intravenous or intramuscular medication must be administered by appropriate nursing or physician personnel.

REFERENCE

American Electroencephalographic Society. Guidelines for laboratory accreditation. *J Clin Neurophysiol* 1986;3:85–92.

GUIDELINE FIVE: RECOMMENDATIONS FOR WRITING JOB DESCRIPTIONS FOR TECHNOLOGISTS AND SAMPLES

The field of EEG has progressed into a whole new dimension, encompassing a variety of different job skills and responsibilities. This change has been further demonstrated in the name change from EEG Technologist to Electroneurodiagnostic Technologist, which reflects our current scope of practice.

These guidelines for writing job descriptions and the job description examples were developed through the perceived need to provide the electroneurodiagnostic community with a resource of standards that the American Society of Electroneurodiagnostic Technologists (ASET) felt should be met by the individuals employed in the field today.

Our goal is to create standards that will reflect the qualifications and abilities required of the profession and to gain recognition for the Electroneurodiagnostic Technologist.

This guideline was originally published as 'How to write job descriptions: recommendations for writing job descriptions and samples.' Carroll, IA: American Society of Electroneurodiagnostic Technologists, 1992, 32 pp. Copyright ©1992 American Society of Electroneurodiagnostic Technologists, Inc. Reprinted with permission of the copyright holder.

Address correspondence and reprint requests to American Society of Electroneurodiagnostic Technologists, Inc., 204 West 7th, Carroll, IA 51401–2317, U.S.A.

OBJECTIVE

These guidelines are designed to provide hospitals, clinics, and physician offices with some direction on how to write job descriptions. They also include example job descriptions that have suggested standards of competence. ASET feels these standards of competence should be met by technologists employed in the field today.

The job descriptions can be adapted to fit the varying needs of individual laboratories and should reflect and be consistent with federal mandates.

FEDERAL LEGISLATION CONSIDERATIONS

The Americans with Disabilities Act (ADA) of 1990 and the Civil Rights Act of 1991 make accurate and complete job descriptions imperative. Your Human Resources or Personnel Department is a valuable and integral resource with regard to these federal mandates.

Quoting from the ADA Title I, Section 101,8:

For the purposes of this title, consideration shall be given to the employer's judgement as to what functions of a job are essential, and if an employer has prepared a written description before advertising or interviewing applicants for the job, this description shall be considered evidence of the essential functions of the job.

Under the Equal Employment Opportunity ruling and guidelines, voluntary credentials cannot be required if there are no state statutes that govern licensure or certification in a field. The job description can state that registry[1] is preferred. However, if the job function and responsibility (e.g., monitoring in the operating room) command a significant degree of knowledge and skill for performance of the job, the content of a Registry examination may serve as a means of documenting a reasonable measure of competent performance.

If your job description is not accurate and detailed as to the qualifications, skills, physical requirements, and functions necessary to successfully perform the job, the employer is more susceptible to wrongful discharge claims and employee litigation. The Civil Rights Act allows compensatory and punitive damages for victims of discrimination based on sex, religion, and disability.

Disability includes: a physical or mental impairment that substantially limits one or more of the major life activities; *or* a record of such impairment (which is now inactive or cured – alcoholism, drug abuse, cancer, etc.); *or* being regarded as having such an impairment. Mental impairment is a difficult area and a highly litigated area.

STATE REGULATIONS

In any state, there may be specific regulations regarding job functions and employee/employer relations that must be considered in writing job descriptions. Your Human Resources or Personnel Department should be your resource regarding state employment regulations.

WRITING JOB DESCRIPTIONS FOR ELECTRONEURODIAGNOSTIC PERSONNEL

Any laboratory that performs electroneurodiagnostic procedures is an integral part of the hospital or clinic organization. It is important to the function of this organization to obtain the best possible people to fill the positions. The first step in this process is the job description. So what is a job description and how do you write one?

Job description A job description is an organized, factual statement of the

---

[1] Registry (registration) is the term used to indicate a technologist has successfully passed national examinations, both written and oral. For EEG and evoked potential technologists, the national examination is conducted by the American Board of Registration of Electroencephalographic and Evoked Potential Technologists, Inc. (ABRET), which awards the R.EEGT. and R.EPT. credentials. Until its cessation in 1990, board examinations were also given by the American Board of Certified and Registered Electroencephalographic Technicians and Technologists (ABCRET), which awarded the CMET, CRET, and CRNT status to its certificants.

duties and responsibilities of a specific job. In brief, it should tell what is to be done, how it is done, and why. It is a standard of function, in that it defines the appropriate and authorized content of a job (Flippo, 1984).

The first step in the process of writing job descriptions is to determine what the job consists of and what skills and abilities are required for the position. One of the best ways to determine this is to perform a *job analysis.*

Job analysis Job analysis is the process of studying and collecting information relating to the operations and responsibilities of a specific job (Flippo, 1984).

The job analysis process involves collection of data that will differentiate a job from other jobs. Helpful information may include work activities, required behavior, machines or equipment used, expected performance, work conditions and personnel requirements (Mathis and Jackson, 1982). Keep in mind what skills, formal training, aptitude, licensing, and experience apply to the job. There are four ways in which you can approach this task: (1) *questionnaires,* (2) *written narratives,* (3) *observation,* and (4) *interviews* (Flippo, 1984).

The questionnaire method is widely used. A survey instrument is developed and given to employees and supervisors to complete. At least one employee per job should complete the questionnaire and return to the supervisor for review. The advantage to the questionnaire is that the data on a large number of jobs can be collected in a short period of time. Follow-up observation and discussion will be required to clarify incomplete questionnaires and interpretation problems.

The narrative method would require the employee and supervisor to keep a daily log or diary of duties performed and the time each is started and finished. This method can be of material assistance to the human resources specialist in defining the requirements of a job, but must be followed up with observation or interview to provide supportive documentation.

In the observation method, the supervisor observes the individual performing the job and makes notes to describe the tasks performed. This method is most useful in repetitive-type jobs.

The interview method requires the supervisor or human resources specialist to visit the job site and talk to the individual performing the job. A structured interview form is used to record the data. The interview method can be very time-consuming (Mathis and Jackson, 1982).

The disadvantages to the questionnaire and narrative methods are unorganized, incomplete, and at times incoherent data. The observation and interview methods provide complete and accurate data and better time utilization. In the electroneurodiagnostic field, the interview coupled with observation provides the best source of information. The job analysis may be done by a staff specialist from the Human Resources Department. This process could also be undertaken by the supervisor of the laboratory. In either case, the following guidelines may be used to insure accurate and complete information (Flippo, 1984):

1. Introduce yourself so that the worker knows who you are and why you are there.
2. Show a sincere interest in the worker and the job being analyzed.
3. Do not try to tell the employee how to do the job.
4. Try to talk to the employees and supervisors in their own language.
5. Do not confuse the work with the worker.
6. Do a complete job study with the objectives of the program.
7. Verify the job information contained.

The product of the job analysis process is the job description.

THE JOB DESCRIPTION

The job description is basically descriptive and summarizes the information obtained from the job analysis. Job descriptions must be accurate, readable, and understandable and the job facts should be organized into some logical order. The job descriptions can be written into three basic sections: identification, general summary, and specific duties. In this case, the identification section should include the job title, department, and reporting relationships. A job code, number of employees holding this position and current pay scale may be included. The general summary describes the general responsibilities

and components that make this job different from others. The specific duties section contains clear, concise statements on tasks, duties, and responsibilities performed. This section will be the most time-consuming when writing job descriptions (Mathis and Jackson, 1982).

A more detailed job description contains sections about working conditions and machines or materials used. A suggested format is (Flippo, 1984):

1. Job identification
2. Job summary
3. Duties performed, including physical requirements
4. Supervision given and received
5. Relation to other jobs
6. Machines, tools, and materials
7. Working conditions
8. Definitions of unusual terms
9. Comments that add to and clarify the above

The identification section should include the job title, department and, if applicable, a division and code number for the job.

The purpose of the job summary is to provide a definition that is useful as additional information when the job title is not sufficient and to orient the reader toward understanding the information that will follow.

The duties-performed section tells what is being done, how it is done, and the purpose of each task. The duties should be arranged in chronological order with an estimate as to the percentage of time spent on each task. There is a suggested writing style for the duties-performed section. It should be direct, giving the impression of action. There are many rules such as: (1) start each sentence with an action verb; (2) use present tense; and (3) use the word 'may' when only some workers perform the duty and the word 'occasionally' when all workers perform at irregular intervals.

The supervision section tells the degree of supervision given such as close or general supervision and may list job titles immediately over and under the job.

The relation to other-jobs section identifies vertical relationships to promotion and the relationship of work flow and procedures. The machines, tools, and materials section describes the types of equipment used and the trade name if needed.

A checklist format may be used to describe the working conditions such as hot, cold, noisy, etc. Hazardous conditions should especially be noted. Any technical or unusual words should be listed and defined in a glossary (Flippo, 1984). A final statement should be included to cover any abnormal or unusual circumstances pertaining to the job that may arise. Such a statement is used to prevent employees from saying, 'It's not in my job description' (Mathis and Jackson, 1982).

The Joint Commission on Accreditation of Healthcare Organizations (JCAHO) does not have any specific standards on writing job descriptions; however, the JCAHO requires that each employee must have a job description, and an annual performance appraisal must be done in reference to this job description. For further definition of these guidelines, refer to the 1992 JCAHO Accreditation Manual for Hospitals. The chapter entitled 'Management and Administrative Services,' which begins on page 46, outlines the specific standards regarding periodic evaluations based on the job description.

Reference should be made to Standard MA.1.4 and Subsection MA.1.4.4. Furthermore Standard MA.1.4.4.1 addresses the ages of patients being served. This standard is defined in order to insure that the employee has the expertise to deal with the various age ranges of the population being served by the institution. For further clarification of the above-mentioned standards, consult the JCAHO Accreditation Manual for Hospitals.

The following examples of job descriptions are provided to serve as a basis for writing job descriptions for employees in EEG laboratories in hospital or clinic settings. Alterations in format or wording may be needed to fit your individual situation.

REFERENCES

Flippo EB. *Personnel management.* New York: McGraw-Hill, 1984.
Mathis RL, Jackson JH. *Personnel, contemporary perspectives and applications*, 3rd ed. St. Paul, MN: West Publishing, 1982.

This section contains sample job descriptions for nine different jobs within a neurology/electroneurodiagnostic laboratory. The Executive Committee and Board of Trustees of ASET has endorsed this document and the job descriptions that follow.

These sample job descriptions are intended only as generic samples and do not reflect the new federal regulations under the ADA or Civil Rights Act, nor do they address any state employment regulations.

All federal, state, local, and institution-specific regulations must be addressed in adapting the following job descriptions to fill the need of your particular employer and laboratory situation.

SAMPLE JOB DESCRIPTIONS

Introduction

The trainee positions for Electroneurodiagnostic Technologist, Evoked Potential Technologist, and Polysomnographic Technologist are written for someone with no previous experience in the field of electroneurodiagnostics. This position does require a high school diploma, and it is a recommended prerequisite that college level courses in anatomy and physiology, basic electronics, and medical terminology have been completed. At the end of the appointed training period, the trainee should pursue the Part I (written) examination for registration in his/her specialty area. Through experience and demonstrated competence, there is growth potential to the Technologist I level of the specialty area.

The Electroneurodiagnostic Technologist I level is written as an entry level position. This would be appropriate for a recent graduate of an EEG technology program. There is potential for growth to Technologist II level through experience and demonstrated competence.

The Electroneurodiagnostic Technologist II is a midlevel position with potential growth through experience and demonstrated competence into a chief technologist or supervisory position.

The Electroneurodiagnostic Technologist III level is written as a chief technologist position. Depending on the organizational structure of your hospital or clinic, this position may serve as the supervisor of the laboratory. The person at this level has the capabilities to supervise a laboratory. If the Technologist III is used as the supervisor, you can make wording changes in the following job description to reflect the supervisory capacity the person will hold. In such a case, the Technologist III or chief technologist would probably be responsible to someone in administration, for example Vice-President, Associate Hospital Administrators, or Program Care Managers.

The Evoked Potential Technologist I level is written as an entry-level position when technologists are employed to perform only evoked potentials. There is growth potential through experience and demonstrated competence.

The Evoked Potential Technologist II level is a midlevel position written for technologists who are employed to perform evoked potentials only. This person would serve as the senior staff member of the evoked potential laboratory if your department is divided into an EEG section and an evoked potential seciton. This person would report to the department supervisor.

The Polysomnographic Technologist I is written as an entry level position when the technologist is employed to perform only polysomnographic studies. For technologists who are also responsible for performing other EEG-related studies in addition to polysomnograms, the Electroneurodiagnostic Technologist II job description may be more appropriate.

The Polysomnographic Technologist II serves as the senior staff member for the laboratory. This position may serve as the supervisor of the laboratory if the laboratory is not under the direction of the Neurodiagnostics Laboratory/Department. For technologists who are also responsible for performing other EEG-related studies in addition to polysomnograms, the Electroneurodiagnostic Technologist III job description may be more appropriate. This position would report to the Neurodiagnostic Department supervisor or medical director, whichever is applicable to the situation.

The Surgical Monitoring Technologist position is written for technologists who are employed to perform operating room (OR) monitoring duties. This is a highly specialized position that requires a significant level of knowledge, skill, and responsibility. Registry is necessary and 1–2 years of technical experience monitoring EEG/EPs in the OR.

The Long-Term Monitoring Technologist position is written for the technologists who perform video/EEG monitoring on an epilepsy unit and other specialized studies involved with epilepsy research, and who may monitor during electrocorticography or other specialized surgical procedures for epilepsy. This highly specialized position requires a significant level of knowledge, skill, and responsibility. Registry is necessary and 1–2 years experience in long-term monitoring on an epilepsy unit.

The Electroneurodiagnostic Laboratory Supervisor or Technical Director is written for hospitals or clinics whose organizational structure provides for such a position. In this case, you may not have Technologist III (chief technologist) level personnel who serve in a first-line supervisory capacity. The supervisor would be capable of the job skills of a Technologist III level and in addition would handle administrative duties. This person would also be responsible to someone such as Vice-President, Associate Hospital Administrator, or Program Care Manager.

Job title: Electroneurodiagnostic Technologist Trainee
Department: Neurodiagnostic Laboratory
Job summary: Under the direct supervision of the laboratory supervisor, learns to perform routine inpatient and outpatient EEGs.

Education/experience: High school graduate. No previous EEG experience required. Recommended prerequisite: college-level courses in anatomy and physiology, basic electronics, and medical terminology.

Skills and responsibilities:

1. Demonstrates positive interpersonal skills with patients, patient families, EEG laboratory staff, physicians, and other members of the hospital staff.

2. Explains the test procedure to the patient.

3. Learns to obtain an accurate and concise patient history. Notes pertinent information, such as seizure types, date of last seizure, and other neurologic symptomatology, and any medications taken by the patient.

4. Learns to measure and apply EEG electrodes using the 10–20 international system in an accurate and efficient manner.

5. Learns to calibrate, evaluate, and adjust the EEG instrument to proper technical standards with emphasis on sensitivity, time axis, and mechanical and electrical baselines in order to obtain top-quality EEG recordings.

6. Learns to record EEG activity using standard montages. Labels all pertinent machine settings and clinical observations on the EEG tracing.

7. Learns to recognize, monitor, and/or eliminate electrode artifacts such as high-impedance leads, muscle artifact, eye movements, respiration artifact, and/or EKG in order to obtain an adequate test.

8. Learns to implement alternative nonstandard montages and machine settings in order to better define abnormalities. This may include the application of additional electrodes.

9. Learns to perform routine activation procedures such as hyperventilation and photic stimulation.

10. Removes electrodes and cleans the patient's scalp.

11. Learns to properly clean the electrodes, and, if necessary, prepares them for sterilization techniques.

12. Maintains work area in an organized and sanitary fashion by cleaning the patient room including changing the linen for the next test.

13. Learns to prepare an EEG worksheet, including a technical description of the EEG, with emphasis on clinical observations in order to assist the neurologist with the final interpretation.

14. Reviews all EEG tracings with the laboratory supervisor. Receives and implements all suggestions for improving the quality of future EEG recordings.

15. Learns to recognize normal patterns, normal variants, and abnormal patterns.

16. Learns various medical and pharmacological conditions that influence the EEG. Learns the clinical correlation of abnormal EEG patterns with various disease states.

17. Takes and passes examinations given by the laboratory supervisor/instructor.

18. Learns to adequately clean and adjust the EEG instrumentation.

19. Learns to log EEG records and fill out charge documents.

20. Learns to accurately file records and reports.

21. Learns to answer telephone inquiries regarding appointments and test information.

22. Attends EEG record-reading sessions and in-service training sessions.

23. Attends scientific courses and seminars on electroneurodiagnostic testing, with special emphasis on basic EEG, for continuing education.

24. Takes and passes, at the end of the training period, Part I (written) examination for registration by ABRET.

Responsible to: Laboratory Supervisor
Promotion to: Technologist I

Job title: Electroneurodiagnostic Technologist I
Department: Neurodiagnostic Laboratory
Job summary: Under the supervistion of the laboratory supervisor, performs EEGs in the laboratory and at the bedside of critically ill patients in intensive care units.

Education/experience: High school graduate and graduate of an accredited electroneurodiagnostic technology program accredited by the Committee on Allied Health Education and Accreditation or equivalent formal training. Some college level course work is preferable. Eligible for/or successful completion of the Part I (written) examination for registration by ABRET and/or 1–3 years experience in EEG.

Skills and responsibilities:

1. Measures and accurately applies electrodes in a timely manner, according to the international 10–20 system. Ensures that electrode impedances meet laboratory standards.

2. Writes a comprehensive patient history gathering appropriate information from patient, patient's record, and family members to include seizure types, date of last seizure, other neurological symptomatology and medications. Explains test procedure to patient and family members present.

3. Performs EEG record according to the standards of the laboratory (routine, sleep, bedside, and electrocerebral silence recordings).

4. Implements alternative methods or adjusts controls to obtain optimal recording. This may include appropriate control setting changes on the machine, use of extra electrodes, extra montages, and use of activation procedures.

5. Recognizes artifact (patient or environmental). Documents, eliminates, or takes proper measures to monitor the artifact.

6. Knowledge of appropriate actions to take during patient emergency situations and insures patient safety (electrical) at all times.

7. Knowledge of basic infection control standards relating to patient and equipment including electrodes.

8. Keeps equipment clean and in proper working order. Knowledge of appropriate calibrations and how to make adjustments. Ability to troubleshoot equipment problems and repair them or report to supervisor promptly.

9. Demonstrates positive interpersonal skills with patients,

patient families, laboratory staff, physicians, and other members of the hospital staff.

10. Knowledge of neuroanatomy and physiology, basic electronics and electrical safety, general knowledge of EEG instrumentation, pattern recognition, and various medical and pharmacological conditions that influence the EEG.

11. Learns to perform intraoperative EEGs and learns at least one modality of evoked potentials under the supervision of a staff member at the Technologist III level.

12. Participants in conferences and technical meetings.

13. Performs other duties as assigned.

Responsible to: Laboratory Supervisor
Promotion to: Technologist II

Job title: Electroneurodiagnostic Technologist II
Department: Neurodiagnostic Laboratory
Job summary: Under the general supervision of the laboratory supervisor, performs EEGs and evoked potential studies in the laboratory and at the bedside of critically ill patients in intensive care units. Under supervision, performs video/EEG monitoring, ambulatory monitoring, routine topographic brain mapping studies, routine polysomnograms, and multiple sleep latency tests (MSLT), and less complicated intraoperative monitoring (i.e., during carotid endarterectomy or Harrington rod placement).

Education/experience: High school graduate and graduate of an Electroneurodiagnostic technology program accredited by the Committee on Allied Health Education and Accredita-

tion or equivalent formal training. Preferred – Registry (see footnote on registry on page 16) in EEG by ABRET and registry eligible in evoked potential studies and/or 3–5 years' experience in EEG and evoked potentials.

Skills and responsibilities:

1. Performs all the duties of the Electroneurodiagnostic Technologist I (see Tech I description).

2. Performs at least two modalities of evoked potentials with high-quality results in both the laboratory and intensive care unit.

3. Capable of recording EEG or evoked potentials intraoperatively as during carotid endarterectomy or Harrington rod placement.

4. Performs special procedure EEGs or evoked potentials, such as neonatal recordings in the intensive care nursery, nasopharyngeal leads, and electrocerebral inactivity recordings.

5. Performs long-term video monitoring or ambulatory recordings (if applicable).

6. Evaluates during scanning process digital EEG or ambulatory EEG for hard-copy printout.

7. Performs advanced neurodiagnostic procedures to include digital EEG, topographic mapping of EEG/evoked potential data, MSLT, and routine polysomnograms (if applicable) and NCVs.

8. Administers sedative medications as prescribed by the patient's physician.

9. Under general supervision of laboratory supervisor or technologist III sends and receives telephone transmission

EEG recordings. Follows recommended guidelines for telephone transmission of EEGs (if applicable).

10. Participates in conferences and technical meetings. Assists junior staff members.

11. Learns to perform advanced EEG/evoked potential recordings during special studies or neurosurgical intraoperative cases.

12. Attends scientific courses and seminars on electroneurodiagnostic testing, with emphasis on conduction velocity procedures, electroretinography, and electronystagmography (if applicable).

13. Performs other duties related to the laboratory as required.

Responsible to: Laboratory Supervisor
Promotion to: Technologist III

Job title: Electroneurodiagnostic Technologist III
Department: Neurodiagnostic Laboratory
Job summary: Under minimal supervision of the laboratory supervisor, performs a wide variety of neurodiagnostic studies to include EEG, evoked potentials, and specialized studies in the laboratory, at the bedside of critically ill patients in the intensive care units, and in the operating room.
Education/experience: High school graduate and a graduate of an electroneurodiagnostic technology program accredited by the Committee on Allied Health Education and Accreditation or equivalent formal training. At least 2 years of college is preferable. Preferred – Registry (see footnote on reg-

istry on page 16) in EEG by ABRET and/or a minimum of 5 years' experience in EEG and evoked potentials.

Skills and responsibilities:

1. Performs all the duties of the Electroneurodiagnostic Technologist II (see Tech II description).

2. Performs all three modalities of evoked potentials with high-quality results in the laboratory, intensive care units, and the operating room.

3. Performs advanced EEG/evoked potential recordings during special studies.

4. Performs EEG and evoked potential monitoring on patients with intracranially placed electrodes and/or grids.

5. Perform EEG/evoked potential recordings during neurosurgical intraoperative studies.

6. Sends and receives telephone transmission EEG recordings. Follows AEEGS recommended guidelines for telephone transmission of EEGs (if applicable).

7. Assists or performs clinical research procedures.

8. Participates in conferences and technical meetings. Assists junior staff members.

9. Assumes responsibilities of the laboratory supervisor in their absence.

10. Assists in establishing and maintaining department procedures and protocols.

11. Performs other duties as assigned.

Responsible to: Laboratory Supervisor
Promotion to: Laboratory Supervisor

Job title: Evoked Potential Technologist Trainee

Department: Neurodiagnostic Laboratory

Job summary: Under the direct and constant supervision of the laboratory supervisor, learns to perform routine inpatient and outpatient evoked potentials.

Education/experience: High school graduate. No previous evoked potential experience required. Recommended prerequisite college level courses in anatomy and physiology, basic electronics, and medical terminology.

Skills and responsibilities:

1. Demonstrates positive interpersonal skills with patients, patient families, laboratory staff, physicians, and other members of the hospital staff.

2. Explains the test procedure to the patient.

3. Learns to obtain an accurate and concise patient history; notes pertinent information such as visual, sensory, and auditory symptomatology.

4. Learns to determine appropriate method of testing for the patient's evaluation and diagnosis.

5. Learns to prepare the patient for testing by measuring and applying electrodes according to established guidelines (AEEGS minimal technical guidelines for evoked potentials).

6. Learns to calibrate, evaluate, and adjust the evoked potential instrument to proper technical standards to insure a top-quality evoked potential recording.

7. Learns to operate and control settings of the averaging computer to include stimulus level, time base, stimulus rate, sensitivity, and display gain.

8. Learns to identify and eliminate electrode and excessive stimulus artifact in order to obtain optimal responses.

9. Learns to display and print the evoked potential waveforms in order to obtain a valid study following established laboratory guidelines.

10. Learns to measure, calculate, and log evoked potential information, such as latencies, voltages, and conduction times for proper interpretation.

11. Learns to label completely all printouts including patient's name, age, and sex, test date, stimulus type and rate, polarity convention used, sensitivity, and time axis scale.

12. Learns to implement alternative methods such as variations of stimulus parameters in certain situations outside of the normative range in order to better define any abnormalities.

13. Removes the electrodes and cleans the patient's scalp.

14. Learns to properly clean the electrodes and if necessary prepares them for sterilization techniques.

15. Learns to maintain work area in an organized and sanitary fashion by cleaning the patient room, including changing the linen for the next test.

16. Learns to prepare an evoked potential worksheet, including a technical description of the evoked potentials, with emphasis on the clinical observations in order to assist the neurologist with the final interpretation.

17. Reviews all evoked potential tracings with the laboratory supervisor. Receives and implements all suggestions for improving the quality of future evoked potential recordings.

18. Learns to recognize normal patterns, normal variants, and abnormal patterns; understands the various medical and pharmacological conditions that influence evoked potentials; understands the clinical correlations between abnormal evoked potentials and various disease states.

19. Takes and passes examinations given by the laboratory supervisor.

20. Learns to adequately clean and adjust the evoked potential instrumentation.

21. Learns to log evoked potential records and fill out charge documents.

22. Learns to accurately file records and reports.

23. Learns to answer telephone inquiries regarding appointments and test information.

24. Attends evoked potential record reading sessions and in-service training sessions.

25. Attends scientific courses and seminars on electroneurodiagnositc testing, with special emphasis on evoked potentials, for continuing education.

26. Takes and passes, at the end of the training period, Part I (written) examination in evoked potentials for registration by ABRET.

Responsible to: Laboratory Supervisor
Promotion to: EP Technologist I

Job title: Evoked Potential Technologist I
Department: Neurodiagnostic Laboratory
Job summary: Under the supervision of the laboratory supervisor or the senior technologist, performs routine evoked potentials in the laboratory and at the bedside of critically ill patients in intensive care units.

Education/experience: High school graduate and a graduate of an accredited electroneurodiagnostic technology program accredited by the Committee on Allied Health Education and Accreditation or equivalent formal training. Some college level course work is preferable. Eligible for or successful completion of the Part I (written) examination for registration by ABRET and/or 1–3 years' experience in evoked potentials.

Skills and responsibilities:

1. Measures and applies electrodes in a timely manner, according to established guidelines (AEEGS Minimal Technical Guidelines for Evoked Potentials). Ensures that electrode impedances meet laboratory standards.

2. Writes a comprehensive patient history gathering appropriate information from patient, patient's record, and family members to include any visual, sensory, and auditory symptomatology. Explains test procedure to patient and family members present.

3. Performs evoked potential records according to the standards of the laboratory (routine and bedside recordings).

4. Implements alternative methods or adjusts controls to obtain optimal recordings. This may include appropriate control setting changes on the machine, use of extra electrodes, extra montages, and use of additional stimulation techniques.

5. Recognizes artifact (patient or environmental).

6. Knowledge of appropriate actions to take during patient emergency situations and to insure patient safety (electrical) at all times.

7. Knowledge of basic infection control standards relating to patient and equipment including electrodes.

8. Keeps equipment clean and in proper working order. Knowledge of appropriate calibrations and how to make adjustments. Ability to troubleshoot equipment problems and repair them or report to supervisor promptly.

9. Demonstrates positive interpersonal skills with patients, patient families, laboratory staff, physicians, and other members of the hospital staff.

10. Knowledge of neuroanatomy and physiology, basic electronics and electrical safety, general knowledge of electroneurodiagnostic instrumentation, pattern recognition, and various medical and pharmacological conditions that influence evoked potentials.

11. Learns to perform intraoperative evoked potentials.

12. Participates in conferences and technical meetings.

13. Performs other duties as assigned.

Responsible to: Laboratory Supervisor
Promotion to: EP Technologist II

Job title: Evoked Potential Technologist II
Department: Neurodiagnostic Laboratory
Job summary: Under the general supervision of the laboratory supervisor, performs evoked potentials in the laboratory, at the bedside of critically ill patients in intensive care units, and during intraoperative monitoring.

Education/experience: High school graduate and graduate of an accredited electroneurodiagnostic technology program accredited by the Committee on Allied Health Education and Accreditation or equivalent formal training. At least 1 year of college is preferable. Preferred – Registry (see footnote on page 16) by ABRET and/or 3–5 years' experience in evoked potentials.

Skills and responsibilities:

1. Performs all the duties of the Evoked Potential Technologist I (see Tech I description).

2. Performs evoked potential intraoperative monitoring as during Harrington rod placement.

3. Administers sedative medications as prescribed by the patient's physician.

4. Participates in conferences and technical meetings. Assists junior staff members.

5. Learns to perform advanced evoked potential recordings during special studies or neurosurgical intraoperative cases as during arteriovenous malformation resections and aneurysm clippings.

6. Assists or performs clinical research procedures.

7. Assumes responsibilities (when applicable) of the laboratory supervisor in their absence.

8. Performs other duties as assigned.

Responsible to: Laboratory Supervisor
Promotion to: Laboratory Supervisor

Job title: Polysomnographic Technologist Trainee

Department: Neurodiagnostic Laboratory

Job summary: Under the direct supervision of the laboratory supervisor, learns to perform routine polysomnographic studies including nocturnal penile tumescence (NPT) studies and MSLT.

Education/experience: High school graduate. No previous polysomnographic experience required. Recommended prerequisite, college level courses in anatomy and physiology, basic electronics, and medical terminology.

Skills and responsibilities:

1. Demonstrates positive interpersonal skills with patients, patient families, laboratory staff, physicians, and other members of the hospital staff.

2. Explains the test procedure to the patient.

3. Learns to administer patient questionnaire to obtain an accurate and complete history.

4. Learns to apply electrodes with collodion. Apply EEG, EOG, EKG, and EMG electrodes in an accurate and efficient manner.

5. Learns to apply appropriate transducers to monitor respiratory effort, airflow, and oxygen saturation.

6. Learns to calibrate, evaluate, and adjust the instrumentation.

7. Learns to monitor the patient throughout the night, observing cardiac rhythm and respiration for abnormalities.

8. Learns to contact a staff physician when indicated.

9. Attends to the personal needs of the patient throughout the night.

10. Learns to perform NPT studies: (a) explains the study to the patient in detail and responds to any questions or concerns; (b) calibrates the gauges and equipment; (c) places mercury gauges to measure NPT circumference changes; (d) measures NPT buckling pressure at the appropriate time; and (e) obtains patient photographs related to the NPT study.

11. Learns to perform MSLT.

12. Learns to administer oxygen and nasal continuous positive airway pressure (CPAP) as directed by the staff physician.

13. Learns to instruct the patient in the proper use and care of nasal CPAP equipment in the home.

14. Removes electrodes and cleans the patient as needed.

15. Learns to clean and maintain the equipment and testing room in an organized and sanitary fashion.

16. Learns to score the polysomnographic record; reviews all tests with the laboratory supervisor.

17. Receives and implements all suggestions for improving the quality of future polysomnographic recordings.

18. Learns to recognize abnormal sleep, respiratory, and cardiac patterns.

19. Takes and passes examinations given by the laboratory supervisor.

20. Learns to log polysomnograms and fill out charge documents.

21. Learns to accurately file records and reports.

22. Learns to answer telephone inquiries regarding appointments and test information.

23. Attends polysomnographic record-reading sessions and in-service training sessions.

24. Attends cardiopulmonary resuscitation certification (CPR) training sessions.

25. Attends scientific courses and seminars on polysomnographic testing.

26. Takes and passes, at the end of the training period, the written portion of the examination for registration by the Board of Registered Polysomnographic Technologists.

Responsible to: Laboratory Supervisor

Promotion to: Polysomnographic Technologist I

Job title: Polysomnographic Technologist I

Department: Neurodiagnostic Laboratory

Job summary: Under the supervision of the laboratory supervisor or senior technologist, performs routine polysomnographic studies in the laboratory.

Education/experience: High school graduate and graduate of an accredited electroneurodiagnostic technology program accredited by the Committee on Allied Health Education and Accreditation or equivalent formal training. Certified in CPR; some college-level course work is preferable. Eligible for/or successful completion of the written portion of the examination for registration by the Board of Registered Polysomnographic Technologists and/or 1–3 years' experience in polysomnography.

Skills and responsibilities:

1. Measures and accurately applies electrodes in a timely manner, according to laboratory standards. Ensures that electrode impedances meet laboratory standards.

2. Writes a comprehensive patient history gathering appropriate information from patient, patient's record, and family members to include any sleep disturbances. Explains test procedure to patient and family members present.

3. Performs polysomnograms according to standards of the laboratory: routine recordings, NPT, and MSLT.

4. Administers oxygen and nasal CPAP as prescribed by the patient's physician. Instructs the patient in the proper use and care of nasal CPAP equipment in the home.

5. Recognizes artifact (patient or environmental). Documents, eliminates, or takes proper measures to monitor the artifact.

6. Knowledge of appropriate actions to take during patient emergency situation and insure patient safety (electrical) at all times.

7. Knowledge of basic infection control standards relating to patient and equipment including electrodes.

8. Keeps equipment clean and in proper working order. Knowledge of appropriate calibrations and how to make adjustments. Ability to troubleshoot equipment problems and repair them or report to supervisor promptly.

9. Demonstrates positive interpersonal skills with patients, patient families, laboratory staff, and other members of the hospital staff.

10. Knowledge of neuroanatomy and physiology, basic electronics, and electrical safety, general knowledge of polysomnographic instrumentation pattern recognition and various medical and pharmacological conditions that influence the polysomnogram.

11. Learns to score polysomnograms.

12. Participates in conferences and technical meetings.

13. Performs other duties as assigned.

Responsible to: Laboratory Supervisor

Promotion to: Polysomnographic Technologist II

Job title: Polysomnographic Technologist II

Department: Neurodiagnostic Laboratory

Job summary: Under the general supervision of the laboratory supervisor, performs a wide variety of polysomnographic studies in the laboratory. Analyzes data, scores polysomnograms, and compiles data into a report for physician review.

Education/experience: High school graduate and graduate of an accredited electroneurodiagnostic technology program accredited by the Committee on Allied Health Education and Accreditation or equivalent formal training. Certified in CPR. At least 2 years of college is preferable. Preferred – Registry by the Board of Registered Polysomnographic Technologists and/or 3–5 years' experience in polysomnography.

Skills and responsibilities:

1. Performs all the duties of the Polysomnographic Technologist I (see Tech I description).

2. Performs any special polysomnographic studies as ordered.

3. Compiles data from scored polysomnograms and additional studies into a report for physician review.

4. Administers unit dose medication as ordered by the patient's physician.

5. Assists in establishing and maintaining department procedures and protocols.

6. Assists or performs clinical research procedures.

7. Participates in conferences and technical meetings. Assists junior staff.

8. Provides patient and family education regarding use of CPAP and Bi-PAP equipment and accessories. Also provides patient and family education for troubleshooting problems with equipment used at home.

9. Assumes responsibilities of the laboratory supervisor in their absence (when applicable).

10. Performs other duties as assigned.

Responsible to: Laboratory Supervisor

Promotion to: Laboratory Supervisor

Job title: Surgical Monitoring Technologist

Department: Neurodiagnostic Laboratory

Job summary: Under minimal supervision of the laboratory supervisor, performs EEGs, evoked potentials, and/or topographic brain mapping recordings in the operating room. Monitors during vascular, orthopedic, and neurological cases when the system is at risk for injury. Performs electrocorticograms (ECoG) from the exposed cerebral cortex in the operating room.

Education/experience: High school graduate and a graduate of an electroneurodiagnostic technology program accredited by the Committee on Allied Health Education and Accreditation or equivalent formal training. At least 2 years of college is preferable. Registry (see footnote on registry on page 16) by ABRET; a minimum of 5 years' experience in EEG/evoked potentials; a minimum of 1–2 years' experience monitoring EEG/evoked potentials in the operating room.

Skills and responsibilities:

1. Performs duties of the EEG Tech III and/or EP Tech II as assigned.

2. Monitors EEG, evoked potentials, and/or topographic brain mapping during vascular, orthopedic, and neurosurgical operative procedures.

3. Performs electrocorticograms from the exposed cerebral cortex in the operating room.

4. Applies troubleshooting methods, repairs, and/or replaces instrument parts as needed.

5. Provides in-service training sessions for EEG/evoked potential staff technologists in proper intraoperative monitoring techniques.

6. Assists in establishing and maintaining department EEG/evoked potential monitoring procedures and protocols.

7. Assists or performs clinical intraoperative research procedures.

8. Prepares presentations and contributes at conferences relating to electroneurodiagnostic testing, with special emphasis on intraoperative EEG/evoked potential monitoring, for continuing education.

Responsible to: Laboratory Supervisor
Promotion to: Laboratory Supervisor

Job title: Long-term Monitoring Technologist
Department: Neurodiagnostic Laboratory
Job summary: Under minimal supervision of the laboratory supervisor, performs long-term video/EEG monitoring on patients with scalp and intracranially placed electrodes on an epilepsy unit and performs ECoG in the operating room, cortical stimulation studies, and special studies such as sodium amytal (Wada) testing.

Education/experience: High school graduate and a graduate of an electroneurodiagnostic technology program accredited by the Committee on Allied Health Education and Accreditation or equivalent formal training. At least 2 years of college is preferable. Registry (see footnote on registry on page 16) by ABRET; a minimum of 5 years' experience in EEG/evoked potentials; a minimum of 1–2 years' experience in long-term monitoring on an epilepsy unit.

Skills and responsibilities:

1. Performs duties of the EEG Tech III and/or EP Tech II as assigned.

2. Performs long-term video/EEG monitoring on an epilepsy unit.

3. Performs EEG and EP monitoring on patients with

scalp and intracranially placed electrodes (depth electrodes and/or grids).

4. Transcribes digital EEG data to hard-copy printouts and correlates video of ictal events, making appropriate notations on the tracing.

5. Assists and records during direct cortical stimulation studies.

6. Performs EEG recordings during special studies such as sodium amytal (Wada) testing, positron emission tomography, and sodium pentothal studies.

7. Performs ECoG from the exposed cerebral cortex in the operating room.

8. Applies troubleshooting methods, repairs, and/or replaces instrument parts as needed.

9. Provides in-service training sessions for electroneurodiagnostic staff technologists in proper long-term monitoring techniques.

10. Assists in establishing and maintaining department long-term epilepsy monitoring procedures and protocols.

11. Assists or performs clinical epilepsy research procedures.

12. Prepares presentations and contributes at conferences relating to electroneurodiagnostic testing, with special emphasis on long-term epilepsy monitoring, for continuing education.

13. Performs other duties as assigned.

Responsible to: Laboratory Supervisor
Promotion to: Laboratory Supervisor

Job title: Electroneurodiagnostic Laboratory Supervisor
Department: Neurodiagnostic Laboratory

Job summary: Under the general supervision of the laboratory medical director and/or hospital administrator, manages the day-to-day operations and activities of the neurodiagnostic laboratory, supervises technical and clerical staff, prepares operating and capital budgets annually, orders equipment and supplies.

Education/experience: Graduate of an electroneurodiagnostic technology program accredited by the Committee on Allied Health Education and Accreditation or equivalent formal training. An Associate Degree from an accredited college is preferred (a Bachelor's Degree is desirable), registry (see footnote on registry on page 16) by ABRET in EEG and evoked potentials is preferred, and/or a minimum of 5 years' experience in EEG and evoked potentials, demonstrated leadership, administrative, supervisory, and teaching skills.

Skills and responsibilities:

1. Assigns all technical and clerical staff to achieve optimum patient service, appropriate division of labor, and an expeditious work flow.

2. Interviews, hires, and evaluates the EEG staff.

3. Formulates and updates policy and procedure manuals.

4. Maintains productivity figures.

5. Monitors expenditures to ensure compliance to approved budgets.

6. Prepares operating and capital budgets annually in collaboration with the medical director.

7. Investigates patient and physician complaints and recommends to the medical director a corresponding course of action.

8. Arranges for equipment repair and servicing.

9. Maintains and reports on total quality assurance program.

10. Orients and trains EEG personnel in laboratory policies and procedures.

11. Provides in-service training sessions and reviews, compiles and distributes pertinent resource materials for staff development.

12. Arranges for staff attendance and participation in continuing education courses and seminars on electroneurodiagnostic testing.

13. Attends scientific courses and seminars on electroneurodiagnostic testing, with special emphasis on managerial and teaching skills, for continuing education.

14. Performs duties of an electroneurodiagnostic technologist as needed.

Responsible to: Laboratory Medical Director or Hospital Administrator

Promotion to: Administrator

Acknowledgements: Special thanks to Mary Jane Wilkerson, Tim Fields, Dee Quinonez, Wendi Nugent, Lillian Scott, Melisse LeWeck, Nancy Thompson, as well as all the ASET Board members who kindly sent us job descriptions used in their laboratories. These job descriptions were used as a basis for writing the new job descriptions. Thanks to the Executive Committee and the 1992 ASET Board of Trustees for their review of the draft. Thanks also to American Electroencephalographic Society's Dr. C.W. Erwin for review of the job descriptions and Mr. Cameron Harris, APT President, for review of the polysomnography job descriptions. I would also like to thank my fellow committee member, Walt Banoczi, for working with me on this project via many phone calls through three time zones.

GUIDELINE SIX: RECOMMENDATIONS FOR TELEPHONE TRANSMISSION OF EEGs

1. Basic standards

The basic standards and technical specifications for clinical EEG, defined in Guideline One: 'Minimum Technical Requirements for Performing Clinical Electroencephalography,' and Guideline Four: 'Standards of Practice in Clinical Electroencephalography,' should be followed in the transmission, interpretation, and preservation of clinical EEGs by telephone (Bennett and Gardner, 1970; Barlow et al., 1974; Frost and Barlow, 1976; Roy, 1976; Committee on Standards, 1983). Within these specifications, recordings at the transmitting and receiving sites should be essentially identical.

1.1 Manufacturers should provide frequency response, noise, and crosstalk data under operating conditions, so that consumers can make intelligent comparisons. Periodic checks of equipment at both the transmitting and the receiving laboratories should be carried out.

1.2 'Fail-safe' indication of difficulties due to line losses or other transmission or receiving problems should be included in the transmitting-receiving system itself. (Assistance from telephone companies with general information concerning the identification of artifacts generated within the telephone systems could be most helpful.)

1.3 Signal checks of equipment at both the transmitting and receiving laboratories should be introduced preceding and following each recording, i.e., prior to the initial calibration and subsequent to the final calibration.

1.4 The identification appearing on the original (transmitted) and the received record should be adequate to identify the latter as being a copy of the former. Identification should include patient ID, all calibrations, and changes in instrument controls and montages.

1.5 The EEG should be recorded both at the transmitting and receiving ends of the circuit, so that the technologists can correlate EEG events with behavior changes or activities of the patient and can determine whether artifacts are present. The preferable method of transmission is to utilize a paper record at both the transmitting and receiving end. Whether paper or alternate methods are used, equipment at both ends should permit simultaneous real-time review of the activities from all recorded channels, should permit reassessment of the activity recorded over the previous minutes of the recording,

This material originally appeared in *J Clin Neurophysiol* 1986;3(Suppl 1):23–5.
© 1994 American Electroencephalographic Society, Vol. 11 (1): 28–29.

and should allow comparison of different segments of the record.

Relevant patient behavior and activity should be noted (see Guideline One: 'Minimum Technical Requirements for Performing Clinical Electroencephalography'). Voice or other signaling capabilities should be incorporated in the telephone–EEG system, from transmitting to receiving stations, to identify EEG–clinical correlations as they occur, with minimal interference with the EEG record. Such on-line correlation will assist in avoiding misinterpretation (e.g., muscle artifact being regarded as spikes, etc.). The use of a standard code for transmitting such information should be required.

1.6 The EEG at both ends should be stored (whether on paper or utilizing an alternate method such as tape or disk). The EEG at the transmitting site should be available when necessary for backup comparison and, to ensure quality control, recordings from both ends should be compared regularly.

2. Technologist qualifications

The statements set forth in Guideline Five are reaffirmed for telephone transmission of EEGs. These standards define the basic level of competence of the EEG technologists at the transmitting and at the receiving sites. Under no circumstances should the technologist at the transmitting laboratory be less qualified than one who works independently under a laboratory director who is based outside of a hospital. Indeed, the responsibilities falling upon the EEG technologist staffing a telephone transmitting laboratory are greater than those of a technologist working under relatively direct supervision in a hospital or office laboratory.

2.1 The technologist at the transmitting laboratory, because of its remoteness from the receiving center, should be well trained, especially in telephone transmission EEG, irrespective of any limited utilization because of size of referral load. This technologist should also be acquainted with the receiving laboratory. In view of the isolation of the transmitting laboratory, provisions for continued education and updating of information are essential to maintaining the skill of the transmitting technologist.

2.2 Technologists staffing a receiving facility should be skilled and experienced, should be specifically trained in telephone transmission EEG, and should particularly be familiar with the recognition of artifacts that are peculiar to this technology. A program of continuing education should be available for the technologist at the receiving laboratory.

2.3 A qualified electroencephalographer should interpret the received EEG and supervise the technologists at both the transmitting and receiving ends (see Guideline Four).

3. Ethical considerations

Provided that all of the above and previously approved procedures are followed, no ethical problem in the use of telephone systems for expediting interpretation of EEGs should arise.

If the procedures in this and in previously adopted guidelines are not followed, and if users are not aware of the characteristics of ancillary equipment used in telephone transmission of EEGs, the installation of a telephone transmission system may well cause a degradation of the quality of practice of clinical EEG.

4. Brain death

At the present time, telephone transmission of EEG cannot be used for determination of electrocerebral silence in the diagnosis of brain death because of the inherent and unpredictable electrical noise present in telephone networks relative to the very low signal amplitudes in the EEG recording itself in this situation (see Guideline Three, 'Minimum Technical Standards for EEG Recording in Suspected Cerebral Death').

REFERENCES

Barlow JS, Kamp A, Morton HB, Ripoche A, Shipton H. EEG instrumentation standards: report of the Committee on EEG Instrumentation Standards of the International Federation of Societies for Electroencephalography and Clinical Neurophysiology. III. EEG telephone (telephone transmission of EEG data). *Electroencephalogr Clin Neurophysiol* 1974;37:552.

Bennett DR, Gardner RM. A model for the telephone transmission of six-channel electroencephalograms. *Electroencephalogr Clin Neurophysiol* 1970;29:404–8.

Committee on Standards of Clinical Practice of EEG and EMG. Telephone transmission. In: *International Federation of Societies for Electroencephalography and Clinical Neurophysiology: Recommendations for the practice of clinical neurophysiology.* Amsterdam: Elsevier, 1983:52–3.

Frost JD Jr, Barlow JS. Telephone transmission of EEGs–practical aspects. In: Frost JD Jr, Barlow JS, eds. *Graphic and magnetic-tape recording of bioelectrical phenomena.* Amsterdam: Elsevier, 1976:3B20–3. (Handbook of electroencephalography and clinical neurophysiology; vol 3, part B.)

Roy OZ. Biotelemetry and telephone transmission. In: Broughton RJ, ed. *Acquisition of bioelectrical data: collection and amplification.* Amsterdam: Elsevier, 1976:3A46–66. (Handbook of electroencephalography and clinical neurophysiology; vol 3, part A.)

GUIDELINE SEVEN: A PROPOSAL FOR STANDARD MONTAGES TO BE USED IN CLINICAL EEG

INTRODUCTION

A great diversity of montages exists among different EEG laboratories, and many of these montages fail to display the EEG adequately or are inordinately complex. Moreover, this diversity impedes interchange of information among electroencephalographers, to the ultimate detriment of patients.

Recognizing the need for improving this aspect of EEG practice, the montages listed in this Guideline are recommended for standard use by clinical laboratories. This proposal should not be construed as an attempt to limit the total number of montages used by any EEG laboratory. Indeed, depending on individual recording circumstances, additional montages may be necessary for an adequate EEG examination and for the solution of particular problems. The proposed montages are intended to constitute a basic minimum, not a maximum, for general-purpose use. If these recommendations are adopted widely, communication among electroencephalographers should be facilitated.

Further, the proposed montages are not designed for special purposes, such as for neonatal EEGs, recording with nasopharyngeal or sphenoidal leads, all-night sleep recordings, or for verification of electrocerebral inactivity.

1. Montage designations

1.1 The class of montage is designated as follows: longitudinal bipolar (LB), transverse bipolar (TB), or referential (R).

1.2 The numeral to the left of the point indicates the number of channels. Montages are designed for four types of instruments: 8, 10, 16, and 18 channels.

1.3 The numeral 2 or 3 to the right of the point indicates an alternative montage of the same class for a particular size of instrument (e.g., LB-16.2 and LB-16.3 are alternative for LB-16.1). The number of alternatives has been limited to a maximum of three.

1.4 A small letter to the right of the point (for 8- and 10-channel instruments) indicates a montage that is to be used in conjunction with at least one other for adequate area coverage (e.g., R-10.1a and R-10.b).

This material originally appeared in *J Clin Neurophysiol* 1986;3(Suppl 1):26–33.© 1994 American Electroencephalographic Society, Vol. 11 (1): 30–36.

2. Recommendations governing selection of the proposed montages with explanatory notes

2.1 The Committee *reaffirms* the statements pertaining to montages set forth previously in the Guidelines of the American Electroencephalographic Society and that are paraphrased as follows:

(a) that no less than 8 channels of simultaneous recording be used, and that a larger number of channels be encouraged,

(b) that the full 21 electrode placements of the 10–20 system be used,

(c) that both bipolar and referential montages be used,

(d) that the electrode connections for each channel be clearly indicated at the beginning of each montage,

(e) that the pattern of electrode connections be made as simple as possible and that montages should be easily comprehended,

(f) that the electrode connections (bipolar) preferentially should run in straight (unbroken) lines and the interelectrode distances kept equal,

(g) that tracings from the more anterior electrodes be placed above those from the more posterior electrodes on the recording page, and

(h) that it is very desirable to have some of the montages comparable for all EEG laboratories.

Table 1. *Number of montages recommended*[a]

No. channels per instrument	Longitudinal bipolar	Transverse bipolar	Referential	Total
18	1 (3)	1 (2)	1 (3)	3
16	1 (3)	1 (3)	1 (3)	3
10	2 (6)	3 (3)	2 (4)	7
8	2 (2)	3 (3)	2 (4)	7

[a]Figures in parentheses refer to the number of alternative montages proposed.

2.2 The Committee recommends a 'left above right' order of derivations, i.e., on the recording page left-sided leads should be placed above right-sided leads for either alternating pairs of derivations or blocks of derivations.

This recommendation coincides with the prevailing practice of the vast majority of EEG laboratories in North America and by laboratories in some, but not all, other countries.

2.3 A maximum number of electrodes should be represented in each montage, within limitations imposed by the number of recording channels, to ensure adequate coverage of head areas.

2.4 Three classes of montage should be represented in each recording: LB, TB, and R.

2.5 For 16- and 18-channel recording, one montage from each of the three classes will be needed. For 8- and 10-channel recording, seven montages (2 LB, 3 TB, and 2 R) will be needed (see Table 1).

501

For adequate mapping of electrical fields, additional montages may need to be devised that include LB and TB chains recorded simultaneously.

In the montages listed for R recording, leads on the mandibular angles may be substituted for the leads on the earlobes if the change is duly noted.

Potential pitfalls in referential recording are numerous, and caution should be exercised if unwanted activity appears in a reference lead. In such instances, another reference should be chosen and the change should be clearly noted in the recording.

2.6 A logical order of arrangement should prevail in each montage and in comparable montages designed for instruments of different sizes.

Recognizing the fact that experienced electroencephalographers differ for valid reasons in their approach to the display of EEG activity, alternative sets of montages have been included in the recommendations. Further details about the principles of montage design and the different preferences by members of this Committee have been published (*Am J EEG Technol*, 17:Nos. 1 and 2, 1977).

In general, the LB.1 and the R.1 series consist of leads grouped in anatomical proximity and extending sequentially across the head from the left to the right. In this system, hemispheric differences are readily appreciated. In the LB.2 and LB.3 series, blocks of homologous derivations are compared (LB.2 extending from the midline sagittal region laterally, LB.3 extending from lateral regions medially). In the R.2 and R.3 series, homologous derivations are juxtaposed in adjacent channels to facilitate comparison of localized regions (R.2 extending from the midline sagittal region laterally and R.3 extending from the lateral regions medially). The alternative montages in the TB series depend, in part, on the extent of polar coverage.

Minor modifications of the recommended montages may be instituted during part of the recording, especially for monitoring other physiologic variables, if the modifications do not infringe upon the principles set froth in these Recommendations

Longitudinal Bipolar Montages

Channel No.	LB-18.1	LB-18.2	LB-18.3
1	Fp1-F7	Fz-Cz	Fp1-F7
2	F7-T3	Cz-Pz	F7-T3
3	T3-T5	Fp1-F3	T3-T5
4	T5-O1	F3-C3	T5-O1
5	Fp1-F3	C3-P3	Fp2-F8
6	F3-C3	P3-O1	F8-T4
7	C3-P3	Fp2-F4	T4-T6
8	P3-O1	F4-F4	T6-O2
9	Fz-Cz	C4-P4	Fp1-F3
10	Cz-Pz	P4-O2	F3-C3
11	Fp2-F4	Fp1-F7	C3-P3
12	F4-C4	F7-T3	P3-O1
13	C4-P4	T3-T5	Fp2-F4
14	P4-O2	T5-O1	F4-C4
15	Fp2-F8	Fp2-F8	C4-P4
16	F8-T4	F8-T4	F4-O2
17	T4-T6	T4-T6	Fz-Cz
18	T6-O2	T6-O2	Cz-Pz

Channel No.	LB-16.1	LB-16.2	LB-16.3
1	Fp1-F7	Fp1-F3	Fp1-F7
2	F7-T3	F3-C3	F7-T3
3	T3-T5	C3-P3	T3-T5
4	T5-O1	P3-O1	T5-O1
5	Fp1-F3	Fp2-F4	Fp2-F8
6	F3-C3	F4-C4	F8-T4
7	C3-P3	C4-P4	T4-T6
8	P3-O1	P4-O2	T6-O2
9	Fp2-F4	Fp1-F7	Fp1-F3
10	F4-C4	F7-T3	F3-C3

Channel No.	LB-16.1	LB-16.2	LB-16.3
11	C4-P4	T3-T5	C3-P3
12	P4-O2	T5-O1	P3-O1
13	Fp2-F8	Fp2-F8	Fp2-F4
14	F8-T4	F8-T4	F4-C4
15	T4-T6	T4-T6	C4-P4
16	T6-O2	T6-O2	P4-O2

Channel No.	LB-10.1a	LB-10.1b	LB-10.2a	LB-10.2b	LB-10.3a	LB-10.3b
1	Fp1-F7	Fp1-F3	Fz-Cz	Fz-Cz	Fp1-F7	Fp1-F3
2	F7-T3	F3-C3	Cz-Pz	Cz-Pz	F7-T3	F3-C3
3	T3-T5	C3-P3	Fp1-F3	Fp1-F7	T3-T5	C3-P3
4	T5-O1	P3-O1	F3-C3	F7-T3	T5-O1	P3-O1
5	Fz-Cz	Fz-Cz	C3-P3	T3-T5	Fp2-F8	Fp2-F4
6	Cz-Pz	Cz-Pz	P3-O1	T5-O1	F8-T4	F4-C4
7	Fp2-F8	Fp2-F4	Fp2-F4	Fp2-F8	T4-T6	C4-P4
8	F8-T4	F4-C4	F4-C4	F8-T4	T6-O2	P4-O2
9	T4-T6	C4-P4	C4-P4	T4-T6	Fz-Cz	Fz-Cz
10	T6-O2	P4-O2	P4-O2	T6-O2	Cz-Pz	Cz-Pz

Channel No.	LB-8.1a	LB-8.1b
1	Fp1-F3	Fp1-F7
2	F3-C3	F7-T3
3	C3-P3	T3-T5
4	P3-O1	T5-O1
5	Fp2-F4	Fp2-F8
6	F4-C4	F8-T4

Channel No.	LB-8.1a	LB-8.1b
7	C4-P4	T4-T6
8	P4-O2	T6-O2

Transverse Bipolar Montages

Channel No.	TB-18.1	TB-18.2
1	F7-Fp1	Fp1-Fp2
2	Fp1-Fp2	F7-F3
3	Fp2-F8	F3-Fz
4	F7-F3	Fz-F4
5	F3-Fz	F4-F8
6	Fz-F4	A1-T3
7	F4-F8	T3-C3
8	T3-C3	C3-Cz
9	C3-Cz	Cz-C4
10	Cz-C4	C4-T4
11	C4-T4	T4-A2
12	T5-P3	T5-P3
13	P3-Pz	P3-Pz
14	Pz-P4	Pz-P4
15	P4-T6	P4-T6
16	T5-O1	O1-O2
17	O1-O2	Fz-Cz
18	O2-T6	Cz-Pz

Channel No.	TB-16.1	TB-16.2	TB-16.3
1	F7-Fp1	Fp1-Fp2	F7-Fp1
2	Fp1-Fp2	F7-F3	Fp2-F8
3	Fp2-F8	F3-Fz	F7-F3

505

(continued)

Channel No.	TB-16.1	TB-16.2	TB-16.3
4	F7-F3	Fz-F4	F3-Fz
5	F3-Fz	F4-F8	Fz-F4
6	Fz-F4	A1-T3	F4-F8
7	F4-F8	T3-C3	T3-C3
8	T3-C3	C3-Cz	C3-Cz
9	C3-Cz	Cz-C4	Cz-C4
10	Cz-C4	C4-T4	C4-T4
11	C4-T4	T4-A2	T5-P3
12	T5-P3	T5-P3	P3-Pz
13	P3-Pz	P3-Pz	Pz-P4
14	Pz-P4	Pz-P4	P4-T6
15	P4-T6	P4-T6	T5-O1
16	O1-O2	O1-O2	O2-T6

Channel No.	TB-10.1a	TB-10.1b	TB-10.1c
1	F7-Fp1	F7-F3	A1-T3
2	Fp1-Fp2	F3-Fz	T3-C3
3	Fp2-F8	Fz-F4	C3-Cz
4	T3-C3	F4-F8	Cz-C4
5	C3-Cz	A1-T3	C4-T4
6	Cz-C4	T3-C3	T4-A2
7	C4-T4	C3-Cz	T5-P3
8	T5-O1	Cz-C4	P3-Pz
9	O1-O2	C4-T4	Pz-P4
10	O2-T6	T4-A2	P4-T6

506

Channel No.	TB-8.1a	TB-8.1b	TB-8.1c
1	F7-Fp1	F7-F3	T3-C3
2	Fp1-Fp2	F3-Fz	C3-Cz
3	Fp2-F8	Fz-F4	Cz-C4
4	C3-Cz	F4-F8	C4-T4
5	Cz-C4	T3-C3	T5-P3
6	T5-O1	C3-Cz	P3-Pz
7	O1-O2	Cz-C4	Pz-P4
8	O2-T6	C4-T4	P4-T6

Referential Montages

Channel No.	R-18.1	R-18.2	R-18.3
1	F7-A1	Fz-A1	F7-A1
2	T3-A1	Pz-A2	F8-A2
3	T5-A1	Fp1-A1	T3-A1
4	Fp1-A1	Fp2-A2	T4-A2
5	F3-A1	F3-A1	T5-A1
6	C3-A1	F4-A2	T6-A2
7	P3-A1	C3-A1	Fp1-A1
8	O1-A1	C4-A2	Fp2-A2
9	Fz-A1	P3-A1	F3-A1
10	Pz-A2	P4-A2	F4-A2
11	Fp2-A2	O1-A1	C3-A1
12	F4-A2	O2-A2	C4-A2
13	C4-A2	F7-A1	P3-A1
14	P4-A2	F8-A2	P4-A2
15	O2-A2	T3-A1	O1-A1
16	F8-A2	T4-A2	O2-A2
17	T4-A2	T5-A1	Fz-A1
18	T6-A2	T6-A2	Pz-A2

Channel No.	R-16.1	R-16.2	R-16.3
1	F7-A1	Fp1-A1	F7-A1
2	T3-A1	Fp2-A2	F8-A2
3	T5-A1	F3-A1	T3-A1
4	Fp1-A1	F4-A2	T4-A2
5	F3-A1	C3-A1	T5-A1
6	C3-A1	C4-A2	T6-A2
7	P3-A1	P3-A1	Fp1-A1
8	O1-A1	P4-A2	Fp2-A2
9	Fp2-A2	O1-A1	F3-A1
10	F4-A2	O2-A2	F4-A2
11	C4-A2	F7-A1	C3-A1
12	P4-A2	F8-A2	C4-A2
13	O2-A2	T3-A1	P3-A1
14	F8-A2	T4-A2	P4-A2
15	T4-A2	T5-A1	O1-A1
16	F6-A2	T6-A2	O2-A2

Channel No.	R-10.1a	R-10.1b	R-10.2a	R-10.2b
1	Fp1-A1	Fp1-A1	Fp1-A1	Fp1-A1
2	F3-A1	F7-A1	Fp2-A2	Fp2-A2
3	C3-A1	T3-A1	F3-A1	F7-A1
4	P3-A1	T5-A1	F4-A2	F8-A2
5	O1-A1	O1-A1	C3-A1	T3-A1
6	Fp2-A2	Fp2-A2	C4-A2	T4-A2
7	F4-A2	F8-A2	P3-A1	T5-A1
8	C4-A2	T4-A2	F4-A2	T6-A2
9	P4-A2	T6-A2	O1-A1	O1-A1
10	O2-A2	O2-A2	O2-A2	O2-A2

(continued)

Channel No.	R-8.1a	R-8.1b	R-8.2a	R-8.2b
1	F3-A1	Fp1-A1	F3-A1	Fp1-A1
2	C3-A1	F7-A1	F4-A2	Fp2-A2
3	P3-A1	T3-A1	C3-A1	F7-A1
4	O1-A1	T5-A1	C4-A2	F8-A2
5	F4-A2	Fp2-A2	P3-A1	T3-A1
6	C4-A2	F8-A2	P4-A2	T4-A2
7	P4-A2	T4-A2	O1-A1	T5-A1
8	O2-A2	T6-A2	O2-A2	T6-A2

GUIDELINE EIGHT: GUIDELINES FOR WRITING EEG REPORTS

These guidelines are not meant to represent rigid rules but only a general guide for reporting EEGs. They are intended to apply to standard EEG recordings rather than to special procedures. When reporting on more specialized types of records (e.g., neonatal records, records for suspected electrocerebral silence), description of technical details should be more complete than in the case of standard recordings. However, if the technique used is the one recommended for those special procedures in the 'Guidelines in EEG,' (American Electroencephalographic Society, 1980), a sentence to that effect should be sufficient (Guidelines 3, 'Minimum Technical Requirements for Performing Clinical EEG' (MTR); 4, 'Minimum Technical Standards for EEG Recording in Suspected Cerebral Death'; and 6, 'Minimal Technical Standards for Pediatric Electroencephalography').

1. *The printed forms for reporting EEGs should provide for a minimum of information about the patient, which could be copied from the Basic Data Sheet (MTR, Sec. 6.1) by the person who types the report. It should be, therefore, unnecessary for the electroencephalographer to repeat in the report the age, sex,* etc., *of the patient. However, in order to avoid confusion, the name of the patient and the EEG identification number should be included.*

2. *The report of an EEG should consist of three principal parts: (A) Introduction, (B) Description of the record, and (C) Interpretation, including (a) impression regarding its normality or degree of abnormality, and (b) correlation of the EEG findings with the clinical picture.*

3. **Introduction.** *The introduction should start with a statement of the kind of preparation the patient had, if any, for the recording session.* The initial sentence should state whether the patient received any medication or other preparation, such as sleep deprivation, as well as the patient's state of consciousness at the onset of the record. If the patient was fasting, this should be stated.

If the printed form used for the report does not provide a space for the regular medication the patient is receiving, as distinguished from medication given specifically for the recording, any medication that could influence the EEG should be included in the electroencephalographer's report.

If the number of electrodes used is not the standard 21 of the 10–20 system or if monitoring of other physiologic parameters is used, this should be stated in the Introduction. Reporting

This material originally appeared in *J Clin Neurophysiol* 1986;3 (Suppl 1):34–7.
© 1994 American Electroencephalographic Society, Vol. 11 (1): 37–39.

the total recording time is also advisable if for some special reason this is significantly shorter or longer than recommended in the American Electroencephalographic Society Guidelines (MTR, Sec. 7.1).

4. **Description.** *The description of the EEG should include all the characteristics of the record, both normal and abnormal, presented in an objective way, avoiding, as much as possible, judgment about their significance.*

The aim is to produce a complete and objective report that would allow another electroencephalographer to arrive at a conclusion concerning the normality or degree of abnormality of the record from the written report, without the benefit of looking at the EEG. This conclusion could conceivably be different from that of the original interpreter, since it is by necessity a subjective one.

The description should start with the background activity,[1] beginning with the dominant activity, its frequency, quantity (persistent, intermittent), location, amplitude, symmetry or asymmetry, and whether it is rhythmic or irregular. The frequency should be given preferably in hertz or cycles per second. For the purpose of standardizing the report, while recognizing that any decision on this point must be arbitrary,

it is recommended that the amplitude of this activity be determined in derivations employing adjacent scalp electrodes placed according to the 10–20 system. It is desirable but not mandatory that the estimated mean amplitude be given in microvolts. This will obviate the need for defining terms such as 'low', 'medium', and 'high'.

Enumeration of nondominant activities with their frequency, quantity, amplitude, location, symmetry or asymmetry, and rhythmicity or lack of it should follow, using the same units as for the dominant frequency.

Response to opening and closing eyes as well as to purposeful movement of the extremities when appropriate, should then be described. The response should be described as symmetric or asymmetric, complete or incomplete, sustained or unsustained.

Abnormal records, infants' records, or records limited to sleep may not have clearly dominant frequencies. In those cases, the different activities with their amplitude, frequency, etc., should be described, in any order. When the record shows a marked interhemispheric asymmetry, the characteristics of each hemisphere should be described separately (i.e., dominant, nondominant frequency, etc., of one hemisphere first, followed by those of the other).

The description of the background activity should be followed by description of the abnormalities that do not form part of this background activity. This should include a description of the type (spikes, sharp waves, slow waves), distribution (diffuse or focal), topography or location, symmetry,

_____
[1]The term 'background activity' is used here as defined by the International Federation of Societies of EEG and Clinical Neurophysiology Committee on Terminology (Chatrian GE, et al.: A glossary of terms most commonly used by clinical electroencephalographers. *Electroencephalogr Clin Neurophysiol* 1974;37:538–48).

synchrony (intra- and interhemispheric), amplitude, timing (continuous, intermittent, episodic, or paroxysmal), and quantity of the abnormal patterns. Quantity has to be expressed in a subjective fashion, since in clinical, unaided interpretation of the EEG, no exact quantities or ratios can be given.

When the abnormality is episodic, attention should be given to the presence or absence of periodicity[2] between episodes and to the rhythmicity or irregularity of the pattern within each episode. The range of duration of the episodes should be given.

In the description of activation procedures, a statement should be included pertaining to their quality (e.g., good, fair, or poor hyperventilation, duration of sleep, and staged attained). The type of photic stimulation used (i.e., stepwise or glissando) should be stated and the range of frequencies given. Effects of hyperventilation and photic stimulation should be described, including normal and abnormal responses. If hyperventilation or photic stimulation are not done, the reason for this omission should be given. If referring clinicians know that these procedures are used routinely, they may expect results even if they have not been specifically requested.

There is no point in including in the description the absence of certain characteristics, except for the lack of normal features, such as low-voltage fast frequencies, sleep spindles, etc.

---

[2]For definition of 'periodic' see Chatrian GE, et al. quoted in footnote 1. Acceptance 2 applies in this instance.

Phrases such as 'No focal abnormality' or 'No epileptiform abnormality' have a place in the impression when the clinician has asked for it either explicitly or implicitly in the request form. They have no place in the description.

Artifacts should be mentioned only when they are questionable and could represent cerebral activity, when they are unusual or excessive (eye movements, muscle) and interfere with the interpretation of the record, or when they may provide valuable diagnostic information (e.g., myokymia, nystagmus, etc.).

5. **Interpretation**.

(a) Impression. *The impression is the interpreter's subjective statement about the normality or abnormality of the record.* The description of the record is directed primarily to the electroencephalographer who writes it for review at a later date, or to another expert, and should be detailed and objective. The impression, on the other hand, is primarily written for the referring clinician and should, therefore, be as succinct as possible. Most clinicians know that their information will not significantly increase by reading the detailed description and hence limit themselves to reading the impression. If this is too long and seemingly irrelevant to the clinical picture, the clinician will lose interest and the report of the record becomes less useful.

If the record is considered abnormal, it is desirable to grade the abnormality in order to facilitate comparison between successive records for the person who receives the report. Since this part of the report is largely subjective, the grading will vary from laboratory to laboratory, but the different grades should be properly defined and the definitions consistently adhered to in any given laboratory.

After the statement regarding normality or degree of abnormality of the record, the reasons upon which the conclusion is based should be briefly listed. When dealing with several types of abnormal features, the list should be limited to the two or three main ones; the most characteristic of the record. If all the abnormalities are enumerated again in the impression, the more important ones become diluted and emphasis is lost. If previous EEGs are available, comparison with previous tracings should be included.

(b) Clinical correlation. *The clinical correlation should be an attempt to explain how the EEG findings fit (or do not fit) the total clinical picture. This explanation should vary, depending on whom it is addressed to. More careful wording is necessary if the recipient is not versed in EEG or neurology.*

If an EEG is abnormal it is *indicative* of cerebral dysfunction, since EEG is a manifestation of cerebral function. However, the phrase 'cerebral dysfunction' may sound too strong to some and it should be used only when the abnormality is more than mild and when enough clinical information is available to make the statement realistic within the clinical context. Otherwise, a sentence like, 'The record indicates minor irregularities in cerebral dysfunction,' may be appropriate.

Certain types of EEG patterns are *suggestive* of more or less specific clinical entities; a delta focus may suggest a structural lesion in the proper clinical context; certain types of spikes or sharp waves suggest potential epileptogenesis. If the EEG abnormality fits the clinical information containing the diagnosis or the suspicion of the presence of a given condition, it may be stated that the EEG finding is *consistent* with or supportive of the diagnosis.

In EEG reports, the term 'compatible with' is frequently found. Strictly speaking, any EEG is compatible with practically any clinical picture. Therefore, the term is not helpful and should not be used.

In cases in which the EEG is strongly suggestive of a certain condition that is not mentioned in the clinical history, it is prudent to mention the fact that such EEG abnormalities are frequently found in association with the clinical condition but are not necessarily indicative of it.

An EEG can be said to be *diagnostic* of a certain condition only in the rare cases in which there is a clinical manifestation present at the time of the recording of an EEG and the record shows an electrical abnormality known to the generally associated with the specific clinical manifestation. Such a case would be one in which a patient presents a typical absence concomitant with a bilaterally synchronous 3/s spike-and-wave burst.

In situations in which the diagnostic clinical impression seems at odds with the EEG findings, some possible reasons for the apparent discrepancy should be offered in the EEG report. These reasons should be presented cautiously, trying to avoid any impression of criticism of the clinical diagnosis, or to appear apologetic for an apparent failure of the EEG as a supplemental diagnostic test.

If an EEG is abnormal, but the abnormal features could be produced, at least in part by medication or other therapeutic interventions such as recent electroconvulsive treatment, it should be so stated.

Under no circumstances should the electroencephalographer suggest changes in medication or other clinical approaches. However, the clinical correlation statement could be followed by a recommendation pertaining to further EEGs with different added procedures, e.g., 'In view of the clinical picture a sleep record could be useful,' or 'Since the record was taken shortly after a clinical seizure, a follow-up EEG may be helpful in determining whether the slow wave focus present in this record is of permanent or of only transitory nature.'

A normal record does not, in general, require further explanation. However, when the clinical information suggests a serious question between two conditions, such as hysteria and epilepsy, a statement should be added that might prevent the clinician from jumping to a wrong conclusion. Such a statement could be: 'A normal record does not rule out a convulsive disorder. If the clinical picture warrants, a recording with (some type of activation) may be helpful.'

GUIDELINE TWELVE: GUIDELINES FOR LONG-TERM MONITORING FOR EPILEPSY

I. INTRODUCTION

Long-term monitoring for epilepsy (LTME) refers to the simultaneous recording of EEG and clinical behavior over extended periods of time to evaluate patients with paroxysmal disturbances of cerebral function. LTME is used when it is important to correlate clinical behavior with EEG phenomena. EEG recordings of long duration may be useful in a variety of situations in which patients have intermittent disturbances that are difficult to record during routine EEG sessions. However, as defined here, LTME is limited to patients with epileptic seizure disorders or suspected epileptic seizure disorders. These guidelines do not pertain to extended EEG monitoring used in critical care, intraoperative, or sleep analysis setting.

Although LTME can, in general, be considered to be longer than routine EEG, the duration varies depending on the indications for monotoring and the frequency of seizure occurrence. Since the intermittent abnormalities of interest may occur infrequently and unpredictably, the time necessary to document the presence of epileptiform transients or to record seizures cannot always be predetermined and may range from hours to weeks. Diagnostic efficacy requires the ability to record continuously until sufficient data are obtained. Consequently, 'long-term monitoring' refers more to the *capability* for recording over long periods of time than to the actual duration of the recording.

New technological developments have made prolonged recording of EEG and associated clinical behavior more practical than could be possible using standard EEG techniques. LTME can be performed in numerous ways with various types of equipment. At present, there is no single approach that can be considered best for all purposes. Since LTME is a dynamic field is which new methods are rapidly being introduced, these guidelines will not attempt to specify equipment or protocols that must. be used; rather, the available technologies and methods will be discussed in terms of relative strengths and weaknesses, and recommendations will be made concerning the indications for which each is best suited.

Descriptions of various approaches to LTME in the literature have been inconsistent, and a standard terminology is recommended. Other acceptable generic terms that have been used are 'long-term neurodiagnostic monitoring for epilepsy'

© 1994 American Electroencephalographic Society, *J Clin Neurophysiol* Vol. 11 (1): 88–110.

and, where video monitoring is used, 'long-term video EEG monitoring.' Within this broad category of diagnostic tests, there are many specific subcategories. EEG can be recorded from extracranial, or from intracranial, electrodes, and may be transmitted by direct cable or telemetry. There can be video monitoring, but this is not always the case. Ambulatory cassette recording requires separate considerations. Consequently, it is recommended that the term 'EEG,' when used alone, should imply extracranial (scalp and sphenoidal if used) recording with direct cable transmission. If intracranial electrodes and/or telemetry, and/or video are used, they should be so specified. Therefore, the following terminology for broad categories of long-term monitoring is recommended:

- *Long-term EEG monitoring:* scalp/sphenoidal electrodes, direct cable, no video.
- *Long-term intracranial EEG monitoring:* depth, subdural, epidural, or foramen ovale electrodes, direct cable, no video.
- *Long-term EEG with video monitoring:* scalp/sphenoidal electrodes, direct cable, video.
- *Long-term intracranial EEG with video monitoring:* depth, subdural, epidural, or foramen ovale electrodes, direct cable, video.
- *Long-term EEG telemetry:* scalp/sphenoidal electrodes, radio or cable telemetry, no video.
- *Long-term intracranial EEG telemetry:* depth, subdural,

epidural, or foramen ovale electrodes, cable or radio telemetry, no video.
- *Long-term EEG telemetry with video monitoring:* scalp/sphenoidal electrodes, cable or radio telemetry, video.
- *Long-term intracranial EEG telemetry with video monitoring:* depth, subdural, epidural, or foramen ovale electrodes, cable or radio telemetry, video.
- *EEG ambulatory cassette recording:* scalp/sphenoidal electrodes, ambulatory cassette recording.

Note: If desired, it would also be permissible to use more specific modifiers, e.g., depth electrode EEG cable telemetry with video monitoring or scalp/sphenoidal EEG telemetry.

II. INDICATIONS FOR LTME

This listing of indications is not meant to be all-inclusive, since special circumstances may warrant additional considerations.

A. Diagnosis

1. Identification of epileptic paroxysmal electrographic and/or behavioral abnormalities in patients with normal or equivocal routine EEG studies. These include epileptic seizures, overt and subclinical, and documentation of interictal epileptiform discharges. EEG and/or behavioral abnormalities may assist in the differential diagnosis between epileptic

disorders and conditions associated with intermittent symptoms due to nonepileptic mechanisms (e.g., syncope, cardiac arrhythmias, transient ischemic attacks, narcolepsy, other sleep disturbances, psychogenic seizures, other behavioral disorders).

2. Verification of the epileptic nature of the new 'spells' in a patient with previously documented and controlled seizures.

B. Classification/characterization

1. Classification of clinical seizure type(s) in a patient with documented but poorly characterized epilepsy.

2. Characterization (lateralization, localization, distribution) of EEG abnormalities, both ictal and interictal, associated with seizure disorders. Characterization of epileptiform EEG features, including both ictal discharges and interictal transients, is essential in the evaluation of patients with intractable epilepsy for surgical intervention.

3. Characterization of the relationship of seizures to specific precipitating circumstances or stimuli (e.g., nocturnal, catamenial, situation-related, activity-related). Verification and/or characterization of temporal patterns of seizure occurrence, either spontaneous or with respect to therapeutic manipulations (e.g., drug regimens).

4. Characterization of the behavioral consequences of epileptiform discharges as measured by specific tasks.

C. Quantification

1. Quantification of the number of frequency of seizures and/or interictal discharges and their relationship to naturally occurring events or cycles.

2. Quantitative documentation of the EEG response (ictal and interictal) to a therapeutic intervention or modification (e.g., drug alteration).

3. Monitoring objective EEG features is useful in patients with frequent seizures, particularly with absence and other seizures having indiscernible or minimal behavioral manifestations.

III. QUALIFICATIONS AND RESPONSIBILITIES OF LTME PERSONNEL

A. Chief or medical supervisor of LTME laboratory

Qualifications

1. A physician with appropriate qualifications to be chief of an EEG laboratory [e.g., as outlined in *Guidelines for Laboratory Accreditation, Standard I,* published by the American Electroencephalographic Society (AEEGS)].

2. Certification by the appropriate national certifying group in EEG if one exists.

3. Special training in the operation of LTME equipment, which is typically more complex than that used for routine EEG recording. Special knowledge of the technical aspects

of data recording, storage, and retrieval is required, and formal training or equivalent experience in electronics and/or computer science is strongly recommended.

4. Special training in the interpretation of EEG and video data generated in an LTME laboratory. Experience beyond routine EEG interpretation is necessary, since much of the analysis involves complex ictal and interictal features, as well as artifacts, seldom encountered in a standard EEG laboratory. Long-term monitoring systems can utilize methods of data display [e.g., cathode-ray tube (CRT)] or formats of data review (e.g., discontinuous segments), which are different from the paper tracing of routine EEG. The analysis of LTME data requires as well the simultaneous interpretation and correlation of EEG data and behavioral events.

5. As a minimum, it is recommended that experience in the practical use of specialized LTME equipment and in data interpretation be gained by working in a major LTME laboratory, preferably under the direction of an individual who meets the qualifications for chief or medical supervisor of an LTME laboratory.

Responsibilities

1. The chief or medical supervisor of an LTME laboratory should have the same responsibilities and authority as the chief of an EEG laboratory.

2. Additional responsibilities include the final interpretive synthesis of LTME data with diagnostic and pathophysiological formulations.

B. Physician LTME electroencephalographer

Qualifications

1. A physician with the qualifications to be a clinical electroencephalographer (e.g., as outlined in *Guideline Four: Standards of Practice in Clinical Electroencephalography*, published by the AEEGS).

2. Specialized training and experience in the use of LTME equipment and in the interpretation of LTME data are necessary, preferably under the direction of an individual who meets the qualifications for chief or medical supervisor of an LTME laboratory.

3. When collected, data can be reviewed in several formats (e.g., paper tracings and rapid video playback of ambulatory EEG); training and experience utilizing each technique are necessary.

Responsibilities

1. Responsibilities include the analysis of, at minimum, pertinent segments of collected electrographic and behavioral data reviewed in all appropriate formats, the writing of LTME reports, and the final interpretive synthesis of LTME data with diagnostic and pathophysiological formulations in the absence or in lieu of the chief or medical supervisor.

C. Nonphysician LTME electroencephalographer

Qualifications

1. A Ph.D. degree in a field of neuroscience, computer science, electrical engineering, or a related physical science with additional formal training or equivalent experience in neuroscience.

2. Three or more years of experience in clinical EEG under the supervision of a qualified electroencephalographer.

3. Specialized training and experience in the use of LTME equipment and in the interpretation of LTME data are necessary, preferably under the direction of an individual who meets the qualifications for chief or medical supervisor of an LTME laboratory.

Responsibilities

1. A nonphysician electroencephalographer may have the same responsibilities and authority as an LTME electroencephalographer as listed above, with the exception of rendering a final clinical interpretation of LTME data.

2. A descriptive report of LTME may be given, but the clinical correlation should be made under the direct supervision of a physician LTME electroencephalographer.

3. Due to the complex technology required for some forms of long-term monitoring, a nonphysician electroencephalographer may provide an essential bridge between technical and medical personnel.

D. LTME EEG technologist I–III

Qualifications

1. A technologist with the minimal qualifications of an EEG technologist as set forth by the appropriate national body (e.g., as outlined in *Guideline Five: Recommended Job Description for Electroencephalographic Technologists*, published by the AEEGS).

2. Special training in the use and routine maintenance of LTME equipment in the laboratory of employment, with particular emphasis on techniques for monitoring the integrity of data recording.

3. Special training and resultant expertise in the recognition of ictal and interictal electrographic patterns and in their differentiation from artifacts.

4. Special training and resultant expertise in the management of clinical seizures and seizure-related medical emergencies. Successful completion of training in cardiopulmonary resuscitation is necessary.

Responsibilities

1. LTME technologists I–III should have the same responsibilities and authority as EEG technologists (e.g., as outlined in *Guideline Two: Recommended Job Description for Electroencephalographic Technologists,* published by the AEEGS).

2. Additional responsibilities include the technical operation of LTME studies (e.g., patient preparation, equipment

set-up, and data recording). Overall management of these is the responsibility of a technologist III.

3. Under the supervision of the electroencephalographer in charge, data retrieval and reduction operations may be performed and EEG records prepared in a form suitable for interpretation, by LTME technologists II and III. This may include a prescreening of EEG and behavioral data to define segments for later analysis.

E. Monitoring technician

Qualifications

1. Special training with resultant expertise in recognition of clinical ictal behavior and interaction with patients during seizures to elucidate specific ictal symptoms.

2. Special training and resultant expertise in aspects of use of monitoring equipment dependent on specific functions of technician (e.g., video monitoring and intercommunication system, CRT EEG monitor).

3. If direct patient observation is involved, special training and resultant expertise in the management of clinical seizures, seizure-related emergencies, and cardiopulmonary resuscitation are necessary.

Responsibilities

1. Patient observation (direct or several patients at a time via video monitoring) to identify and note ictal events and interact with patients during seizures and to alert appropriate personnel (e.g., physician, EEG technologist, nursing staff) to the occurrence of each seizure.

2. Depending on specific training and requirements, the monitoring technician may also adjust video cameras to keep patient in view and in focus, oversee the adequate function of EEG recording equipment, administer or monitor continuous performance tasks, and otherwise maintain the integrity of the monitoring procedure, calling appropriate personnel to assist when problems occur.

3. Due to the need for continuous observation during most LTME procedures, monitoring technicians provide essential specialized services that do not require the expertise of physicians, nurses, or EEG technologists, but medical and technical personnel must be immediately available when called by the monitoring technician.

IV. LONG-TERM MONITORING EQUIPMENT AND PROCEDURES

The following is a discussion of the EEG equipment that is available for long-term neurodiagnostic monitoring and the variety of ways it may be used. Unless otherwise stated, these are not meant to be strict requirements, but only guidelines to appropriate usage.

A. Electrode types

Scalp

1. Disk
   a) Used for scalp LTME and ambulatory EEG recording.
   b) Electrodes should be applied with collodion/gauze for effective long-term results.
   c) Electrode with hole in top is best, since it permits periodic rejelling.
2. Needle, electrode cap – not recommended for long-term recordings.

Basal extracranial electrode positioning

1. Nasopharyngeal locations are used to record epileptiform activity from the mesial aspect of the temporal lobe. Because these electrodes cause local irritation, their use is not recommended for long periods of time, but they can be used for hours to 1 day. Cannot be used unattended or in an ambulatory patient. Lateralization of transients is poor with nasopharyngeal electrodes, since recording tips are close together and connected by wet mucous membrane.

2. Sphenoidal locations are used to record epileptiform activity from the mesial or anterior aspects of the temporal lobe in the region of the foramen ovale. Solid needle or wire construction is not recommended; fine flexible braided stainless steel wire, insulated except at the tip, is best and can be used for periods of days to weeks.

3. Other locations, such as nasoethmoidal, supraoptic, and auditory canal electrode positions, have also been employed under special circumstances to better record focal discharges; however, the indications for these placements are not well defined. These electrodes are not recommended for routine use.

4. There is increasing evidence to suggest that earlobe or T1, T2 placements may be at least as good as nasopharyngeal electrodes when used in the appropriate montage arrangement (see Section VI F3). However, simultaneous recording from multiple basal electrodes may provide additional information about the field of EEG transients.

Intracranial

1. Epidural and subdural electrodes are used to record over the surface of the brain. Electrode 'grids' are made of small platinum or stainless steel disks that are embedded into soft silastic. Each grid has 4–64 contact points, a few millimeters to about 1 cm apart. Grids are placed epi- or subdurally over the cerebral cortex and require a craniotomy. Electrode 'strips' consist of a row of disks embedded in silastic, or a bundle of fine wires, each tip of which is a recording point. Strips are usually inserted through a burr hole.

2. Intracerebral electrodes are used to record from within the brain. Procedures and types of electrodes used vary widely. Two major types include rigid and flexible probes. Most probes are 'multi-contact' with up to 16 recording points arranged along the shaft, constructed of either stainless steel or magnetic-resonance-imaging-compatible metals such as nichrome.

3. Foramen ovale electrodes are used to record from mesial temporal structures without requiring penetration of the skull. A 1- to 4-contact flexible electrode is placed in the ambient cistern with the aid of a needle inserted through the foramen ovale. These electrodes are not as close to hippocampal structures as intracerebral electrodes and do not allow as large a recording field as grids and strips but detect mesial temporal EEG discharges better than sphenoidal and scalp electrodes. When extracranial recordings are equivocal, foramen ovale electrodes offer a less invasive alternative to a more complete intracranial evaluation or can be used in association with grids and strips. Foramen ovale electrodes may also be constructed from MRI-compatible metals.

B. EEG amplifiers

1. It is recommended that EEG amplifiers, including those for ambulatory cassette systems, comply with the equipment standards for performance and safety as established previously for routine clinical EEG amplifiers and set forth elsewhere in the international guidelines.

2. It is recognized that to achieve the goals of the LTME, small size and low power may be required features, and certain compromises in standards may have to be made. These should not, however, detract from the essential properties required to record an EEG.

3. The following are recommended performance specifications:

a) Low-frequency response of at least 0.5 Hz.
b) High-frequency response of at least 70 Hz.
c) Noise level less than 1 μV rms.
d) Input impedance of at least 1 MΩ.
e) Common mode rejection of at least 60 dB.
f) Dynamic range of at least 40 dB.

4. Frequency filters and gain of the recording system should be set up to obtain maximum information, rather than clean tracings, when these recordings can be modified as necessary upon replay of recorded EEGs.

5. Certain specifications of existing commercial ambulatory EEG systems, such as high-frequency response, may diverge from the above standards. These differences are recognized and considered acceptable with this recording technique for recommended indications.

6. Newly introduced LTME instrumentation should equal or surpass the specifications of existing systems to be acceptable.

C. Amplifier locations

EEG amplifiers for LTME may be located in a variety of positions relative to the patient. In general, the closer the amplifier is to the signal source (i.e., the shorter the electrode leads), the less opportunity there is for intrusion of artifact.

The following is a list of possible amplifier locations, with the advantages and disadvantages associated with each.

1. Scalp (glued to) (no longer available from major manufacturers)
   a) Advantages – shortest leads, most secure.
   b) Disadvantages – time-consuming attachment of each pre-amp, complexity of connections with increasing channel numbers, montages usually fixed,[1] since channels derived at the preamplifier.
2. Head (mount upon)
   a) Advantages – easy and fast to mount.
   b) Disadvantages – longer leads, not as secure, weight or size can be a problem on head, fixed[1] montages.
3. Body (carried on)
   a) Advantages – easy and fast to attach, weight and size less of a problem.
   b) Disadvantages – longer leads, greater potential for lead movement artifact, montages usually fixed[1].
4. Remote
   a) Advantages – flexibility of operation (gain, filtering, montage selectable).
   b) Disadvantages – long leads and cables, increased potential for lead movement artifact.

---

[1]It is possible to use a fixed recording montage utilizing a single common reference and replay data recorded from active electrodes in any desired montage.

D. EEG transmission

The following is a list of techniques by which EEG signals are transmitted from amplifiers to recording apparatus or, in the case of remote amplification, from patient to amplifiers. Advantages and disadvantages associated with each are given.
1. Standard cable (one wire for each electrode)
   a) Advantages – simplest, widely available, least expensive, no additional equipment over standard EEG, operational flexibility of remote amplication.
   b) Disadvantages – impaired patient mobility, increased nonphysiological artifact, inconvenience of separate leads to jackbox, one wire for each electrode is required within cable.
2. Local record (ambulatory cassette)
   a) Advantages – maximum patient mobility, no cable, simple.
   b) Disadvantages – fixed montage, inability to visualize EEG during recording.
3. Cable telemetry (only one wire for multiplexed signal)
   a) Advantages – simple, low interference, inexpensive.
   b) Disadvantages – patient mobility relatively limited, inconvenience of cable.
4. Radio telemetry
   a) Advantages – no cable necessary, increased patient mobility.
   b) Disadvantages – susceptible to interference and signal dropout, limited range, more complicated at transmis-

sion and reception sites, more expensive, more power required.

5. Infra-red telemetry
   a) Advantages – same as radio telemetry.
   b) Disadvantages – same as radio telemetry, uncommonly used.

6. Multiplexers, demultiplexers. Unlike standard cable transmission in which one wire is required for each electrode position or at best for each channel, telemetry usually involves signal multiplexing, which eliminates the need for multiwire cables or multiple radio transmission channels. Most multiplex systems are analog, but digital multiplex systems are becoming more practical. The latter offer advantages of very high signal quality without transmission degradation.
   a) Advantages – multiplexers can combine a number of EEG signals, typically 16–64, into one channel and thus greatly reduce the total number of individual wires in the transmission cable or the number of transmission channels necessary in radio telemetry. Demultiplexers separate out the component EEG signals before or after recording.
   b) Disadvantages – multiplexing adds to the complexity of the required electronics and, if multiplexed signal is recorded rather than merely transmitted, a higher-frequency response of the recording apparatus is required.

E.   EEG recording and storage

The method of EEG recording/storage need not be dependent on the technique used in data transmission, except in the case of ambulatory EEG where transmission and storage are initimately linked.

Listed below are recognized methods and their associated advantages and disadvantages.

1. Continuous paper writeout
   a) Advantages – simple operation involving traditional EEG machine, data easy to interpret and immediately accessible, no added equipment cost over standard EEG machine, easy to implement, records EEG data with appropriate frequency response and noise level.
   b) Disadvantages – requires qualified attendant during the recording, record bulky and expensive when long-term, interpretation lengthy, paper copy cannot be reproduced or modified, cannot utilize computer data reduction or analysis.

2. Discontinuous paper writeout (pages) using electrostatic, heat-sensitive, laser, or ink jet methods
   a) Advantages – high-resolution (300 dots/inch) word-processing printout formats provide multichannel EEG traces (up to 128 channels with variable time base).
   b) Disadvantages – only suitable for epoch-type events, requires computer equipment.

3. Analog magnetic tape (instrumentation or video)
   a) Advantages – allows continuous unattended recording (typically 6–10 h/tape), tapes can be reused, less expensive than paper if tapes reused, less bulky storage, video recorders relatively inexpensive, data can be modified upon replay, records EEG data with appropriate frequency response and noise level above a given tape speed, data can be subjected to computerized reduction or analysis.
   b) Disadvantages – instrumentation tape recorder relatively expensive, typical recorder may not have sufficient channels unless multiplexed data are recorded, recording of multiplexed data requires faster tape speeds (shorter recording times, increased wear), data not directly accessible, replay onto paper copy or CRT necessary for visual analysis.
4. Analog magnetic tape (ambulatory cassette)
   a) Advantages – allows continuous unattended recording for up to 24 h per tape, tapes can be reused, easy storage, data can be modified upon replay, computerized data reduction or analysis possible.
   b) Disadvantages – channel number usually limited to four or eight with continuous recording, high-frequency response may be reduced, data not directly accessible, on-line visualization of signal not possible, replay necessary onto video or paper copy for visual analysis. For at least one system, two 8-channel recorders can be electronically linked so data can be transferred to computer disk and printed out as 16 synchronous channels on a polygraph.
5. Audio channel on videotape
   a) Advantages – EEG data recorded on same tape as behavioral information, EEG and behavioral data synchronized, video recorder relatively inexpensive, recording times up to 8 h/tape unattended, tapes can be reused, easy storage, data can be modified upon replay, records EEG data with appropriate frequency response and noise level.
   b) Disadvantages – only one channel (audio 1 or 2) available to record EEG data, multiplexing and demultiplexing necessary (frequency response or recording time compromised), data not directly accessible, replay necessary or CRT or paper copy for visual analysis.
6. EEG reformatter
   a) Advantages – EEG data transformed to video and recorded on same video image as behavior, data necessarily synchronized, video recorder relatively inexpensive, recording times up to 8 h/tape unattended, tapes can be reused, easy storage.
   b) Disadvantages – reformatter relatively expensive, usual EEG writeout cannot be obtained from taped record, resolution of video image of EEG and duration of visible signal insufficient for official interpretation, data accessible only by replay of video.

7. Digital tape
   a) Advantages – data stored in a format suitable for additional computer analysis, others as above (E3).
   b) Disadvantages – computer equipment necessary, may be complex and expensive, data not directly accessible, replay necessary.
8. Digital disk
   a) Advantages – data stored in format suitable for additional computer analysis, fixed disk (Winchester-type) can store up to 24 h and optical disks over 40 h of 16-channel EEG, specific locations on disk can be rapidly accessed, others as above (E3); WORM (write once, read many) optical disks may provide an alternative permanent archival medium.
   b) Disadvantages – standard removable disks can store less than 1 h of 16-channel EEG, no permanent storage on fixed disks, since must be reused with new data, computer equipment necessary, data not directly accessible, replay necessary.
9. Digital code within video signal
   a) Advantages – 6 h of 64-channel simultaneous EEG, video and audio can be stored on a single inexpensive videotape, others as above (E3).
   b) Disadvantages – part of the video image is lost.
10. Selective EEG storage – computer-assisted
   a) Advantages – storage of only pertinent EEG segments selected by triggering from patient push-button or automatic computer programs that detect seizures and interictal epileptiform events, time delay available to allow recording of onset of seizure detected by either means, less storage capacity required, data analysis simplified and shortened, unattended operation.
   b) Disadvantages – record is not continuous, automated computer detection programs are not completely accurate, causing false-positive detections and failure to detect some genuine ictal or interictal events, patient must have warning for push-button trigger, computer equipment, and detection programs necessary, periodic sampling may not allow identification of infrequent interictal abnormalities.
11. Selective EEG storage – event recording/epoch sampling ambulatory cassette
   a) Advantages – less storage capacity required, since only a few minutes before and following patient push-button trigger, or periodic samplings of the EEG, are recorded, data analysis simplified and shortened, increased ber of channels (16 or 24) and better recording characteristics obtainable.
   b) Disadvantages – record is not continuous, onset of seizures can be missed with triggering by patient, seizures without warning or auras may be missed unless witnessed by an observer, subclinical seizures not recorded, shorter time delay than computer-assisted system and periodic sampling may not allow identification of infrequent interictal abnormalities.

12. Selective EEG storage – portable take-home computer
   a) Advantages – same as 10, plus it is small enough to be taken home by patient to be recorded overnight at bedside.
   b) Disadvantages – same as 10, plus it is not ambulatory.

F. EEG retrieval and review

1. Complete review of EEG – continuous paper recording
   a) Advantages – immediately accessible and interpretable by traditional means, subclinical seizures and interictal abnormalities can be identified.
   b) Disadvantages – lengthy analysis, data cannot be replayed to allow modifications in filter or gain settings, montages, and paper speed, cannot be subject to computer-assisted data reduction or analysis.
2. Complete review of EEG – rapid video/audio playback
   a) Advantages – rapid review (20–60 × real time) of long monitoring records, subclinical as well as clinical seizures and interictal abnormalities can be identified, selective writeout of EEG as paper copy, sound output for auditory analysis of EEG; rapid video playback is commonly used with ambulatory cassette monitoring, but can be applied to other systems as well.
   b) Disadvantages – requires additional review skills, minor abnormalities may be overlooked at fastest review rate, difficulty of review increases with number of channels; requires expensive equipment.
3. Selective review of EEG – clinical events
   a) Advantages – review time shortened, since only EEG associated with clinical seizures necessarily transcribed onto paper from tape, seizure located on tape or recording only initiated by event marker activated by patient or observer.
   b) Disadvantages – assessment of clinical seizures for which event marker was not activated, subclinical seizures, and interictal abnormalities dependent upon random sampling.
4. Selective review of EEG – computer-assisted recognition
   a) Advantages – automated recognition of clinical and subclinical ictal and interictal events can be used online to record only selected segment, can be used offline with tape- or disk-recorded EEG to select segments for review, shortens analysis time, only selected segments written out on paper copy; EEG available for review on high-resolution computer display (F5).
   b) Disadvantages – automated computer detection programs not completely accurate, false-positive detections and failure to detect some genuine ictal or interictal events, computer equipment and detection program necessary.
5. Selective review of EEG – high-resolution computer display
   a) Advantages – digital recordings can be reproduced

on high-resolution computer monitor in any montage, gain or filter setting desired; movable time markers, spike maps, and high resolution make interpretation possible with or without hard copy.

b) Disadvantages – requires more physician training.

V. EQUIPMENT AND PROCEDURES FOR LTME OF BEHAVIOR AND CORRELATION WITH EEG

A major objective of LTME is the correlation of behavior with EEG findings. Behavioral and EEG data are truly complementary. Bizarre ictal behaviors that are not easily recognized as seizures are appropriately identified by a simultaneous epileptiform discharge on EEG. Conversely, videotaped evidence of classic behavioral manifestations of a seizure may be sufficient to diagnose epilepsy even in the absence of a clearly defined epileptiform EEG abnormality during such an episode.

A variety of techniques for behavioral monitoring and its correlation with EEG may be employed. This section will discuss the advantages and disadvantages of each and provide recommendations as to their proper use.

A. Types of behavioral monitoring

1. Self-reporting
   a) Features – a daily diary or log in which the patient notes the occurrence of behavioral episodes in question. This is the principal form of behavior monitoring in ambulatory cassette EEG recording and an adjunct to inpatient LTME. A more advanced form of self-reporting includes the use of a push-button event marker on the ambulatory EEG recorder or by the bedside for the patient to signal the occurrence of an episode.
   b) Advantages – simple, requires little special equipment, easy to implement, practical way to monitor patients with infrequent seizures for which they have warning or memory. When used with ambulatory cassette recordings, it can provide information regarding the effect of circadian cycles, environmental factors, and antiepileptic drug fluctuations on seizure activity.
   c) Disadvantages – correlation is subjective, record of behavior not available for detailed visual analysis, temporal correlation may be inaccurate even when event marker is used, not possible with seizures for which the patient has no warning or memory, ictal descriptions usually not obtained, not suitable for final correlation in a presurgical workup, but, with 16–24-channel ambulatory cassette recording. It may provide preliminary data that can minimize inpatient monitoring.
2. Observer reporting
   a) Features – observer reporting complements self-reporting in daily diaries. Observer reporting by trained hospital personnel can be objective and in-

cludes the use of standardized checklists of information to be recorded, direct interaction with the patient to assess mental function (level of consciousness, language function, memory) and neurological deficits. A push-button event marker, activated by a family member, friend, or LTME staff, can provide temporal correlations of clinical episodes on ambulatory cassette or inpatient EEG recordings. This is a major form of behavior monitoring in ambulatory cassette EEG recording, particularly in young children or in mentally retarded patients who cannot reliably self-report. It is also used in inpatient settings when personnel are available to monitor patient activity. Data in these instances are recorded on the EEG if a continuous hard copy is being produced or on an audio channel of a tape-recorded EEG.

b) Advantages – simple and inexpensive, requires little specialized equipment, easy to implement interactive assessments provide critical information about functional deficits accompanying episodes. Since it can be used with seizures for which the patient has no warning or memory, it provides a practical way to monitor patients with infrequent seizures.

c) Disadvantages – correlation is subjective, record of behavior not available for detailed visual analysis, temporal correlation may be inaccurate even when event marker used, not sufficient for presurgical evaluations. Seizures may be missed if observer is not continuously observing patient.

3. Video/audio tape recording

a) Features – principal and most effective means of behavior monitoring in inpatient setting. Patient behavior is continuously recorded on videotape simultaneously with EEG, which is recorded by one of several techniques. Behavioral and EEG data temporally correlated by means of synchronized time code generators or by recording both on the same tape. Observations of LTME personnel, self-reporting by patients, or automated computer analysis of EEG identify episodes that are potentially seizures that require detailed analysis. Direct assessment of neurological function of patient by LTME staff adds to other recorded data.

b) Advantages – objective record of behavior, available for replay and associated direct EEG correlation, temporal correlations accurate when synchronization achieved with time code generators or same tape recording, useful in seizures of all types even if minimal behavioral manifestations are initially unrecognized, since permanent record allows subsequent review of behavior associated with EEG changes. The interaction between monitoring personnel and the patient, when properly structured, defines the events more explicitly than other mechanisms.

c) Disadvantages – specialized equipment required, can

be time-consuming to implement. When recording without personnel present, interactive assessments of neurological function are unavailable. A major problem is that freedom of movement is limited by the necessity for the patient to stay in view of the camera. Autotracking techniques are being developed to deal with this, although they are not yet generally available (see 4d).

4. Polygraphic and reaction time monitoring. A variety of approaches can be used to record aspects of ictal behavior along with the EEG. Monitoring of specific physiological functions such as eye movement of electromyography (EMG) may provide useful information for characterizing the behavioral manifestations of ictal events. Cognitive disturbances can be documented by reaction time tasks, with stimulus and response times recorded on an event marker channel. This technique can also be used to demonstrate that discharges that would ordinarily be thought of as interictal can interfere with cognitive processing on a transient basis. Selection of appropriate tasks that can be maintained for prolonged periods, recorded, and quantified allows time indexing to the EEG and, in essence, may extend the definition of what is ictal for a given patient.

B.   Equipment – behavioral data acquisition

1. Video cameras
   a) Standard monochrome (black and white) – requires illumination of 0.5 footcandle, satisfactory for daylight monitoring conditions, unsatisfactory for nocturnal monitoring under reduced lighting conditions.
   b) Low light level monochrome – allows monitoring in only 0.03 footcandles of illumination, particularly sensitive to red light, useful for nocturnal monitoring under reduced lighting conditions, automatic iris needed to compensate for sudden increases in light level, especially focal, which can cause 'blooming'.
   c) Silicon intensified target ('starlight') – effective in as little as 0.000025 footcandles of illumination, image intensifier technology, high resolution for nocturnal monitoring, expense is substantial, value for increased resolution is not established.
   d) Color – requires 25 footcandles of illumination, better resolution of facial features than black and white, valuable for perceiving certain autonomic changes (e.g., blushing, pallor), not suited to nocturnal monitoring but continuous auto-white balance improves resolution during changes in ambient light, exclusive color systems may be impractical.
   e) Low-light level color – requires 1–10 footcandles of illumination, can be used for nocturnal monitoring with small night light, increased expense, value unestablished in nocturnal conditions except to attempt exclusive use of color cameras.
   f) Solid-state sensor monochrome – longer lasting than tube cameras, good resolution, no 'blooming' and no

image retention ('burn in'), tolerates difficult lighting conditions, is available with built-in infrared illuminators for night monitoring.

2. Video camera lenses – irises
   a) Standard – iris requires manual adjustment for changing light conditions, inconvenience may lead to neglect of this factor, minimally acceptable for LTME.
   b) Automatic – iris automatically adjusts to changing light conditions, facilitates prolonged monitoring under varying conditions, 'blooming' may still occur with a sudden focal increase in light (such as from a match), manual override can compensate for unusual light conditions.

3. Video camera lenses – field of view
   a) Standard – size of viewing field fixed relative to distance between camera and object.
   b) Fixed wide-angle – increases the area monitored at the expense of detail, patient more easily keep within field of view.
   c) Remote zoom – allows personnel to obtain close-up view of area of particular interest (e.g., motor onset of simple partial seizure), utilizes separate 6-V AC power unlike 24-V AC power to camera and remote pan/tilt.
   d) Remote zoom wide-angle – allows variable area to be monitored depending on clinical situation, 15-mm focal length preferred.

4. Video camera mobility
   a) Fixed position camera – requires that the patient remain within the camera's unchangeable field of view; this degree of restriction of patient mobility difficult to maintain over long monitoring periods, particularly if close-up of face is required.
   b) Mobile or portable camera – provides a changeable field of view to allow some patient mobility, necessitates intrusion into monitoring room and physical repositioning of camera by personnel for each change.
   c) Remote pan/tilt device – allows personnel to keep patients in view of the camera as they move about the room by moving camera side to side or up/down; recommended for permanent monitoring rooms, separate remote control panel may activate combined focus, zoom, and pan/tilt functions of camera.
   d) Auto tracking – one system is available that allows automatic tracking of the patient by the camera. The patient wears a radio frequency transmitter, which is picked up by receivers mounted on the camera. The signals are used to maneuver a remote pan-tilt-zoom device that follows the patient as he/she moves about the room. Two additional systems are being developed. One uses a coded pulse of infrared light, with the source located on the camera. The patient wears a reflecting strip. A detector, also located on the camera, picks up the reflected light pulses. This is fed into a personal computer that controls the pan-tilt-zoom

mechanism to maintain the camera of the patient. The other system uses multiple cameras, which surround the patient. The patient is, thus, always on some camera. The cameras that are viewing the patient are directed to the recording device by a computer that senses contrast. These all work for maintaining focus on the patient's body but do not yet maintain focus on the face.

5. Special effects generator

Images of the body as a whole and an image restricted to the face can be accomplished and may be necessary for some cases. Maintaining a tight focus currently requires intensive and constant effort by monitoring personnel and is difficult to maintain for prolonged periods.

    a) Forms a composite video image from two or more video sources by dividing the screen into several distinct areas; vertical splitting into two halves is a simple example.

    b) Component video sources must have the same camera synchronization signal, which is supplied by a synchronization generator.

    c) Various types of input are commonly mixed in a split-screen composite (e.g., two views of the patient, one wide angle and one close up; both monochrome or color or one of each); one view of the patient and one view of an ongoing EEG paper writeout; or two views of the patient plus one of the EEG writeout – the lat-

ter also provides a means for synchronizing EEG with behavior.

    d) Resolution of the EEG in a split-screen video presentation is poor; viewing more than eight channels results in an unacceptable loss of detail and only a short segment of the record is visible at a time.

6. Waveform-to-TV reformatter (see also IV E6)

    a) Transforms analog-amplified EEG signals directly onto a video image that can be recorded simultaneously with patient behavior in a split screen or overlay format, provides synchronization of EEG and behavioral data.

    b) Eight- and 16-channel reformatting is available, the latter requiring a 19-inch monitor for adequate display; special effects generator and EEG paper writeout not required to visualize the EEG on the video screen.

    c) Reformatted EEG does not provide adequate or sufficiently long segments of recording to make official EEG interpretations; reformatted EEG cannot be transcribed back into analog signals for paper writeout; separate EEG recording facilities are also required for most purposes.

7. Video time/date generator

    a) Creates a video image of a running digital clock (with date and other information), which is transposed on the image of the patient and/or EEG being recorded to give it a temporal signature.

b) Means by which specific bahavioral events are located in the review process.

8. Time code generator

a) Provides an electronic pulse code, usually binary, which may be placed in synchronized fashion on the beginning of each video frame as well as the EEG data to allow accurate time correlation upon replay and analysis. Code readout accurate to the second is available upon video playback and may be transposed with the EEG onto a paper copy. Various forms of time writeout exist, both coded binary and alphanumeric. Either is acceptable; the latter is more convenient to use.

b) Appropriate temporal correlation between EEG and behavior is necessary in order to conclude a causal relationship. This is particularly important in attempts to localize the origin of EEG abnormalities during presurgical evaluation.

c) Split-screen techniques for recording both behavior and EEG, including the use of a reformatter, may not provide adequate resolution for accurate correlations. Event markers or imprecisely synchronized separate clocks are inadequate for the most demanding purposes, such as presurgical evaluation.

9. Alphanumeric character generator

a) Allows additional information to be written onto the video image online or offline after editing (e.g., patient identification, seizure type, purpose of recording, etc.).

10. Audio – microphones. In addition to the video image of patient behavior, it is important to have an audio record of clinical episodes, which includes not only the patient's verbalizations, but also a description of behavior and neurological function as assessed and related by LTME personnel attending to the patient during the episode.

a) Unidirectional – picks up only sound coming from directly in front of the microphone head, eliminates extraneous noise, requires readjustment with patient movement, usually attached to video camera, which is aimed at patient, unsatisfactory for recording nearby LTME personnel.

b) Omnidirectional – picks up sound in roughly a spherical distribution around the microphone, eliminates need for directional readjustment, subject to interference from extraneous sounds, recommended as a minimal standard.

c) Pressure zone – mounts to flat surfaces for reduced echo-reverberation, but picks up extraneous sound; discrete and less vulnerable to handling.

d) Sound mixer – combines multiple audio sources into a single signal for recording on videotape; unidirectional and omnidirectional microphone inputs may be combined to obtain improved audio recording capability.

C. Equipment – behavioral data storage and retrieval

1. Videotape recorders – formats
   a) Reel to reel – more durable than cassette recorder for continuous use, but higher initial cost, tape must be rewound or new tape threaded to reuse, loss of approximately 10% of recording time on rewind unless second unit available to record, being phased out in favor of cassette recorders except for 1-inch video production recorders.
   b) Cassette – provides simple and rapid exchange of tapes during monitoring with minimal loss of recording time, widespread availability of playback capability. Only high-grade tapes should be employed, 0.75-inch cassette systems offer better resolution than 0.50-inch systems, but longer recording times available with 0.50-inch format (6–8 h). S-VHS cassette systems now offer better resolution than 0.75-inch or standard VHS systems and have 6–8 h capability. On well-maintained equipment, 6-h tapes have a lifespan of 500 replays without excessive wear, but 8-h tapes are less reliable.
   c) Digital – provides more reliable storage with no degradation of copies. Cost is currently prohibitive for the majority of facilities.
2. Videotape recorders – control options
   a) Rapid scan – provides a faster forward or backward movement of the videotape with preservation of the video image, time passage is proportionately speeded up, useful in locating a behavioral episode when the exact time of occurrence is not known or in scanning through a video sequence faster than in real time.
   b) Slow motion – provides a slower forward movement of the videotape on replay, time passage is proportionately slowed, useful in characterizing the sequence of complex behavior and/or in defining accurately the onset of a particular behavior.
   c) Freeze frame – provides the ability to stop the forward movement of the videotape during replay and maintain the integrity of the video image, useful in the detailed analysis of a video image and in defining accurately the time of onset of a particular behavior.
   d) Automatic time search – provides the ability to automatically search through a video (or instrumentation) tape and find a particular time or event as defined by a recorded time or event code, useful in locating a behavioral episode (or EEG feature), which occurred at a known time or which was noted by the patient or an observer by activating an event marker.
   e) Time lapse – records video frames at slower rate, recording times per tape lengthened, but resultant video playback is jumpy, resolution of subtle behavior is unsatisfactory, EEG–behavior correlations become difficult; not acceptable for presurgical evaluations.
3. Video monitors
   a) Monochrome – perceived optical resolution is 525

line pairs, satisfactory for LTME, higher optical resolution of up to 1000 line pairs available in some monitors, resolution limiting factor is usually video recorder, however.

b) Color – perceived optical resolution of 250 line pairs, minimal acceptable standard for LTME.

D. Equipment – impending developments

High-definition video is currently being developed. A standard format has not yet been determined, and this capability is currently experimental. Combination of this with digital storage will potentially allow recording of large areas (entire body) and playback of smaller areas (face) with minimal image degradation.

E. Behavioral data storage protocols

1. Storage for initial analysis
   a) All video/audio monitoring data as well as associated EEG recordings should be saved until appropriately analyzed and reduced by trained personnel.
   b) When long-term monitoring is only for the purpose of recording clinical episodes, partial data reduction can be performed online. Tapes containing no episodes may be erased and reused.
   c) If a clinically significant event has occurred, the tape

should be stored for later analysis along with a brief description of the episode, time of occurrence, tape location number, and number of corresponding EEG tape or paper record.

2. Archival storage
   a) When it has been determined upon analysis that a behavioral episode is clinically relevant, video-recorded data should be copied onto a master tape for long-term storage.
   b) Edited data to be stored should include a short period (approximately 2 min) prior to and after the event, as well as the entire episode. A log of the contents of all edited tapes should be maintained.

F. Behavioral data analysis and correlations with EEG

1. Event analysis
   a) Using the appropriate videotape recorder control options, a detailed characterization of the temporal sequence of the patient's behavior during each clinical episode should be accomplished under the direct supervision and review of the LTME electroencephalographer.
   b) Attention should be paid to the sequence and character of motor activity, verbalizations, responsiveness to stimuli, and any other noteworthy features.
2. Correlation of behavior and EEG
   a) EEG that is temporally concurrent with the clinical

episode in question should also be analyzed in detail for significant change of progression in pattern, with particular emphasis on those that are ictal in character.

b) The progression of behavioral alterations as outlined in the event analysis can be correlated to any EEG changes by utilizing synchronous time codes recorded on each. Time codes should be accurate to less than 0.5 s.

VI. TECHNICAL AND METHODOLOGICAL CONSIDERATIONS

A. Electrode locations

1. Use of the international 10–20 system with supplementary positions is suggested in order to maintain standardization.

2. Atypical electrode positions such as T1, T2, and Nz (nose tip), as well as special electrodes such as sphenoidal may be used, depending on the clinical indications.

3. Intracranial electrode placements (epidural, subdural, intracerebral, foramen ovale) are used in candidates for surgical resection of an epileptic lesion. They are indicated to answer specific questions about the localization of discharges determined to be of focal origin by surface-recording techniques, but insufficiently defined to direct surgical interventions. Use of nonferrous metals such as platinum and nichrome allows MRI verification of electrode location. In these instances of intracorporeal recording sites, the guidelines for patients with in-dwelling devices should be followed in the United States, UL, Type A patient). They are not appropriate when surface EEG recordings provide no clues to the presence or location of a focal lesion. Due to the diversity of the techniques in use, specific recommendations concerning electrical and mechanical safety precautions are beyond the scope of this discussion.

B. Electrode application/insertion

1. Disk – collodion technique is currently the only method that will insure a stable long-term recording. Application by electrode paste alone is not recommended. Collodion should be dried slowly to make a film over the electrode, which prevents the electrode jelly from drying out. This may be facilitated by the use of a hair dryer or low pressure air. Underlying skin should not be unduly abraded when electrodes are to remain in place several days. Electrode jelly that is used should not contain irritants or dry out quickly. A felt pad may be used under a disk electrode to prevent pressure breakdown of the skin.

2. Nasopharyngeal – two electrodes are usually inserted without anesthetic by an electroencephalographer or trained technologist through each nostril to rest on the posterolateral wall of the nasopharynx. The length of electrode extending beyond the nose is minimized by bending it toward the cheek

at the nostrils. Electrode wires are secured to the cheeks with adhesive tape. Electrodes may have to be repositioned when the recording is contaminated by various artifacts. Because these electrodes cause local irritation and offer no documented advantage over other basal electrodes for detection of epileptiform activity, they are not recommended for long-term use. Additional useful information may be obtained concerning the electrical field of EEG transients, however, when nasopharyngeal electrodes are used in association with other basal electrodes for limited periods of time.

3. Sphenoidal – inserted bilaterally through the skin below the zygomatic arches in the direction of the foramen ovale by an electroencephalographer or qualified physician, with or without local anesthetic. Flexible wire electrodes are placed 3–4 cm deep, within or alongside a needle, and the needle is then removed. The external wire should be coiled, to relieve tension, and fixed to the cheek with collodion and/or tape at the point of exit from the skin.

4. Epidural and subdural – inserted during a neurosurgical procedure. Epidural and subdural electrode grids are directly placed over accessible areas of the cerebral cortex through a craniotomy. Strip electrodes are usually placed freehand through burr holes.

5. Intracerebral – inserted stereotactically into bilateral temporal and/or extratemporal sites.

6. Foramen ovale – inserted bilaterally through the skin using an approach similar to that for percutaneous trigeminal rhizotomy, by a qualified neurosurgeon. A 1–4-contact flexible electrode remains in the ambient cistern after the insertion needle is withdrawn.

C. Electrode maintenance

1. Disk – recording characteristics of electrodes should be checked every day so that electrode contact deterioration can be detected and corrected without interruption of the recording. Impedance should be checked periodically, and if recording characteristics change. Rejelling should be performed as necessary to maintain low impedance. Scalp irritation can usually be avoided if the patient uses a strong anti-dandruff shampoo before the electrodes are applied.

2. Nasopharyngeal – should be inspected periodically and repositioned when artifacts interfere with the recording.

3. Sphenoidal – care must be taken to relieve stress on the recording wires. External wires should be inspected periodically to insure proper fixation to the skin and minimize the possibility of breakage or accidental removal. The status of the electrode will be apparent from the recording.

4. Epidural, subdural, intracerebral, foramen ovale – once inserted for chronic recording, electrode malfunction cannot be corrected, although its condition can be assessed through the quality of the recording. The special connectors used with these electrodes are liable to cause problems and must be inspected periodically.

D. Electrode impedance

1. Disk – impedance should be measured at the beginning, periodically during, and with ambulatory EEG at the end of the recording. Initial impedance should be less than 5000 Ω. During inpatient LTME, attempts should be made to maintain this level.

2. Nasopharyngeal sphenoidal – impedance can be measured in routine fashion and may be of help in verifying the cause of a change in recording characteristics.

3. Epidural, subdural, intracerebral, foramen ovale – impedance measurements can be safely performed with currents in the range of 10 nA for electrodes inserted intracranially. Electrode conductivity and integrity of insulation should be checked prior to sterilization of the electrodes.

E. Calibration

1. EEG machines should be calibrated according to previously established standards.

2. Tape- or disk-recording systems – analog, video, digital
   a) In addition to recording calibration signals appropriate to EEG, calibration procedures appropriate for the specific instruments should be performed as suggested by the manufacturer.
   b) Before beginning LTME and periodically during the monitoring, the integrity of the entire recoding system from electrode to storage medium should be checked by observing ongoing EEG, tapping electrodes or connectors, and/or by having the patient generate physiological artifact. The resultant signals should be examined online and offline and compared to baseline recordings.

3. Ambulatory cassette EEG recorders
   a) A 10–15-s period of all channel calibration using a 50–100-μV square wave or pulse should be recorded at the beginning of each tape.
   b) Initial calibration signals should be reviewed from tape on video playback or monitored on-line by EEG writeout to assess the functioning of the system prior to beginning the EEG recording.
   c) A similar period of calibration at the end of a recording is recommended. This will test for problems that may have developed during the recording.
   d) Recorder amplifier sensitivity may have to be decreased in those patients with high-amplitude baseline rhythms or previously recognized paroxysmal abnormalities in order to prevent amplifier blocking.
   e) At the beginning and again at the end of a monitoring session, an on-line EEG writeout from recorder outputs should be obtained to check the integrity of the system. An artifact-screening procedure, as noted above in 2b, should be performed at the onset. The resultant record of common activity artifacts in that particular patient (e.g., eye movements, swallowing,

chewing, talking) may be useful in their later differentiation from electrographic abnormalities.

F. Recording techniques

1. Number of channels – standard LTME
   a) Telemetered EEG long-term monitoring requires a minimum eight channels, similar to the guideline for routine clinical EEG. Twelve or more channels are routinely used and are in particular necessary for accurate localization when nasopharyngeal or sphenoidal electrodes are employed.
   b) A large number of EEG channels are essential for obtaining accurate localization, as is required in a presurgical evaluation. Sixteen- to 64-channel recordings are recommended for this purpose. Two or more EEG machines may be necessary for the simultaneous writeout of these data, although usually such volumes of data are multiplexed and/or digitized and recorded on tape or computer disk.
2. Number of channels – ambulatory cassette EEG
   a) Fewer than three EEG channels are usually not sufficient for a primary EEG evaluation. In certain circumstances with a previously well-characterized abnormality, quantitative information concerning its occurrence may be provided by a lesser number of channels. The same may be true in situations in which only information concerning baseline rhythms or sleep-wakefulness cycles is required.
   b) In ambulatory EEG recordings of three or four channels, separate electrodes for each input grid of the preamplifiers are recommended. Electrodes with bifurcated leads that supply input to two adjacent channels in a linked montage are discouraged, since artifact in or loss of one electrode can confound one-half to two-thirds of the available EEG data.
   c) Electrodes with bifurcated leads are more appropriate with six or more ambulatory EEG channels.
   d) Three EEG channels can effectively be used for the detection and six for lateralization of EEG abnormalities; however, characterization requires the improved spatial resolution of a larger number of channels.
3. Montages – extracranial recordings
   a) Montages should be appropriate for the abnormalities anticipated and should be determined on the basis of previously documented EEG findings.
   b) When using bipolar montages with basal electrodes (e.g., nasopharyngeal, sphenoidal, earlobe, T1, T2), it is useful to simultaneously record standard lateral temporal bipolar chains as independent bipolar chains utilizing the basal electrode sites. Normal values such as small sharp spikes and 14 and 6/s positive spikes can be very difficult to differentiate from true epileptic transients otherwise. Inclusion of central electrodes in the basal electrode chain will also help

identify cancellation between lateral and mesial temporal sites.

Separating basal derivations with an electrode at the tip of the nose (Nz) aids in lateralization, although connected basal electrodes may at times demonstrate the direction of propagation when both sites record an epileptiform transient. Both configurations could be used. Another alternative used in some laboratories is to record each electrode of interest with respect to a single reference distant from the area(s) of interest. This also allows the data to be redisplayed into any desired montage.

Examples of basal electrode (PG) montages that are independent from lateral temporal derivations:

16 Channels	12 Channels	
Fp1-F7	Fp1-F7	
F7-T3	F7-T3	
T3-T5	T3-T5	
T5-O1	T5-O1	
Fp2-F8	Fp2-F8	
F8-T4	F8-T4	
T4-T6	T4-T6	or
T6-O2	T6-O2	C3-PG1
C3-T3	T3-PG1	C3-PG1
T3-PG1	PG1-PG2	PG1-PG2
PG1-Nz	PG2-T4	PG2-C4
Nz-PG2	ECG	ECG
PG2-T4		
T4-C4		
C4-Cz		
ECG		

Example of a basal electrode montage that is not independent from the lateral temporal derivations:

Fp1-F7
F7-PG1
PG1-T3
T3-T5
T5-O1
Fp2-F8
F8-PG2
PG2-T4
T4-T6
T6-O2

  c) Simultaneous electrocardiographic (ECG) recording is recommended, since cardiac arrhythmias may produce artifacts that mimic epileptiform EEG transients.

4. Montages – intracranial recordings
  a) Montages depend upon the type and location of the implanted electrodes.
  b) Common approaches include linking adjacent contact points in a linear bipolar chain to survey a large area, defining well a small area with closely spaced bipolar derivations or referring all contact points to a least active point to obtain a referential recording.
  c) Montages may include some scalp derivations to assure adequate characterization of abnormalities.

5. Montages – ambulatory cassette EEG
  a) Montage selection for a given patient should be

540

guided by previously documented abnormalities on routine EEG and by clinical history.

b) General screening montages should provide sampling of both hemispheres in a symmetrical fashion.

c) Montages designed in a chain-linked or near-linked fashion are recommended.

d) Preferential sampling of the frontal and temporal regions is suggested in those situations of limited channel numbers.

e) Montages designed to display data from both hemispheres in a mirror image, as well as symmetrical, fashion may enhance perception of lateralized or focal abnormalities on rapid video review. Because of the goals of ambulatory recordings and the restricted number of channels, montages appropriate for this use differ from those used in the clinical laboratory.

f) Examples of commonly used ambulatory EEG montages include (asterisks indicate audio-multichannel audio now available):

3 Channels
T5-T7, F5-F6*, F8-T6
T5-T1, F7-F8*, T2-T6
P3-F3, F7-F8*, F4-P4

4 Channels
T5-T3, F7-F3*, F4-F8*, T4-T6
T5-T1, F7-F1*, F2-F8*, T2-T6

5 Channels
F3-T5, T5-F7, F5-F6*, F8-T6, T6-F4

6 Channels
T5-T3*, T3-F7, F7-F3*, F3-F4, F4-F8*, F8-T4, T4-T6*

7 Channels
T5-T3*, T3-F7, F7-F3*, F3-F4, F4-F8*, F8-T4, T4-T6*

8 Channels
T5-T3*, T3-F7, F7-F3*, F3-C3, C4-F4, F4-F8*, F8-T4, T4-T6*
F3-C3, T5-T3*, T3-F7, F7-F3*, F4-F8*, F8-T4, T4-T6*, C4-F4

g) Montages recommended for extracranial EEG LTME (F3) are appropriate for ambulatory EEG recordings of more than eight channels, as are modifications of these montages to provide increased sampling in the frontal and temporal regions and mirror image symmetry.

6. Use of filters and sensitivity – EEG signals

a) When recording on tape or disk, low linear filters and sensitivity settings should be adjusted to prevent blocking, but it is best to record information in as wide a frequency band as possible and selectively filter the signals, as necessary upon playback.

b) Filter settings in most cases are the same as those used in standard laboratory EEG, i.e., high linear frequency filter at 70 Hz and low linear frequency filter at 1 Hz (time constant, 0.1 s). More selective filtering may enhance the information obtained from intracranial recording.

c) Certain environments may require the use of a 50–60-Hz notch filter. Under certain unavoidable conditions, more restrictive filtering than that above may improve the recording, particularly with nasopharyngeal electrodes.

d) Sensitivity settings for extracranial recording should be equal among channels and follow the recommendations for routine EEG. For intracranial recordings, equal sensitivity settings are recommended, if possible, as when using equally spaced chain linkage bipolar or common reference montages. Sensitivity can be set independently for each channel to obtain the best relative signal when closely or irregularly spaced bipolar intracerebral derivations are used.

7. Monitoring of other physiological parameters

a) Recording of the ECG, electro-oculogram (EOG), EMG, or respiration may be indicated for particular clinical situations. Recording techniques are the same as in standard polygraphy.

b) In 4-channel ambulatory EEG systems, the use of more than one channel for other physiological monitoring will significantly limit the usefulness and validity of the EEG data.

G. Special considerations for reviewing ambulatory cassette EEG

1. Use of filters and sensitivity

a) The use of a high-frequency filter on video playback is discouraged, since the recording and replay characteristics of most ambulatory EEG systems utilizing ultra-slow tape transport and paginated video display have a natural bias against high-frequency signals and a limited upper frequency range.

b) Shorter time constants (0.1–0.05 s) may be used on video playback to compensate for the disproportionately enhanced slow-wave activity.

c) Sensitivity should be equal among equivalent channels and otherwise follow the recommendations for routine EEG. Gain should be varied during video playback as necessary to view ongoing activity clearly and avoid visual clutter.

2. Video playback parameters

a) A review speed of 40–60 times real time may be used in scanning for ictal events. Such high rates of review are not recommended for the detection of isolated interictal discharges. Slower scanning rates of 20–40 times real time are more appropriate for perceiving isolated and focal transients.

b) Analysis of individual electrographic waveforms, particularly the differentiation of epileptiform discharges from normal transients and artifacts, can be more accurately performed at a 30 mm/s video display. A time compression of 15 mm/s or less may be useful during rapid review, particularly for ictal events.

3. Audio monitoring
   a) Simultaneous monitoring of the audio reproduction of the EEG is recommended when video scanning. Seizures, interictal transients, and artifacts all have characteristic sounds that can be used for event detection and differentiation.
   b) In order to monitor both hemispheres effectively, at least one channel from each side or at minimum one channel derived in a transverse fashion across the head should be reproduced for aural analysis. When available, a stereo audio mixer and headphones should be used to monitor more than one channel from each hemisphere. Listening to nonadjacent channels is suggested in order to avoid audio cancellation of focal activity. Only events occurring in the channels selected for audio monitoring will be detected by this means.

H. Artifacts

The differentiation of artifacts and normal EEG transients from EEG abnormalities poses an increased problem in LTME, particularly in ambulatory EEG recordings with a limited number of channels. Unusual artifacts not seen in standard laboratory EEG recording are commonly encountered.

1. Biological
   a) In addition to the normally recognized eye movements, blinking, muscle tension, ECG, respiration, sweating, and tremor, activities such as chewing, talking, and teeth brushing can produce EMG, glossokinetic, and/or reflex extraocular movement potentials and result in potentially confusing patterns.
   b) Standard disk electrode recordings are very susceptible to biological artifact. Nasopharyngeal electrode monitoring is in addition particularly prone to respiration, pulsation, and pharyngeal muscle contraction artifacts. Sphenoidal electrodes are associated with much less artifact. Intracranial electrode recordings are usually free of biological artifacts, except for pulsation and respiration.

2. Mechanical or external
   a) The main mechanical artifacts of telemetry originate from altered electrode/scalp contact or intermittent lead wire disconnection induced by body movement. Direct connection with standard cable imposes additional artifacts from movement of the cable itself.
   b) Artifacts produced by rubbing or scratching of the scalp and other rhythmic movements of head or extremity can, in association with accompanying biological artifact, result in particularly confusing patterns that must be differentiated from ictal discharges.

c) The most common external artifact in surface recordings is 50- or 60-Hz interference. Electromagnetic fields due to nearby fans, air conditioning, or ballasts of fluorescent lights can produce interference of 50- or 60-Hz plus harmonics. Electrostatic potentials due to nearby movement of persons with dry clothing or telephone ringing may produce spurious transients.

d) In intracranial recording, mechanical artifacts due to body movement are usually negligible and those due to electrical interference are usually less than with extracranial electrodes.

3. Instrumental

a) Any part of the recording and playback system, e.g., electrodes, wires, amplifiers, receivers, switches, reformattters, tape recorders, oscillographs, can be a source of artifact.

b) Common sources of spurious transients are electrode popping, faulty switches or connectors, or touching of dissimilar metals. Rhythmic slow waves can be due to chipped silver–silver chloride coating, instability of the electrode scalp interface, and electrode wire movement.

4. Recognition/interpretation

a) A conservative interpretation of unusual or equivocal EEG events is mandatory in LTME, particularly in instances in which the patient's activity at that moment cannot be verified for possible artifact production.

b) Personnel should familiarize themselves with the common artifacts of active wakefulness and EEG transients of normal sleep. Recognition of the instrumental artifacts of a particular laboratory or recording arrangement is equally necessary to insure reliable differentiation from cerebrally generated events.

c) In ambulatory EEG monitoring, all common biological and mechanical artifacts should be produced by the patient and/or technologist at the beginning or the end of the recording, where they can serve as a reference for confusing transients noted on review of that particular tape.

d) When simultaneous video-recorded behavior is available, artifacts due to biological and mechanical disturbances, particularly rhythmic ones, can usually be verified by review of the videotape.

e) When patient behavior is not being video recorded, identification of a rhythmic discharge as an epileptic seizure can be made by recognition of well-formed epileptiform spike-and-wave patterns with a believable field and typical ictal progression (for partial and convulsive seizures, the ictal discharge usually begins with low-voltage fast activity and becomes slower with higher amplitude), as well as postictal slowing, appropriate interictal abnormalities in other portions of the record, and an appropriate episode noted in the patient's diary or by an observer.

f) Interictal epileptiform EEG abnormalities should be identified as recurrent independent transients in artifact-free portions of the record, such as quiet wakefulness or sleep. Sharp waveforms noted only during active wakefulness should be interpreted as abnormal with caution.

I. Baseline EEGs and LTME quality assurance

1. Routine laboratory EEG studies should be performed to determine the need for any form of LTME and to select proper montages.

2. An EEG recording should always be performed at the beginning of LTME, not only to provide information on the patient's baseline EEG status, but to establish the integrity of the system. Using the electrodes placed for LTME, an EEG should first be run directly to an EEG machine set at the LTME montage, and then through whatever telemetry system, recording tape, or disk is to be used. The resultant two EEGs should be similar. During both recordings, each extracranial electrode should be tapped or rubbed in the sequence in which they are utilized in the montage and the output used to verify the montage setting.

3. Periodic checking of the status of ongoing EEG recording is essential and should be performed at least once a day. A paginated video review of ambulatory EEG data is sufficient.

In nonambulatory LTME settings, on-line monitoring of EEG data should be available by means of an oscilloscope, microprocessor-based digital display, video playback system, or EEG writeout.

VII. RECOMMENDED USES OF SPECIFIC LTME SYSTEMS

Although the large numbers of different EEG and behavior monitoring components create the possibility of many combinations that could comprise an LTME system, there are only a small number of configurations in general use. Listed below are recommended basic system configurations along with indications (refer to Section II) for which each is appropriate and not appropriate. Combinations of these systems are commonly used.

A. Monitoring with paper writeout only

1. EEG transmission – 'hard wire' (standard cable) or telemetry (cable or radio)
2. EEG recording/storage – continuous paper writeout
3. EEG review/analysis – complete manual review
4. Behavior monitoring – self, observer, and video
5. Clinical indications
   a) Appropriate – documentation, characterization, and quantification of clinical and subclinical ictal events and interictal EEG features over a period of hours.

Assessment of their relationship to behavior, performance tasks, naturally occurring events or cycles, or therapeutic intervention.

b) Comment – an on-line EEG record allows observer interaction during subclinical as well as clinical events and provides continuous feedback as to quality and content of data recorded. Long-term monitoring of this type is relatively labor-intensive and becomes progressively cumbersome with duration. At least 16 channels of EEG data and synchronized video monitoring are required for presurgical localization of epileptogenic regions.

c) Not appropriate – evaluations benefiting from a freely moving patient or when continuous monitoring lasts for days.

B. Monitoring with continuous storage on tape

1. EEG transmission – cable or radio telemetry
2. EEG recording/storage – analog or videotape
3. EEG review/analysis – selective writeout of clinical ictal events, random sampling writeout for subclinical ictal and interictal events
4. Behavior monitoring – self, observer, and video
5. Clinical indications
   a) Appropriate – documentation, characterization, and quantification of clinical ictal episodes and their EEG features over days to weeks and assessment of their

relationships to behavior, performance tasks, naturally occurring event or cycles, or therapeutic intervention.

b) Comment – at least 16 channels of EEG data and synchronized video monitoring are required for presurgical localization of epileptogenic regions. Radio telemetry provides more mobility than cable telemetry; however, video monitoring becomes difficult or impossible when this degree of mobility is required.

c) Not appropriate – for the quantitative analysis of subclinical ictal or interictal features and for evaluation benefiting from complete freedom of movement.

C. Computer-assisted selective monitoring

1. EEG transmission – cable or radio telemetry
2. EEG recording/storage – digital tape/disk, computer-assisted selective storage
3. EEG review/analysis – selective writeout of clinical and computer-recognized ictal and interictal events
4. Behavior monitoring – self, observer, and video
5. Clinical indications
   a) Most appropriate – documentation, characterization, and quantification of ictal (clinical and subclinical) and interictal EEG features and assessment of their relationship to behavior, performance tasks, naturally occurring events or cycles, or therapeutic intervention.

b) Comment – computer recognition programs have not been perfected and are subject to a variable amount of false-negative and false-positive error. At least 16 channels of EEG data and synchronized video monitoring are required for presurgical localization of epileptogenic regions. Radio telemetry provides more mobility than cable telemetry; however, video monitoring becomes difficult or impossible when this degree of mobility is required.

c) Not appropriate – evaluations benefiting from complete freedom of movement.

D. Ambulatory cassette (4 channels)

1. EEG transmission – ambulatory cassette (4 channels)
2. EEG recording/storage – analog cassette tape
3. EEG review/analysis – rapid paginated video review, selective writeout of ictal (clinical and subclinical) and interictal events
4. Behavior monitoring – self, observer
5. Clinical indications
   a) Appropriate – documentation and quantification of ictal (clinical and subclinical) and interictal EEG features and assessment of their relationship to reported behavior, naturally occurring events or cycles, or therapeutic intervention, when the data are most likely to be obtained outside the hospital or laboratory environment.

b) Comment – also applicable in an inpatient setting, particularly when mobility is of benefit. Differentiation of seizures from artifacts during active wakefulness may be difficult. The absence of EEG changes during a reported episode is not helpful in ruling out an epileptic condition.

c) Not appropriate – detailed characterization of EEG features as is required in presurgical evaluation, classification of seizure types, or characterization of behavioral/performance manifestations.

E. Ambulatory cassette (8 channels)

1. EEG transmission – ambulatory cassette (8 channels)
2. EEG recording/storage – same as D
3. EEG review/analysis – same as D
4. Behavior monitoring – same as D
5. Clinical indications
   a) Appropriate – same as D
   b) Comment – also applicable in an inpatient setting, particularly when mobility is of benefit.

Characterization of abnormal EEG features is improved over 4 channels such that differentiation from artifact is less of a problem.

   c) Not appropriate – detailed characterization of EEG features as is required in presurgical evaluation.

F. Ambulatory cassette – selective event recording/epoch sampling

1. EEG transmission – ambulatory cassette (16–24 channels)
2. EEG recording/storage – analog cassette tape, event recording/epoch sampling (periodic or after trigger)
3. EEG review/analysis – epoch writeout
4. Behavior monitoring – self, observer
5. Clinical indications
   a) Appropriate – documentation, characterization, and quantification of EEG features of seizures for which there are auras of behavioral changes that allow the patient or an observer to trigger the recording; assessment of their relationship to reported behavior, naturally occurring events or cycles, or therepeutic intervention, when the data are most likely to be obtained in an outpatient setting.
   b) Comment – also applicable in an inpatient setting.
   c) Not appropriate – identification of interictal EEG features or seizures for which the patient has no warning, characterization of behavioral manifestations, final presurgical evaluations (although useful as a triage step between routine EEG and inpatient monitoring)

G. Ambulatory cassette – selective, computer assisted

1. EEG transmission – ambulatory cassette (16–24 channels)
2. EEG recording/storage – analog cassette tape, epoch sampling, computer-assisted selective storage onto digital disk
3. EEG review/analysis – selective writeout of computer-recognized ictal and interictal events
4. Behavior monitoring – self, observer
5. Clinical indications
   a) Appropriate – same as F, except that seizures without an obvious behavioral change may be detected.
   b) Comment – same as F, but not truly ambulatory, since portable computer must be plugged into electrical outlet.
   c) Not appropriate – evaluations benefiting from complete freedom of movement, characterization of behavioral manifestations, final presurgical evaluations (although useful as a triage step between routine EEG and inpatient monitoring).

VIII. MINIMUM STANDARDS OF PRACTICE FOR SPECIFIC INDICATIONS

When inpatient LTME is performed, an EEG technologist, monitoring technician, epilepsy staff nurse, or other qualified personnel must observe the patient, record events, and maintain recording integrity.

A.   Presurgical evaluations

The most exacting evaluation in LTME is the attempt to localize, by means of surface and/or intracranial electrodes, a region of epileptogenic brain tissue that is the site of origin of recurrent seizures and that is amenable to surgical removal. The following are minimum acceptable standards.

1. EEG transmission – standard cable ('hard wire') or telemetry EEG with at least 16 channels of EEG data. Cable telemetry is the most common technology. Ambulatory EEG is not acceptable for final evaluation, but may serve a useful triage function.

2. EEG recording storage – continuous paper writeout with time code is adequate. Continuous or computer-assisted selective tape (analog instrumentation, video cassette, or digital) or disk (digital) recording EEG with a synchronized time code and subsequent selective playback on paper or other high-quality display is preferable.

3. EEG review/analysis – detailed visual analysis of all seizures and representative interictal abnormalities from a paper writeout or other high-quality display is adequate. Repeat analyses of seizures recorded on tape or disk with variations in playback parameters are preferable. Additional computer analyses of EEG abnormalities (temporal and distribution characteristics) may be beneficial.

4. Behavior monitoring – continuous video recording with a time code synchronized to EEG. Observer or self-reporting of behavior is not sufficient. Time-lapse video recording is discouraged.

B.   Diagnosis of nonepileptic seizures

Minimum standards of practice in the differentiation of nonepileptic seizures from epileptic seizures are the same as above, although 8 channels of EEG data can be adequate to identify most epileptic events. Regardless of the number of channels, however, absence of clear ictal EEG abnormalities during a behavioral event must be interpreted with reference to the complete clinical evaluation before a diagnosis of nonepileptic seizures can be made.

C.   Classification and characterization of epileptic events

Although 4-channel ambulatory EEG is adequate for documentation of certain interictal and ictal electrographic abnormalities, only systems with eight or more channels can provide basic characterization of epileptic EEG events. Classification and characterization of epileptiform EEG features are enhanced by an increased number of EEG channels and at least 12, preferably 16 or more, channels of EEG are needed for detailed analyses.

Classification of epileptic seizures usually requires video documentation of the behavioral features, synchronized with

EEG data. Characterization of the relationship of epileptic events to specific precipitating factors may require video recording or ambulatory capability, depending on features of the provocative stimuli or circumstances.

D. Quantification of electrographic abnormalities

Four-channel ambulatory EEG is adequate to quantify the frequency of occurrence of recognizable electrographic inter-ictal or ictal events. In order to differentiate clinical from subclinical seizures, however, video monitoring is essential.

IX. GUIDELINES FOR WRITING REPORTS ON LTME

A. General considerations

1. Formal typewritten reports at frequent intervals are recommended when the physician interpreting LTME data is not the same physician caring for the patient. These reports should document the intent, scope, technical features, and performance of inpatient LTME and serve as timely portrayals of their salient findings and clinical significance. Also, these reports should explain the basis for changes in LTME procedures (altering antiepileptic medication dosage, changes in montages or derivations selected for paper writeout, advisability of performing ancillary studies on any given day, etc.). A final summary at the end of LTME outlines salient features and states the final diagnosis and/or conclusions.

2. LTME reports should be produced at intervals according to the clinical situation, in particular the frequency with which events of interest are occurring. These intervals are usually 24 h, but may be as long as the patient's entire hospitalization, if few or no abnormalities are recorded.

3. Daily handwritten preliminary reports should be entered into the patient's chart to briefly summarize pertinent findings in rapidly evolving situations and circumvent possible delays in typing of final reports.

4. Reports of LTME should include the following identifying information: patient name, age, hospital number, date(s), times and/or duration of observations, source of referral, name of the attending physician, unit or clinic to which the reports should be sent, LTME procedure number, type and duration of study performed, and the name of the interpreter.

5. The LTME report should consist of four principal parts.
   a) In the initial report, a statement of the clinical problem and overall intent of LTME and, in subsequent reports, documentation of relevant clinical, behavior, and electrographic concerns as they arise.
   b) An explanation of technological aspects of the recording.
   c) A description of the findings.
   d) An interpretation, stating the overall impressions gained from, and clinical significance of, the electrographic and behavioral correlations.

B. Interval reports

1. *Clinical problem and intent of LTME.* Background information should include a brief summary of the clinical history and physical findings, the reasons for referral and a brief review of current medications and other existing conditions that might alter recorded EEGs or behavior. The purpose of the LTME (e.g., diagnostic study, presurgical evaluation) should be clearly stated.

2. *Technological aspects of the recording.* Technological considerations, such as number of channels of EEG recorded, type and location of electrodes (e.g., scalp, sphenoidal, intracranial, multiple EMG, ECG, etc.) and the use of manual and/or automated seizure and/or discharge detection should be documented initially and after changes in these. The use of random, continuous and/or selected paper writeout of the EEG and/or continuous fast review should be documented. Special observations (oximetry, sleep assessment, blood pressure or cardiac arrhythmia monitoring) are indicated. Activation procedures (drug injection, suggestion, hyperventilation, exercise, re-enactment of precipitating events), testing of reaction times, etc., should be fully described. The reduction of medications, especially those intended to increase or decrease the incidence of seizures, is described. Serum levels of antiepileptic drugs, serum prolactin levels, etc., are noted in this section. When multiple reports are generated during one hospitalization, this section need not always be as comprehensive as in the first, but it should include a description of significant changes as the LTME progresses.

3. *Description (findings).* A statement concerning waking and sleeping EEG patterns, magnitude and location of non-epileptiform abnormalities, and the presence of artifacts that might reflect upon the overall quality of the recording are reported. The frequency of occurrence, character, topographic distribution and propagation of interictal epileptiform discharges should be reported. Behavioral and electrographic ictal events should be emphasized and described in detail; however, a full description of each of a series of similar episodes is not always needed. Instead of the latter, relevant differences among them should be given. A suggested format presents the number and time of occurrence of each seizure followed by the statement 'A. Clinically, ...' and a description of clinical events. Then after 'B. Electrographically, ...' the EEG features are described. As needed, after the statement 'C. Special observations ...' results of ancillary studies are detailed. Descriptions of patient behavior should include portrayal of activity immediately preceding the attack, characteristic features of the onset, course, and termination of the episode, and ictal and postictal behavior evident spontaneously, as the result of examination, and as supplemented by reports of observers. Specifically, responsiveness, orientation, language, memory, motor activity, and other neurological functions are to be reported. The electrographic findings to be reported should include descriptions of background activity and epileptiform discharges preceding the seizure, the

mode, pattern, and location of onset of ictal activity, the propagation and termination of seizure discharges, and postical charges. The durations, relative times of onset, and significant changes in clinical and electrographic ictal events should be presented. The temporal relationship between behavioral manifestations and ictal electrographic events should be noted.

4. *Interpretations.* This portion of the report should be an interpretive synthesis rather than a reiteration of the description. Seizures should be classified on the basis of behavioral, electrographic, and ancillary observations according to the International Classification of Epileptic Seizures (*Epilepsia* 1981;22:489–501). Overall pathophysiological and diagnostic formulations should include reference to available data on the quantitative and topographic features of interictal epileptiform and nonepileptiform, as well as ictal, abnormalities. Inferences as to the site of origin and propagation of seizures should be made when this is justified by the findings. Suggestions for subsequent studies are stated.

C. Summary reports

1. A brief summary serves as a useful supplement to formal interval reports when these are made, or a more detailed overall summary of LTME should be provided at the end of the monitoring period.

2. The summary should contain brief statements of the clinical problems, goals of LTME, technological features, and type of studies performed and significant EEG and behavioral findings during LTME. The results of earlier standard EEGs and previous LTME studies can be outlined as background to present observations. All ictal events, epileptiform patterns, nonepileptiform abnormalities and other observations of interest leading to the final diagnosis and/or conclusions are summarized. Based on the overall perspective offered by LTME, the summary interpretation offers inferences regarding the pathophysiological nature of recorded events, a final clinical–electrographic correlation, and a classification of the observed ictal events. A concluding statement indicates whether or not and/or the extent to which the goal of LTME was attained. The direction of future LTME studies is suggested. In addition to this EEG impression, when the individual writing the report is involved in the patient's care, a clinical impression is also appropriate. In this case, the results of other diagnostic tests, including imaging, and the conclusions of multidisciplinary discussions, can be incorporated into a final statement.

GUIDELINE THIRTEEN: GUIDELINES FOR STANDARD ELECTRODE POSITION NOMENCLATURE[1]

These guidelines propose a method for combining a slight modification of the international 10–20 system with a slight modification of a strict combinatorial rule that allows for an extension of the present 10–20 system to designate the 10% electrode positions that are currently unnamed.

This report is divided into the following sections: (1) desirable characteristics of an alphanumeric nomenclature; (2) head diagram of proposed 'modified combinatorial nomenclature'; (3) explanation of modification of the 10–20 nomenclature within the modified combinatorial system; (4) explanation of the deviation from a strict combinatorial nomenclature in the modified system proposed herein; and (5) extension of combinatorial nomenclature to positions inferior to those demonstrated in Fig. 1.

---
[1]Prepared by the Electrode Position Nomenclature Committee.

Address correspondence and reprint requests to American Electroencephalographic Society, One Regency Drive, P.O. Box 30, Bloomfield, CT 06002, U.S.A.

© 1994 American Electroencephalographic Society, *J Clin Neurophysiol* Vol. 11 (1) 111–113.

I. DESIRABLE CHARACTERISTICS OF AN ALPHANUMERIC NOMENCLATURE

1. The alphabetical part should consist preferably of one but no more than two letters.

2. The letters should be derived from names of underlying lobes of the brain or other anatomic landmarks.

3. The complete alphanumeric term should serve as a system of coordinates locating the designated electrode according to the following rules.

a. Each letter should appear on only one coronal line. (In standard 10–20 terminology, the only outstanding exception to this rule are the 'T' (temporal) names that appear on both the central and parietal coronal lines. For reasons explained in Section III, this exception is replaced by a more consistent terminology within the nomenclature recommended by the Committee. For emphasis, this modification is displayed on the head diagram in Section II with white lettering on a black background.)

b. Each number should designate a sagittal line so the same postscripted number identifies all positions lying on that sagittal line. (Again, the only outstanding exception to this rule in the current 10–20 system is in the 'T' numbering. For example, this results in the F7, T3, and T5 designations all appearing on a single sagittal line. This exception is also elimi-

MODIFIED COMBINATORIAL NOMENCLATURE

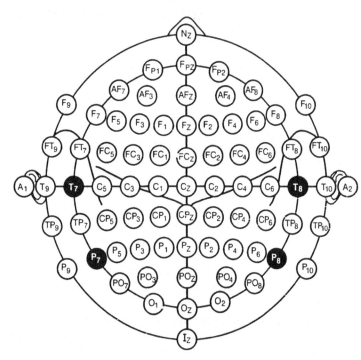

Fig. 1. Modified combinatorial nomenclature.

nated within the recommended nomenclature. Once more for emphasis, this modification is displayed in the head diagram in Fig. 1 with white lettering on a black background.)

II. HEAD DIAGRAM OF PROPOSED 'MODIFIED COMBINATORIAL NOMENCLATURE'

In Fig. 1, the modifications of the current 10–20 terminology, instituted for reasons explained in Section III, are emphasized by displaying them with white lettering on a black background.

III. EXPLANATION OF THE MODIFICATION OF THE 10–20 NOMENCLATURE WITHIN THE MODIFIED COMBINATORIAL SYSTEM

The modified combinatorial terminology replaces the inconsistent T3/T4 and T5/T6 terms with the consistent T7/T8 and P7/P8. The head diagram in Fig. 1 emphasizes consistency of the terms T7/T8 and P7/P8 by showing them with white lettering on black circles. The value of this becomes evident when inspecting the head diagram, which shows that, except for Fp1/Fp2 and O1/O2, all electrode positions along the same sagittal line have the same postscripted number and that all electrodes designated by the same letter(s) lie on the same coronal line. Thus, the alphanumeric nomenclature for each electrode specifies its coordinate location within the 10–20 grid system. Once this is done, the positions *10% infe-*

rior to the standard frontotemporal electrodes are easily designated as F9/F10, T9/T10, and P9/P10, respectively.

As indicated above, the straightforward designation of an electrode's coordinate localization by its nomenclature requires replacement of the inconsistent T3/4 by T7/8, which is a readily understandable modification. A more radical modification replaces T5/6 by P7/8. However, even with this more radical departure, P can easily be recognized as representing parietal when it is associated with a postscripted number with a value of 6 or less, whereas it can be readily recognized as implying posterior temporal if P is associated with a number with a value of 7 or greater.

However, even though T7/8 and P7/8 in the head diagram *emphasize the internally consistent logic* of the system, it would clearly be *an acceptable alternative* to continue to use T3/4 and T5/6 without detracting from the logic of the remaining system.

IV. EXPLANATION OF THE DEVIATION FROM A STRICT COMBINATORIAL NOMENCLATURE IN THE MODIFIED SYSTEM PROPOSED HEREIN

The current 10–20 system does not name electrode positions forming the four 10% intermediate coronal lines lying between the five standard coronal lines containing currently named electrode positions. The strict combinatorial system designates the currently unnamed positions by combining the names or letters for the two standard electrode positions that surround a currently undesignated 10% intermediate electrode position.

Thus, positions in the second intermediate coronal line are designated as either the frontotemporal positions (FT) or the frontocentral positions (FC), depending on their location as noted in the head diagram.

The electrode positions in the third intermediate coronal line are designated as temporal-posterior temporal (TP) or centroparietal (CP) as noted in Fig. 1.

The positions in the fourth and final intermediate coronal line are designated as posterior temporo-occipital (PO) or parieto-occipital (PO).

The *only proposed deviation* from the strict combinatorial rule discussed above is in naming the first intermediate transverse positions as anterior frontal (AF) electrodes rather than frontopolar-frontal electrodes. The latter terminology would designate the electrodes with either three letters (FpF) or the same two letters (FF). Since neither of these letter designations is desirable (the first because it uses three letters and the second because it uses the same letter twice), the Committee proposes using the readily understandable anterior frontal (AF) designation displayed in Fig. 1.

Once the above letters are assigned to the currently unnamed 10% intermediate positions, then their alphanumeric designation is completed by postscripting the letters assigned to an electrode by the number designating the sagittal line upon which the electrode lies. For example, in Fig. 1 AF3,

FC3, CP3, and PO3 all lie on the same sagittal line designated by the number 3.

When this is done, each new alphanumeric designation not only is directly related to a slight modification of the currently accepted 10–20 terminology but serves as an internally consistent coordinate system that locates each newly designated electrode position at the intersection of a specified coronal (identified by the prefixed letter) and sagittal (identified by the postfixed number) line.

V. EXTENSION OF COMBINATORIAL NOMENCLATURE TO POSITIONS INFERIOR TO THOSE DEMONSTRATED IN FIG. 1

Positions posterior to electrodes displayed in the ninth and tenth rows would be designated as PO9 (10% inferior to PO7), PO10 (10% inferior to PO8), O9 (10% inferior to O1), and O10 (10% inferior to O2). Electrodes 10% inferior to the ninth row would be designated with the postscripted number 11 (F11, FT11, T11, TP11, P11, PO11, O11), and those 10% inferior to the tenth row would be designated with a postscripted number 12 (F12, FT12, T12, TP12, P12, and O12).

GUIDELINE FOURTEEN: GUIDELINES FOR RECORDING CLINICAL EEG ON DIGITAL MEDIA

INTRODUCTION

With digital systems becoming widely available and relatively inexpensive, it has become practical to record EEG onto magnetic or optical long-term storage media. Such recording has several advantages. It can help reduce the space problem of storing original paper rercords over many years. It also allows review of selected portions of an EEG record using montages, filters, vertical scaling (gain or sensitivity), and horizontal scaling (e.g., paper speed) selected after the original recording. Finally, digital recording allows the possibility of further digital processing after the fact.

These recommendations describe only minimal technical standards for recording clinical EEG on digital media. Standardization of the structure and format of the data recorded, for free exchange of compatible recordings among EEG laboratories, is addressed separately by the American Electroencephalographic Society (AEEGS) document, 'Standard Specification for Transferring Digital Neurophysiological Data Between Independent Computer Systems.'

© 1994 American Electroencephalographic Society, *J Clin Neurophysiol* Vol. 11 (1): 114–115.

PATIENT INFORMATION

The electronically recorded information should include the patient's name and date of birth, date on which the test was run, and relevant patient and laboratory identification numbers. In addition, all the routine information that would normally be written onto the facesheet of the EEG should be recorded electronically along with the EEG signals. Preferably, the EEG report will also be stored and merged with the EEG signal after review of the record by a physician. Correction of errors or omissions in the patient-identifying information should be possible after the recording.

IDENTIFYING INFORMATION DURING THE RECORDING

Calibration signals should be recorded at the beginning and end of each recording, in the manner already conventional for EEG. Biocalibration signals should also be run at the beginning of the record. The time of day should be recorded along with the EEG data, as well as any other information that could be used for finding events in the stored record. The recording should contain all of the technologist's comments since they would ordinarily be written onto a conventional EEG paper record. The technologist should be able to enter event codes and comments even after the EEG is recorded. Codes recorded with the data can represent common events such as eyes closed or eyes open, beginning and end of hyperventilation, details of photic stimulation, or notation of the patient's alert, drowsy, or asleep state. Free text comments should be able to be entered by keyboard as well and stored along with the EEG data on the recording medium. In addition, there should be provisions for automatically recording information, such as filter settings, gain, montage selections, and other technical amplifier control settings at the start of the recording, and any changes made during the recording should be immediately recorded with the data.

RECORDING

Acquisition of EEG data onto a digital storage medium should occur at a minimum sampling rate three times the high-frequency filter setting, e.g,, 100 samples/s for 35-Hz high filter and 200 samples/s for 70-Hz high filter. Higher rates are preferable. The sample rate needs to be sufficient to prevent aliasing. Digitization should use a resolution of at least 11 bits per sample including any sign bit. A resolution of 12 or more bits is preferable, since the recording should be able to resolve EEG down to 0.5 μV and record potentials up to plus or minus several millivolts without clipping. For example, with a 0.5-μV resolution and a 12-bit analog-to-digital conversion, the maximum allowed excursion would be ± 1.023 mV. Interchannel crosstalk should be less than 1%, i.e., 40 dB down or better. Common mode rejection ratio should be at least 80 dB, preferably better, for each of the channels. Additional noise in the recording should be less than 2 μV peak-to-peak, at any frequency 0.5–100 Hz, including 60 Hz.

RECORDING MEDIA

At the present time, several magnetic and nonerasable and erasable optical storage devices seem adequate for routine long-term recording and storage of EEG records. We recognize the uncertainty about durability, especially regarding magnetic recording media. We also recognize uncertainty regarding the availability of commercial transcription devices to replay the stored EEG years into the future. The present lack of standards for commercial nonerasable optical disk storage results in incompatability between various commercially available devices and may lead to the impossibility of reading, repair, or replacement of some optical disk recordings and drives within a few years. Newly emerging standards for erasable optical media may make this type of storage less prone to this problem. At present, magnetic tapes can replay EEG adequately after 5 years of storage. However, degradation of the magnetic tape may become a serious problem by 10 years.

Note is made of the existence of statutes governing medical records in each of the individual states, as well as existence of local or hospital statutes regarding EEG record storage. These govern the duration of storage, and in some instances they may also dictate whether magnetic or optical storage is to be allowed.

DISPLAY

A recording system for clinical use should have the capability to review recorded EEG data on a video display or on paper, preferably with both types of displays available. Overall, review on paper or on a screen should approximate the temporal and spatial resolution of traditional analog paper recordings. Montages available for review should be consistent with those in standard use in the laboratory and with previous AEEGS recommendations, preferably allowing additional user flexibility. This should be done using bipolar or referential reconstruction techniques. Post hoc digital filtering should also be available. Playback systems should be able to display channel (montage) designations, gain or filter settings where appropriate, technologist comments, and event markers along with the raw or transformed EEG data. A time stamp on each screen or page of EEG data is essential.

A standard horizontal scaling should be available in which 1 s occupies between 25 and 35 mm with a minimum resolution of 100 data points/s on screen and 200 data points/s on paper. Other more compressed and more expanded horizontal scales should also be available, including scaling differing from standard by a factor of 2, e.g., 7.5, 15, 30, or 60 mm/s. Vertically, appropriate channel spacing between the baseline of each channel depends on the number of channels displayed. A standard vertical scaling with a minimum spacing of 10 mm per channel should be used for a display of up to 21 channels. Other choices for vertical scaling may be provided too. Larger gaps can be introduced where necessary to separate blocks of channels and increase readability. Occasional overlap of data between channels is acceptable. An adequate screen and paper display should have a minimum of 2 pixels resolution per vertical millimeter. The horizontal and vertical scales on screen and paper should be indicated on the display. For purposes of comparison between different devices, important considerations are the maximum number of channels and the maximum number of seconds that could be displayed on a single screen or on a piece of paper, using the standard scaling as defined above.

The system should allow simultaneous display of multiple segments of EEG, allowing side-by-side visual comparison of different segments within one recording as well as different segments from different recordings obtained on different days. If the playback system has hard-copy capabilities, however, one could also compare different EEG segments by printing them individually. Continuous, fan-folded paper is generally preferable for most EEG applications displaying long segments or the entire record.

GUIDELINE FIFTEEN: GUIDELINES FOR POLYGRAPHIC ASSESSMENT OF SLEEP-RELATED DISORDERS (POLYSOMNOGRAPHY)

1. INTRODUCTION

1.1 The role of clinical neurophysiology laboratories in the diagnostic evaluation of sleep and sleep-related disorders

Polygraphic recordings during sleep for the evaluation of sleep-related disorders are routine procedures offered by many clinical neurophysiology laboratories. The assessment of such disorders requires a polygraphic approach, in which multiple physiologic parameters, in addition to EEG, are recorded over prolonged periods in order to document specific relationships that may have diagnostic value. The technique is referred to as 'polysomnography' (PSG), although many individuals prefer the more simple term, 'sleep study.'

1.2 Indications for sleep monitoring

Many individuals who have significant sleep disorders may have no symptoms or complaints about their nocturnal sleep patterns or may be unaware of episodes of sleep at inappropriate times. The most common reasons for referral for sleep monitoring are to evaluate: (a) episodes of sleep at inappropriate times, (b) difficulty sleeping during scheduled sleep periods (insomnia), (c) difficulty staying awake during scheduled awake periods (hypersomnia), (d) atypical behavioral events occurring during sleep (e.g., sleepwalking, loud snoring, respiratory difficulties, excessive movements, possible seizures), and (e) the effectiveness of various therapeutic regimens that may be instituted for the management of sleep disorders.

1.3 Patient referral dynamics

PSG is usually carried out within one or two existing administrative structures: (a) the sleep laboratory, which is an entity analogous to an EEG laboratory; patients are primarily physician-referred, and their subsequent care is the responsibility of the referring physician; and (b) the sleep clinic or center, in which patients are either self- or physician-referred,

Address correspondence and reprint requests to American Electroencephalographic Society, One Regency Drive, P.O. Box 30, Bloomfield,CT 06002, U.S.A.
© 1994 American Electroencephalographic Society, *J Clin Neurophysiol* Vol. 11 (1): 116–124.

and in which complete clinical evaluation and treatment plans are formulated and implemented, in addition to PSG. These guidelines relate only to the recording and interpretation of laboratory procedures for the diagnostic evaluation of sleep and sleep-related disorders, regardless of the setting; they do not address the management of patients with sleep disorders.

1.4 The scope of polygraphic monitoring and its goals

A PSG study allows events occurring in a variety of physiologic systems, across a spectrum of neurophysiologic states, to be observed simultaneously. Much of its diagnostic utility depends on the ability to correlate specific changes or abnormalities of one physiologic parameter with specific conditions defined by another parameter or parameters (e.g., a cardiac arrhythmia occurring coincidentally with an episode of obstructive apnea, or myoclonic jerks of the limbs occurring during Stage 2 sleep). Consequently, it is a significantly more powerful and complex tool than could be provided by individual and independent measurements of each variable. This advantage, however, is offset by a number of inherent difficulties related to optimal graphic display of the disparate parameters and the means for reliably detecting and documenting a multitude of possible patterns of diagnostic value among these variables.

These guidelines attempt to address the issues cited above in a systematic manner, by considering both the methods and requirements for recording each of the variables and their in-

tegration within the diagnostic protocols. The guidelines also address the basic principles of interpretation and the qualifications of those performing and interpreting the procedures.

2. RECORDING TECHNIQUES

2.1 Physiologic parameters measured and equipment parameters

2.1.1 Routine variables

2.1.1.1 EEG. The earliest descriptions of the electrophysiologic activity associated with sleep were derived from EEG recordings; the EEG remains the primary variable for the staging of sleep [1]. The EEG also provides crucial information regarding the presence or absence of epileptiform activity, interhemispheric asymmetries, focal abnormalities, drug effects, and other abnormal patterns associated with neurologic disease.

A single central channel (e.g., C3-A2 or C4-A1) is sufficient for basic sleep staging. However, additional channels are required to provide redundancy and to permit adequate assessment of other EEG characteristics (e.g., seizures and other epileptiform activity, asymmetries). Consequently, it is recommended that six or more channels of cortical activity be used routinely and that the montage includes, at a minimum, combinations of the following electrode placements: Fp1, Fp2 (or other left and right frontal positions), C3, C4, O1, O2, T3, and T4.

The electrode types, methods of application, and other recommendations stated in the American Electroencephalographic Society (AEEGS) Guidelines in EEG should be followed [2,3]. After use, electrodes should be cleaned according to institutional protocols for infection control. All other recommendations for recording EEG as related to amplifiers, frequency response, calibration, etc., must also follow the recommendations of the AEEGS Guidelines in EEG [2,3]. Although the standard chart or paper speed for PSG is 10 mm/s [1], higher paper speeds (15 mm/s or 30 mm/s) may be necessary to facilitate EEG interpretation.

2.1.1.2 Electro-oculography (EOG). EOG recording provides information regarding sleep onset (i.e., slow, rolling eye movements that occur with transition to Stage 1) and, most important, is essential for the recognition of REM (rapid eye movement) sleep. At least two channels of EOG are recommended. One channel may record from an electrode placed 1 cm lateral to and 1 cm above the outer canthus of the other eye. An ear–mastoid position may be used as a reference for each channel. A backup ear–mastoid site on the other side can be utilized if the initial reference electrode malfunctions. With these montages, most conjugate eye movements produce out-of-phase voltage deflections in the two channels, whereas co-existing EEG activity is usually in phase. Should a distinction between vertical and lateral eye movements be required, additional EOG montages, using a supranasion reference electrode that produces deflections in phase with vertical eye movements, may be employed. A supranasion reference electrode alone, however, may result in the integration of EEG activity with extraocular movement potentials. Consequently, other reference locations may be required for specific circumstances. Recordings can be performed using differential AC amplifiers with a time constant setting at 0.3 s and a sensitivity at 7 μV/mm.

2.1.1.3 Submental electromyography (EMG). Submental EMG activity is used for determining the level of muscle tone, which is significantly decreased during REM sleep. This channel also provides supplemental information regarding patient movements and may be useful in evaluating artifacts in other channels.

A single channel is sufficient; electrodes are placed under the chin, in the submental region. Two standard silver-cup surface disk electrodes of the type used for scalp EEG recording are routinely used and may be applied with collodion glue and/or adhesive tape. Other types of miniature stick-on electrodes may also be used. The recording is obtained through standard EEG amplifiers (bandpass typically 10–70 Hz) with the sensitivity adjusted to provide an adequate baseline EMG level during wakefulness (typically 20 μV/cm).

2.1.1.4 Electrocardiography (ECG). The electrocardiogram serves as a monitor of heart function and can reflect the severity of cardiorespiratory dysfunction, such as in sleep apnea. Alterations in the rate may be quite dynamic, with prolonged bradycardia, extrasystoles and/or asystole, suggesting a severe disease condition and the risk of sudden death.

A single ECG channel is sufficient for PSG monitoring;

electrode placement is not critical but should be carefully documented. Typically, two electrodes are placed: one in the sternal area and the other at a lateral chest location. Alternatively, an arm or leg placement, referred to the shoulder or other derivation, may be used. The amplifier setting should allow for faithful reproduction of activity between 5 and 70 Hz. The gain used is generally less, by a factor of 10 or more, than that required for EEG.

If nocturnal angina or other specific cardiac disease is suspected as a cause of the patient's sleep disturbance, a more extensive and specific ECG recording is warranted, or, if home assessment is needed, a Holter or ambulatory monitoring study with several ECG channels may be desired.

2.1.1.5 Respiration (measures of respiratory effort and airflow). The monitoring of respiration during PSG is specific for the detection of apneas and hypopneas of a central or obstructive nature. Other breathing abnormalities, including bradypneas and tachypneas as well as respiratory arrhythmias and other conditions of a potentially lethal nature, may be associated with significant sleep disturbances.

It is important to record at least three respiratory parameters: (a) air exchange through both the mouth and nose; (b) respiratory effort as manifested by expansion and relaxation of the thorax and abdomen; and (c) level of oxygen saturation in the peripheral blood (see Section 2.1.1.6 below).

Monitoring of the air exchange may be accomplished by a variety of transducers, but the use of thermistors or thermocouples is widely accepted. It is important that all three orifices (both nostrils and the mouth) be monitored at all times, individually or simultaneously, because air exchange can occur through a combination of any of the three orifices.

Monitoring of thoracic and abdominal movements associated with breathing may also be accomplished by several methods, including measurement of intercostal EMG, thoracic and abdominal impedance, or, more commonly, by means of strain gauge devices that permit differentiation between abdominal and thoracic motions.

Both respiratory effort and airflow can be monitored with AC amplifiers; however, long time constants (1 s or more) are preferred for adequate reproduction of the responses. The sensitivity settings are directly related to the type of transducer used and are usually set empirically to provide the desired degree of excursion. The resultant recording will register excursions in relation to expansion and contraction of the abdomen and thorax and a corresponding oscillation of the tracing(s) recording air exchange. Respiratory rates are easily detected and calculated, as are the amplitudes of the respiratory effort and air exchange indicators. The absence of respiratory effort, and consequently lack of evidence of air exchange, indicates central apnea. When respiratory effort is present, but no air exchange is detected, the phenomenon is indicative of obstructive apnea. When respiratory effort is present, but no air exchange is detected, the phenomenon is indicative of obstructive apnea. When the apneic episode begins with a central component and then evolves into an obstructive component, it is designated to be of mixed type. Thoracic and abdominal motions during obstructive apnea are typically of opposite phase (paradoxical respiration). Respiratory pauses are considered to be apneic if they persist at least 10 s. Oxygen saturation may decrease significantly, usually in direct relation to the lengths of the apneic episodes.

Ongoing monitoring of respiratory parameters may demonstrate episodes of decreased effort to breathe, with a resultant decreased volume of air exchange and, consequently, a drop in oxygen saturation (central hypopnea). When ongoing adequate effort to breathe occurs in the presence of decreased air exchange (partial obstruction), the condition is referred to as obstructive hypoventilation (or hypopnea) and is typically associated with a paradoxical respiratory pattern. These conditions may result in significant oxygen desaturation.

Because apneas and hypopneas frequently trigger arousals and interrupt the normal sleep cycle phenomena, it is most important that other parameters of sleep, including EEG, EMG, and EOG, be recorded to allow for the development of a sleep profile with which the breathing abnormality can be plotted and correlated.

2.1.1.6 Blood oxygenation (P_{O_2} or O_2 saturation). The diagnosis most often established by PSG is sleep apnea or another form of sleep-related breathing disorder. Continuous monitoring and display of blood oxygen levels are mandatory because they provide crucial information regarding the severity of the respiratory dysfunction. Pulse oximetry, a noninvasive and relatively inexpensive technique, is recommended. The technique does have some limitations, such as errors due

to the presence of carbon monoxide (as may be seen in smokers).

Commercially available oximeters can be easily interfaced with the polygraphic recorder. The sensors of the pulse oximeter usually fit either the fingertip or earlobe and can be attached easily, with good mechanical contact. Calibration of each apparatus differs, and the newer units are self-calibrated. The outputs of the oximeter must be recorded through a DC-coupled amplifier and displayed simultaneously with other pertinent PSG variables.

Although most laboratories use pulse oximetry as their index of tissue oxygenation, transcutaneous P_{O_2} recording can be carried out as well. In this technique, a Clark oxygen electrode is attached directly to the skin and heated to 43–45°C. This device measures the transpired P_{O_2}, which fairly accurately reflects the tissue P_{O_2}. This technique has found widespread use in the monitoring of neonates in an intensive care setting. In adults, it is accurate only in patients with good tissue perfusion. The transcutaneous P_{O_2} technique has an inherently longer time constant than oximetry and thus may not accurately reflect the transient decreases of O_2 saturation seen in association with episodes of apnea.

2.1.1.7 Expired CO_2. The recording and display of the expired carbon dioxide level (capnography) is another useful means for evaluating respiratory function; it may be readily used in the sleep laboratory. During inspiration, essentially no carbon dioxide is present. During expiration, as alveolar air is expelled, the partial pressure of CO_2 rises to the end of expiration, where it closely approximates intra-alveolar P_{CO_2}. In the sleep laboratory, this provides two types of information. First, it shows that air exchange is, in fact, taking place, and the patient is not obstructed; second, it reveals the partial presence of CO_2 in the alveoli, which will rise during an apneic phase and fall back to baseline levels after several successive breaths. It is also useful for detecting and evaluating underlying pulmonary disease, which, if present, may modify the interpretation of observed respiratory variables.

Sampling is accomplished by taping the end of a piece of small-diameter plastic tubing that leads from the instrument to an area beneath either nostril or near the mouth. A mild degree of suction is applied by the instrument in order to draw air continuously into the analysis chamber. In practice, three lengths of tubing are usually used: one placed below each nostril and the other placed at the mouth. Provision is made to permit any of the tubes to be switched into the analysis device, thereby allowing the technologist to direct the sampling to whichever orifice presents adequate airflow.

2.1.1.8 Body/limb movement. Common causes of sleep disturbances are the restless legs syndrome (RLS) and periodic myoclonus in sleep (PMS). These movements are often visually detectable if the patient is videotaped. Quantification of these events during the night is one means of detecting disturbed sleep; this may be accomplished either indirectly by registration of EMG activity from the limbs, or directly by visual detection of limb movement. Electrodes placed on the right and left anterior tibial muscles provide a sensitive measure of myoclonic activity that may be so subtle as to be unnoticed by the external observer.

Minimal technical requirements include one channel of EMG derived from an electrode placed over the anterior tibial muscles on the left side; referred to a similar placement on the right side. Standard EEG electrodes are sufficient for surface recording of the EMG, although long leads are necessary to allow the patient adequate mobility. Amplifier settings can be established at the outset of the PSG recording, but, in general, gains will be significantly less than required for a routine EEG. Reproduction of physiologic data between 5 and 70 Hz is required.

Another method is to use accelerometers, which give a quantitative index of the amount of movement and hence the potential for sleep disruption caused by myoclonic activity. Accelerometry may also be useful if the patient has a movement disorder such as tremor, which may disrupt sleep. Most movement disorders are prominent in the waking state and relatively suppressed in sleep, so sensitivities can be adjusted at the beginning of the recording as required.

It is recommended that videotaping of the patient be included, along with the observation of the patient by the technologist. Unusual or complex movements, or even seizure activity, may occur unexpectedly. The technical requirements for this type of monitoring are discussed in Section 2.1.1.9 below.

2.1.1.9 Audio/video monitoring and behavioral observation. The capability to observe the patient's behavior directly and to monitor any vocalization or snoring during sleep is a crucial and integral part of the PSG procedure. This is most easily implemented through closed-circuit television, with on-line display through a video monitor located within view of the technologist, and with preservation of the information on videotape to allow later detailed review of any abnormal events. This audio/video monitoring is particularly important for assessment of the patient's body position in relation to snoring and other respiratory dysfunctions, for detection and specification of body and limb movements during sleep, for characterization of arousal disorders (e.g., night terrors, sleep-walking), and for assessment of suspected seizures.

The video camera should be mounted in the patient recording room, so as to provide a full-body view of the reclining subject. The camera should be capable of producing a high-quality image with very low or absent visible high levels. This commonly requires installation of a suitable source of low-level infrared or ultraviolet light, which remains on when the normal room lights are extinguished at bedtime. Addition of a remote-controlled zoom lens to the camera is recommended, since this will permit the technologist to provide closeup views of events (e.g., facial muscle twitches, limb movements) that might not be visible with a fixed whole-body view. Addition of a remote-controlled pan-and-tilt mechanism to the camera mount is also required to allow positioning during closeup views. Microphone placement is less critical but should provide distinct pickup of even low-level vocalizations or respiratory sounds. The videotape recorder, video monitor, and all camera controls should be located in the technologists' work area, proximate to the polygraphic recorder, so that on-line correlations are possible between the audio–video information and other recorded variables. The capability to obtain precise off-line time synchronization of the recorded audio/video signals and the polygraphic record is also crucial, and suitable time-code generators that provide simultaneous outputs to both systems should be used (see Section 2.1.1.10 below).

2.1.1.10 Time. The times of recording onset and cessation should be noted on all recordings. If the recording is interrupted for any reason, the times at interruption and resumption should be noted, together with the reason for interruption. Finally, when paper records are obtained, the paper speed should be noted; and, when data are obtained electronically, the time relationships of the recorded data should be specified.

When both video and polygraphic data are obtained, it is essential that the time relationships between the two be assessable with precision. This requires the use of a single time-code generator, which can imprint the same time information simultaneously on both records. Separate clocks are not satisfactory because of a gradual drift between the two timers that usually will occur over a period of hours.

Although split-screen techniques are useful means of displaying clinical behaviors and physiologic data, they may not provide adequate resolution for accurate correlation. Split-screen techniques should not be considered a substitute for precise display of the physiologic data.

A number of methods of displaying time data on the video

and physiologic records are available. Any one of these is satisfactory, as long as the principles noted above are observed. The technical details of time stamping of recordings are also discussed in 'Guidelines for Long-Term Neurodiagnostic Monitoring in Epilepsy' [4].

2.1.2 Optional/special-purpose variables

Under special circumstances, monitoring of other parameters may be required during sleep such as: (a) esophageal pH on patients suspected of having regurgitation of stomach contents, related or unrelated to obstructive apneas, (b) determination of core temperature via a temperature probe used rectally or as a swallowed capsule may be necessary in cases of sleep/wake-schedule disorders, and (c) nocturnal penile tumescence measurements used in the evaluation of male impotence in order to differentiate organic and psychogenic causes.

Because of the variety of equipment suitable for such monitoring, specific hookups to the polygraphic equipment, as well as amplifier requirements and settings, must follow manufacturers' recommendations.

2.2 Recording protocols

2.2.1 Routine for standard nocturnal study

PSG is designed to obtain the maximum clinically relevant physiologic information with the least disruption of the patient's normal sleep patterns. The study must be carried out as close as possible to the patient's normal sleep time and must be conducted in a quiet, comfortable room that resembles a bedroom or hotel room. Intrusive equipment should be kept to a minimum. Recording apparatus should be physically separated from the patient, with appropriate shielding of light and sound. Interruptions through the night for adjustment of the monitors should be kept to a minimum. 'Backup' electrodes and sensors can be helpful wherever feasible.

Details of the study must be planned in advance, based on the questions PSG is asked to answer. The design of the montage should be clearly established with the professional and technical staff before the patient's arrival at the laboratory. Detailed clinical information about the patient's sleep-related problems and general medical problems is necessary, because the patients are often relatively incapacitated, and technologists are required to make minute-to-minute judgments in relation to the patient's health and safety. After the electrodes have been applied and the apparatus calibrated, the lights should be turned off as close as possible to the patient's usual bedtime. The time of 'lights out' should be marked on the record. The technologist should continuously monitor the patient's clinical status and position in bed and record changes either on the record, in a log, or both. Any entry by the technologist into the patient's room should be recorded. Patient vocalizations or other activities should also be noted on the record or in the log. 'Lights on' should take place as close as possible to the patient's usual time of arising, although this may be slightly modified for patient convenience or for laboratory scheduling purposes. Ideally, 8 h of recording from 'lights out' to 'lights on' should be obtained. However, a minimum of 6.5 h is required for a nocturnal study. After the electrodes have been removed, the patient should have access to appropriate shower and bathroom facilities. The patient should be instructed before leaving the laboratory as to the procedure for obtaining the results of the study and/or information regarding follow-up studies.

All laboratories should have established procedures to handle life-threatening situations, such as severe sleep-disordered breathing, dangerous cardiac arrhythmias, changes in the patient's sensorium or clinical state, or other serious clinical changes. These policies should be established well in advance and carefully conveyed to the technical and professional staff.

2.2.2 Evaluation of daytime sleepiness

The multiple sleep latency test (MSLT) is a standardized test of daytime sleepiness [5,6]. Adherence to a protocol provides a reproducible measure of sleepiness as well as a measure of the effectiveness of drugs and other treatments for hypersomnolence. As a measure of sleepiness, the MSLT is influenced by drugs the patient takes and by sleep deprivation. Consequently, it is important to minimize or stabilize drug use for 2 weeks before the test and to perform MSLT the day after an overnight PSG examination, so that the quality of overnight sleep preceding the study can be established and the presence of any sleep pathology documented.

The patient should be prepared for the test with timely instructions regarding drugs and sleep prior to the examination.

The patient may be required to discontinue certain or all medications and drugs for an appropriate period before the test. The electrode application should be completed well before the scheduled onset of testing. The patient should be prepared to spend the day relaxing in or near the laboratory.

Four or five sleep latency tests are performed at 2-h intervals throughout the day. The usual times are 10 a.m., noon, 2 p.m., 4 p.m., and 6 p.m. For night-shift workers who are entrained to other sleep schedules, the study should start 2 or 3 h after the normal awakening time for each particular patient. Each sleep latency test is performed in bed, in the sleep monitoring room described above (Section 2.2.1). The recording system is checked for integrity; then the patient is instructed to rest quietly, or preferably to sleep. The room should be dark, and the time should be marked on the record. The test continues for 20 min if the patient does not sleep, or for 15 min after the first epoch of sleep. If unquestionable REM sleep is documented, the test may be terminated immediately. Then the patient is aroused and must be kept awake until the next latency test. Supervision by laboratory personnel or family is desirable between testing periods.

The critical parameters are sleep-onset latency for each test period and REM latency, if it occurs after sleep onset. Sleep onset latency is measured as the time from lights out until the first occurrence of any sleep stage. The average of the sleep latency over the four or five periods provides a measure of sleepiness. Two or more short latency REM episodes (i.e., onset of REM sleep during the 15-min sleep period on two occasions) indicate a disturbance of REM sleep and may be diagnostic of narcolepsy. The number of such REM episodes and their latencies are reported.

In the maintenance of wakefulness test (MWT), the patient is requested to remain awake for specified periods of time [7]. This procedure permits evaluation of the degree of alertness and detection of a tendency to sleep at inappropriate times.

The PSG montage used for MSLT and MWT testing should include, at a minimum, EOG, submental EMG, and central and occipital EEG activity. Accurate staging is essential.

2.2.3 Extralaboratory monitoring

Monitoring in the home or in other settings outside the laboratory has, in certain circumstances, proved to be a useful adjunct to conventional monitoring. It must be recognized, however, that ambulatory monitoring is prone to the same artifacts as occur in the laboratory, along with the added potential for artifacts due to a more mobile patient, while not providing the full array of monitoring possibilities. The results of extralaboratory recordings must therefore be assessed with great care. In many cases, previous recordings in the laboratory can help direct the focus and purpose of the extralaboratory investigation.

Extralaboratory monitoring devices should include the number of channels of data required to answer the specific clinical questions for the particular patient. The technical details of extralaboratory (ambulatory) monitoring are discussed in greater detail in 'Guidelines for Long-Term Neuro-diagnostic Monitoring in Epilepsy' [4]. The technical details outlined there are reaffirmed for this application. Subsequent experience has emphasized the importance of recognizing artifact and obtaining an adequate number of channels of data.

3. INTERPRETATION: DATA ANALYSIS AND REPORTING

The results of a sleep monitoring procedure must be presented in the form of a comprehensive, but concise, report that summarizes all the observations. This document must also provide an integrated interpretation conveying the medical significance of the findings to the referring physician and/or others involved in the management of the patient's problem. Consequently, the report is the single most important element of the PSG examination, and, as such, its preparation should involve a systematic and thorough approach. The following sections delineate the minimal information that shuold be included in the report and provide suggestions regarding the overall organization.

3.1 Patient identification

The report should be clearly labeled on each page with the patient's full name and the inclusive date(s) of the study. The report should also include the patient's age and any identification numbers required for retrieval of filed supplementary information (e.g., samples of the polygraphic record, videotapes, technologists' logs). If the patient has been studied previously in the same laboratory, this fact should be indicated and the dates provided.

3.2 History

The report should contain sufficient historical information to document the reason why the study was recommended, any significant existing medical conditions, prior major medical problems, relevant medications used during the preceding 30 days (e.g., hypnotics, stimulants, antidepressants), and any special therapy the patient is receiving (e.g., use of supplemental O_2 at night, continuous positive airway pressure). Any special procedures the patient has had that might influence the study (e.g., tracheostomy, UPPP) should also be listed.

3.3 Recording conditions

The report should document the exact periods of time the patient was monitored during the overall study period and should indicate the conditions of each session (e.g., 'an 8-h nocturnal monitoring session with the patient in bed and lights out, beginning at 23:05; an MSLT beginning at 10:00'). The physiologic parameters actually recorded during each monitoring session should also be listed (see Section 2.1.1 and 2.1.2 above). If multiple channels are used for some measures (e.g., EEG, EOG, respirations), these should be specified. When significant, the type of sensor used and its ana-

tomic location should also be documented (e.g., O_2 saturation by ear oximeter, leg movement by accelerometer).

3.4 Technical description

A concise description of the polygraphic characteristics of each monitoring session should be provided. Subsections of this description include the following.

3.4.1 Sleep statistics

The report should provide a complete summary of the sleep parameters, including total time in bed, duration of interspersed wakefulness, total sleep time [absolute and/or percentage of total time in bed (sleep efficiency)], sleep latency, REM latency, number of awakenings, and the actual, and percentages of, time spent in each stage of sleep.

Presentation of this information is facilitated by the inclusion of a sleep stage versus time graphic plot and a table listing quantitative values of the sleep parameters. This description should delineate values considered to be outside the normal range and should include comments regarding any atypical characteristics of the sleep architecture.

3.4.2 Respiratory characteristics

The report should summarize the result of analysis of the respiratory characteristics with respect to sleep state. Information should be provided concerning the respiratory rate awake and asleep, the presence or absence of snoring, the presence of a paradoxical respiratory pattern, the number and types of apneic episodes and/or hypopneic events, the frequency and degree of O_2 desaturation, and the occurrence of end-tidal Pco_2 elevation (if recorded). Atypical events should be characterized with respect to both sleep state and body position. Presentation of these data is facilitated by computer-generated plots or histograms showing selected parameters.

3.4.3 ECG/heart rate

Typical heart rate values awake and asleep (REM and NREM) should be provided, and the report should document extreme values occurring transiently. Arrhythmias should be documented with respect to frequency of occurrence and type. It is particularly important to describe the occurrence of heart rate changes or arrhythmias with respect to the ongoing respiratory characteristics such as O_2 desaturation. Any associated alteration of other physiologic variables should be carefully documented (e.g., EEG slowing following pronounced bradycardia or asystole, epileptiform EEG activity preceding or accompanying cardiac arrhythmias).

3.4.4 Myoclonus/leg movements

Myoclonic activity recorded from the extremities must be evaluated in terms of frequency of occurrence and periodicity, sleep/wake status, and presence or absence of subsequent arousal. Movements that follow EEG signs of arousal (often seen with termination of apneic events or accompanying nor-

mal spontaneous arousals), movements that clearly precede and cause arousal from sleep (true nocturnal myoclonus), and movements that occur in the absence of any alterations in sleep, respiration, or other parameters must be clearly differentiated. When myoclonus is present, any associated epileptiform EEG events should be documented.

3.4.5 Behavioral observations

Any unusual or atypical behavioral events documented by the technologist (and/or by video monitoring) should be described and discussed in terms of associated polygraphic variables.

An attempt should be made to determine the probable cause of each awakening from sleep (e.g., relationship to respiratory dysfunction, myoclonus, seizure); the absence of any obvious cause should also be noted, particularly in the case of patients who have frequent arousals. Episodes of sleep talking or coordinated motor behavior during sleep should be reported. Seizures or other unusual events should be described and correlated with ongoing EEG characteristics and other physiologic variables.

3.4.6 EEG characteristics

Careful and accurate EEG interpretation is essential. A summary of the EEG characteristics should be provided, including basic characterization of the awake and asleep background patterns and a description of any abnormal features. Asymmetries and focal features should be noted. Care should be taken to determine any correlation between EEG alterations and changes in other physiologic parameters.

3.4.7 Optional/special-purpose variables

If any optional physiologic variables (see Section 2.1.2 above) have been recorded, a description should be included that summarizes the observations and relates the observed changes in those parameters to both sleep state and other recorded measures.

3.5 Summary

While not essential, it is extremely helpful to the referring physician if a brief summary of the key objective findings of the study is provided at the end of the report, prior to the impression. This section should include the essential findings from all areas of the report and should represent the factual basis for the impression.

3.6 Impression

The impression section should be as concise as possible and should relate the objective findings of the study to recognized diagnostic entities within the context provided by the patient's history. Thus, a clear statement (or statements) should be made by the interpreter describing the normality or abnormality of the study and including the basis for his judgment. Whenever possible, a more definitive statement should be made, suggesting specific clinical diagnoses with which the findings are consistent. The impression is most useful if it also provides an estimation of the severity of any problem(s) identified. If the patient has been studied previously, the impression should include a comparison with the earlier results.

4. STANDARDS OF PRACTICE

4.1 Qualifications of individuals interpreting test results

Individuals interpreting PSG studies should be qualified as follows.

1. They should be able to demonstrate the minimal qualifications of a clinical electroencephalographer as outlined in 'Guideline Four: Standards of Practice in Clinical Electroencephalography' [8].

2. They should be able to document supervised experience in clinical PSG of at least 6 months' duration.

4.2 Qualifications of technologists

Individuals performing PSG studies should be qualified as follows.

1. They should be able to demonstrate familiarity with the polygraphic recording instrumentation, including knowledge of operating procedures, calibration methods, and routine troubleshooting as outlined in 'Guideline Five: Recom-

mended Job Descriptions for Electroencephalographic Technologists' [9].

2. They should be proficient in basic EEG technology, including knowledge of the techniques of electrode application, the international 10–20 electrode placement system, impedance testing, and electrical safety rules.

3. They should be familiar with the classification of sleep disorders and with the polygraphic characteristics of each.

4. They should be familiar with the normal EEG characteristics of adults and children and should be able to recognize the various sleep stages.

5. They should be trained in basic cardiopulmonary resuscitation and should be familiar with the normal ranges of the polygraphic parameters recorded.

6. They should have a minimum of 6 months' supervised experience in a sleep laboratory before serving in an unsupervised setting, regardless of prior training or experience in other areas.

4.3 Laboratory organization and record-keeping

A procedure manual should be developed and maintained, indicating all laboratory procedures as outlined above. Equipment, electrodes, and recording procedures should meet the standards set forth in this and other guidelines for performing clinical procedures.

The organization of the laboratory should be in compliance with Guideline Four of the AEEGS [8].

Storage of recorded data should be in compliance with statutes in the locality in which they are obtained. In the case of physiologic data, it is preferable that the entire record be saved. If this is not practical, an acceptable alternative is storage of the report describing the complete record, together with samples of actual data representing important physiologic events. In the case of behavioral (i.e., video) data, an edited version that preserves recorded events is acceptable, but both physiologic and behavioral data should be time-stamped, to allow correlation with one another. If behavioral events occur semicontinuously, preservation of the video record of representative events, together with a description of the entire night's recording, is a satisfactory alternative. It should be recognized that advances in storage technologies may, at some point, make storage of larger amounts of data more practical than it is now. Notwithstanding such advances, storage as described would be satisfactory to meet the needs of patient care.

REFERENCES

1. Rechtschaffen A, Kales A, eds. *A manual of standardized terminology, techniques and scoring system for sleep stages of human subjects.* Washington, DC: U.S. Government Printing Office, 1968.
2. American Electroencephalographic Society Guidelines in EEG and Evoked Potentials 1986. Guideline One: Minimum technical requirements for performing clinical electroencephalography. *J Clin Neurophysiol* 1986;3(Suppl 1):1–6.

3. American Electroencephalographic Society Guidelines in EEG and Evoked Potentials 1986. Guideline Two: Minimum technical standards for pediatric electroencephalography. *J Clin Neurophysiol* 1986;3(Suppl 1):7–11.
4. American Electroencephalographic Society Guidelines in EEG and Evoked Potentials 1986. Guidelines for long-term neurodiagnostic monitoring in epilepsy. *J Clin Neurophysiol* 1986;3(Suppl 1):93–126.
5. Richardson GS, Carskadon MA, Flagg W, van den Hoed J, Dement WC, Mitler MM. Excessive daytime sleepiness in man: multiple sleep latency measurement in narcoleptic and control subjects. *Electroencephalogr Clin Neurophysiol* 1978;45:621–7.
6. Carskadon MA, Dement WC, Mitler MM, Roth T, Westbrook PR, Keenan S. Guidelines for the Multiple Sleep Latency Test (MSLT): a standard measure of sleepiness. *Sleep* 1986;9:519–24.
7. Mitler MM, Gujavarty KS, Browman CP. Maintenance of wakefullness test: a polysomnographic technique for evaluating treatment efficacy in patients with excessive somnolence. *Electroencephalogr Clin Neurophysiol* 1982;53:658–61.
8. American Electroencephalographic Society Guidelines in EEG and Evoked Potentials 1986. Guideline Four: Standards of practice in clinical electroencephalography. *J Clin Neurophysiol* 1986;3(Suppl 1):18–9.
9. American Electroencephalographic Society Guidelines in EEG and Evoked Potentials 1986. Guideline Five: Recommended job descriptions for electroencephalographic technologists. *J Clin Neurophysiol* 1986;3(Suppl 1):20–2.

Transmission of infection during routine EEG recording procedures is almost unheard of except under special conditions, such as depth electrode placement in patients with spongiform encephalopathy (Bernoulli et al., 1977). The publication of guidelines for handling patients with Creutzfeldt–Jakob disease (CJD) (Gajdusek et al., 1977) or acquired immunodeficiency syndrome (AIDS) (Conte et al., 1983) led us to consider the necessity of developing our own guidelines for handling patients with infectious diseases during EEG recording. Such guidelines are important not only for correct care of infectious patients but also for protection of other patients and personnel in the EEG laboratory from possible exposure to infection.

The EEG is an important part of the clinical evaluation of patients with infectious diseases (Radermecker, 1977), particularly in those with infections such as CJD and subacute sclerosing panencephalitis, or with dementia or seizures as a possible symptom of infectious disease.

Infections can be transmitted by any of four routes: contact, air, a common vehicle (food or water), or a vector (mosquito, flea, tick, mite, or louse) (American Hospital Association,

Revised from the report in *J Clin Neurophysiol* 1986;3(Suppl 1):38–42.
© 1994 American Electroencephalographic Society, Vol. 11 (1) 128–132.

1979). In the EEG laboratory, the major concern is to prevent contact and airborne transmission of infection. Contact transmission may occur from inadequate cleaning of electrodes and equipment. Airborne transmission may be caused by inadequate cleaning of the laboratory, a poor ventilation system, or inappropriate handling of patients or staff members who cough and sneeze.

In hospital environments in which patients may be immunocompromised as a result of anticancer therapy, or organ transplantation, appropriate care must be exercised to prevent exposure of patients to seemingly banal, but potentially life-threatening, infections such as varicella-zoster (chickenpox, 'shingles').

CREUTZFELDT–JAKOB DISEASE AND VIRAL HEPATITIS

CJD and viral hepatitis need special attention because viruses in these diseases are resistant to many conventional sterilizing agents or techniques.

The CJD virus resists inactivation by boiling, ultraviolet irradiation, 70% alcohol, formaldehyde vapor, 4% formaldehyde, and β-propiolactone. The virus has been found in some human organs, with the highest titer in the brain, the spinal cord, and cerebrospinal fluid. It is not yet known whether blood, serum, leukocytes, urine, feces, sputum, saliva, tracheal aspirates, semen, and hair follicles are infectious; in a limited number of experiments they have not been. No special ward isolation is recommended. How early in the preclinical stage a case of CJD becomes infectious is also unknown. At this time, it is recommended that blood and cerebrospinal fluid should be considered potential sources of infection, whereas exposure to breath, saliva, nasopharyngeal secretions, urine, or feces should not be cause for special concern. In the latter types of exposure, thorough washing of hands or other exposed parts with a detergent or soap is sufficient, but vigorous scrubbing with a brush such as to cause skin abrasion should be avoided. Great caution should be exercised to avoid accidental puncture of skin with a contaminated needle (Gajdusek et al., 1977). However, there has been no increased risk of infection among medical personnel, including neuropathologists, who have come in direct contact with brain tissue from patients having died from CJD.

There are at least three types of viral hepatitis: A (infectious), B (serum), and non-A, non-B (serum). It is now known that the enteric route is the principal mode of transmission of hepatitis A virus, but maximal levels of hepatitis A virus excretion occur before the onset of jaundice. Infected blood is the principal mode of transmission of hepatitis B virus. Non-A, non-B hepatitis is similar epidemiologically to hepatitis B. Thus, a major precaution in caring for patients with viral hep-atitis is to prevent contamination from infected blood (Favero et al., 1979).

The hepatitis A virus is not inactivated by ether, temperatures of $-20°C$ or $37–60°C$ for 39 min, or acid pH, but is inactivated by ultraviolet irradiation or boiling for 1 min (Krugman et al., 1978). An extraordinary degree of isolation and precaution is not justified for the patient with hepatitis A infection, but rather the same precautions for handling feces from all other hospitalized patients, which should include wearing gloves when handling bedpans or fecal material, should be observed (Favero et al., 1979).

For hepatitis B virus (Bond et al., 1977; Favero et al., 1979), the vast majority of infections result from overt (transfusion, tattooing, ear piercing, acupuncture, accidental needle puncture) or inapparent exposure to contaminated blood (minor abrasions of the skin, toothbrushes, razors, hangnails, simply scratching or rubbing the skin, accidental splashes in the eyes with infective serum or plasma, contaminated baby bottles, toys, coffee cups, rubber gloves). The hepatitis B virus is still viable after storage for 15 years at $-20°C$, 6 months at room temperature, 4 h at $60°C$, and after exposure to ultraviolet irradiation, triple ether, β-propiolactone, benzalkonium chloride, or alcohol. However, the hepatitis B virus is inactivated by boiling for 1 min or heating at $60°C$ for 10 h.

A 5% sodium hypochlorite solution has been found efficacious in sterilizing both CJD and hepatitis B virus (Bond et al., 1977; Gajdusek et al., 1977) but is not suitable for sterilizing metal instruments because it is corrosive (Bond et al.,

1977; Hoeprich, 1977). Glutaraldehyde is an excellent disinfectant for hepatitis B virus, but the sterilization process using this agent takes about 10 h (Bond et al., 1977). Glutaraldehyde has no effect on CJD virus (Asher et al., 1977). The effective method of choice for sterilizing CJD and hepatitis virus is steam autoclaving: the CJD virus is completely inactivated at 121°C and 15 psi for at least 1 h (Brown et al., 1990) and hepatitis B virus at 121°C and 15 psi for 15 min (Asher et al., 1977).

The effective method of choice for sterilizing CJD and hepatitis virus is steam autoclaving: the CJD virus is completely inactivated at 132°C for at least 2 h (Brown et al., 1990) and hepatitis B virus at 121°C and 15 psi for 15 min (Bond et al., 1977).

ACQUIRED IMMUNODEFICIENCY SYNDROME

AIDS is characterized by severe suppression of the cellular immune system, and patients are susceptible to the development of Kaposi's sarcoma and some other cancers and to a variety of opportunistic infections. The disease is associated with a high incidence of neurologic complications, particularly involving the central nervous system (Snider et al., 1983), and has an extremely high probability of a fatal outcome.

AIDS is an infectious disease caused by the human T-cell lymphotrophic virus type-III/lymphadenopathy-associated virus (HTLV-III/LAV). The main route of transmission is sexual contact. Blood-borne transmission also has been implicated in certain groups of patients, such as hemophiliacs, intravenous drug abusers, and recipients of blood transfusions and blood products. There is no evidence of transmission through household contacts (Friedland et al., 1986) or saliva (Groopman et al., 1984). Hospital workers, in frequent contact with AIDS patients or their blood, have been seronegative for HTLV-III/LAV (Hirsch et al., 1985). Surveillance of health-care workers with documented injuries from needles or sharp instruments contaminated with blood or other body fluids of AIDS patients suggests a very low transmission rate, but the findings are not conclusive (McCray, 1986). A significant portion (40%) of these exposures probably could have been prevented if the workers had followed recommended precautions for infection control. There is a well-documented case of AIDS virus transmission following a deep intramuscular needle stick injury (Stricoff and Morse, 1986).

The AIDS virus is inactivated by alcohol, hypochlorite, the detergent NP-40 (but not Tween-20), hydrogen peroxide, phenolics, and paraformaldehyde at concentrations well below those usually formulated for use as a disinfectant (Martin et al., 1985).

ROLE OF THE EEG LABORATORY STAFF

The staff should be sensitive about infectious diseases. This information usually is supplied on the EEG request form or in the medical record. If there is some uncertainty, the laboratory staff should consult the referring physician or the electroencephalographer.

When the presence of infection is known or suspected, the laboratory staff should inform the electroencephalographer, and the necessary sterile technique or isolation procedure should be followed. In the hospital, the sterile technique or isolation procedure is easily obtained from the patient's nursing staff or from the institution's Infections Control Committee. If infection is suspected but unconfirmed, the laboratory staff should assume that the suspected infection is definite and exercise the prescribed precautionary measures. All laboratory staff should be familiar with handling of patients with CJD, viral hepatitis, and AIDS.

The need to prevent transmission of blood-borne pathogens led the Centers for Disease Control to formulate Universal Precautions. The premise of these recommendations is that all individuals should be managed as if known to be a potentially contagious carrier of HIV.

1. *Gloves* should be worn for touching blood and body fluids, mucous membranes, or nonintact skin of all patients including skin that has been abraded for reduction of impedance while placing conventional disk electrodes, for handling items or surfaces soiled with blood or body fluids and for performing vascular access procedures and placement of electrodes.

2. *Hands* and other skin surfaces should be washed immediately and thoroughly if contaminated with blood or other body fluids. Hands should also be washed immediately after gloves are removed.

3. *Gowns* or plastic aprons are indicated if blood spattering is likely, such as in the operating room.

4. *Mask and protective goggles* should be worn if aerosolization or splattering are likely to occur, such as in surgical procedures including placement of invasive electrodes.

5. To minimize the need for emergency mouth-to-mouth resuscitation, mouthpieces, resuscitation bags, or other ventilation devices should be strategically located and available.

6. Sharp objects should be handled in such a manner to prevent accidental cuts or punctures. Used needles should not be bent, broken, reinserted into their original sheath or handled unnecessarily. They should be discarded intact immediately after use into an impervious needle disposal box, which should be readily accessible. All needlestick accidents, mucosal splashes, or contamination of open wounds with blood or body fluids should be reported immediately to designated infection control specialist or officer.

7. All patient blood specimens or other potentially contaminated body fluids, such as cerebrospinal fluid, should be considered biohazardous.

8. Health-care workers with exudative skin lesions should refrain from all direct patient care.

9. Pregnant health-care workers are *not* known to be at greater risk of contracting HIV infection; however, if a pregnant health-care worker contracts HIV infection during pregnancy, the infant is at risk of infection resulting from perinatal transmission. Because of risk, health-care workers who may

become pregnant should be especially familiar with and adhere to precautions to minimize the risk of HIV transmission.

Knowledge of the following procedures may be important (American Hospital Association, 1979):

1. *Enteric precautions:* Preventing spread of infection due to contamination with urine and feces.

2. *Respiratory precautions:* Preventing spread of infection due to contamination of air or dust with secretions.

3. *Strict isolation:* This is undertaken when high virulence and great communicability of the infecting agent are suspected.

4. *Compromised host precautions:* To protect a patient who has a defective immune mechanism.

To effect the above precautions, the following actual procedures are used in various combinations, depending on which precaution is to be effected: wearing of gown, mask, and gloves; hand washing; cleaning of equipment and supplies; and cleaning of the laboratory floor or any other horizontal surfaces (Centers for Disease Control, 1986, 1987).

CLEANING RECORDING EQUIPMENT AFTER USE

EEG machine and related equipment

EEG equipment other than electrodes usually imposes no significant hazard of infection transmission. However, after its use on a patient with an infectious disease, the EEG machine should be wiped with 70–90% ethyl alcohol or isopropyl alcohol, phenol, or other noncorrosive disinfectant. EEG equipment can be handled and cleaned similarly in most of the infectious diseases. Only when the EEG machine is contaminated with secretions or blood should it be wiped with hypochlorite solution (Safai, 1985; Committee on Health Care Issues, 1986).

Electrodes

Disk electrodes. Placing disk electrodes on the patient's scalp exposes the EEG laboratory staff to direct contact with infected patients. It is recommended that rubber gloves be worn when placing electrodes on a patient with suspected or known infectious disease. Special attention must be paid to patients with CJD, hepatitis, or AIDS. In these patients, scratching or abrasion of the scalp should be avoided because blood or secretion from the scalp may be potentially infectious. If abrasion with blunted needles is necessary, however, handling and cleaning of the electrodes should be done as described below. Blunted needles used for injecting conductive jelly should be treated the same as disk electrodes, but those used for scratching and abraiding should be bagged, autoclaved, and then discarded.

For all types of infectious diseases, disk electrodes should first be cleaned with gauze, tap water, or ideally with a mechanical cleaner (ultrasonic cleaner) (Conte et al., 1983) to remove particulate matter. They should be immersed in 2% glutaraldehyde solutions for at least 30 min or other noncor-

579

rosive disinfecting agents (phenols, iodophors, alcohol, 5% sodium hypochlorite). If the method of decontamination is in doubt, however, the electrodes should be immersed in disinfecting solution and then autoclaved at 132°C for 2 h.

In patients with CJD, viral hepatitis, or AIDS, disk electrodes should be handled with gloves, especially if the EEG staff member has any break of the skin on his/her hands. Immediately after removal, the electrodes should be placed in a disinfectant solution (Dakin solution) for several hours, then rinsed with tap water. Visible residue can be removed by gentle scrubbing or by a mechanical cleaner. Thereafter, the electrodes should be steam-autoclaved at 132°C for 2 h (Brown et al., 1990). The autoclaving temperature must be below 350°F (177°C) so as not to damage the insulation of the electrode (Grass and Grass, 1977).

Needle electrodes. Needle electrodes should not be used in patients with dementia, CJD, hepatitis, or AIDS.

Nasopharyngeal electrodes. Nasopharyngeal electrodes should be constructed so as to be autoclavable at 132°C for 2 h and should be autoclaved after each use. Nasopharyngeal electrodes that are not autoclaved are not recommended.

Depth electrodes. The reuse of depth electrodes is discouraged. If they are reused, they must be soaked in 5% or 1:5 dilution of sodium hypochlorite solution and then steam-autoclaved at 132°C for 3 h. At the present time, the reuse of depth electrodes used in patients with dementia, CJD, or AIDS is not recommended. However, when alternative electrodes are unobtainable and the situation requires the im-

mediate use of depth electrodes, such electrodes may be reused only after they are autoclaved twice at 121°C and 15 psi with immersion in a warm detergent solution between autoclaving (D.C. Gajdusek, personal communication, 1982).

REFERENCES

American Hospital Association. *Infection control in the hospital,* 4th ed. Chicago: American Hospital Association, 1979.

Asher DM, Gibbs CJ, Gajdusek DC. Slow virus: safe handling of the viruses of subacute spongiform encephalopathy. In: *Manual of laboratory safety.* American Society for Microbiology, 1977.

Benoulli C, Siegfried J, Baumgartner G, Regli F, Rabinowicz T, Gajdusek DC, Gibbs CJ Jr. Danger of accidental person-to-person transmission of Creutzfeldt–Jakob disease by surgery. *Lancet* 1977;1:478–9.

Bond WW, Peterson NJ, Favero MS. Viral hepatitis B: aspects of environmental control. *Health Lab Sci* 1977;14:235–52.

Brown P, Liberski P, Wolff A, Gajdusek D. Resistance of scrapie infectivity to steam autoclaving after formaldehyde fixation and limited survival after ashing at 360 degrees C: practical and theoretical implications. *J Infect Dis* 1990;161:467–72.

Brown P, Rohwer RG, Gajdusek DC. Sodium hydroxide decontamination of Creutzfeldt–Jakob disease virus. *N Engl J Med* 1984;310:727.

Centers for Disease Control. Recommendations for preventing transmission of infection with human T-lymphotrophic virus type-III/lymphadenopathy-associated virus during invasive procedures. *Morbid Mortal Weekly Rep* 1986;35:221–3.

Centers for Disease Control. Recommendations for prevention of HIV transmission in health care setting. *Morbid Mortal Weekly Rep* 1987;36 (Suppl), No. 25.

Committee on Health Care Issues. American Neurological Association. Precautions in handling tissues, fluid, and other contaminated materials from patients with documented or suspected Creutzfeldt-Jakob disease. *Ann Neurol* 1986;19:75–7.

Conte JE Jr, Hadley WK, Sande M. University of California, San Francisco. Task Force on the Acquired Immunodeficiency Syndrome. Special report. Infection-control guidelines for patients with the acquired immunodeficiency syndrome (AIDS). *N Engl J Med* 1983;309:740–4.

Favero MS, Maynard JE, Leger RT, Graham DR, Dixon ER. Guidelines for the care of patients hospitalized with viral hepatitis. *Ann Intern Med* 1979;98:872–6.

Friedland GH, Saltzman BR, Rogers MF, Kahl PA, Lesser ML, Mayers MM, Klein RS. Lack of transmission of HTLV-III/LAV infection to household contacts of patients with AIDS or AIDS-related complex with oral candidiasis. *N Engl J Med* 1986;314:344–9.

Gajdusek DC, Gibbs CJ, Asher DM, Brown P, Diwan A, Hoffman P, Nemo G, Rohwer R, White L. Precautions in medical care of, and in handling materials from, patients with transmissible virus dementia (Creutzfeldt-Jakob disease). *N Engl J Med* 1977;297:1253–8.

Grass AM, Grass ER. *Electrode maintenance and infection control in the EEG laboratory*. Quincy, MA: Grass Instrument Company, 1977.

Groopman JE, Salahuddin SZ, Sarngadharan MG, Markham PD, Gonda M, Sliski A, Gallo RC. HTLV-III in saliva of people with AIDS-related complex and healthy homosexual men at risk for AIDS. *Science* 1984;226:447–9.

Hirsch MS, Wormser GP, Schooley RT, et al. Risk of nosocomial infection with human T-cell lymphotrophic virus III (HTLV-III). *N Engl J Med* 1985;312:1–4.

Hoeprich PD. Sterilization, disinfection and sanitization. In: Hoeprich PD, ed. *Infectious diseases: a modern treatise of infectious processes*, 2nd ed. Hagerstown, MD: Harper & Row, 1977.

Krugman S, Grocke DJ. Viral hepatitis. In: Smith LH Jr, ed. *Major problems in internal medicine,* vol 15. Philadelphia: Saunders, 1978.

Martin LS, McDougal JS, Loskoski SL. Disinfection and inactivation of the human T lymphotrophic virus type III/lymphadenopathy-associated virus. *J Infect Dis* 1985;152:400–3.

McCray E, the Cooperative Needlestick Surveillance Group. Special report: occupational risk of the acquired immunodeficiency syndrome among health care workers. *N Engl J Med* 1986;314:1127–32.

Radermecker FJ. Infections and inflammatory reactions, allergy and allergic reactions: degenerative diseases. In: Rémond A, ed. *Handbook of electroencephalography and clinical neurophysiology*, vol 15. Amsterdam: Elsevier, 1977.

Safai B. Safety precautions for dealing with AIDS. In: DeVita VT Jr, Hellman S, Rosenberg SA, eds. *AIDS: etiology, diagnosis, treatment and prevention.* New York: JB Lippincott, 1985.

Snider WD, Simpson DM, Nielsen S, Gold JWM, Metroka CE, Posner JB. Neurological complications of acquired immune deficiency syndrome: analysis of 50 patients. *Ann Neurol* 1983;14:403–18.

Stricoff RL, Morse DL. HTLV-III/LAV seroconversion following a deep intramuscular needlestick injury. *N Engl J Med* 1986;314:1115.

Appendix III

CLINICAL AND ELECTROENCEPHALIC CLASSIFICATION OF EPILEPTIC SEIZURES: DEFINITION OF TERMS*

Each seizure type will be described so that the criteria used will not be in doubt.

Partial seizures

The fundamental distinction between simple partial seizures and complex partial seizures is the presence or the impairment of the fully conscious state.

Operationally in the context of this classification, *consciousness* refers to the degree of awareness and/or responsiveness of the patient to externally applied stimuli. *Responsiveness* refers to the ability of the patient to carry out simple commands or willed movements and *awareness* refers to the patient's contact with events during the period in question and its recall. A person aware and unresponsive will be able to recount the events that occurred during an attack and his inability to respond by movement or speech. In this context,

*Adapted from *Epilepsia*, 1981, 22: 489–501. © 1981 The International League Against Epilepsy.

unresponsiveness is other than the result of paralysis, aphasia or apraxia.

(A)   Partial seizures
(1) *With motor signs.*   Any portion of the body may be involved in focal seizure activity depending on the site of origin of the attack in the motor strip. Focal motor seizures may remain strictly focal or they may spread to contiguous cortical areas producing a sequential involvement of body parts in an epileptic 'march'. The seizure is then known as a Jacksonian seizure. Consciousness is usually preserved; however, the discharge may spread to those structures whose participation is likely to result in loss of consciousness and generalized convulsive movements. Other focal motor attacks may be versive with head turning to one side, usually contraversive to the discharge. If speech is involved, this is either in the form of speech arrest or occasionally vocalization. Occasionally a partial dysphasia is seen in the form of epileptic pallilalia with involuntary repetition of a syllable or phrase.

Following focal seizure activity, there may be a localized paralysis in the previously involved region. This is known as

583

Todd's paralysis and may last from minutes to hours.

When focal motor seizure activity is continuous it is known as epilepsia partialis continua.

(2) *Seizures with autonomic symptoms* such as vomiting, pallor, flushing, sweating, piloerection, pupil dilatation, boborygmi, and incontinence may occur as simple partial seizures.

(3) *With somatosensory or special sensory symptoms.* Somatosensory seizures arise from those areas of cortex subserving sensory function, and they are usually described as pins-and-needles or a feeling of numbness. Occasionally a disorder of proprioception or spatial perception occurs. Like motor seizures, somatosensory seizures also may march and also may spread at any time to become complex partial or generalized tonic-clonic seizures as in A.1 of Table 16.1. Special sensory seizures include visual seizures varying in elaborateness and depending on whether the primary or association areas are involved, from flashing lights to structured visual hallucinatory phenomena, including persons, scenes, etc. (see A.4.f., Table 16.1). Like visual seizures, auditory seizures may also run the gamut from crude auditory sensations to such highly integrated functions as music (see A.4.f., Table 16.1). Olfactory sensations, usually in the form of unpleasant odors, may occur.

Gustatory sensations may be pleasant or odious taste hallucinations. They vary in elaboration from crude (salty, sour, sweet, bitter) to sophisticated. They are frequently described as 'metallic'.

Vertiginous symptoms include sensations of falling in space, floating, as well as rotatory vertigo in a horizontal or vertical plane.

(4) *With psychic symptoms* (disturbance of higher cerebral function). These usually occur with impairment of consciousness (i.e., complex partial seizures).

(a) *Dysphasia.* This was referred to earlier.

(b) *Dysmnesic symptoms.* A distorted memory experience such as distortion of the time sense, a dreamy state, a flashback, or a sensation as if a naive experience had been experienced before, known as déjà vu, or as if a previously experienced sensation had not been experienced, known as jamais vu, may occur. When this refers to auditory experiences these are known as déjà entendu or jamais entendu. Occasionally as a form of forced thinking, the patient may experience a rapid recollection of episodes from his past life, known as panoramic vision.

(c) *Cognitive disturbances* may be experienced. These include dreamy states; distortions of the time sense; sensations of unreality, detachment, or depersonalization.

(d) *With affective symptomatology.* Sensation of extreme pleasure or displeasure, as well as fear and intense depression with feelings of unworthiness and rejection may be experienced during seizures. Unlike those of psychiatrically induced depression, these symptoms tend to come in attacks lasting for a few minutes. Anger or rage is occasionally experienced, but unlike temper tantrums, epileptic anger is apparently unprovoked, and abates rapidly. Fear or terror is the most frequent symptom; it is sudden in onset, usually unprovoked,

Table I

Proposal for revised seizure classification*

I. Partial (focal, local) seizures

Partial seizures can be classified into one of the following three fundamental groups:

A.   Simple partial seizures
B.   Complex partial seizures
    1.   With impairment of consciousness at onset
    2.   Simple partial onset followed by impairment of consciousness
C.   Partial seizures evolving to generalized tonic-clonic convulsions (GTC)
    1.   Simple evolving to GTC
    2.   Complex evolving to GTC (including those with simple partial onset)

Clinical seizure type	EEG seizure type	EEG interictal expression
A. *Simple partial seizures* (consciousness not impaired)	Local contralateral discharge starting over the corresponding area of cortical representation (not always recorded on the scalp)	Local contralateral discharge

1. With motor signs
    (a) Focal motor without march
    (b) Focal motor with march (Jacksonian)
    (c) Versive
    (d) Postural
    (e) Phonatory (vocalization or arrest of speech)		

2. With somatosensory or special-sensory symptoms (simple hallucinations, e.g., tingling, light flashes, buzzing)
    (a) Somatosensory
    (b) Visual
    (c) Auditory
    (d) Olfactory
    (e) Gustatory
    (f) Vertiginous		

*   Adapted from *Epilepsia*, 22: 498–501, 1981.

TABLE I *(continued)*

Clinical seizure type	EEG seizure type	EEG interictal expression
3. With autonomic symptoms or signs (including epigastric sensation, pallor, sweating, flushing, piloerection and pupillary dilatation)		
4. With psychic symptoms (disturbance of higher cerebral function). These symptoms rarely occur without impairment of consciousness and are much more commonly experienced as complex partial seizures (a) Dysphasic (b) Dysmnesic (e.g., déjà vu) (c) Cognitive (e.g., dreamy states, distortions of time sense) (d) Affective (fear, anger, etc.) (e) Illusions (e.g., macropsia) (f) Structured hallucinations (e.g., music, scenes)		
B. *Complex partial seizures* (with impairment of consciousness; may sometimes begin with simple symptomatology) 1. Simple partial onset followed by impairment of consciousness (a) With simple partial features (A.1.–A.4.) followed by impaired consciousness (b) With automatisms 2. With impairment of consciousness at onset (a) With impairment of consciousness only (b) With automatisms	Unilateral or frequently bilateral discharge, diffuse or focal in temporal or frontotemporal regions	Unilateral or bilateral generally asynchronous focus; usually in the temporal or frontal regions

TABLE I *(continued)*

Clinical seizure type	EEG seizure type	EEG interictal expression
C. *Partial seizures evolving to secondarily generalized seizures* (This may be generalized tonic-clonic, tonic, or clonic) 1. Simple partial seizures (A) evolving to generalized selzures 2. Complex partial seizures (B) evolving to generalized seizures 3. Simple partial seizures evolving to complex partial seizures evolving to generalized seizures	Above discharges become secondarily and rapidly generalized	

II. Generallized seizures (con-vulsive or non-convulsive)

Clinical seizure type	EEG seizure type	EEG interictal expression
A. 1. *Absence seizures* (a) Impairment of consciousness only (b) With mild clonic components (c) With atonic components	Usually regular and symmetrical 3 Hz but may be 2–4 Hz spike-and-slow-wave complexes and may have multiple spike-and-slow-wave complexes. Abnormalities are bilateral	Background activity usually normal although paroxysmal activity (such as spikes or spike-and-slow-wave complexes) may occur. This activity is usually regular and symmetrical

587

TABLE I *(continued)*

Clinical seizure type	EEG seizure type	EEG interictal expression
(d) With tonic components (e) With automatisms (f) With autonomic components (b through f may be used alone or in combination)		
2. *Atypical absence*	EEG more heterogeneous; may include irregular spike-and-slow-wave complexes, fast activity or other paroxysmal activity. Abnormalities are bilateral but often irregular and asymmetrical	Background usually abnormal; paroxysmal activity (such as spikes or spike-and-slow-wave complexes) frequently irregular and asymmetrical
May have: (a) Changes in tone that are more pronounced than in A.1 (b) Onset and/or cessation that is not abrupt		
B. *Myoclonic seizures* Myoclonic jerks (single or multiple)	Polyspike and wave, or sometimes spike and wave or sharp and slow waves	Same as ictal
C. *Clonic seizures*	Fast activity (10 c/s or more) and slow waves; occasional spike-and-wave patterns	Spike-and-wave or polyspike-and-waves discharges
D. *Tonic seizures*	Low voltage, fast activity or a fast rhythm of 9–10 c/s or more decreasing in frequency and increasing in amplitude	More or less rhythmic discharges of sharp and slow waves, sometimes asymmetrical. Background is often abnormal for age.

TABLE I *(continued)*

Clinical seizure type	EEG seizure type	EEG interictal expression
E *Tonic-clonic seizures*	Rhythm at 10 or more c/s decreasing in frequency and increasing in amplitude during tonic phase, interrupted by slow waves during clonic phase	Polyspike and waves or spike and wave, or, sometimes, sharp and slow wave discharges
F *Atonic seizures* (Astatic) (combinations of the above may occur, e.g., B and F, B and D)	Polyspikes and wave or flattening or low-voltage fast activity	Polyspikes and slow wave

III. Unclassified epileptic seizures

Includes all seizures that cannot be classified because of inadequate or incomplete data and some that defy classification in hitherto described categories. This includes some neonatal seizures, e.g., rhythmic eye movements, chewing, and swimming movements.

IV. Addendum

Repeated epileptic seizures occur under a variety of circumstances:

(1) as fortuitous attacks, coming unexpectedly and without any apparent provocation; (2) as cyclic attacks, at more or less regular intervals (e.g., in relation to the menstrual cycle, or the sleep–waking cycle); (3) as attacks provoked by: (a) nonsensory factors (fatigue, alcohol, emotion, etc.), or (b) sensory factors, sometimes referred to as 'reflex seizures'.

Prolonged or repetitive seizures (status epilepticus). The term 'status epilepticus' is used whenever a seizure persists for a sufficient length of time or is repeated frequently enough that recovery between attacks does not occur. Status epilepticus may be divided into partial (e.g., Jacksonian), or generalized (e.g., absence status or tonic-clonic status). When very localized motor status occurs, it is referred to as epilepsia partialis continua.

and may lead to running away. Associated with the terror, there are frequently objective signs of autonomic activity, including pupil dilatation, pallor, flushing, piloerection, palpitation, and hypertension.

Epileptic or gelastic seizure laughter should not, strictly speaking, be classed as an affective symptom because the laughter is usually without affect and hollow. Like other forms of pathological laughter it is often unassociated with true mirth.

(e) *Illusions.* These take the form of distorted perceptions in which objects may appear deformed. Polyoptic illusions such as monocular diplopia, distortions of size (macropsia or micropsia) or of distance may occur. Similarly, distortions of sound, including microacusia and macroacusia, may be experienced. Depersonalization, as if the person were outside his body, may occur. Altered perception of size or weight of a limb may be noted.

(f) *Structured hallucinations.* Hallucinations may occur as manifestations or perceptions without a corresponding external stimulus and may affect somatosensory, visual, auditory, olfactory, or gustatory senses. If the seizure arises from the primary receptive area, the hallucination would tend to be rather primitive. In the case of vision, flashing lights may be seen; in the case of auditory perception, rushing noises may occur. With more elaborate seizures involving visual or auditory association areas with participation of mobilized memory traces, formed hallucinations occur and these may take the form of scenery, persons, spoken sentences, or music. The character of these perceptions may be normal or distorted.

(B) Seizures with complex symptomatology

Automatisms. These may occur during both complex partial and absence seizures. In the *Dictionary of Epilepsy* (Gastaut, 1973), automatisms are described as more or less coordinated adapted (eupractic or dyspractic) involuntary motor activity occurring during the state of clouding of consciousness either in the course of, or after an epileptic seizure, and usually followed by amnesia for the event. The automatism may be simply a continuation of an activity that was going on when the seizure occurred, or, conversely, a new activity developed in association with the ictal impairment of consciousness. Usually, the activity is commonplace in nature, often provoked by the subject's environment, or by his sensations during the seizure; exceptionally, fragmentary, primitive, infantile, or antisocial behavior is seen. From a symptomatological point of view the following are distinguished: (a) eating automatisms (chewing, swallowing); (b) automatisms of mimicry, expressing the subject's emotional state (usually of fear) during the seizure; (c) gestural automatisms, crude or elaborate; directed toward either the subject or his environment; (d) ambulatory automatisms; (e) verbal automatisms.

Automatisms may also occur as a postictal phenomenon, particularly following tonic-clonic seizures, and are usually associated with confusion.

Ambulatory seizures again may occur either as prolonged automatisms of absence, particularly prolonged absence continuing, or of complex partial seizures. In the latter, a patient may occasionally continue to drive a car, although may contravene traffic light regulations.

There seems to be little doubt that automatisms are a common feature of different types of epilepsy. While they do not lend themselves to simple anatomic interpretation, they appear to have in common a discharge involving various areas of the limbic system. Crude and elaborate automatisms do occur in patients with absence as well as complex partial seizures. The EEG is of cardinal localizational importance here.

Drowsiness or somnolence implies a sleep state from which the patient can be aroused to make appropriate motor and verbal responses. In stupor, the patient may make some spontaneous movement and can be aroused by painful or other vigorously applied stimuli to make avoidance movements. The patient in confusion makes inappropriate responses to his environment and is disoriented as regards place or time or person.

Aura.   The aura is that portion of the seizure which occurs before consciousness is lost and for which memory is retained afterwards. It may be that, as in simple partial seizures, the aura is the whole seizure. Where consciousness is subsequently lost, the aura is, in fact, the signal symptom of a complex partial seizure.

An aura is a retrospective term which is described after the seizure is ended.

Generalized seizures

(A) Absence seizures

The hallmark of the absence attack is a sudden onset, interruption of ongoing activities, a blank stare, possibly a brief upward rotation of the eyes. If the patient is speaking, speech is slowed or interrupted; if walking, he stands transfixed; if eating, the food will stop on its way to the mouth. Usually the patient will be unresponsive when spoken to. In some, attacks are aborted when the patient is spoken to. The attack lasts from a few seconds to half a minute and evaporates as rapidly as it commenced.

(1) *Absence with impairment of consciousness only.* The above description fits the description of absence simple in which no other activities take place during the attack.

(2) *Absence with mild clonic components.*   Here the onset of the attack is indistinguishable from the above, but clonic movements may occur in the eyelids, at the corner of the mouth, or in other muscle groups which may vary in severity from almost imperceptible movements to generalized myoclonic jerks. Objects held in the hand may be dropped.

(3) *Absence with atonic components.* Here there may be a diminution in tone of muscles subserving posture as well as in the limbs leading to drooping of the head, occasionally slumping of the trunk, dropping of the arms, and relaxation

of the grip. Rarely, tone is sufficiently diminished to cause this person to fall.

(4) *Absence with tonic components.* Here during the attack tonic muscular contraction may occur, leading to increase in muscle tone which may affect the extensor muscles or the flexor muscles symmetrically or asymmetrically. If the patient is standing the head may be drawn backward and the trunk may arch. This may lead to retropulsion. The head may tonically draw to one or another side.

(5) *Absence with automatisms.* (See also prior discussion on automatisms.) Purposeful or quasipurposeful movements occurring in the absence of awareness during an absence attack are frequent and may range from lip licking and swallowing to clothes fumbling or aimless walking. If spoken to the patient may grunt or turn to the spoken voice and when touched or tickled may rub the site. Automatisms are quite elaborate and may consist of combinations of the above-described movements or may be so simple as to be missed by casual observation. Mixed forms of absence frequently occur.

(B) Tonic-clonic seizures

The most frequently encountered of the generalized seizures are the generalized tonic-clonic seizures, often known as grand mal. Some patients experience a vague ill-described warning, but the majority lose consciousness without any premonitory symptoms. There is a sudden sharp tonic contrac-

tion of muscles, and when this involves the respiratory muscles there is stridor, a cry or moan, and the patient falls to the ground in the tonic state, occasionally injuring himself in falling. He lies rigid, and during this stage tonic contraction inhibits respiration and cyanosis may occur. The tongue may be bitted and urine may be passed involuntarily. This tonic stage then gives way to clonic convulsive movements lasting for a variable period of time. During this stage small gusts of grunting respiration may occur between the convulsive movements, but usually the patient remains cyanotic and saliva may froth from the mouth. At the end of this stage, deep respiration occurs and all the muscles relax, after which the patient remains unconscious for a variable period of time and often awakes feeling stiff and sore all over. He then frequently goes into a deep sleep and when he awakens feels quite well apart from soreness and frequently headache.

Generalized tonic-clonic convulsions may occur in childhood and in adult life; they are not as frequent as absence seizures, but vary from one a day to one every three months and occasionally to one every few years.

Very short attacks without postictal drowsiness may occur on occasion.

Myoclonic seizures

Myoclonic jerks (single or multiple) are sudden, brief, shock-like contractions which may be generalized or confined to the face and trunk or to one or more extremities or even to individual muscles or groups of muscles. Myoclonic jerks may be rapidly repetitive or relatively isolated. They may occur predominantly around the hours of going to sleep or awakening from sleep. They may be exacerbated by volitional movement (action myoclonus). At times they may be regularly repetitive.

Many instances of myoclonic jerks and action myoclonus are not classified as epileptic seizures. The myoclonic jerks of myoclonus due to spinal cord disease, dyssynergia cerebellaris myoclonica, subcortical segmental myoclonus, paramyoclonus multiplex, and opsoclonus-myoclonus syndrome must be distinguished from epileptic seizures.

Clonic seizures

Generalized convulsive seizures occasionally lack a tonic component and are characterized by repetitive clonic jerks. As the frequency diminishes the amplitude of the jerks do not. The postictal phase is usually short. Some generalized convulsive seizures commence with a clonic phase passing into a tonic phase, as described below, leading to a 'clonic-tonic-clonic' seizure.

Tonic seizures

To quote Gowers, a tonic seizure is 'a rigid, violent muscular contraction, fixing the limbs in some strained position. There is usually deviation of the eyes and of the head toward one side, and this may amount to rotation involving the whole body (sometimes actually causing the patient to turn around, even two or three times). The features are distorted; the color of the face, unchanged at first, rapidly becomes pale and then flushed and ultimately livid as the fixation of the chest by the spasms stops the movements of respiration. The eyes are open or closed; the conjunctiva is insensitive; the pupils dilate widely as cyanosis comes on. As the spasm continues, it commonly changes in its relative intensity in different parts, causing slight alterations in the position of the limbs'.

Tonic axial seizures with extension of head, neck, and trunk may also occur.

Atonic seizures

A sudden diminution in muscle tone occurs which may be fragmentary, leading to a head drop with slackening of the jaw, the dropping of a limb or a loss of all muscle tone leading to a slumping to the ground. When these attacks are extremely brief they are known as 'drop attacks'. If consciousness is lost, this loss is extremely brief. The sudden loss of postural tone in the head and trunk may lead to injury by projecting objects. The face is particularly subject to injury. In the case of more prolonged atonic attacks, the slumping may be progressive in a rhythmic, successive relaxation manner.

(So-called drop attacks may be seen in conditions other than epilepsy, such as brainstem ischemia and narcolepsy cataplexy syndrome.)

Unclassified epileptic seizures

This category includes all seizures that cannot be classified because of inadequate or incomplete data and includes some seizures that by their natures defy classification in the previously defined broad categories. Many seizures occurring in the infant (e.g., rhythmic eye movements, chewing, swimming movements, jittering, and apnea) will be classified here until such time as further experience with video-tape confirmation and electroencephalographic characterization entitles them to subtyping in the extant classification.

Epilepsia partialis continua

Under this name have been described cases of simple partial seizures with focal motor signs without a march, usually consisting of clonic spasms, which remain confined to the part of the body in which they originate, but which persist with little or no intermission for hours or days at a stretch. Consciousness is usually preserved, but postictal weakness is frequently evident.

Postictal paralysis (Todd's paralysis)

This category refers to the transient paralysis that may occur following some partial epileptic seizures with focal motor components or with somatosensory symptoms. Postictal paralysis has been ascribed to neuronal exhaustion due to the increased metabolic activity of the discharging focus, but it may also be attributable to increased inhibition in the region of the focus, which may account for its appearance in non-motor somatosensory seizures.

REFERENCES

Gastaut, H. (1970) Clinical and electroencephalographic classification of epileptic seizures. Epilepsia 11: 102.

Gastaut, H. (1973) Definitions. In: Dictionary of Epilepsy. Part I. World Health Organization, Geneva.

Jackson, J.H. (1931) In: J.A. Taylor (Ed.), Selected Writings of J. Hughlings Jackson, Vol. I: On Epilepsy and Epileptiform Convulsions. Hodder and Staughton, London.

Index of Subjects

Readers may also refer to the Glossary of Terms most commonly used by clinical EEGers, pp. 439–456

Italic bold numbers indicate that the corresponding keyword (or chain of keywords) refers to a headline

597

607